Basic Clinical Surgery
for Nurses and Medical Students

Second Edition

Basic Clinical Surgery

for Nurses and Medical Students

Second Edition

Edited by

John McFarland, MD, ChM, FRCS

*Consultant Surgeon, Royal Liverpool Hospital;
Clinical Lecturer in Surgery, University of Liverpool;
formerly Member of the Court of Examiners and
Hunterian Professor, Royal College of Surgeons*

Nursing Adviser

Diana Smither, SRN, DN, RNT
Nurse Tutor, Royal Liverpool Hospital School of Nursing

With Forewords by

Lord Smith of Marlow, KBE, Hon.DSc, MS, FRCS, Hon.FRACS, Hon.FRCSE,
Hon.FACS, Hon.FRCS (Can), Hon.FRCS (I), Hon.FDS
Past President, Royal College of Surgeons

Muriel Skeet, SRN, FRCN
*Formerly Chief Nursing Officer and Adviser, The British Red Cross Society;
Chairman, Nursing Advisory Committee, League of Red Cross Societies, Geneva;
and President and Chairman of Executive Board, Nurses' Commonwealth
Federation*

BUTTERWORTHS
London and Boston
Sydney—Wellington—Durban—Toronto

The Butterworth Group

United Kingdom	**Butterworth & Co (Publishers) Ltd** London: 88 Kingsway, WC2B 6AB
Australia	**Butterworth Pty Ltd** Sydney: 586 Pacific Highway, Chatswood NSW 2067 Also at Melbourne, Adelaide and Perth
Canada	**Butterworth & Co (Canada) Ltd** Toronto: 2265 Midland Avenue, Scarborough, Ontario, M1P 4S1
New Zealand	**Butterworths of New Zealand Ltd** Wellington: T & W Young Building, 77—85 Customhouse Quay, 1, CPO Box 472
South Africa	**Butterworth & Co (South Africa) (Pty) Ltd** Durban: 152—154 Gale Street
USA	**Butterworth (Publishers) Inc** Boston: 10 Tower Office Park, Woburn, Mass. 01801

First published 1973
Reprinted 1975
Reprinted 1979
Second edition 1980

ISBN 0 407 80101 4

© Butterworth & Co (Publishers) Ltd 1980

British Library Cataloguing in Publication Data

*Basic clinical surgery for nurses and medical
students.* — 2nd ed.
  1. Surgery
I. McFarland, John

617'.002'4613   RT65   80—40102

ISBN 0—407—80101—4

Typeset by Butterworths Litho Preparation Department
Printed in England by Page Bros Ltd, Norwich, Norfolk

*To all those who
have helped their
children learn to
care for the sick*

Contents

Contributors to this volume

Paul Atkins, MS, FRCS
Consultant Surgeon, Royal Liverpool Hospital and Walton Hospital, Liverpool; Clinical Lecturer in Surgery, University of Liverpool

B. J. Bickford, FRCS
Formerly Consultant Cardiothoracic Surgeon, Royal Liverpool Children's Hospital and Broadgreen Hospital, Liverpool; Clinical Lecturer in Cardiothoracic Surgery, University of Liverpool

Roger Brearley, ChM, FRCS
Consultant Surgeon, Whiston and St Helens Hospitals, Mersey Region; Research Associate, Department of Surgery, University of Liverpool

R. B. Crosbie, BSc, ARIC, FRCS
Consultant Surgeon, Wirral Area Hospitals, Mersey Region

A. H. Cruickshank, MD, PhD, MRCPath
Formerly Reader in Pathology, University of Liverpool and Honorary Consultant Pathologist, Liverpool Area Health Authority (Teaching)

J. E. Dalby, MA, FRCR
Consultant in Radiotherapy and Oncology, Mersey Regional Centre for Radiotherapy and Oncology; Clinical Lecturer in Radiotherapy, University of Liverpool

Charles de Boer, FRCS, FRCOG
Consultant Obstetrician and Gynaecologist, Royal Liverpool Hospital, Women's Hospital and Liverpool Maternity Hospital; Clinical Lecturer in Obstetrics and Gynaecology, University of Liverpool

N. V. Freeman, FRCS, FRCSE
Senior Lecturer in Paediatric Surgery, University of Southampton; Consultant Paediatric and Neonatal Surgeon, Wessex Regional Centre for Paediatric Surgery, Southampton

A. A. Gilbertson, FFARCS
Consultant Anaesthetist and Director of the Intensive Therapy Unit, Royal Liverpool Hospital; Clinical Lecturer in Anaesthesia, University of Liverpool

R. M. Jameson, MB, BS, FRCS
Consultant Urological Surgeon, Regional Urological Centre, Royal Liverpool Hospital and Regional Spinal Injury Centre, Southport; Postgraduate Clinical Lecturer in Urology, University of Liverpool; Member of the Board of Examiners in Applied Physiology, Royal College of Surgeons

Richard Jeffreys, MChir, FRCSE
Consultant Neurological Surgeon, Mersey Regional Department of Medical and Surgical Neurology, Walton Hospital, Liverpool; Clinical Lecturer, Associated Unit of Neurological Sciences, University of Liverpool

John McFarland, MD, ChM, FRCS
Consultant Surgeon, Royal Liverpool Hospital; Clinical Lecturer in Surgery, University of Liverpool

D. O. Maisels, FRCSE, FRCS
Consultant Plastic Surgeon, Regional Burns and Plastic Surgery Unit, Whiston Hospital, Mersey Region; Clinical Lecturer in Surgery, University of Liverpool

Averil O. Mansfield, ChM, FRCS, FRCSE
Consultant Surgeon, Royal Liverpool Hospital; Clinical Lecturer in Surgery, University of Liverpool

C. J. E. Monk, MChOrth, FRCS, FRCSE
Consultant Orthopaedic Surgeon, Royal Liverpool Hospital and Royal Liverpool Children's Hospital; Clinical Lecturer in Orthopaedic Surgery, University of Liverpool

T. R. Preston, MA, FRCS, FRCSE
Consultant Surgeon, Whiston and St Helens Hospitals, Mersey Region

C. B. Sedzimir, MD, FRCSE
Consultant Neurological Surgeon, Mersey Regional Department of Medical and Surgical Neurology, Walton Hospital, Liverpool; Chairman, Associated Unit of Neurological Sciences, University of Liverpool

Robert Sells, FRCS, FRCSE
Consultant Surgeon and Director of the Renal Transplant Unit, Royal Liverpool Hospital; Clinical Lecturer in Surgery, University of Liverpool

Robert Shields, MD, FRCS, FRCSE
Professor of Surgery, University of Liverpool; Honorary Consultant Surgeon, Royal Liverpool Hospital and Broadgreen Hospital, Liverpool; Member of the Court of Examiners, Royal College of Surgeons

P. M. Stell, ChM, FRCS, FRCSE
Professor of Oto-Rhino-Laryngology, University of Liverpool; Honorary Consultant ENT Surgeon, Royal Liverpool Hospital and Broadgreen Hospital, Liverpool

J. E. Utting, FFARCS
Professor of Anaesthesia, University of Liverpool; Honorary Consultant Anaesthetist, Royal Liverpool Hospital

Foreword

The last two decades have seen enormous scientific and technological advances affecting the whole of Medicine. In common with every other specialty, the practice of surgery has been profoundly altered by these advances and new scientific aids to diagnosis abound as well as advanced equipment capable of providing and monitoring new and better methods of treatment.

The medical student or nurse anxious to understand modern surgery might very well be excused for losing their way amongst all this technology and for leaving out of their calculations, or at least underestimating, the importance of the clinical aspects of surgery. The availability of science as an aid to surgery does not reduce the need for taking an accurate history from a sick patient, for carrying out a proper physical examination, and for monitoring the progress of an illness by repeated examinations as well as through the use of scientific aids and laboratory investigations.

The authors of this timely book are deserving of much praise for insisting upon the importance of this aspect of surgery. The title they have chosen 'Basic Clinical Surgery' is a good one provided that it is clearly understood that in this context the word 'Basic' has no temporal connotation, implying that clinical skills are learnt first as a preliminary to moving on to the more important examinations of modern technology. 'Basic' means basic to the understanding of surgery, a foundation of knowledge which is indispensable.

One cannot make a start in surgery without this knowledge and indeed at a later stage in a surgical career a surgeon who allows himself to lose touch with the clinical aspects of disease will find that his standards will inevitably decline. That is why this book, aimed primarily at the young, should be read by surgeons of all ages, for the experienced will find its attractive style and presentation hold the interest while it is salutary to be reminded from time to time that one's memory i basic clinical aspects of Medicine can be fallible.

Rodney Smith

Foreword

It is now six years since this work was first published and for members of the health professions in this country they have been six turbulent years.

Perhaps today, even more than at that time, health practitioners as well as students, need to pause and consider certain fundamental issues such as professional standards, ethical behaviour and even the very reason for our existence as doctors and nurses. Certainly this publication affords us opportunities to do so.

When we read, for example, 'hospitals are for ill people. . . all of us who work in them have one common aim: it is to relieve suffering. . .' we cannot but reflect that we have been in danger sometimes of losing sight of this as our priority objective. Those of us who have worked in surgical wards and operating theatres for several years and regard the tasks we perform there as so much routine, will find it useful to be reminded that 'for most people, a surgical operation will be one of the most severe physical and psychological tests in their lives'. And for those who hold the awesome responsibility of taking decisions which affect the length of a patient's life, there is the gentle reminder that 'death may be dreaded, hoped for, or simply accepted, but everyone will die. It is his right to be allowed to do so with dignity'.

Surgery is one method of treating a patient. It can also represent — as it obviously does to John McFarland and his colleagues in Liverpool — practical compassion. And although, as the Editor says in one of his own contributions, 'compassion, a quality fundamental to medicine (and nursing), cannot readily be instilled by the printed word', succinct truths such as some of those contained in this textbook help to put compassion back into the frightening and technological procedures which many of our patients often face during their stay in hospital. Nurses learn to channel their inevitable emotional involvement with an ill patient into providing practical help for him This help may take several forms but in today's busy, complex and sometimes understaffed wards, it is more necessary than ever before. To quote the text once more. . . 'the help which a doctor or nurse can give in such simple ways as taking the time to explain to him what is happening, or letting him appreciate that, although he may feel that a hospital is a strange and frightening place, he is amongst friends, cannot be measured'.

This book not only gives complete coverage of the surgical syllabus for the State Final Examination of the General Nursing Councils of this country, it is a well-written classic expressing practical concern for patients and a renewal of belief in the value of those precious relationships which can exist among patients and their doctors and nurses.

I hope that future generations of nurses will know that happiness which so many of us have derived from caring for surgical patients and will delight in a true understanding, as well as in the practice, of what is written within these pages.

Muriel Skeet

Preface

On the occasion of a second edition of *Basic Clinical Surgery* it is appropriate to ask whether a re-definition of the readership is needed. The original intention was 'to help all those students, whether of nursing or of medicine, who are starting their work in the wards of a hospital'. This has remained our aim, although not without some debate, for it has been evident that the book has had a major appeal to nurses and has indeed been recommended as a standard text in many centres. Nonetheless the spirit of the first edition has been maintained both by ensuring that the syllabus for nurses in training is fully covered and that information on every aspect of the work they will encounter in the surgical wards is readily and clearly available, and also by extending the text to give coverage at a basic level of all clinical surgery of interest to medical students. For the former, the guidance of the nursing adviser, Miss Diana Smither, who has been involved at every point from the planning stage onwards, has been crucial.

The rewriting has been very extensive. There is one completely new chapter on 'Gynaecology' and others have been greatly enlarged so that branches of surgery dealt with in a limited way in the first edition have been expanded into chapters on 'Neurosurgery', 'Thoracic Surgery' and 'Orthopaedic Surgery and Traumatology'. To avoid the volume being unduly large some compression in other areas has been called for. I am most appreciative of the effort, whether in expanding or compressing, that each author has taken. I welcome Charles de Boer and Richard Jeffreys to a largely unchanged team.

The language of medicine cannot be immediately accessible. Terms intended to improve communication may initially be a hindrance, requiring a specialized dictionary for complete elucidation. Nonetheless, in this book every possible effort has been made for the contents to be clear to the reader coming to the subject for the first time. Hence the marginal definitions, which are repeated in the Glossary, of every word or concept (other than anatomical terms) that could possibly cause difficulty. A consideration new to this edition has been with regard to units of measurement, for Système International Units (SI Units) were adopted in the United Kingdom in

1975. These have been used throughout but usually the previous nomenclature (e.g. mg/100 ml) has also been indicated.

In the production of a book which is the work of so many people many others have been involved. Their help may not have been recorded but it has been appreciated. Recognition of my gratitude is, however, due to Lord Smith of Marlow and to Miss Muriel Skeet who have both written such generous Forewords, to Mr Eric Parry for particular help with a difficult chapter; to my secretary, Mrs Veronica Gibson; to the artist, Mr John Booth and to the editorial staff of Butterworths. My mother, Dr Ethel McFarland, has read every word in proof and her help has been untiring and invaluable.

It is pleasant to recall that many others have given constructive criticism. I hope that they will forgive the absence of individual mention but will regard the incorporation of their advice into the second edition as the most sincere acknowledgement. Two who cannot do this but who took a particular interest were Lord Cohen of Birkenhead and Professor Norman Capon. I salute their memory as I do that of Sir John Bruce and Miss Anne White who wrote the Forewords to the first edition.

None of these friends has hesitated in his support for the original principle of this book that 'The professions of medicine and nursing are uniquely linked and their common objective needs the teamwork that can flourish only in an atmosphere of mutual trust and affection' and neither do I. This is why I am so proud to be again associated with a venture which is dedicated to this ideal.

John McFarland

1

Surgery: perspectives, diagnosis, management and rehabilitation

John McFarland

Surgery is one method of treating a patient. There are many other methods, and very many diseases in which there is no place for surgical treatment. Furthermore, there are medical treatments, for example those suppressing cell division or altering endocrine activity, which may cause a more profound change in the body and even in the human spirit than would follow a major operation. Thus the validity of designating hospital units as medical or surgical could be questioned. Surgery is, however, a large and important part of medical practice and it is evident that, of all treatments, a surgical operation arouses the greatest popular interest and concern. There are good reasons for this: for the patient – apprehension about suffering, and the fear of the unknown; for the surgeon – a particular feeling of responsibility for someone on whom he has operated. Also the management of the patient undergoing an operation and the support of the surgeon who performs it does require a special concentration of knowledge, technique and organization. This book is about the understanding of these skills which are fundamental to the practice of surgery.

This chapter takes an overall look at the principles of clinical surgery largely from the point of view of a student entering the wards of a hospital for the first time. It is important, first of all, that he or she has some grasp of the general scheme of referral for a surgical opinion, the relative frequency of conditions amenable to surgical treatment and the way both of these fit into the overall pattern of medical care. This problem is discussed in the section on Perspectives. Under the heading Diagnosis, a consideration of the underlying principles is followed by an outline of the practical stages involved. Under the heading Management the nature of non-operative and operative treatment is described. Finally, there is a section on Rehabilitation, describing the measures necessary to help the patient progress as quickly as possible from operation to full recovery.

1

PERSPECTIVES

Everyone is aware that illness usually starts outside the hospital and may require a visit to the family doctor (general practitioner – GP) or a request that the doctor makes a home visit. The problem is likely to be one with which the GP can readily deal. If he wishes to have a second opinion or considers that an operation may be necessary, what are the next steps and what is the relationship between the general practitioner and hospital care of the patient?

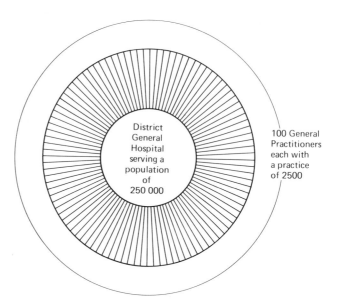

District General Hospital serving a population of 250 000

100 General Practitioners each with a practice of 2500

Figure 1.1. The numerical relationship between hospital and general practice. (Data based on Fry, 1966)

Some idea of the relative roles of the family doctor and hospital may be gained from *Figure 1.1,* illustrating the possible concentration in hospital of referred patients and showing that the hospital experience may be 100 times greater than that of each general practitioner. From *Figure 1.2* it may be seen that only about one-fortieth of all sick people come to hospital. There are important extensions of these principles within the hospital. Broadly speaking, about 60 per cent of referred patients are seen in surgical clinics (*Figure 1.3*) and the same percentage of admissions is to the surgical wards (*Figure 1.4*). These are not, of course, the same group, but the figure represents an overall proportion of patients seen for the first time in the surgical department of a hospital; about 1.7 per cent of all disease (*see Figure 1.2*).

It follows from these considerations that relatively common disorders such as dyspepsia (a symptom) and peptic ulceration (one of the causes) will be familiar to doctors within or without hospital. Thus, if in an average practice of 2500 some 250

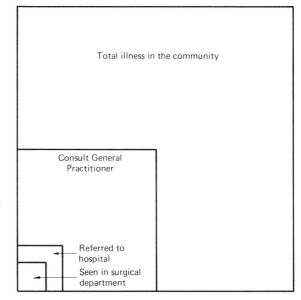

Figure 1.2. The large square represents all the disease occurring in a community. The general practitioner's advice is sought for about one-quarter of this and he refers one-tenth of these patients to hospital. Two-thirds of these are seen in a surgical department which thus deals with about one-sixtieth (1.7 per cent) of all disease. (Data based on Fry, 1966)

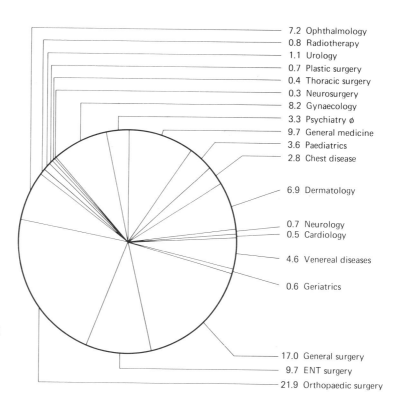

Figure 1.3. New patients seen in hospital clinics. The figures are for referrals for 1 year (1977) to all hospitals in the Mersey Region and are expressed as percentages

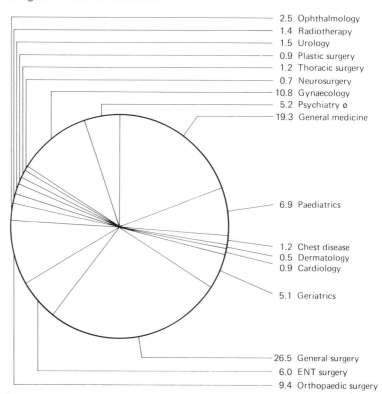

2.5 Ophthalmology
1.4 Radiotherapy
1.5 Urology
0.9 Plastic surgery
1.2 Thoracic surgery
0.7 Neurosurgery
10.8 Gynaecology
5.2 Psychiatry ø
19.3 General medicine

6.9 Paediatrics

1.2 Chest disease
0.5 Dermatology
0.9 Cardiology

5.1 Geriatrics

26.5 General surgery
6.0 ENT surgery
9.4 Orthopaedic surgery

Figure 1.4. In-patients according to specialty. The figures are for the numbers of patients discharged or dying in 1 year (1977) from all the hospitals in the Mersey Region and are expressed as percentages

people consult their doctor each year with dyspepsia about 62 (2.5 per cent) of these will arrive in hospital, and about 42 (1.7 per cent) will be seen in the surgical unit.

In the case of an extremely rare condition the situation is different. A good example of this is that of a phaeochromocytoma, a tumour of the adrenal medulla which releases large amounts of a vasoconstrictor chemical (noradrenaline) into the blood stream with a resultant serious increase in the patient's blood pressure. The incidence of this condition has been thought to be in the order of 1 new case for 1.5 million people per year. A general practitioner with a practice of 2500 would have a theoretical chance of seeing 1 of these patients in 600 years! Even in a hospital with a catchment area postulated above, only 1 such patient would be seen in 6 years. Treatment of this condition is by surgical removal of the adrenal gland containing the tumour. The operation and the associated management of the patient is difficult and unless there is some concentration of such patients no one surgeon (or even group of surgeons) is likely to gain the necessary expertise to do this really well — much less to advance knowledge of the condition. The pathway of referral for such a case is indicated in *Figure 1.5.*

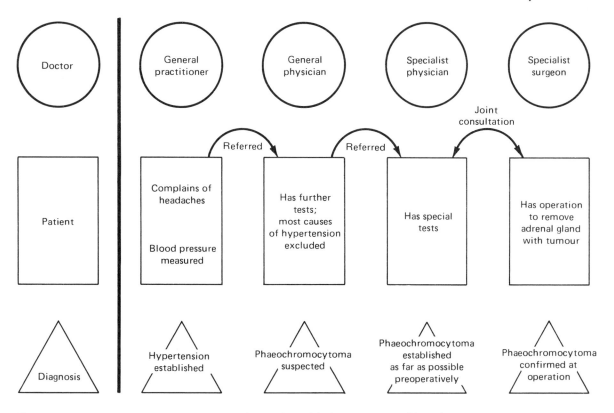

Figure 1.5. Pathways of diagnosis and treatment for a patient with the very rare condition of phaeochromocytoma

Most conditions for which patients are admitted to general surgical departments of a hospital fall within these two extremes.

An idea of the relative frequency of conditions for which an operation is undertaken may be gained from studying *Figure 1.6*. It is important for anyone, such as the student or nurse in training, spending a relatively short time in each ward, to appreciate these proportions and consider them in conjunction with the overall spectrum of illness. Otherwise, quite false impressions of the incidence of diseases and their treatment may be gained. The situation is further complicated by the separation of surgery into several specialities, such as orthopaedic, thoracic, plastic and neurosurgery, all of which are now clearly demarcated and practised separately from general surgery. Furthermore, many clinicians with a general surgery practice develop a special interest in one aspect of their work and from this it follows that one clinic may see only patients with thyroid problems or one unit accept a very high proportion of patients with liver disease.

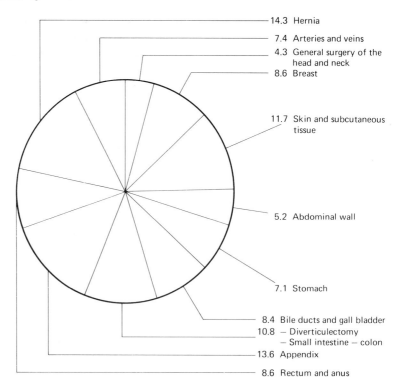

14.3 Hernia
7.4 Arteries and veins
4.3 General surgery of the head and neck
8.6 Breast
11.7 Skin and subcutaneous tissue
5.2 Abdominal wall
7.1 Stomach
8.4 Bile ducts and gall bladder
10.8 — Diverticulectomy
— Small intestine — colon
13.6 Appendix
8.6 Rectum and anus

Figure 1.6. Relative frequency of major operations. The figures are of principal operations performed in all hospitals of the Mersey Region during 1977 on in-patient residents of the Mersey Region

Appreciation of the proportional incidence of disease is equally important to the doctor. If he works in a general practice or a general clinic, he will accept that the majority of illness will have an 'ordinary' diagnosis but he must be alert to the possibility of something unusual. The super-specialist will be attuned to dealing constantly with what is 'unusual' for others, but will be aware that the diagnosis, and the remedy, may at times be quite simple. Students are sometimes warned against too readily diagnosing a rarity by the question: 'In a flock of birds eating crumbs on a lawn, how often would you expect to see a canary?' But one may be there, just as a sparrow may slip into a cage!

A fallacy highlighted by such an analysis of actual figures is that of personal impressions. As has been stated, a student may have a wrong impression by seeing a non-representative grouping of patients. Similarly, factors other than the incidence of disease may naturally make a great impression on the doctor (for example, personal association). Memory for these may be vivid and possibly result in undue weighting of diagnostic or treatment factors.

I am conscious that this discussion of the perspectives of medical care is based on practice in the United Kingdom, a small part of Western Europe. Some other parts of the world are fortunate enough to have similar cover; some are not. I have a vivid picture in my mind of a 30-bedded hospital which I visited some 20 years ago. It was situated very near the point where the borders of Kenya, Ethiopia and Somaliland meet. No one recalled a previous visit by a doctor. The patients were looked after by an African nursing orderly, who had had 4 years' training in Nairobi. The facilities were extremely meagre and his assistants had been recruited and trained locally. I still recall with humility his real devotion to the work and the remarkable degree of his success.

DIAGNOSIS

It would appear self-evident that diagnosis is an essential stage in the care of a patient. What exactly does the term mean and how does one set about establishing a diagnosis?

The meaning of diagnosis

Diagnosis means 'thorough knowledge' and, in the medical sense, 'determination of the nature of a diseased condition'. 'A complete diagnosis must tell us where disease is, what functional disturbances are present and how these have arisen' (Cohen, 1943). For example, if it is considered that the patient has a defective heart valve, we will be aware that this may explain the various features of his disease (congestion of the lungs, peripheral oedema) that follow the anatomical defect. But we must realize that, although such an analysis has increased our understanding of the diseased condition, it has not completed it. We should ask, 'How did the damage occur? Was it inflicted by genetic or environmental circumstances?'. If the evidence suggests the latter, the nature of the causative agent should be sought, inflammatory, traumatic, neoplastic or other. Perhaps the damaging agent can be shown to be inflammation arising from bacterial invasion. But where do the bacteria come from? How do they gain entry? What gives them their power to damage? Why does this occur in this situation?

Until these questions can be answered, the diagnosis has not truly been made. But here a practical point arises. An ill patient must be treated. For this it may be necessary to know (in the above example) only that the heart valve is fibrosed. Anatomical correction can be done by surgery and physiological function restored, or, if there is still active inflammation due to the presence of bacteria, these may be isolated and appropriate antibacterial drugs given. Diagnosis up to this point may allow help to be given to this particular patient. It may be called a 'diagnosis for treatment'.

Fibrosis The development of fibrous tissue in a part or an organ.

Furthermore there is another aspect of diagnosis of the greatest practical importance. In essence it is the identification of the needs — in the widest sense — of an individual patient that allows the nursing staff to work out and implement a detailed plan of care. This has been called *the nursing process* and is referred to again a little later in this chapter.

Answers to the further questions (where? when? what? why?) may not be of immediate importance to the individual patient. They should, however, lead to a greater understanding of the disease process. Furthermore, it will be evident that the greatest possible degree of accuracy is necessary if worthwhile information is to be gained for scientific analysis. For example, if a study of treatment for duodenal ulcer is being made, it is pointless if patients with duodenal ulcer, gastric ulcer or gastritis are included indiscriminately in the analysis. The knowledge gained from answering such questions and analysing such information may eventually lead to the fundamental goal — prevention.

The diagnostic process

How is a diagnosis made? The process may be relatively simple, as when the clinician recognizes something he has seen before or of which he has had a clear account. The pitfalls for the inexperienced are evident; nonetheless, a great many conditions may be diagnosed in this way. This is particularly so when the lesion can be inspected; examples commonly seen in a surgical clinic are sebaceous cyst, Dupuytren's contracture, inguinal hernia, pilonidal sinus and so on.

In the more complex situation there are several degrees, which may be called suspicion, consideration, and confirmation, to which must be added labelling or naming.

Suspicion

His assessment of the symptoms he has been told and the signs he has detected should lead the clinician to suspect the diagnosis. This exercise of his skill and knowledge is critical. If he has missed some feature of the story or some physical clue or is unaware of their significance, the diagnosis may escape him.

Consideration

This is the pause to assess whether the facts he knows would also fit another diagnosis or indeed several. He may make a list of possibilities — a so-called differential diagnosis. As a greater number of facts becomes known, so the differential diagnosis list becomes shorter.

Additional facts may be of the same physical order, and here time can be of the greatest importance; a fever or a palpable swelling may be absent one day but evident the next. Or the facts may be of a different order; usually the results of special tests. Specimens from the patient (blood, urine, faeces and so on) have undergone analysis in the laboratory. The patient has been to special departments for radiography, **electrocardiography** or other studies. An accurate assessment of the diagnostic possibilities has enabled the clinician to decide which special tests are necessary.

Confirmation

This is the point at which the results of tests are available to the clinician and the possible alteration of physical signs by time may be taken into account. If the facts fit, a diagnosis for treatment should be possible. However, treatment itself can have some place in diagnosis. A cough is a symptom for which simple medical treatment may be given. If this is enough to relieve the patient, treatment plus a degree of diagnosis (i.e. that there is no serious cause for the cough) may have been achieved. Expert knowledge, judgement and caution are required.

It is clearly of the greatest importance that such symptomatic treatment does not simply depress the symptoms to the point where the diagnosis is obscured or delayed. The management of pain is a very important instance of this. A patient may be in great distress with acute severe abdominal pain which it is quite possible to relieve by an injection of morphia. If this is done before the diagnosis (at least to the point of the decision to operate) has been made, the eventual consequence for the patient may be disastrous. Another example is when chronic pain in the presence of **carcinoma** is being treated. The too facile assumption that extension of pain means spread of carcinoma may be made. Accuracy is essential, for corrective treatment may be possible. Palliation also requires that the diagnosis is as clear-cut as it can be.

Naming

Naming should clearly and briefly describe the known situation. For example, in the case described above, in which the patient had a defective heart valve, the original diagnosis will be 'mitral valve stenosis'. This may later be qualified, in this case probably as 'secondary to rheumatic fever'.

Decisions regarding treatment must be based on the most accurate diagnosis possible but, as has been seen, it may be necessary for treatment to be started before a diagnosis

Electrocardiography The recording of the electrical potentials generated by the activity of the heart.

Carcinoma A malignant tumour arising from epithelial cells; a more precise term than 'cancer' which may also be used, more loosely, to describe any malignant growth.

(other than at a very simple level) has been made. This may, in fact, be so vague as to be simply a label. For example, a lump in a woman's breast may be assessed before operation as a carcinoma or as a simple cyst. The experienced clinician is not usually wrong in such a diagnosis if the physical signs are definite enough; but he may be. While a definite carcinoma or a definite cyst is diagnosed with relative confidence, there is a stage in between when even the experienced observer admits that he cannot tell. A label is then given of 'lump in the breast'. The making of the diagnosis is, in effect, delayed until the operation affords the opportunity for the lump to be handled and cut and examined microscopically (this would usually be by frozen-section histology — a technique which allows tissue sections to be hardened, sliced and examined within minutes). The surgeon can then make his decision with the fullest possible knowledge of the facts. It can be appreciated, however, that he has to decide his course of action more quickly and with less opportunity for consultation than if a firm and correct preoperative diagnosis had been made.

A situation not unlike the above is the emergency abdominal operation when the preoperative 'diagnosis' has been 'acute abdomen'. This is a label which means that the surgeon cannot decide on the exact nature of the abdominal condition but considers that urgent operation (laparotomy — opening the abdomen) is necessary. The question of the definitive treatment faces the surgeon after the abdomen has been opened. Decision and action must be prompt.

Practical stages in diagnosis

A person's awareness of discomfort may be the first of several steps leading to the diagnosis of his disease. For example, he may be troubled by an unduly persistent or recurring pain, a normal bodily function such as regular bowel action may change, a skin ulcer or a deeper lying lump may appear, or he simply feels unduly tired and 'run down'. Possibly the first signs are seen by someone else. This is often so when jaundice or anaemia develop. It is also quite usual when the subject is a child for his mother to notice that he is limping, is eating poorly or is vomiting.

In the case of small children the inability or difficulties of direct communication lend a special aspect to this stage of the diagnostic process. The general principles involved may best be understood if the situation is considered when an adult consults his doctor about a specific problem.

In the National Health Service, the first consultation will be with the patient's general practitioner who will refer the patient to a hospital consultant (for example, a general physician or a general surgeon) if this is necessary. In some cases this may be followed by further reference to another consultant who is a specialist in a particular field (for example, a neurologist or a neurosurgeon). The principles of case history taking and clinical examination are the same at all stages, although the GP may tend to be more brief, and the specialist more specific, than the general consultant physician or surgeon. The GP's referral may be straight to the 'super-specialist' but both will be aware of how important it is that the overall general assessment of the problem is not forgotten.

The case history

The doctor will initially give the patient the opportunity of talking freely about the problem and the associated circumstances which seem important. This information is particularly useful but it is likely that soon the conversation must be guided by the doctor. The patient, eager to impart all possible information, sometimes finds it difficult to do this in a logical way and even if he has special training (for example, a doctor) the story begins to lack direction and repetition creeps in. This guided account is the second stage of the interview when the doctor persuades the patient to elaborate on his symptoms still in his own words and avoiding the imposition of a preconceived pattern. The third stage is more formal. Here, by direct questioning, the doctor will seek to 'fill in the gaps' in the patient's account and supplement this with background information about his previous illnesses, personal circumstances and family health.

The clinical examination

Following the interview the doctor undertakes a physical examination of the patient. Clearly, the history he has obtained may have suggested certain diagnoses and this will allow him to concentrate his attention initially on that aspect. For example, an account of a probable groin hernia would lead to this area being inspected early in the examination. In some instances the account itself may be particularly illuminating and the doctor may suspect that clinical examination will give little further lead towards the diagnosis. Such a situation is the rule with a patient who has a chronic duodenal ulcer. Nonetheless, a complete physical examination is necessary in cases such as these or any others where a diagnosis is sought or active treatment contemplated.

The clinician will first examine physically — by sight, touch and sound (described more formally as inspection, palpation/ percussion and **auscultation**). This will be followed, when appropriate, by examination employing instruments such as

Auscultation Listening to sounds produced in any part of the body.

the **sphygmomanometer** to measure the blood pressure, or the **ophthalmoscope** to inspect the retina through the lens of the eye.

The case record
The case history and the findings at clinical examination will be recorded by the doctor at the time. Notes taken throughout the interview will allow it to be recorded in a standard way such as follows:

presenting complaint: summarized in a line or two;
previous illnesses: and list of operations with dates;
previous history: job (precise description) and home circumstances, habits with regard to alcohol and tobacco;
family history: significant illnesses in blood relations;
history of the present complaint: a detailed account of the problems and related circumstances.

The examination findings will also be clearly and logically recorded; general comments are noted first, followed by the system in question: general (height, weight and other physical characteristics); respiratory system; vascular system (central and peripheral); nervous system (central and peripheral); gastrointestinal tract; urinary system; locomotor system and special senses.

The doctor will usually indicate his provisional diagnosis and note the laboratory, radiological and other specialized investigations he has requested. Subsequently, the reported results of these tests will be appended to the case record. The patient's progress and the significance of the test results will be commented on by the doctor who may then modify his diagnosis. The findings at operation and the procedure carried out will be recorded with particular care as will the **histological** characteristics of any tissue removed.

A disease process has been likened to a cine film of which the observer can look at the one current frame. A good case history can capture this impression with surprising vividness.

An example of the stages in diagnosis
The following is a brief account of the diagnostic process in a patient with jaundice. This somewhat complex problem is discussed more fully in Chapter 24.

The symptom of jaundice will be evident to the patient. The association of this with dark (bile-stained) urine and pale (bile-free) faeces will lead the clinician to conclude that the fault lies in the liver or the biliary duct system. If he cannot palpate a distended gall bladder, further diagnostic progress cannot be made until the results of biochemical liver function tests are known. They may exclude serious liver disease, indicating that the cause must be obstruction of the bile duct

Sphygmomanometer An instrument for measuring arterial blood pressure.

Ophthalmoscope An instrument for inspecting the interior of the eye.

Histology The study of anatomy through the microscope.

system. The level of jaundice precludes useful radiology and the diagnosis cannot be pressed further without operation. When this is done it may be found that the obstruction is caused by gall-stones in the bile duct. These can be removed and the patient cured. Alternatively it may be found that the duct is compressed by a hard mass judged to be secondary carcinoma in lymph nodes. Material is taken for histology which confirms the malignancy. The primary cancer is in the stomach but the situation is too far advanced for resection and a by-pass procedure is done to relieve the jaundice. A histological diagnosis has been made but only complete postmortem examination could fully assess the extent of the malignant process.

The place of the computer

Up to this point it has been considered how the exercise of selecting the relevant figures and weighing their importance is done by an individual with an expert knowledge of the subject. It will be clear that this may become essentially a mathematical exercise. In principle, the greater the range and depth of information held as a basis for decision, the greater the accuracy of decision in individual cases. The principle may be simple (and not of a different order from diagnosis by clinical judgement) but the calculations involved would be far too time-consuming to be undertaken without using a computer. Such computer-based analysis is not likely to take over from the doctor but can help as a guide, both in general management of a patient and in individual diagnosis and prognosis (forecasting further progress).

MANAGEMENT

The nursing process

In recent years a notable attempt has been made to specify in quite a formal way the individual needs of a patient from the nursing point of view so that a rational system of care may be developed. For this the term 'The Nursing Process' has been coined and although it may be seen as but a logical extension of Florence Nightingale's dictum that 'the nurse's primary concern is for the person who is ill, rather than the illness itself' (1860) the implications of the principle are quite subtle. For example, it is based on the compilation of a 'nursing history' which, as it seeks to identify how *overall* help may best be given, may look at circumstances a little differently from the 'case history' described earlier. A good account is given in the monograph (Crow, 1977) listed at the end of this chapter.

Resection Surgical removal of a part of the body or a tumour. ('Excision' is used with the same meaning.)

Management by the surgeon and surgical management are not, of course, the same thing. A surgical ward may be largely occupied by patients who have been admitted for an operation but will also contain those who have been admitted for diagnostic tests or who are receiving drugs or other non-operative forms of treatment. One can appreciate the feelings, in such a situation, of the two small boys in adjacent beds who were overheard asking the following. 'Are you medical or surgical?' 'What d'you mean medical or surgical?' 'Well, were you ill when you came in or did they do it to you?'

Non-operative management

A patient is usually referred to the surgical department of a hospital because it seems that an operation is likely to form part of the treatment. This is not always so. There may be a local situation where a particular clinician has an interest and good reputation in the management of all aspects of a problem. Such could be a surgeon with a special interest in colitis and other large bowel disease. It must be admitted that tradition may sometimes play a part; in one area problems of leg ulceration are seen by a surgeon, in another by a derma-tologist. The referral of patients with varying degrees of dyspepsia is a good example of the apparently random way people are sent for a second opinion when either medical or surgical treatment may be indicated. Even when the dyspepsia can be shown to be due to definite duodenal ulceration, operation is not mandatory unless there are complications. Non-operative supervision can be undertaken by physician or surgeon, and there is a good case for them working closely together, perhaps in a joint clinic. There are many similar situations (notably in thyroid disease, renal disease, heart disease and so on). Clearly the closest co-operation between surgeon and radiotherapist is essential.

In certain conditions rational treatment requires not only a proper understanding of the disease process but, in addition, an appreciation of the progression of the condition if untreated and how this is modified by treatment. This is the natural history of the disease, and in a society such as ours, where early treatment is the rule, it may not be readily observable. However, the concept is extremely important, as many disease processes have natural remissions which may be either permanent or for a limited period. A new form of treatment, however excellent it may seem, must be matched against already accepted practice and the results assessed by a clinician not concerned with administering the treatment. This is best done by means of a controlled clinical trial, in which different types of treatment are compared prospectively by randomly assigning each patient to a group undergoing one of the two (or more) types of treatment. It is clearly possible for treatment by a drug (but not by an operation) to be tested against no treatment. The patient in the latter group will receive a placebo, that is tablets which are inactive although apparently identical to the active ones. If neither the patient nor the doctor knows which are the active tablets and which the placebo, the trial is known as a double blind one.

Operative management

The scope of this book does not call for detailed consideration of operative surgical techniques either here or in the chapters that follow. The principles of each procedure are described and the circumstances preceding, during (particularly the anaesthesia) and following the operation are outlined in the relevant chapters. However, some general points are important and may conveniently be discussed here.

The operating department
In very many hospitals (particularly in the United Kingdom) this is known as the 'operating theatre'. Indeed, to some extent the parallel to a theatrical situation is inescapable. In other hospitals (particularly in North America) 'operating room' is the customary name.

The general circumstances are well known. The patient on the operating table is the central figure. At one side stands the surgeon; opposite to him is his assistant. At the surgeon's side is the scrub nurse, who may also have an assistant, with the instruments and equipment for the operation suitably laid out. She is supported from the theatre floor by the circulating nurse. At the head end of the table is the anaesthetist with his equipment and medical and technical assistants. The patient is covered by drapes, allowing exposure only of the area of the operation. This is brilliantly lit from above by a specially designed lamp.

What is less well known is the series of events necessary to produce these circumstances, that is to say, the principles of timing and decision essential to each procedure, the place of anaesthesia and the basic rules of every surgical operation.

Timing of an operation
Operations are commonly thought of as elective or emergency. It is helpful to consider also a third category, the urgent operation. It will be appreciated that the decision when to operate may be no less difficult than the decision whether to operate. It is most unfortunate that in recent times of

'industrial unrest' the degree of urgency of an operation has been given a political significance. This is to be deplored and such considerations have no place in this account of clinical practice.

Elective operation Elective operation is the so-called 'cold' operation for which the patient's admission to hospital is planned and the operation done at a time convenient to the patient, the surgeon, the anaesthetist and the operating theatre staff. Usually this is one of a list of operations planned for that day. The patient has been prepared both physically and mentally for the operation, and the publication of the list sufficiently well ahead has allowed the anaesthetist to make a careful additional assessment of the situation. If any difficulties arise or it is considered that the patient's condition could be improved by further medical treatment, the operation is postponed.

Emergency operation The timing of the emergency operation is quite different. This must be done as soon as possible. For example, one most urgent procedure is the clearance of the main airway for respiration. Usually, if there is a blockage in the trachea, a tube may be passed through it; if not, the operation of tracheostomy must be done. If respiratory obstruction is complete, there will not be time to move the patient to theatre. The arrest of massive haemorrhage may be nearly as urgent. If the site of the bleeding is peripheral, as from a lacerated artery, compression may suffice initially. If it is thoracic or abdominal (as may happen in an ectopic pregnancy), this cannot be done; blood must be replaced as rapidly as possible by transfusion and the patient taken to the operating theatre for operation as soon as possible.

Next to these and other thoracic situations (such as, tension pneumothorax) the emergency is usually one of degree. That is to say, although a perforated duodenal ulcer, strangulated intestine or acute appendicitis call for emergency operation, there is adequate time for the patient to be prepared. The decision regarding the time that may be spent in resuscitation of the patient (by fluid replacement, drugs and so on), balanced against the delay in operating necessitated by this, may be a very difficult one calling for experience and fine judgement. An important point is that when the decision to operate has been made, strong **analgesics** need not be withheld.

Urgent operation The need for urgent operation occurs in clinical situations, such as complete obstruction of urine flow, or intestinal obstruction without strangulation, when

Analgesic A drug or technique which reduces pain without inducing unconsciousness

operation may be deferred for a matter of days (in prostatic obstruction with urine drainage by fine catheter, in intestinal obstruction with intestinal suction and intravenous fluid replacement).

Other circumstances may increase the urgency of an operation. For example, appendicitis perforation without localization of pus is more likely in children than in adults. Operation is correspondingly more urgent. Spontaneous cessation of bleeding is less likely from an elderly patient, with haemorrhage from erosion of a sclerotic artery in the base of a gastric ulcer, than if the same bleeding occurs in a young patient. Also the elderly patient is less able to stand the blood loss. All these factors may cause the surgeon to operate sooner, although he is aware that, generally, the risks of operation for the older patient are greater.

Type of operation

Operations may, in principle, be classified by type, but there are limitations and it will be clear that more than one sort of procedure may be used during an operation. For example, excision will usually be followed by some form of reconstruction, however simple. Nonetheless, some understanding of the way surgeons work may be gained by considering operative procedures under these two headings and also Opening, Alteration of function, Support and Transplantation.

Opening Opening may be into a body cavity (-otomy) for removal of blood, pus or other abnormal fluid; for example, the procedure of craniotomy to evacuate a blood clot arising following trauma to the skull, or a thoracotomy to remove pus from the pleural cavity. It may also be into a body cavity such as the peritoneal cavity to inspect the viscera lying there when the exact diagnosis is in doubt. A simple opening, or cut (incision), may be made into an abscess or blood clot in a tissue for evacuation and drainage of the contents.

Excision An area of the body known to be diseased is removed (-ectomy). An organ which is the site of a primary cancer may be resected in, for example, **mastectomy, gastrectomy, cystectomy**. Or there may be other reasons such as removal of a gall bladder which contains stones or is inflamed (**cholecystectomy**) or removal of an inflamed appendix (**appendicectomy**).

Alteration of function The type of procedure which aims to alter function rather than form is based on a knowledge of normal and altered physiology. An example is the division of

Appendicectomy The surgical removal of the appendix. By convention this always refers to the vermiform appendix (opening off the caecum) rather than any of the other numerous appendices in the body. 'Appendectomy' is the American term for the same operation. The suffix 'ectomy' is derived from the Greek *ectome* = a cutting out, hence it is used with the appropriate prefix to indicate, in a word, the removal of an organ (e.g. mastectomy — of the breast; gastrectomy — of the stomach etc.).

B

the vagus nerves in the abdomen with a resultant fall in the level of gastric acid secretion, a circumstance favourable to the healing of a duodenal ulcer. The slowing of gastric emptying is an unwanted effect which must be overcome by a 'gastric drainage' procedure designed to hasten this (*see* page 487). Another example is the removal of the adrenal glands (also an excision operation — adrenalectomy) to take away a source of circulating oestrogen which may be aiding growth of secondary breast carcinoma. An unwanted effect here is the removal of the source of cortisone; this must be replaced in drug form.

Support Damaged or weakened tissues require support for which the body's own tissue or an implant of foreign material is used. Thus a poorly healed fractured bone may be supported by a bone graft or a metal bar; a bad hernia may be repaired using adjacent fascia, or it may be necessary to use a foreign material (e.g. a plastic). It is important that foreign material used in this way should be practically inert, i.e. it must not promote any reaction to its presence by the body tissues.

Reconstruction A simple form of reconstruction is the suturing in continuity of the two ends of bowel after a segment has been removed. Sometimes reconstruction is more complex as after resection of the head of the pancreas when biliary, pancreatic and gastrointestinal continuity must be restored (*see* page 532). In certain situations, there are alternate procedures such as when, after partial gastrectomy (*see* page 487), when reconstruction may be in continuity (Billroth I) or end-to-side (Billroth II; Polya).

Transplantation Tissues may be transplanted from one site to another; split skin grafting is a good example. Tissues or organs may be transplanted from one body to another. If the effect does not depend on the tissue being revascularized and retaining the identical pre-transplant form, for example, a bone graft which serves mainly as a basis for new bone formation, the rejection phenomenon is immaterial. This does, however, assume great importance when an organ such as a kidney is transplanted and, unless the donor is genetically identical to the recipient (identical twins), some form of repression of the immune mechanism responsible for the rejection process, is necessary. This subject is discussed in much greater detail in Chapter 11.

Anaesthesia
Anaesthesia, or loss of feeling, may be either general, in which case the patient undergoing operation is also relaxed

and may require assisted respiration, or local, when the area of operation alone is rendered insensitive to pain. The subject is considered fully in Chapter 3.

The basic rules of an operation

Operative surgery should be safe, clean and sound in technique and system.

Safety There is some hazard in every operation but many dangers are avoidable. The strictest attention to routine precautions is essential if errors are to be prevented. Hospitals will usually have procedural instructions for these. Points of particular importance are:

(1) complete identification and labelling of each patient;
(2) unambiguous marking of the site, limb or digit for operation when this is appropriate — this is best done at the time the patient signs the consent for operation form;
(3) correct preoperative preparation and premedication of the patient;
(4) meticulous counting and recording of all swabs and instruments at the start and finish of every operation;
(5) correct insulation of diathermy apparatus and positioning of the electrode pad; and
(6) correct earthing of apparatus and full antistatic precautions to avoid any possible ignition of an inflammable vapour.

Asepsis In many operative situations, such as, for example, when gut is opened or internal sepsis is present, this may be relative. However, the principle of asepsis (that is, avoiding the introduction of any bacteria into the operative field) must be rigorously applied by:

(1) the sterilization of instruments — usually by heat;
(2) the surgeon and his assistants' hand and arm 'scrubbing' followed by 'gowning up' in sterile gown and gloves; and
(3) skin preparation for the site of the incision and a wide surrounding area — usually soap and water washing in the ward (at which time all body hair is shaved) and spirit solution cleaning at the start of the operation.

Technique At the most basic level, operating in general surgery involves the use of the following three manoeuvres, in themselves quite simple. The surgeon (1) cuts with a knife or scissors, (2) helps arrest the bleeding, mainly by pressure, either widely on the bleeding area as with a pack, or locally to an individual vessel which is clamped and tied, or in some cases coagulated by diathermy. This sounds easy and usually it is; but not always. Also the word 'helps' is used advisedly. For arrest of haemorrhage to be maintained effectively, the body's haemostatic mechanisms must function soundly; they are complex and the possibilities of interference numerous. If natural haemostasis is defective, the surgeon's job may be very difficult; if it is absent, bleeding will not stop. (3) The surgeon sews. The suture material, if it is catgut or similar, will later be absorbed or, if it is nylon or silk for example, will be permanent.

System By the term 'system' is meant the surgeon's systematic approach to the problem — incision, exploration, procedure, closure. The following account indicates briefly how it would be applied in an abdominal operation for persistent unexplained abdominal pain.

(1) Incision: the surgeon elects for an approach giving good access to the abdominal cavity and being capable of extension. A right paramedian approach would be suitable. In this procedure the abdominal skin, subcutaneous tissues and muscle sheath are incised in a vertical line just to the right of the umbilicus. The edges of the wound and the surrounding skin are then covered with water-repellent cloth or plastic drapes. The muscle (rectus abdominis) is pulled to the side and the posterior muscle sheath and peritoneum incised in the same line.

(2) Exploration: the omentum is eased to one side and the surgeon may readily find that several inches of the lower end of the small intestine are caught up in fibrous tissue that has possibly followed inflammation several years earlier. This would explain the abdominal pain, but the surgeon still proceeds carefully to palpate and, where possible, examine all the other abdominal viscera.

(3) Procedure: it is necessary for a short length of small intestine to be resected. This is done using light non-crushing clamps to avoid bowel content spillage. The two ends are anastomosed, being held together by absorbable sutures.

(4) Closure: the abdominal cavity is closed. Three layers are sutured: peritoneum with posterior muscle sheath, anterior sheath, and finally skin.

If this analysis of the surgeon's art should seem unduly prosaic, let me quote from Lord Moynihan's (1920) tribute to the American surgeon, J. B. Murphy:

> He believed in safe and thorough work rather than in specious and hazardous brilliance. He was infinitely careful in preparation, and compared with many was inclined to be slow; but every step in every operation which I ever saw him do was completed deliberately, accurately, once for all. It led inevitably to the next step, without pause, without haste; that step completed, another followed.

REHABILITATION

No operation and no treatment is likely to be considered a success by the patient unless his suffering or disability is relieved. It is his hope that within a reasonable time he will have regained the health that should be his and the ability and enthusiasm to live fully. The process associated with an operation or other appropriate treatment leading to this aim is rehabilitation.

Such a definition is very general, but I believe that it is most important for rehabilitation to be seen in this way. It is clearly in the national interest for men who have been injured to be enabled to return to work as soon as possible and, therefore, the provision of full facilities for rehabilitation is essential. There is, rightly, concern that their application is in no way limited regarding age or sex; nor is the principle of rehabilitation confined to any one aspect of disease, such as, the effects of an injury. A businessman who has had half his stomach removed, a housewife after a mastectomy, a pensioner following a mid-thigh amputation; each requires individual advice, possibly guidance about prostheses and, certainly, encouragement.

To direct such rehabilitation after an operation, except if this is of the simplest type, is a most important role of the surgeon and the nurse, with support, when necessary, from the physiotherapist and occupational therapist. Nor must it be forgotten that the process should, if possible, be started before the operation and begin with a simple and sympathetic explanation to the patient of what is likely to happen. What else may be done in a more specific way?

General approach

The operation is best regarded simply as one incident, albeit important, during the patient's stay in hospital. He should not be admitted further ahead than is necessary for essential preoperative investigation and treatment. There is usually no cause for him to be confined to bed during this period. Afterwards, a start towards normal activity should be made as soon as possible. For example, a patient should get out of bed, at least to sit on a chair, the morning after a gastrectomy operation. Intravenous fluid lines and other tubing to which he is attached may limit his mobility. This support may be essential at first but it should not be extended unnecessarily. When the patient is mobile, self-help must be insisted on. Modern hospital wards will be designed for progressive care of the patient which means that he should graduate as quickly as he reasonably can from total dependence on nursing care to independence.

Events in the postoperative period are of great importance and are discussed in some detail later in the book: the relatively smooth postoperative progress of the patient in Chapter 4, and the complex problems that require intensive therapy unit care in Chapter 5. At this time the surgical team should be particularly aware of how much help their patient can be given by the physiotherapy department. But the nurse is closest of all to the patient and therefore best able to give him a positive attitude to recovery.

Special problems related to amputation and trauma

If an active person has sustained a serious injury, it may be suspected initially, and agreed eventually, that he cannot fully return to the life and work that was his before the accident. Therefore, the final stages of his rehabilitation, which may be lengthy, are directed towards the best use of the function he has regained. This will usually mean a different type of job or even a sheltered occupation. However, the initial stages present problems which differ according to the type of injury.

Amputation of a leg

As soon as his amputation stump has healed, the patient is referred to the artificial limb and appliance service for the area. Even before this, correct bandaging will have helped to form a good stump shape for an artificial limb. This will initially be of a temporary type (pylon) while the individual artificial limb is made. An elderly patient may stay in hospital until he is walking well on this.

Bone or joint injury

Enforced rest leads to wasting of associated muscles; an excess form of this is disuse atrophy. Active exercises are essential for this to be overcome and if conscious control is defective, muscle contraction may be stimulated electrically. This is done in the physiotherapy department. Without full return of muscle activity complete recovery cannot occur.

Spinal cord injury

The effects of this (**paraplegia** or **quadriplegia**) present one of the major challenges in rehabilitation. A concentration of medical and physiotherapeutic expertise and also specialized apparatus are necessary and these are located in national rehabilitation centres. The possibility of physical recovery may be limited (a wheel-chair life) but given the right support and encouragement man's spirit is wonderfully resilient.

Head injury

The effects of head injuries are enormously variable. A mild concussion may be followed by no detectable ill effects, while the sequelae of prolonged unconsciousness may include extreme cerebral and emotional change. At the more serious end of this spectrum a great deal of support will be necessary and full rehabilitation less likely than with spinal injuries.

Special problems related to the operation

Operations leading to altered function require certain initial adjustments. Examples of this are the adaptation necessary to the change following subtotal **thyroidectomy** for **thyrotoxicosis** or to the alteration in bowel habits that may follow **vagotomy** and **pyloroplasty**. If patients are warned of these possibilities and given the right support, problems are usually minimal.

The effect of an operation altering form can seem severe (mastectomy is a procedure which causes a great deal of anxiety before the operation), yet a sympathetic straightforward approach can help greatly. Furthermore, modern **prostheses** (for example, a special postmastectomy brassiere) are very good.

There is, also, the particular case of a type of operation which has resulted in the permanent diversion of faeces or urine into the abdominal wall. A special appliance is necessary for the collection of waste matter.

Colostomy

The most common operation for which the direction of faeces onto the abdominal wall is done as a permanent procedure is removal of the rectum for cancer. The end of the descending colon is brought out onto the abdominal wall. This operation has a good prognosis in terms of life expectancy and patients usually manage well with a **colostomy**

Paraplegia Paralysis of both legs and the lower part of the body.

Quadriplegia Paralysis of all four limbs.

Thyroidectomy Excision of the thyroid gland.

Thyrotoxicosis A disease caused by excessive thyroid secretion in which there may be weight loss, extreme nervousness, sweating, tachycardia (q.v.), cardiac irregularities and heart failure.

Vagotomy Division of the vagus nerves. The suffix 'otomy' is derived from the Greek *temnein* = to cut, hence it is used with the appropriate prefix to indicate surgical division (e.g. tenotomy – of a tendon; laparotomy – of the abdominal wall, etc.).

Pyloroplasty Surgical reshaping; in the case of the pylorus = enlarging of the opening. The suffix 'plasty' is derived from the Greek *plassein* = to mould. Hence it is used with a suitable prefix to indicate a refashioning (e.g. mammoplasty – of the breast; vesicoplasty – of the urinary bladder).

Prosthesis An artificial part which may be used to replace one which has been removed – either externally (e.g. the breast or a limb, etc.) or internally (e.g. a heart valve or a hip joint etc.).

Colostomy An opening made through the abdominal wall into the colon. The suffix 'ostomy' is derived from the Greek *stoma* = mouth, hence it is used with a single prefix to indicate a surgically made external opening (e.g. ileostomy; ureterostomy etc.) or with a double prefix to indicate an opening fashioned between one internal cavity and another (e.g. gastrojejunostomy, choledochoduodenostomy (choledochus = bile duct) etc.).

for many years. A rhythm of colon emptying of firm faeces is usually established and a belt with a firmly fitting bag that can be emptied regularly is the essential appliance.

Individual advice to patients is available through the Colostomy Welfare Group, 38/39 Eccleston Square (Second Floor), London SW1V 1PB (Telephone: 01-828 5175).

Ileostomy

Total removal of the rectum and colon means that the end of the patient's small intestine must be fashioned into a spout on the abdominal wall. This is less commonly done than a colostomy and more difficult to manage. The problem is that the contents of the bowel at this level remain fluid and pass through at irregular intervals. There must, therefore, be a watertight fit between the neck of the bag and the skin. This is usually done by a special adhesive which allows the retaining flange of the bag to be stuck to the skin.

Considerable help by advice on individual problems can be given by the Ileostomy Association of Great Britain and Ireland, 23 Winchester Road (First Floor), Basingstoke, (Hants RG21 1UE) (Telephone: Basingstoke (STD 0256) 52320). This organization has a large patient membership with divisions throughout the country.

Urinary diversion

Urinary diversion is necessary when there has been total removal of the bladder for cancer or when bladder control is grossly defective. The latter situation occurs particularly in **spina bifida** cases. The most common method is an ileal bladder (more accurately, an ileal conduit, as the ureters are implanted into a short length of bowel which drains the urine to the surface). Management problems are similar to those of an ileostomy.

Special problems related to the patient

The adult of working age will usually return home within a week after his operation. He will expect to spend a period of rest at home and will then start work again. The length of this period depends on several factors, in particular the nature of the operation and the patient's physique. Convalesence in a more formal sense, that is to say a period of two weeks or so spent in a convalescent ward, is not usually indicated, although there are certain situations when this may be valuable. For example, someone living alone would benefit from such an arrangement as would a housewife with unavoidable family responsibilities in her home.

Spina bifida A congenital failure of fusion of the lamina of the vertebra. Usually several vertebrae are affected. There may be nerve damage and thus serious interference with bladder function, locomotion, etc.

Extremes of age can magnify the problem. Most young children adapt well to an operation. For the elderly this is not the rule, and support at home may be necessary for a prolonged period. If such a patient has lived alone, assistance from the local authority is sometimes necessary; this may be by provision of a 'home help' or in an extreme case by finding suitable accommodation, possibly in a hostel.

The follow-up

Once he has returned home, the further medical care of the patient is quite definitely the responsibility of his general practitioner. The surgeon will have forwarded to him an account of the diagnosis and the operation with advice regarding future management. However, it would be surprising if the surgeon felt he had completely discharged his responsibility of the patient at this point, and an appointment is usually made for him to be seen at the follow-up clinic. The surgeon will want to know details of progress following the operation and to examine the patient, particularly the healed wound. Radiological or laboratory checks may be necessary.

In the great majority of cases one such visit, usually about a month after the operation, will suffice. However, certain circumstances, such as cancer problems or rare clinical situations, make further hospital visits advisable. It is essential that there be agreement on this policy and full interchange of information between everyone concerned with the patient.

This chapter was intended to set the scene for this book on clinical surgery. I have referred to several of the chapters that follow and I have tried to fill in the gaps between the topics they cover. In a book such as this it is sometimes difficult to find the right balance between the mechanistic and the humane approach. Compassion, a quality fundamental to the practice of medicine, cannot readily be instilled by the printed word. Furthermore, the help which the doctor or nurse can give to the patient in such simple ways as taking the time to explain to him what is happening or letting him appreciate that, although he may feel that a hospital is a strange and frightening place, he is among friends, cannot be measured. It may do more good than tablets from the pharmacy; who knows?

There are, however, two final points which should be emphasized. Firstly, hospitals are for ill people. All of us who work in them have one common aim: it is to relieve suffering. Secondly, although we work very hard to save life there must eventually be an end. Death may be dreaded, hoped for or simply accepted, but everyone will die. It is his right to be allowed to do so with dignity.

REFERENCES

Cohen, H. (1943). The nature method and purpose of diagnosis. The Skinner Lecture. *Lancet* **1**, 23

Crow, J. (1977). *The Nursing Process.* London: A Nursing Times Publication

Fry, J. (1966). *Profiles of Disease. A Study in the Natural History of Common Disease.* Edinburgh and London: E. and S. Livingstone

Moynihan, B. G. A. (1920). John B. Murphy, surgeon. The first Murphy memorial oration. *Surgery Gynec. Obstet.* **31**, 549

Nightingale, F. (1893). Sick nursing and health. Women's Missionary Services of Congress. In *Philanthropic Work of Women.* Ed. Baroness Burdett Couttes

Organization and Staffing of Operating Departments, The. (1970). Report of a joint sub-committee of the Standing Medical Advisory Committee and the Standing Nursing Advisory Committee. London: H.M.S.O.

Tunbridge, R. (1972). *Report of the Sub-committee on Rehabilitation of the Standing Medical Advisory Committee.* London: H.M.S.O.

2

Preoperative preparation of the patient

J. E. Utting

For most people a surgical operation will be one of the most severe physical and psychological tests in their lives. The purpose of preoperative preparation is to make sure that the patient is in the best possible condition to overcome the challenges which an operation presents.

PREOPERATIVE INVESTIGATION

This can only be done if sufficient is known about the patient; for this reason a case history must be taken, a physical examination performed and frequently investigations will have to be arranged. The results of this whole procedure may suggest that treatment is necessary; it may, for example, be found that the patient is anaemic or diabetic and, therefore, perhaps requires a preoperative blood transfusion or stabilization of his diabetes on insulin. In addition, there are other procedures which may be required such as bathing, shaving and marking the side of the patient to be operated on.

Case history

A full case history should be taken from every patient who is to undergo major surgery; and, indeed, a brief case history from any patient who is presented for operation however trivial.

In addition to information about the patient's current complaint, a full case history will include some details about family background and personal history. A number of questions about non-specific symptoms may also be asked; 'Are you short of breath?' is an example of a question which can yield a great deal of information.

A question on the drugs a patient is taking must always be included in the surgical case history. A number of drugs, e.g. those used in the treatment of hypertension, may affect the

Table 2.1   Some of the drugs which may cause difficulty to the anaesthetist

Drug	Reason for caution
Antibiotics (for example, kanamycin, neomycin)	May cause prolonged paralysis with muscle relaxant drugs
Antihypertensive agents	May cause hypotension and bradycardia during anaesthesia
Corticosteroids	May have caused suppression of adrenal cortex; might result in collapse during or after anaesthesia and surgery
Diuretics	May cause hypopotassaemia which prolongs action of some muscle relaxants
Ecothiopate (eye-drops)	May prolong action of the muscle relaxant suxamethonium
Insulin	May cause hypoglycaemia under anaesthesia
Monoamine oxidase inhibitors	Used in psychiatry; may cause collapse with pethidine or anaesthetic agents

choice of anaesthetic and the way in which it is given. Some of the more important drugs in this respect are shown in Table 2.1.

Physical examination

Preoperative preparation of the patient must include a full physical examination. Usually if there is something wrong, for example with the patient's heart or lungs, this will have become apparent when the history was taken.

This, however, is not always so. Sometimes physical examination will detect some previously unrecognized abnormality. It may be found, for example, that the patient has swelling of the ankles, engorgement of the jugular veins and other signs of cardiac failure when he has given no history to suggest this as a possibility, either because the symptoms are minimal or because he has decided to conceal them.

Preoperative physical examination is mainly concerned with the respiratory and cardiovascular systems since most of the more important complications of anaesthesia are concerned with respiration or with circulation. Thus a patient may go into a state of respiratory failure and be unable to breathe adequately after operation; this may occur in people with a 'bad chest', and if the patient has been shown by his history and physical examination to be a respiratory cripple, then his condition should be carefully assessed and special care taken to avoid this complication.

Engorgement Congestion of a blood vessel or vessels.

In emergency cases in which the patient has lost blood or body fluids the preoperative examination is of especial importance. Here the concern is that the patient's condition has been made as good as possible by transfusion of blood or infusion of fluids, such as saline, in patients who have lost fluid by vomiting, in intestinal fistulas and so on. In these circumstances it is always dangerous, and usually unnecessary, to induce anaesthesia and commence operation till the blood pressure has been restored to acceptable levels and the pulse rate has declined if **tachycardia** was present.

Special investigations

Before undergoing surgery most patients will be subjected to several investigations. Some of these may have been performed before the patient enters hospital. A patient who is suspected of having a peptic ulcer or gastric cancer may have a barium meal investigation carried out in the radiology department before admission. In addition to investigations which are directed towards the diagnosis and evaluation of the patient's surgical condition, other investigations may be indicated to evaluate the patient's fitness for surgery and anaesthesia and will be undertaken before or after the patient comes into hospital depending on circumstances. An investigation is of value because it may reveal that the patient has underlying disease unrelated to his surgical condition; a preoperative electrocardiogram (ECG), for example, may show evidence of unsuspected coronary artery disease.

It is neither practical nor desirable to subject every patient to every investigation, and there has clearly got to be common sense in any approach to this problem. For example, it is unusual to take an ECG recording preoperatively from an apparently fit woman aged 30 years because the chances of finding an abnormality are minute.

Urine analysis is frequently performed as routine on the ward, though a sample is often sent to the laboratory as well. Among the common tests performed are tests for sugar (the presence of which suggests the possibility of **diabetes mellitus**), protein (the presence of which suggests renal disease), and acetone (the presence of which suggests diabetes but which may also be present in dehydration and other conditions). The specific gravity of the urine also gives an estimation of renal function in some circumstances.

The commonly required investigations before operation can be considered in five groups: haematological investigations, biochemical investigations, ECG, chest radiograph and pulmonary function tests. Many others may be required from time to time but these are the main ones.

Tachycardia Fast heart rate.

Diabetes mellitus A common disease associated with a pathologically high blood sugar and a tendency to acidosis. It is caused by a relative or absolute failure to secrete enough insulin.

Haematological investigation

If the patient is thought to be anaemic or is likely to have a blood transfusion, the haemoglobin concentration in the blood should be determined; indeed it is usual to perform this investigation as a routine in patients who are to undergo major surgery.

If the operation is likely to be associated with anything other than a minor degree of blood loss then the patient's blood group must be determined. In some operations (e.g. abdominoperineal resection of rectum) blood transfusion is nearly always required, and blood should be crossmatched before operation. In the cases of some other operations (e.g. abdominal **hysterectomy**) blood transfusion is not usually required, though occasionally it may be necessary. Here the patient's blood group is determined before operation and his serum kept in the laboratory so that if blood be required during operation it can be rapidly crossmatched.

Biochemical investigations

The plasma **electrolyte** and blood **urea** concentrations are commonly determined before surgery if it is suspected that abnormal values may be obtained. This is so in many conditions; for example, after prolonged vomiting and diarrhoea, after failure of adequate fluid intake, after treatment with some diuretics and in various forms of renal failure.

Bacteriological investigation

If the patient is producing sputum, as in chronic bronchitis, an attempt should be made to culture the sputum and determine the antibiotic sensitivities of any pathogenic organisms grown.

Electrocardiogram

It is usual to perform an ECG on patients who are suspected of having a coronary artery disease. As this disease is common, particularly in men, it is frequently decided to have an ECG performed routinely on patients over, say, the age of 50 years. In this way a number of cases of unsuspected coronary artery disease may be detected, and a useful base-line record obtained for subsequent reference after surgery.

Hysterectomy Removal of the whole, or the body, of the uterus.

Electrolyte Any substance which in solution dissociates into electrically charged particles. Refers in the blood to the ionized salts of sodium, potassium, chloride and bicarbonate.

Urea A nitrogenous waste product normally eliminated by the kidney. Urea is produced mainly by metabolism of such substances as proteins.

Chest radiograph

A chest radiograph will be taken if respiratory or cardiovascular disease is suspected, and is often used as a routine investigation in elderly patients presented for major surgery. Most of the more serious pathological conditions involving the lung will be shown up on a chest radiograph and, for example, pneumonia, pulmonary oedema, collapse of the lobe, and even carcinoma of the lung may also be detected in this way. The chest radiograph will also give an indication of the size of the heart which may be enlarged in heart disease.

Pulmonary function tests

The performance of pulmonary function tests may be indicated when such diseases as chronic bronchitis and emphysema are suspected (*see* below). There are many of these tests but, indeed, it can also be a valuable test of pulmonary function just to observe the degree of breathlessness which is caused by normal activities such as undressing.

Of the tests requiring special equipment, the determination of the vital capacity of the lungs is one of the commonest. The vital capacity is the volume of air which can be breathed out after the patient has taken the biggest possible breath in.

However, a vital capacity of such and such a volume does not denote how quickly the patient can breathe out, and this may be important. The vital capacity manoeuvre can be timed; the patient takes a deep breath as before but then tries to breathe out as fast as possible. From a tracing obtained in this way it is possible to work out forced expiratory volume per second (FEV_1), that is the volume of air breathed out in one second. In conditions in which there is obstruction to airflow (for example, asthma, emphysema) the FEV_1 is much reduced.

PREOPERATIVE THERAPY

Preoperative medical treatment

The purpose of taking a case history, examining the patient and studying the results of investigations is twofold. First, it facilitates diagnosis and treatment of intercurrent disease (for example, bronchitis); the patient can thus be made as fit as possible for operation. Secondly, it enables a more accurate prognosis to be made.

The possibility of making the patient as fit as possible for operation can only be judged in the light of the urgency of the operative procedure. It is, for example, of little use suggesting a course of antibiotic treatment and physiotherapy for a patient who has chronic bronchitis and has been admitted with a perforated peptic ulcer. It may, on the other hand, be quite wrong not to undertake such treatment in the case of a patient who is presented for surgical treatment of a chronic duodenal ulcer.

Emphysema A common chronic disease of the lungs characterized by breathlessness due mainly to difficulty in breathing out; it is associated with distension of the small air passages and air sacs in the lung.

There are, of course, many 'medical' conditions which may require assessment and treatment before operation. A few of the more important ones will be mentioned briefly.

Chronic bronchitis and emphysema

Chronic bronchitis and emphysema are probably distinct conditions, but usually coexist and can, for this reason, be conveniently considered together. They are characterized by varying degrees of breathlessness, cough, sputum and wheeze.

Preoperative **antibiotic** therapy should be considered in patients who have purulent sputum. If it has been possible to obtain the sensitivities of the organisms present in the sputum, the antibiotic administered will be chosen with these results in view. Otherwise a broad spectrum antibiotic (for example, ampicillin) may be administered. If, as frequently is the case, there is neither time to await the results of the bacteriological investigations nor time to give a course of antibiotic, then a broad spectrum antibiotic should be given straightaway after a specimen for sputum culture and sensitivity has been taken.

Physiotherapy has much to offer, particularly in the case of the patient with much sputum production. Postural coughing to drain the various parts of the lung of as much sputum as possible can be performed preoperatively. The patient is put in various positions and encouraged and stimulated to cough. Postural drainage consists of keeping the patient in a particular position for some considerable length of time in order to drain sputum from the lobes of the lung above; this procedure is of particular value in patients in whom there is a degree of **bronchiectasis**.

Patients with pure emphysema (who do not produce much sputum) are less susceptible to improvement, though they can benefit from breathing exercises. These are designed to teach the patient to use his abdominal muscles and the diaphragm in breathing, and this helps because the chest wall is capable of only very limited movement.

In chronic bronchitis and emphysema there is obstruction to the airways, especially when the patient breathes out. The obstruction to the flow of air out of the chest may give rise even to an audible wheeze. Sometimes there is a considerable degree of reversible airways obstruction similar to the **bronchospasm** which is seen in asthma; it is probably due to constriction of the muscle in the walls of the air passages and to the swelling of their walls and can be tackled by therapy before operation. In patients with reversible airways obstruction bronchodilator drugs should be used preoperatively in an attempt to reduce the obstruction. Patients with bronchial asthma, of course, may require attention in this way.

Antibiotic Drug obtained from moulds which prevents the growth of, or destroys, bacteria.

Bronchiectasis Severe infection and cavitation of lung tissue.

Bronchospasm Constriction of the muscle of the bronchial tree, usually giving rise to an audible wheeze, as in bronchial asthma.

Finally it must also be remembered that it is common for patients with bronchopneumonia and acute bronchitis to be presented for operation. Their chest infections may merely be a feature of the fact that they are severely ill due to, for example, intestinal obstruction.

Cardiac failure

If there is heart failure present this must be treated. The treatment depends both on the type of failure and its degree. Acute left ventricular failure, for example, will require the intravenous administration of morphine and of a **diuretic** such as frusemide (Lasix). A patient with mild right-sided congestive cardiac failure due to **mitral stenosis** with atrial **fibrillation** will require the administration of digitalis and oral diuretics.

Hypertension

Hypertension should be treated medically where possible before the patient is presented for elective surgery. The antihypertensive drugs block the normal circulatory responses to the administration of anaesthetic agents. There is a tendency for many of the drugs used in anaesthesia to cause mild and temporary cardiac dysfunction and peripheral **vasodilatation**; both these factors frequently lead to a decrease in blood pressure. The body normally attempts to compensate for this mild 'poisoning' by increased activity of the **sympathetic nervous system**. The drugs commonly used in the treatment of hypertension interfere with the sympathetic nervous system and may, therefore, reduce the body's ability to compensate, and can also cause an even greater fall in blood pressure and slowing of the heart by **synergy** with the anaesthetic agents. Nevertheless it is now commonly held that the patient on antihypertensive therapy is better off facing an anaesthetic still on dry therapy than he would be if it were witheld.

Diabetes mellitus

Diabetes is a disease caused by underproduction or diminished effectiveness of the hormone insulin, which is produced by the beta cells of the islets of Langerhans in the pancreas. It is not always caused, as used to be thought, by failure of secretion of insulin but may also occur because of over-production of substances which antagonize the action of the hormone.

The young patient (juvenile-onset type) has to be treated with insulin by injection and will have to go on taking this for the rest of his life and will also have dietary restrictions. He will readily develop **ketoacidosis**. Frequently, however,

Diuretic Drug used to increase the secretion of urine in such conditions as cardiac failure (frusemide, i.e. Lasix).

Mitral stenosis A partial closing down of the mitral valve, on the left side of the heart between the left atrium and ventricle, due to the effects of rheumatic fever. Heart failure eventually results.

Fibrillation A quivering, unco-ordinated movement of muscle (usually the heart).

Vasodilatation An increase in calibre of blood vessels usually associated with an increase in flow of blood.

Sympathetic nervous system A part of the nervous system (autonomic, or functionally independent) which regulates the activity of structures not under voluntary control, e.g. smooth muscle, etc.

Synergy Working together.

Ketoacidosis Increased acidity of the blood due to acids derived from ketones (organic compounds — e.g. acetone — produced by an oxidation process).

diabetes first appears in the middle years of life often in association with obesity (maturity-onset type). In this group of patients the disease can often be controlled by a low carbohydrate diet alone, with or without oral hypoglycaemic agents, but without the need for insulin.

Not only is diabetes mellitus a common condition, but it is also one which has many complications for which the patient may seek surgical advice — peripheral vascular disease (sometimes leading to gangrene of the toes), cataract and infections are among these. Thus patients known to be diabetics, or unsuspected diabetics, are not uncommonly found attending surgical clinics.

The management of patients with diabetes mellitus who are presented for surgery is a difficult problem, and one which cannot be treated fully in a few words. A few basic points must, however, be mentioned.

Hypoglycaemic coma due to too much insulin is a greater hazard to the insulin-taking diabetic undergoing surgery than is hyperglycaemia. Hypoglycaemia comes on quickly and in the conscious patient is associated with agitation, irrational behaviour and eventual loss of consciousness. It is easy to miss hypoglycaemia when the patient is anaesthetized or just recovering from an anaesthetic, and in these circumstances brain damage can occur.

It has become increasingly realized in recent years that many patients who are on even moderately large doses of insulin can be successfully managed for operations of mild or moderate severity by omitting insulin on the day of operation, and even on the day before operation if long-acting insulins are being used. If, on the other hand, insulin is necessary because the patient is a severe diabetic and the operative procedure is of a serious nature, then soluble insulin only must be used. An intravenous infusion is set up and glucose administered to avoid the patient becoming hypoglycaemic. Until relatively recently it was not unusual for patients who were on insulin and who were having insulin to be given breakfast on the morning of operation. All too often this resulted in fatal inhalation of vomit.

Most patients who are taking oral hypoglycaemic agents present no great problem. They will not require to take the drugs during the time of surgery, and can be managed without slipping into diabetic (hyperglycaemic) coma even if they do not take their tablets for a few days.

Preoperative fluid therapy

One of the most important methods of preparing a patient for surgery is by the intravenous administration of blood, saline, or other fluid to correct preoperative deficiencies.

Hyperglycaemia An excessive blood sugar concentration.

Hypoglycaemia A decrease in the blood sugar associated with such symptoms as sweating, anxiety, clouding of consciousness and eventually coma.

The number of different fluids used for intravenous infusion is, of course, legion. Here only a few of the more important ones will be very briefly considered.

Blood

Stored blood, also called 'ACD blood' because the blood from the donor is taken into acid citrate dextrose solution to stop clotting, is used before surgery in two circumstances. First, it is used to restore blood which has been lost acutely as in the case of a patient with, for instance, a bleeding peptic ulcer or after a road traffic accident. Secondly, it may be used to correct anaemia which is due to chronic blood loss or failure of the body to build up new red cells. In some circumstances, such as for example a long-standing and profound anaemia, the ability of the heart to deal with the increased blood volume may be reduced. It is then necessary to give blood very slowly, or to use packed cells, that is a transfusion in which red blood cells are given, but with less total fluid than is the case with ACD blood, the blood stored having been spun down in a centrifuge and some of the supernatant fluid removed. It is now, indeed, common practice to reduce the plasma content of blood before it is given to patients, the plasma removed being stored and used for other patients as indicated below.

It must always be remembered that there are important differences between the blood bank blood which is administered and the blood normally found in vein and artery: ACD blood is cold and acid; it also contains citrate and the plasma of this blood has a higher concentration of potassium than has normal blood. This difference may become important when large volumes of blood are given very rapidly. In these circumstances 'citrate intoxication' may occur. This consists of an acute cardiac failure. The treatment is to give calcium.

Plasma and dextrans

Plasma protein fraction (PPF) is obtained from blood. Some of the clotting factors have been removed, and the resultant is basically a solution of albumin. PPF can be used to restore circulating blood volume; it is especially useful in burns.

The various dextran preparations are also used to keep up the circulating volume; the dextrans of low molecular weight are also used to improve the flow through tissues. None of these preparations have much use preoperatively. Neither plasma nor dextrans, of course, carry oxygen since neither contain haemoglobin.

Dextran A carbohydrate substance, a solution of which can be given intravenously as a substitute for plasma.

Normal saline

Normal **saline** is a solution of 0.9 per cent sodium chloride in water and is **isotonic** with plasma. This means that red blood cells suspended in saline will not absorb water and blow up and burst (as they would if the solution were too dilute) nor yet shrink because water has been drawn out of them and so become wrinkled (as they would if the solution were too concentrated).

Deficiency of sodium chloride occurs in a number of situations. Indeed in surgical patients 'dehydration' caused by fluid loss is usually due not only to loss of water but also of sodium chloride (or better sodium ions and chloride ions). Thus, for example, after vomiting there is a deficiency not only of water but of water plus sodium and chloride (since vomit contains both some sodium ions and chloride ions, though it must be remembered that it contains hydrogen ions as well).

Normal saline may be used to treat dehydration due to vomiting, diarrhoea, loss of fluids from intestinal **fistulae**, and so on. It must, however, be remembered that in these cases potassium is also lost, to a greater or lesser degree, and will often need replacing, either by adding potassium to saline, or using a solution containing potassium, such as Darrow's solution.

Dextrose solution

Saline is a source of water and sodium chloride but 5 per cent dextrose is a source of water only, though stronger solutions provide calories to meet the body's metabolic requirements for energy, and to some extent saves the body from burning up its own substance when other substances are not available because food is not being ingested. The 5 per cent solution, however, is not a useful source of energy since great volumes would be required to give a normal intake of calories; nevertheless, the carbohydrate provided will stop the development of **ketosis**.

Pure water depletion (which would require 5 per cent dextrose for its correction) is not a very frequent finding in clinical practice. Nevertheless there are circumstances in which there has occurred a disproportionate loss of water over sodium chloride and in this case glucose solution is the main fluid required for correction of the condition.

Other fluids containing electrolytes

Darrow's solution has various formulations. It contains potassium and is used as a replacement for extracellular fluid. Some types, used when acidosis is present, contain

Saline Salt solution. In the medical context, unless otherwise stated, saline is a solution of 0.9 per cent sodium chloride.

Isotonic solution A solution in equal pressure balance (due to chemical concentration) with another solution so that fluid transference does not occur. (Usually with reference to normal body fluids.)

Fistula An unnatural communication between the cavity of an organ and the skin or the cavity of another organ.

Ketosis The presence of excessive quantities of ketones (organic compounds — e.g. acetone — produced by an oxidation process) in the blood.

bicarbonate. Hartmann's solution also contains sodium, chloride, potassium and bicarbonate.

If a severe metabolic acidosis is to be treated, sodium bicarbonate or sodium lactate may be used. This may occur, for example, after cardiac arrest when there has been an accumulation of acid metabolites.

Diet

Though frequently patients can be allowed a normal diet before surgery a wide variety of special diets is sometimes required for various reasons. In the ward great care is required to make sure that the patients get the correct diet as mistakes may have unfortunate consequences.

Perhaps the most widely known diet is that used for patients with *diabetes*. Here carbohydrate has to be restricted. In most cases of severe diabetes the food has to be weighed and the diet regulated on an 'exchange' scheme to allow some degree of choice; for example, 20 g of bread contains the same amount of carbohydrate (10 g) as does 120 g of porridge. In the case of mild diabetes (or when the patient is unable to follow a strictly weighed diet) an unmeasured diet may be used.

In such conditions as *peptic ulcer* (and in some cases of malignant disease of the gastrointestinal tract) a bland diet, low in roughage, is required. Milk often forms a conspicuous part of such diets, together with egg, sieved vegetable and so on. When *obstruction* of the gastrointestinal tract appears to be imminent a semi-fluid, low roughage diet may be used ('slops'); in this case the nearest approach to solid food allowed might be an omelette.

The *malabsorption syndrome* has many causes; an obvious one is the removal of a large part of the small intestine at operation; another the destruction of the absorbing surface in regional **ileitis**. In these cases there is a type of starvation and a high protein diet will be required, together with supplements of such substances as calcium. Another reason for giving a high protein diet is the presence of certain types of *liver disease,* such as for example, certain stages of **cirrhosis**. This is not, however, the only diet which may be required for a patient with liver disease: in patients who have more severe liver disease, for example due to infective hepatitis or severe obstructive jaundice, a diet which contains very little fat and a lot of carbohydrate will be preferable.

Obesity is a very important condition in the surgical patient as it greatly increases the risks of anaesthesia and surgery. The treatment of obesity is to reduce the intake of

Ileitis Inflammation of the ileum, or, more usually, a part of it.

Cirrhosis Progressive fibrosis throughout an organ, usually referring to the liver.

food. In many cases this can be done with the patient staying at home, i.e. before admission. Sometimes, however, it may be necessary to admit the patient to the ward and give a diet of, for example, 3780 to 4200 kJ (900—1000 kcal). Living on this diet can be very unpleasant and many patients will exert considerable ingenuity in obtaining other sources of food and drink.

Parenteral nutrition

'Parenteral' nutrition means nutrition by a route other than the intestine; in practice the term is synonymous with 'intravenous feeding'. It may be required before surgery in patients who have been unable to absorb adequately by the usual route and who have suffered a severe degree of starvation as a result. The malabsorption syndrome, mentioned above, is an example of the kind of condition in which parenteral alimentation may, from time to time, be required. For the severely ill, cachexic patient a preoperative period of intravenous feeding may be necessary before surgery for survival.

Unfortunately the nutrients given by vein are all sclerosant, i.e. they tend to cause venous **thrombosis**. For this reason the intravenous line for feeding must be placed in a large vein, such as the superior vena cava, and not in a small peripheral vein, though the latter may be perfectly adequate for short-term administration of 5 per cent dextrose, saline, blood and the like.

The substances used for intravenous feeding consist, basically, of pre-digested preparations of the main foodstuffs, i.e. carbohydrates, proteins and fats. There are innumerable formulations for a good intravenous feeding regimen, and the subject is still much debated. It must be remembered that, not only has the fluid been given to provide nutrition it has also to contain acceptable concentrations of the correct **electrolytes** as well.

The carbohydrate substances used in parenteral nutrition consist of glucose in high concentrations (for example 50%), and laevulose: sorbitol, which is a type of alcohol, is also used to provide calories in basically the same way as carbohydrate. The protein moiety of intravenous feeding consists of such preparations as mixtures of amino acids and sometimes larger particles (in protein hydrolysates). Various preparations of fats are also available, derived from such substances as soya bean oil.

Thrombosis Clotting of blood in blood vessels during life.

Electrolyte Any substance which in solution dissociates into electrically charged particles. Refers in the blood to the ionized salts of sodium, potassium, chloride and bicarbonate.

The care of the patient with a full stomach

Normally if vomiting occurs, the vomitus does not enter the air passages and is cleared from the pharynx by coughing.

During anaesthesia and during recovery from anaesthesia, however, protective reflexes such as coughing disappear, and in these circumstances the patient can die as a result of the vomit entering the trachea and lower air passages. Moreover, when the patient is anaesthetized, stomach contents can come up the oesophagus from the stomach passively (regurgitation) without the active contraction of the abdominal muscles which is associated with vomiting. Thus inhalation of gastric content is one of the commonest causes of death associated with surgical operations. It is also a cause of death which can usually be avoided.

After a meal the stomach empties in about 4 hours, which is a very approximate figure, though for medicolegal reasons it is frequently regarded as being a fixed law. Several factors can slow gastric emptying and result in the presence of food in the stomach a day or more after it has been ingested. The stomach may fill with blood from a bleeding peptic ulcer, from oesophageal **varices** or a bleeding gastric cancer.

It is obvious that the stomach will only empty slowly when there is a **pyloric stenosis** present, but the other factors delaying gastric emptying are also of great importance. After injury (for example in a road traffic accident) there may be gross delay in gastric emptying, though not infrequently the patient vomits and voids all or some of the content. Morphine and other analgesic drugs, too, may delay gastric emptying, though these may also cause vomiting.

In some forms of elective surgery and in some forms of emergency surgery it may be necessary to try to empty the stomach before operation. Unfortunately this is much easier said than done. A small nasogastric (Ryle's) tube is often thought to empty the stomach adequately, but this is not always so. The nasogastric tube may get rid of some of the fluid content, and may precipitate vomiting and so get rid of some solids as well, but it is not possible to remove solid debris reliably in this way. Not infrequently the end of the nasogastric tube is found in a stomach which is tense with blood and blood clots, despite the fact that careful efforts have been made to remove the blood by suction on the tube. A wider bore tube may be passed through the mouth, but though this may be more efficient than the nasogastric tube, passing it is an unpleasant procedure and it may be unwise to do so in the case of a badly shocked patient. Not infrequently, then, the patient may come to surgery with an incompletely empty stomach.

It is usual to allow no fluid by mouth after midnight to patients having an operation in the morning, and merely perhaps a cup of tea and a piece of toast at 6.00 a.m. to patients having an operation after 2.00 p.m.

Varix (pl. varices) A pathologically dilated vein.

Pyloric stenosis Narrowing of the pyloric opening between the stomach and the duodenum.

Mistakes, however, do occur; for example the patient awaiting operation in the afternoon may be given a full breakfast. In these situations it is vitally important that the anaesthetist gets to know about this, and a decision can then be made as to when the operation should be performed.

GENERAL MANAGEMENT

Patients awaiting operation are almost always anxious, and some are terrified. Drugs are frequently given to allay anxiety, and certainly they have a place, but there are other less obvious factors to consider. The behaviour of the staff is important; thus an air of confidence and optimism in those attending the patient can do a great deal. The ill-considered, tactless remark may produce anxiety which no drugs can effectively alleviate.

Night sedation

Patients sleep badly in hospital, and this is especially so of patients on the night before operation. For this reason some sort of drug is usually given. The barbiturates are commonly used but so, too, are others, for example nitrazepam (used to promote sleep by allaying anxiety) and the antihistamine, promethazine. These drugs will be prescribed by the house surgeon and it is important to make sure that they are given.

Premedication

Central nervous depressant drugs
Traditionally morphine has been used as a premedication, administered about an hour before the operation is due. In many patients this does produce a state of calm and sleepy indifference in the last hour before going to the operating theatre, though morphine makes some patients miserable, and many become nauseated. For this reason morphine may be given with an anti-emetic (Chapter 6). Obviously morphine given an hour before operation can only influence the state of anxiety at the last stage before the patient goes to theatre. This may well be the most anxious time but not necessarily so. Papaveretum injection (Omnopon) contains a mixture of opium alkaloids and is commonly used instead of morphine. It is half as potent.

In an attempt to reduce anxiety and apprehension for a longer period before operation than just for an hour or so, use of some of the drugs used in psychiatry to reduce anxiety and promote tranquillity has been tried and of these diazepam

(Valium) has, perhaps, been most popular. It is too early to give a completely authoritative assessment of this sort of premedication.

It must always be remembered that the use of premedication should be viewed against the background of what is safe for the patient. It may be, for example, quite unsafe to use morphine to premedicate a patient with severe respiratory or hepatic disease, no matter how apprehensive the patient may be.

The use of the central depressant drugs, such as morphine, in premedication is mainly to reduce apprehension, but not entirely so. There are other reasons, though with modern anaesthetic techniques these have become less relevant. It used to be said that morphine and similar drugs reduced the patient's metabolic rate which made for an easier induction of anaesthesia. This is probably a very valid point: morphine premedication may well reduce the incidence, duration and severity of the 'struggling' which commonly occurred when anaesthesia was induced with ether. It is doubtful, however, if, with modern techniques of inducing anaesthesia, for example with thiopentone, this is really a considerable advantage.

Anticholinergic drugs

This is only one side of the problem of premedication; there is also another. For many years it has been customary to administer an anticholinergic drug, usually atropine, as well as a central depressant drug such as morphine. These drugs stop the effects of parasympathetic stimulation, such as salivation, lacrimation, **bradycardia**, hypotension, and many more.

There are two main reasons for giving atropine or a similar drug. First, because atropine reduces salivation; this used to be very important when anaesthesia was induced with such agents as ether because the patient tended to salivate excessively and the accumulation of saliva in the mouth could make breathing difficult. The second reason for using atropine is that it helps to stop the undesirable parasympathetic effects of stimulation of the vagus which could take place under anaesthesia; these include bradycardia and even cardiac arrest. It is still very important to administer atropine before using drugs like the muscle relaxant, suxamethonium, which is very likely to cause cardiac arrest in this way.

Modern anaesthetic agents do not cause the excessive salivation which was so common when induction with ether was used, and it is now quite usual not to give atropine (or morphine) in the ward before operation but to give the drug either before or with the agent used to induce anaesthesia

Bradycardia Slow heart rate.

Table 2.2 **Summary of the usually stated advantages of premedication with morphine and atrophine**

Drug	Advantages
Morphine	Alleviates anxiety
	Reduces metabolic rate
	Aids induction
	Diminishes postoperative pain
Atropine	Reduces salivation
	Diminishes effect of vagal stimulation

(for example, thiopentone). This has the virtue of avoiding the injection required to give the premedication in the ward.

The main reasons for using premedicant drugs are summarized in Table 2.2.

Observations before operation

As a routine, immediately after admission to the ward, the patient's weight will be determined, the temperature taken and the pulse rate and blood pressure ascertained. Temperature and pulse rate will, of course, be taken again before surgery as part of the ward routine but if the patient is sick (for example after loss of blood) careful monitoring will be needed and the patient's pulse rate and blood pressure taken frequently.

In normal circumstances a routine urine analysis will be undertaken on the ward as soon as the patient is admitted. This will test for glucose, ketones, protein and blood; in addition to this it is often the rule to send a mid-stream specimen of urine to the laboratory for further investigation.

If the patient is already on intravenous fluid therapy or on diuretics, or being subjected to a twenty-four hour collection of urine, fluid balance charts will often be required. In other circumstances, however, this will not be necessary.

Preparations

Consent
The patient must give informed consent to the operative procedure, that is he must consent and know what he is consenting to. Obtaining consent from the patient is a medical responsibility and the patient will be required to sign a form saying that the operative procedure has been explained to him. The nurse in the ward may well be required to witness this signature.

Identification

It is important for the patient to be sent to the theatre with a name tab on, or with the name written on the arm. The name tab may be put on after the patient has been bathed. It is often put on over the wrist but here it may hinder the anaesthetist when he is attempting venepuncture.

It is also essential to mark the site to be operated on in the ward before the patient goes to theatre. Errors in the side to be operated on are, unhappily, quite frequent: they are indefensible, causing suffering and danger to the patient and they represent a grave medicolegal hazard to the hospital staff. Indicating the site to be operated on is a medical responsibility.

Shaving

It is usual for the abdomen and the genitalia to be shaved for all abdominal operations and those on the upper part of the lower limb. If necessary the lower chest should be shaved for upper abdominal operations. The genital region is also shaved for operations involving cutting in the perineal region, though not always for haemorrhoidectomy. Sometimes, too, the genitalia are shaved before operations for dilatation and curettage of the uterus but not always so.

Shaving the genitalia can be embarrassing. It is usual for a male member of the staff to shave male patients. Many women find genital shaving, even by a sympathetic nurse, quite unpleasant.

Skin preparation

It is usual for patients to have a bath on the day before operation and then don a clean gown and go back into clean sheets. Before the patient is put on the trolley to go to the operating theatre it is often the custom for the part to be operated on to be washed with an antiseptic solution (for example Hibitane) and covered with a sterile towel.

Bowel preparation

It is now not usual to give a routine enema before all operations. However, preparation of the bowel for operations on the colon is very important. The patient is given a low residue diet and then fasted. The bowel is cleansed by enemas (say a soap and water enema for two days) and wash-outs (with warmed water daily for, perhaps, five days) and a suitable antibiotic is given orally.

Operative clothing

The choice of operative clothing is something which is governed by the practice of the hospital. It is essential, however, that the patient must not be allowed to become cold (i.e. normal body temperature should be maintained). There has been a tendency for the long woollen stocking to disappear from hospitals in recent years; no one appears to mourn the loss.

Prostheses

It is very important that the patient's dentures are removed (though it must be remembered that this leaves many patients both very embarrassed and almost inarticulate). Induction of anaesthesia can be hazardous if dentures are present as they can impact in the pharynx and cause asphyxia.

Other prostheses (for example, artificial eyes and limbs) are normally also removed. It is frequently unkind to remove hearing aids from the deaf; they should be allowed to bring them to theatre and, if necessary, they can be kept in theatre till the end of the operation. It is, however, very important that someone is detailed to look after them.

Wedding rings should be covered with plaster. This procedure helps to avoid the risk of burns with diathermy. A ring is a good conductor of electricity and a current will tend to flow through it; plaster partially insulates the metal.

Catheter

Sometimes a urinary catheter has to be passed in the ward though, if possible, it should be passed after anaesthesia has been induced. In these circumstances strict sterile precautions are, of course, necessary as they always are with this procedure. In other circumstances, however, the catheter may be required to be removed before the patient goes to the operating theatre.

Ryle's tube

The Ryle's tube, if possible, is better passed under anaesthesia. Nevertheless in some circumstances the Ryle's tube must be passed in the ward. Those passing the Ryle's tube must remember that it is one of the most unpleasant experiences that the patient will have when visiting the operating theatre. For this reason the greatest possible gentleness and reassurance must be given to the patient during the procedure. The use of a small quantity of water to enable the patient to swallow effectively while the tube is being passed has much to commend it.

Asphyxia Death by obstruction of the respiratory passages.

Diathermy Intense local heat, generated in a blade or needle by a high frequency electric current, which may be used to seal bleeding vessels or cut tissues.

Going to theatre

Finally the actual journey to the operating theatre must be considered. This is usually the culmination of the whole process of preparation. Quite obviously details of how the patient is dealt with at this stage vary from place to place but there are several basic facts to be considered.

Psychological support

The arrival of the trolley for the patient is probably the most unnerving part of the whole visit to theatre. The nurse will recognize this and do her best to allay the anxiety which is felt at this time.

Not infrequently the nurse from the ward has to leave the patient at the door to the operating suite. This, again, can be very unnerving to the patient; it can be very helpful if someone who has met the patient before can receive him into the operating suite when the nurse from the ward has to retire.

The trolley should be moved carefully; it is important that it should not be allowed to knock into objects en route as this is especially unnerving. It is desirable, too, to have the patient with his head away from the direction in which the trolley is travelling as this gives a better feeling of confidence to him. In ideal circumstances a nurse from the ward with whom the patient is familiar would be able to go to the operating theatre and hold the patient's hand while anaesthesia is induced. In most circumstances, however, this is considered to be impossible for reasons of sterility as well as those of nursing routine. In many circumstances a nurse can be sent out of the operating theatre to see the patient before he or she arrives at the operating theatre. When the ward nurse reaches the theatre she can, as it were, hand over to the nurse who has visited the patient in the ward; the patient is thus passed from one nurse whom he knows to another, and the presence of a familiar face in a very frightening situation has a great deal to commend it.

3

Anaesthesia

A. A. Gilbertson

INTRODUCTION

Without the informed co-operation of all the staff concerned, anaesthesia would be a hazardous and frightening experience for the patient. The purpose of this chapter is to outline the basic principles of this subject and to describe how the procedures involved, so completely essential to modern surgery, may be carried out safely and smoothly.

There are more objects of anaesthesia than might appear at first sight. It would not be possible to operate on someone who had been merely 'put to sleep'. Even if the patient did not recover consciousness at the first painful stimulus, he would move reflexly, making precise surgery impossible. An anaesthetic must make surgery comfortable for the patient, it must be safe, and it must also provide good operating conditions for the surgeon.

If an anaesthetic, in fulfilling these functions, renders the patient unconscious, it is called a 'general' anaesthetic.

However, it is often possible to prevent sensation reaching the brain from the part of the body where the surgery is being performed, without making the patient lose consciousness. This is referred to as 'local' anaesthesia. If some sensation can reach the brain from the area of the operation but pain cannot, it is more correct to speak of local analgesia (anaesthesia — no sensation; analgesia — no pain).

GENERAL ANAESTHESIA

All general anaesthetics produce, in varying degrees, three effects on the patient:

(1) unconsciousness — this may range from a light sleep to a deep coma;
(2) analgesia — some anaesthetics produce freedom from pain even before consciousness is lost. With others, the patient will move reflexly in response to pain until he is very deeply unconscious;

(3) muscular relaxation — again there is great variation between different anaesthetic agents. For example, cyclopropane quickly produces well-relaxed muscles, whereas trichloroethylene (Trilene) does not relax muscles well even when the maximum safe concentration is used.

One of the greatest advances in modern anaesthesia has been the introduction of separate drugs to produce just the required degree of relaxation or analgesia so that it is no longer necessary to expose the patient to the ill effects of very deep general anaesthesia in order to obtain good operating conditions.

General anaesthetic agents

Nitrous oxide

Nitrous oxide is a gas and is almost odourless and tasteless. It is stored in cylinders under sufficient pressure to make it liquid (about 4500 kPa), but when the pressure is reduced to about 400 kPa in the anaesthetic machine it becomes a gas again. It is not inflammable.

When a mixture containing equal parts of nitrous oxide and oxygen is inhaled by the patient, he becomes much less sensitive to pain, although consciousness is not lost. If the percentage of nitrous oxide is increased to 80 per cent, with 20 per cent oxygen, all but perhaps the most resistant patients will lose consciousness. However, they will not be relaxed and will move in response to strong stimuli and only minor surgery could be performed under this light anaesthetic.

As it is not safe for the patient to breathe less than 20 per cent oxygen, deeper anaesthesia is not possible with nitrous oxide as the sole agent.

Because nitrous oxide is free from toxic effects, such as damage to the heart, kidneys, liver and so on, it is often used to produce unconsciousness, and it is supplemented by other anaesthetic agents, analgesics and relaxant drugs to produce the required state of anaesthesia.

Ether

There are many different ethers, but anaesthetic ether (*BP*) (diethyl ether) is the one most commonly used. This is a liquid which evaporates easily at ordinary room temperature giving off a vapour which can be inhaled with air or other oxygen-containing gas mixtures (air contains about 20 per cent oxygen and 80 per cent nitrogen).

Ether vapour is irritant to the respiratory tract and causes coughing and choking unless it is given gradually and carefully.

It produces unconsciousness and quickly prevents response to pain. As anaesthesia deepens, the muscles (particularly jaw and abdominal muscles) relax to a useful degree.

The respiratory and cardiovascular systems are not much depressed and to this extent ether is a safe anaesthetic.

Unfortunately patients are often slow to recover after ether anaesthetics, and many feel nauseated and vomit. Moreover, ether vapour is inflammable and so excludes the use of diathermy. For these and other reasons ether is rarely used in this country today, but because it can be given with minimal equipment, and is cheap, it is still frequently used in some parts of the world.

Halothane

Apart from nitrous oxide, halothane (trade name Fluothane) is probably the most commonly used anaesthetic in Great Britain at present. Like diethyl ether, halothane is a liquid which readily evaporates forming a vapour which can be inhaled. Unlike ether vapour, halothane is not inflammable and is less liable to make the patient cough or tend to hold his breath.

Halothane quickly produces unconsciousness and muscular relaxation, but suppression of reflex reaction to pain occurs less readily than with ether.

If too much halothane is given, rapid, shallow, inadequate breathing results owing to depression of the respiratory centre in the brain. The heart muscle is also affected and the tone in the arteries reduced, so that the pulse slows and the blood pressure falls. To regulate the dose of this potent anaesthetic, special vaporizers are used which deliver a known concentration under a wide range of conditions. Usually up to 4 per cent of halothane vapour diluted with a mixture of nitrous oxide and oxygen is given. When the patient is 'deep' enough, the halothane is reduced to 1—2 per cent.

Trichloroethylene

Trichloroethylene (Trilene) is also a liquid which forms a non-inflammable, not too irritating, vapour. It is coloured blue by the addition of a dye. It produces poor relaxation and takes a long time to administer. It has largely been superseded in Great Britain by halothane. However, unlike halothane, trichloroethylene does not increase bleeding from the pregnant uterus. For this reason many anaesthetists prefer trichloroethylene for such operations as evacuation of the uterus.

Cyclopropane

Like nitrous oxide, cyclopropane is a gas, supplied in cylinders in which it is compressed to a liquid. The gas is inhaled in a mixture with oxygen and very rapidly produces deep anaesthesia with analgesia and muscular relaxation. Because it is so potent cyclopropane may be given with a high proportion of oxygen. For this reason, and because it is relatively non-toxic, some anaesthetists use it for administration to frail patients. Unfortunately it is highly explosive and great care has to be taken to eliminate sparks or other sources of ignition from the operating theatre during its use.

Methoxyflurane (Penthrane) is used both as a general anaesthetic and as an inhalational analgesic. Many other substances, including chloroform, Vinesthene (divinyl ether) and ethyl chloride, have been used as anaesthetics but are no longer in general use.

Stages of anaesthesia

As the patient passes from consciousness to deep anaesthesia, certain intermediate stages occur. These stages may be clearly seen when anaesthesia is induced slowly, but with modern methods of induction, particularly by intravenous agents, the patient passes through the stages very quickly and therefore they may be difficult to distinguish.

Stage 1 — the stage of analgesia

Certain anaesthetic drugs, particularly nitrous oxide, tri-chloroethylene (Trilene) and methoxyflurane (Penthrane), relieve pain before the patient becomes unconscious. This stage of analgesia is used in childbirth. The mother breathes from a machine which automatically supplies the requisite concentration of anaesthetic to relieve pain, allowing her to remain conscious and co-operative.

Stage 2 — the stage of reflex excitement

In conscious animals, the cerebral cortex modifies and controls many simple reflex actions. In the second stage of anaesthesia this conscious control is lost, and the patient may pass through an excitement phase in which previously suppressed feelings of fear, pain, or perhaps aggression, may now produce an exaggerated response. Such a patient must be prevented from damaging himself until the tranquillity of the third stage is reached.

Stage 3 — surgical anaesthesia

The beginning of this stage is recognized by the onset of regular respiration, and the pupils become fixed and central.

The patient no longer reacts to mildly painful stimuli and reflex activities are gradually depressed. For example, the cough reflex which protects the lungs by ejecting any material which may be about to soil the trachea, will be lost at the beginning of this stage. The anaesthetist must therefore assume the responsibility of keeping the lungs free of contamination should there be vomit or perhaps blood in the mouth and pharynx.

As anaesthesia is deepened and the patient passes into stage 3, more painful stimuli will be ignored and the anaesthetist must select the correct level of anaesthesia for the operation to be performed. The patient's muscles relax gradually and again the anaesthetist must provide enough relaxation for the surgeon to operate. This is particularly important in abdominal surgery as the muscles must be relaxed so that the assistant can retract them to allow access to the abdominal contents.

Stage 4

If anaesthesia is inadvisedly deepened further, although more analgesia and muscular relaxation may be gained, it will be at the expense of unacceptable toxic effects.

Respiration will be depressed, both because the respiratory muscles will be weakened, and because the parts of the brain which control breathing will be inactivated.

The cardiac output will decrease, and the peripheral blood vessels will relax, leading to inadequate blood flow to vital organs.

The liver and kidneys will cease to function. The liver in particular may be permanently damaged by an overdose of some anaesthetics.

If the depth of anaesthesia is carried still further, the patient will be in danger of death from cardiac and respiratory failure.

Although satisfactory anaesthesia for many operations can be obtained without reaching the depths at which these toxic effects occur, it was in order to achieve good relaxation of muscles without the dangers of deep anaesthesia that the muscle relaxant drugs were developed.

Muscle relaxants

Muscle relaxants are not anaesthetic agents as they do not produce unconsciousness. They are drugs which may be added to a light anaesthetic to produce relaxation or complete muscle paralysis (which may be temporary or prolonged as required for the operation).

The relaxants do not only affect the muscles in the area in which the surgeon is working; they affect all the skeletal muscles including those of respiration. Therefore, when relaxants are used, artificial ventilation of the patient's lungs is usually necessary until the effect of the drug is terminated.

The following are the most commonly used relaxant drugs.

Suxamethonium chloride

Suxamethonium chloride (Scoline, Anectine) produces almost immediate complete paralysis when injected intravenously into an anaesthetized patient. The paralysis lasts for 2 to 3 minutes only, and is useful for relaxing the jaw muscles so that the larynx can be seen with a laryngoscope and an endotracheal tube inserted. The patient's lungs must then be inflated with an oxygen/anaesthetic mixture until the paralysis wears off. Anaesthesia may be continued either by allowing the patient to breathe an inhalational anaesthetic spontaneously, or else a longer-acting relaxant may be injected and artificial ventilation continued throughout the operation.

Tubocurarine chloride

Curare was a South American arrow poison which was found to produce muscular paralysis, and *d*-tubocurarine chloride (Tubarine) is the commercially available purified extract. Its action takes longer to commence than that of suxamethonium – about 1.5 to 3 minutes – and lasts for about 30 minutes. Small supplementary doses can be given to prolong the relaxation for as long as is required.

At the end of the operation the action of *d*-tubocurarine is usually terminated by injecting the antidote – neostigmine methylsulphate. As this drug by itself causes excessive salivation and bradycardia, a suitable dose of atropine is always given with it.

When the *d*-tubocurarine has been reversed in this way, the very light anaesthetic can be discontinued and the patient wakes up in a matter of minutes with the protective reflexes intact. This is in marked contrast to patients whose muscles have been relaxed by deep anaesthesia. These patients may not regain consciousness for many hours after the operation, and may suffer from the toxic effects of the anaesthetic for days. Alcuronium chloride (Alloferin), gallamine triethiodide (Flaxedil), and pancuronium (Pavulon) are drugs with a similar action to *d*-tubocurarine, but without the tendency to produce hypotension and bronchospasm which it sometimes causes. The tachycardia which gallamine causes is a disadvantage which has limited its use.

Intravenous induction agents

The gradual onset of anaesthesia produced by inhalation of gases or volatile anaesthetics may be unpleasant or even frightening for some patients. Certain drugs produce sleep in a few seconds after intravenous injection. These drugs are hypnotics rather than anaesthetics, that is, they produce little analgesia and relaxation. The sleep they induce is of only a few minutes' duration. However, they do so pleasantly, and once the patient is unconscious other agents can be used to produce adequate surgical anaesthesia.

Thiopentone sodium

Thiopentone (Pentothal), an ultra-short-acting barbiturate, has been the most widely used intravenous induction agent since its introduction in 1934. It is a pale yellow powder which is dissolved in water for injection to form a 2.5 per cent solution which will keep for 2 days. It must not be used if it has become cloudy. The usual dose needed to produce sleep in adults is about 250 mg; less in the old and the ill, more in large or resistant patients. Care must be taken that no thiopentone is injected outside the vein as the solution is very irritant to the tissues. Accidental intra-arterial injection may lead to the loss of a limb.

As well as acting on the cortex and reticular formation of the brain to produce sleep, thiopentone also depresses the respiratory centre, the circulatory centres and the heart muscle itself. Thus it may severely depress respiration and cause hypotension and circulatory failure unless it is used with care and understanding, and it should never be given except by persons adequately trained in anaesthesia. The anaesthetist will consider certain patients unfit for thiopentone and may use another drug or indeed avoid intravenous induction completely.

Methohexitone sodium

Methohexitone (Brietal Sodium) is a newer drug with a shorter action than thiopentone. It is also less irritant to the tissues. It is frequently used for inducing anaesthesia for dental extractions, where rapid recovery is desirable. Although the patient may wake up in a few minutes, he should not drive or operate machinery that day, as the brain will not be completely free of the effects of the drug for about 15 hours. Patients should always be escorted home after out-patient anaesthetics.

Propanidid

Propanidid (Epontol) is even shorter acting. As very little 'hangover' follows its administration, it is very often used for short operations. It is not a barbiturate and so it can be used in patients who are allergic to them.

Ketamine

This drug is usually used as an induction agent or as the sole anaesthetic for short surgical procedures. It differs in two important respects from other induction agents: first, ketamine usually *increases* the blood pressure, while other agents may lower it; and second, ketamine can be given either intravenously or intramuscularly. This may be very useful in small children with difficult veins. It may cause unpleasant dreams and delerium during recovery. This may be prevented by correct premedication.

Alphaxalone/Alphadolone (Althesin)

This agent must be given intravenously. Although it is usually used as a pleasant induction agent, it may be used as an intravenous infusion to provide unconsciousness for several days in patients in intensive care units. Unfortunately the incidence of severe allergic reactions to Althesin (and propanidid) may be higher than to the older induction agents.

Diazepam

Diazepam (Valium) is usually used as a tranquillizer, but when injected intravenously it produces sleep. It is slow in action, although patients seem to find it very pleasant. The sleep produced is very light and has to be carefully deepened with other agents. It is of particular value that diazepam has little effect on the circulation even in patients with a damaged or diseased heart.

The anaesthetic machine

Although anaesthetic apparatus can be very simple, it is convenient to have a machine in which gases can be mixed in accurate proportions at convenient pressures, and passed through vaporizers so that the selected vapour may be delivered through flexible tubing to the patient.

The machine, in common use in Great Britain and many other countries, is the Boyle's machine of which there are many models, differing only in detail.

The Boyle's machine (*see Figure 3.1*) consists of the following parts.

(1) A trolley, with a flat working surface on top.
(2) Gas storage cylinders — two oxygen cylinders, two nitrous oxide cylinders, and often one carbon dioxide cylinder and one cyclopropane cylinder. The cylinders

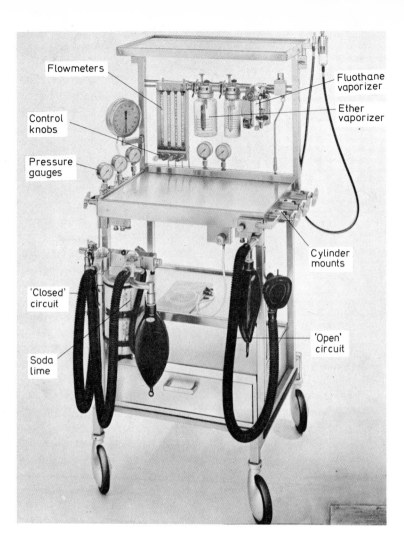

Figure 3.1. A Boyle's anaesthetic machine. (Reproduced by courtesy of The British Oxygen Company Limited)

fit onto special mounting points called yokes, and are made so that it is impossible to fit the wrong type of cylinder to the machine; for example, nitrous oxide will not fit in the oxygen mount, and vice versa.

(3) Reducing valves — these reduce the pressures of nitrous oxide and oxygen from the very high pressure at which they are stored in the cylinders to a reasonable working pressure (now usually 60 lb/in^2).

(4) Mounted behind the table top are the control knobs for the gases: oxygen, nitrous oxide, carbon dioxide and cyclopropane. As these knobs are turned, they operate needle valves which regulate the flow of each gas separately. The rate at which each gas is flowing is continuously indicated by flowmeters.

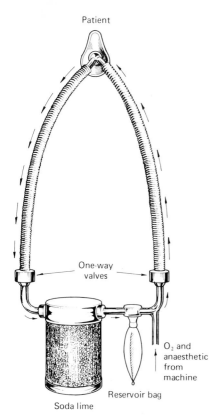

Figure 3.2. Diagram of a closed circuit anaesthetic machine

(5) Flowmeters are vertical glass tubes, slightly wider at the top and marked in millilitres or litres per minute. In each, a bobbin is supported by the gas stream and the level of the top of the bobbin indicates the gas flow. Above the flowmeters there is a mixing chamber in which the gases are mixed before they pass into the vaporizers.

(6) Vaporizers — usually one for halothane and another one which may be for either ether, Trilene or sometimes methoxyflurane. When a vaporizer is turned on the selected mixture of gases passes through it and is mixed with the required vapour.

(7) The 'breathing circuit' transmits the anaesthetic gases and vapours from the machine to the patient. Two main types are used.

(a) The 'open circuit' (*Figure 3.3*) (more directly called Magill attachment or Mapleson type A circuit) consists of a reservoir bag, a length of wide bore corrugated tubing, an expiratory valve and a connector to either a face mask or endotracheal tube. When the patient is breathing from this circuit, he inhales the gas/vapour mixture from the reservoir bag. When he exhales the bag refills with a mixture of fresh gas from the machine and the first part of the exhalation. The last part of the exhalation, which has come from the depth of the lung where it has lost some oxygen and gained carbon dioxide, is discharged to the atmosphere by the expiratory valve. So that the expired gas will not be inhaled by the operating theatre staff, the expiratory valve may be connected to an exhaust tube which carries the waste gases out of the theatre to the open air.

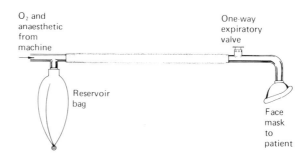

Figure 3.3. Method of delivery of an anaesthetic gas/vapour mixture from the machine to the patient

(b) In the 'closed circuit' (*Figure 3.2*) one tube takes the gases to the patient, and another returns them to the reservoir bag. The exhaled carbon dioxide is removed by passing the gases through a canister containing 'soda lime', which absorbs it. The patient then rebreathes the exhaled gases, which have been 'freshened up' by the addition of a small amount of oxygen and anaesthetic. This system is economical as little of the gas is lost to the atmosphere and it is also a more efficient means of administering artificial respiration.

Originally the gas/vapour mixture from the anaesthetic machine was delivered to the patient's air passages by means of a face mask. However, it is often more convenient to pass

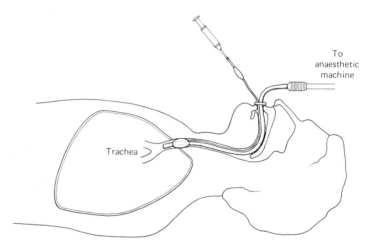

To anaesthetic machine

Trachea

Figure 3.4. Cuffed endotracheal tube *in situ*

a tube into the anaesthetized patient's trachea (*Figure 3.4*) and connect this directly to the breathing circuit. The advantages of endotracheal intubation are as follows.

(1) It facilitates the maintenance of a clear, unobstructed airway.
(2) If the tube is made to fit the trachea exactly (by inflating a cuff around the lower end of the tube) the air passages are protected from contamination by secretions, blood, vomit and so on.
(3) The airtight connection to the machine makes artificial ventilation (for example, by squeezing the reservoir bag to inflate the patient's lungs) very easy.

Anaesthetic sundries

As well as an anaesthetic machine, several instruments and accessories must also be available. These are usually prepared and set out by the nurse or technician. Every nurse should at least know what these instruments look like so that she may pass them to the anaesthetist who may need them urgently.

Airways

Airways are short tubes which are placed in the mouth and extend into the pharynx (not into the trachea) to prevent the tongue of the anaesthetized patient from falling back and obstructing the air passages. It is important to realize that an airway in the patient's mouth does not guarantee that the air passages are clear. The airway may be wrongly placed or be too small (*see* Postoperative period).

There are several types of airways, but the most often used is the Guedel pattern, which is now commonly made of plastic and is disposable (*Figure 3.5*). Several sizes should be available.

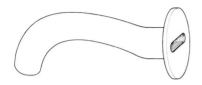

Figure 3.5. Guedel disposable plastic airway

Mouth gags

It occasionally happens that an unconscious patient will reflexively clench his teeth when it is necessary for the mouth to be opened in order to clear excessive secretions, or to place an airway. Mouth gags should always be available. They have small 'jaws' which are placed between the patient's upper and lower teeth. When the handles of the gag are squeezed together the mouth is forced open, taking care not to damage the patient's mouth or teeth. Pressure on anterior teeth, or on loose or heavily filled teeth, should be avoided.

A commonly used pattern is Ferguson's, and the modification with Ackland's jaws, which fit one in front of the other (*see Figure 3.6*), is usually easier to insert in the mouth.

The practice of enclosing the jaws in pieces of 'protective' rubber tubing is dangerous, as these bits of tubing may become detached and enter the bronchi, where they will cause a lung abscess.

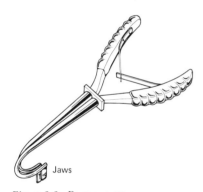

Figure 3.6. Ferguson gag

Instruments for endotracheal intubation

Instruments needed for endotracheal intubation (*Figure 3.7*) are: laryngoscope(s), endotracheal tubes, cuff inflator, or syringe and self-locking forceps, and catheter mount.

Laryngoscope Laryngoscopes are instruments which are passed into the mouth of anaesthetized patients to expose and illuminate the vocal cords in the larynx. The endotracheal tube is then passed between the cords into the trachea. Laryngoscopes used in anaesthesia have a handle which contains batteries, and a blade which presses the tongue down, and carries a light bulb. Two main types are used — Macintosh's which has a curved blade, and Magill's which has a straight one. Special laryngoscopes are used for small children and babies.

Endotracheal tubes It is important to use the largest tube which will fit comfortably and so a range of sizes is available, from the 2.5 mm internal diameter used for neonates up to 9—10 mm used for adults. Endotracheal tubes may be passed through the nose, instead of the mouth, for example, in major dental operations. Special nasal tubes are used for this purpose.

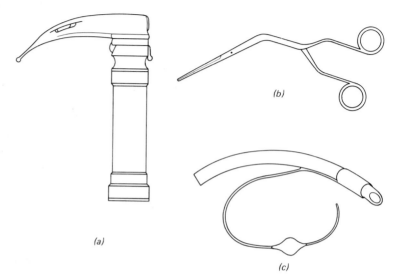

Figure 3.7. Intubation instruments: (*a*) Macintosh laryngoscope; (*b*) Magill forceps; (*c*) Magill tube with cuff

Catheter mounts Catheter mounts are short rubber tubes which connect the breathing attachment of the anaesthetic machine to the endotracheal tube. The catheter mount has at one end a metal connector to fit the breathing attachment and at the other a push-on or plug-in connection to a metal fitting on the end of the endotracheal tube.

Cuff inflator Most endotracheal tubes have a cuff at the end, which is inflated when the tube is in place to form an airtight fit in the trachea. This may be done by a small inflator, which contains a valve to prevent it collapsing again, or by using a 10 ml syringe, and then clipping the inflatory tube with a **haemostat** (e.g. Spencer Wells forceps).

Intubation forceps Special forceps are used for guiding endotracheal tubes — particularly nasal ones — into the larynx, and for placing packs in the pharynx. Their particular feature is that the handles do not obscure the anaesthetist's view down the throat.

Throat packs Throat packs are usually made from damp 2 inch ribbon gauze, and are used for either making uncuffed tubes airtight, or for absorbing blood or secretions from the mouth so that they will not contaminate the trachea or bronchi.

Haemostat Small arterial clip.

LOCAL ANAESTHESIA

Local anaesthetics act on nerve fibres to prevent pain and other sensations reaching the brain. The drug can be applied to the nerve fibres at different points along their pathways so that the patient will feel no pain from the operation.

Methods of administration

Topical analgesia
Strong solutions of local anaesthetic drugs will penetrate membranes to reach the underlying nerve endings. It is possible to anaesthetize the urethra (for **cytoscopy**) or the larynx and trachea (for **bronchoscopy**) in this way. Many operations on the eye may be performed by applying local anaesthetic solution to the conjunctiva.

Infiltration
The nerves supplying a small part of the body may be made insensitive by injecting local anaesthetic solution so that it soaks all the nerves in the area (for example, for removal of a sebaceous cyst). For larger areas, a dangerous amount of anaesthetic would be required.

Nerve block
A relatively small amount of local anaesthetic can block a large nerve. For example, by injecting local anaesthetic around the nerves of the brachial plexus, the whole arm may be made anaesthetic to allow, for example, a fractured radius to be reduced.

Spinal anaesthesia
By injecting the local anaesthetic drug into the spinal canal, the nerves supplying the legs and abdomen can be blocked as they leave the spinal cord. This can be done by two methods.

Epidural anaesthesia 'Epi' is the Greek word meaning 'upon', and in epidural anaesthesia the solution is placed in the bony spinal canal 'upon' the dura mater which surrounds the spinal cord and the nerves leaving it. The epidural space is small and, therefore, practice and care are needed to locate it.

Spinal subarachnoid anaesthesia Spinal subarachnoid anaesthesia (which is what is usually meant by 'a spinal') is produced by injecting the local anaesthetic into the cerebrospinal fluid which surrounds the spinal cord. This is easier to carry out than an epidural injection but has two great disadvantages: it

Cytoscopy The inspection of the interior of the fluid filled urinary bladder through an instrument. The suffix — 'oscopy' is derived from the Greek *skopein* = to watch, hence it is used with a suitable prefix to denote inspection of various body cavities or internal chambers (e.g. ophthalmoscopy — of the eye; arthroscopy — of a joint, etc.).

Bronchoscopy Inspection of the inside of the bronchial tube.

may cause infection (meningitis) unless a very meticulous technique is practised; and very severe postoperative headache is frequently observed (the incidence is less with very fine needles).

The epidural method does not cause headaches and is less likely to cause infection (although scrupulous care must still be taken with asepsis). Epidural anaesthesia is, therefore, tending to supersede subarachnoid in Great Britain.

Local anaesthetic agents

Lignocaine hydrochloride (Xylocaine) is the most commonly used drug for infiltration and nerve blocks. Cocaine, which is the only local anaesthetic which most lay people have heard of, is rarely used today except by some ophthalmologists and ENT (Ear, Nose and Throat) surgeons.

Lignocaine produces complete anaesthesia almost immediately. It is used in several strengths: 0.5–1 per cent solution for infiltration, 1–2 per cent solution for nerve blocks, 1.5–2 per cent solution for epidural anaesthesia, and 4 per cent solution as a spray for topical analgesia (for example, of the larynx).

Adrenaline is often added to produce vasoconstriction. The resultant decrease in blood flow in the anaesthetized area both reduces bleeding and delays absorption of the lignocaine into the bloodstream. Thus more lignocaine can be given without producing toxic effects.

The maximum dose of lignocaine is 200 mg (20 ml of 1 per cent solution) without adrenaline, or 500 mg with adrenaline. The adrenaline itself may be dangerous if any solution enters a blood vessel, and lignocaine with safer vasoconstrictors (for example, orciprenaline) is now available.

When injecting an anaesthetic solution for a subarachnoid ('spinal') anaesthetic, it is necessary to know whether the solution is heavier or lighter than the cerebrospinal fluid. If it is heavier, the analgesic area will spread downward in the sitting patient, and vice versa.

'Heavy' Nupercaine is a 1:200 solution of cinchocaine. It produces good analgesia for about 2½ hours and it can be made to spread up or down the spinal cord by tilting the patient so that the direction of travel is downward from the site of injection.

Prilocaine hydrochloride is longer acting than lignocaine and less toxic, although it can alter haemoglobin to methaemoglobin, which does not transport oxygen.

Bupivacaine (Marcain), a newer anaesthetic, is becoming very popular, particularly for epidural anaesthesia. It is so long-acting that analgesia may persist for several hours after the operation.

Effects of overdose of local anaesthesia

Following an overdose of local anaesthetic the patient may pass through the following phases: pallor, anxiety, nausea, vomiting, confusion, convulsions, hypotension, tachycardia, coma and death.

Treatment consists of maintaining respiration by inflating the lungs with oxygen through an endotracheal tube, controlling convulsions with relaxant drugs, and maintaining adequate cardiac output.

GENERAL CARE OF THE PATIENT

In the anaesthetic room

It is usual and desirable for a nurse from the ward to accompany the patient to theatre. Specific directions may have been given about the journey from the ward to theatre. For example, patients with heart disease may have to travel sitting up, small children may prefer to be carried, underwater chest drains may need to be clamped and so on. The nurse should be aware of the name of the patient, the operation, the type of premedication used and when it was given, and she must check that all the case notes and radiographs are on the trolley. Her attitude to the patient on the way to the theatre can be very helpful (or otherwise). It cannot be overemphasized to the patient that he is an individual whose welfare is of great concern to everyone. Such a comment as 'I'll be back soon to take you to bed' conveys the reassuring inference that the ordeal is not going to last long, and that there is no doubt that the patient will survive it.

The anaesthetist will be assisted in the anaesthetic room by either a nurse or a technician ('operating department assistant'). This invaluable ally will have had more detailed instruction in anaesthesia than is possible to provide here. He will have checked the anaesthetic machine, ensured that all the accessories are available, and will be ready to pass whatever the anaesthetist needs during the anaesthetic. The final responsibility for ensuring that the machine is serviceable and all the equipment is ready must rest with the anaesthetist, but in a well-ordered anaesthetic department his needs will have been anticipated.

Induction of anaesthesia

A typical anaesthetic induction will consist of the injection of an intravenous induction agent, and the assistant will have helped to find the vein. Anaesthesia may be then continued by placing the mask over the patient's face, supporting the chin to maintain the airway and turning on oxygen, nitrous oxide and perhaps halothane. This provides adequate anaesthesia for minor procedures or operations when not much relaxation is required. If better control of the airway or more relaxation is needed, then, after the intravenous induction, a relaxant will be given, the trachea is intubated and the lungs inflated with oxygen and anaesthetic. Machines are usually used if artificial ventilation is needed for more than a few minutes.

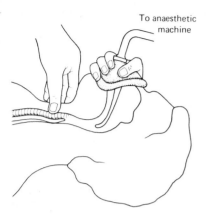

Figure 3.8. Position to exert pressure on cricoid – Sellick's manoeuvre

Sellick's manoeuvre

Sellick's manoeuvre (*Figure 3.8*) is a method of preventing gastric contents entering the lungs during induction of anaesthesia in patients with a full stomach. Anaesthesia may be necessary in these circumstances because the patient is bleeding into the stomach from a peptic ulcer, or because there is a delayed and uncertain emptying of the stomach, as in pyloric stenosis or during labour, or an emergency operation may have to be performed before the patient has digested the last meal.

When anaesthesia is induced the sphincter between the stomach and oesophagus (the cardiac sphincter) relaxes, and may allow gastric contents to run up the oesophagus to the pharynx. Because the anaesthetic has also depressed the cough reflex, acid content from the stomach may then flow down the trachea into the lungs where it may cause severe, even fatal, chemical pneumonia.

To prevent this catastrophe, the cricoid cartilage (just below the thyroid cartilage) may be pressed backwards to compress the oesophagus against the vertebrae which are immediately behind it. If performed properly this technique, which is known as Sellick's manoeuvre, prevents any escape of fluid from the oesophagus. Pressure must be maintained on the cricoid cartilage until the anaesthetist has passed a cuffed endotracheal tube which completely blocks off the trachea and removes any possibility of contamination of the lower respiratory tract.

In theatre the anaesthetist's main task is to keep a careful watch on the patient's condition (which has been aptly described as a carefully controlled coma). He may also be active in setting up intravenous infusion of blood or electrolyte solutions, measuring arterial and venous pressures, monitoring electrocardiograms or blood gases. In some cases the anaesthetist may use cardiopulmonary by-pass equipment to maintain the circulation, while the surgeon stops the patient's heart. His assistants for this work need special training and a high degree of skill.

THE POSTOPERATIVE PERIOD

Immediately following anaesthesia, patients may be in a very vulnerable state and may depend on vigilant and competent medical and nursing care for their very survival. During this period particular attention must be directed to patients' *respiration* and *circulation*.

Respiration

Patients may asphyxiate after anaesthetics because of obstruction to the respiratory tract, depression of the respiratory centre in the brain, or weakness of the muscles of respiration.

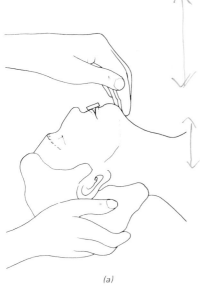

(a)

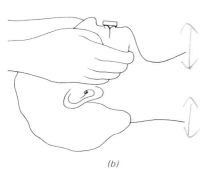

(b)

Figure 3.9. Two methods of maintaining a clear airway: (*a*) lifting the chin, (*b*) lifting the jaw forward from the angle

Obstruction of the respiratory tract

By the tongue During anaesthesia the muscles of the larynx and tongue are almost invariably very relaxed. If the patient is lying on his back, the tongue will fall back and block the larynx. This must be prevented by supporting the lower jaw so that the attachments of the tongue are lifted away from the posterior pharyngeal wall. This may be done as in *Figure 3.9a*, but this is not always effective and the method shown in *Figure 3.9b* will always open the airway. The insertion of an artificial oropharyngeal airway may make the task less arduous but support of the mandible is of prime importance and must be practised by all nurses until practice has made the technique perfect.

By inhalation of material from the pharynx Normally the larynx reacts reflexly to prevent any foreign material entering the trachea. In conscious people the glottis closes and violent coughing expels any material which might be about to enter the trachea. However, in deeply unconscious patients, including those receiving or recovering from anaesthetic, *this reflex is lost* and the trachea must be protected against the possible entry of foreign matter.

Such 'foreign matter' may be either solid, such as vomited undigested food or a throat pack which may have been inadvertently left in the larynx, or liquid, such as vomited or regurgitated gastric contents, or blood after dental operations or tonsillectomy.

After light anaesthesia where relaxants have been used, the patients may appear to have an adequate cough reflex immediately after the operation. It is still wise, however, to assume that the cough mechanism is less effective than usual.

The principal method of protecting the trachea from contamination is to place the patient on his side with the head tilted slightly downwards. All patients recovering from anaesthetics should be in this position if it is at all possible. Any material from the stomach or mouth will then tend to fall out of the mouth rather than into the lungs. Throat packs should always have their ends hanging out of the mouth so that their presence is obvious.

If vomiting is observed or obstruction is suspected, the patient's mouth must be opened, using a mouth gag if necessary, and the pharynx inspected. Any obstructing material should be sucked out. Solid matter (for example, undigested food) may have to be removed with the fingers in an emergency.

Respiratory depression

Respiratory depression may be due to: (1) depression of the respiratory centre caused by anaesthetic agents or drugs used in premedication; or (2) weakness of the muscles of respiration when relaxants have not been fully reversed.

Even the slightest depression may be particularly serious in patients who have chronic respiratory illness and have, therefore, very little functional reserve. Respiratory depression may only become evident after the stimulus of the operation is finished and the anaesthetist has left the patient to the care of the recovery room nurse. If there is the slightest doubt about the patient's colour or the adequacy of his respiratory efforts, the anaesthetist should be called urgently. With modern anaesthesia postoperative respiratory depression should not occur, but the need for vigilance remains.

Circulation

Operation and anaesthesia may impose considerable strains on the circulation, and acute changes may occur in the early recovery period. The nurse must be satisfied that the circulation is adequate by observing the following signs.

(1) Skin colour — which should be pink. **Cyanosis** may be an indication of respiratory or circulatory failure. The signs of adequate respiration should be checked by the nurse while the anaesthetist is being called. Pale skin may indicate circulatory failure (for example, the need for blood transfusion) or it may be the result of the type of anaesthetic technique which has been used. The anaesthetist will be able to tell the nurse how much importance to attach to this sign.

(2) Skin temperature — a warm pink skin is an indication of good blood flow.

(3) Pulse — the nurse can observe the rate and volume of the pulse by feeling the pulse in the carotid artery at

Cyanosis A blue appearance of the skin and mucous membranes due to deficient oxygenation of the blood.

the angle of the jaw. This pulse can be felt by the hand which is holding the chin forward, and in this way every breath and every pulse beat can be felt at this critical time.

(4) Blood pressure and central venous pressure — the anaesthetist will decide how frequently these readings must be recorded and within what limit they should be kept.

As well as observing respiration and circulation the nurse will watch the progress of the patient's return to consciousness. Patients should not be returned to the ward until they are sufficiently awake to respond to simple commands and to maintain a clear airway without help. In many hospitals patients are nursed in a special postoperative recovery ward until they have reached a safe stable state following anaesthesia and surgery.

Position of the patient

A patient should be transported back to the ward lying on his side. In exceptional circumstances this may not be possible, for example certain patients with heart disease may need to sit up. In these cases the anaesthetist will keep the patient in the recovery area until there is no danger of inhalation should the patient vomit.

Certain anaesthetic techniques, particularly spinal subarachnoid and epidural anaesthesia, and controlled hypotensive anaesthesia, may leave the patient's blood vessels unable to contract. If such a patient were to sit up, the blood vessels in the legs would fill up with blood, leaving the heart and brain insufficiently perfused. The anaesthetist will therefore ask for the patient to be kept in a supine position for a prescribed period until control of the blood vessels is regained. If these instructions are not followed, cardiac arrest and brain damage may easily result.

Postoperative analgesia

The amount of pain which patients experience after operations depends partly on the type of surgery, and also very much on the individual patient. Consequently, the analgesic drugs and techniques employed must be related to each patient's requirements. The anaesthetist will prescribe an analgesic which he *expects* will be suitable in each case. He may not be in a position to know whether or not the pain is relieved by his prescription unless the ward nurses inform him, and it is most important that this is done. It must be appreciated, however, that frequently a little reassurance will convince the patient that there is no sinister significance in his pain. This in itself may enable him to regard as minor discomfort what, in his anxiety, he might have considered an unbearable misery.

The degree of pain relief attainable by most analgesics is limited by the respiratory depression which the larger doses produce. For this reason other methods of pain relief have been evolved. For example, continuous postoperative analgesia may be produced by injecting local anaesthetic agents into a catheter introduced into the epidural space. As soon as the analgesia starts to wear off, a further 'topping-up' dose is given aseptically into a special sterile connector at the end of the catheter.

In suitably equipped wards continuous nitrous oxide analgesia may be administered for many hours and provide complete pain relief for the most painful part of the post-operative period.

It must be admitted that many patients suffer more pain after operations than is really necessary. No one should be complacent about this situation and the anaesthetist or doctor in charge should always be informed if pain relief is not adequate.

REFERENCE

Hayward, J. (1975). *Information – A Prescription Against Pain*. London: Whitefriars Press

Postoperative management

T. R. Preston

This chapter deals with the general care of the patient who has undergone a surgical operation. The period of care commences as he leaves the operating theatre and ends when he is discharged from the ward; the first part of the time being spent in an unconscious or semiconscious state recovering from the immediate effects of surgery, the second part as a convalescent when he may develop complications of a general nature or those specific to the particular procedure he has undergone. Most modern hospitals now possess recovery rooms in close proximity to the operating theatres. Here facilities for resuscitation exist — piped oxygen, suction, and the availability of other trained nursing and medical staff should an emergency arise. The patient's immediate postoperative management therefore takes place in the recovery room and when his condition is satisfactory he may return to the ward for further care. If the operation is successful, a large part of the credit will belong to the nursing staff who have tended to the patient's physical and psychological needs during the continuum of care in the preoperative and postoperative periods; if he develops a complication, however, it may have been that a little more attention to detail, a little more knowledge or expertise might have prevented it. Above all it must be recognized that communication is of paramount importance between the nurse and the patient and, indeed, the importance of communication at every level and at every stage can never be overemphasized.

MANAGEMENT IN THE RECOVERY ROOM

While in the recovery room the patient's breathing, blood pressure and pulse rate must be recorded, the area of the wound examined, his position checked and any drains or tubes seen to be functioning satisfactorily. These items will now be discussed more fully.

Respiratory system

Respiration may fail in two ways: either due to obstruction of the airway or due to pulmonary insufficiency. The nurse's

67

first duty lies in the maintenance of a clear airway which can easily become obstructed in the unconscious patient, leading to respiratory difficulty, stridor and cyanosis. Before the patient leaves the operating table the anaesthetist removes all tubes, mouth packs, swabs and connections to the mouth and confirms by direct laryngoscopy that the airway is clear; nevertheless it is not unknown for such articles, and even dental plates, to be left in the mouth. Particularly after operations on the nose or mouth, blood or mucus and sometimes regurgitated vomit may collect in the pharynx, be inhaled, and so cause laryngeal obstruction. The mere contact of these items will readily induce the larynx to go into a state of spasm and the opposed vocal cords will further embarrass the respiration. Perhaps the commonest cause of airway obstruction in the unconscious patient is the tongue which falls backwards into the throat. The airway can also be obstructed from without by clothing drawn tightly around the neck or by bleeding occurring into the soft tissues of the neck causing tracheal compression. Whatever the cause, obstruction of the airway calls for immediate action — the mouth is inspected for foreign bodies and any vomitus, blood or mucus aspirated from the pharynx; the jaw is then held from behind the angle on each side and pushed upwards and forwards. This manoeuvre prevents the tongue falling back into the throat. Any constricting clothes or tapes around the neck are freed and if obstruction still persists, the anaesthetist must be informed immediately.

Respiration may also fail because of insufficiency; normal inspiration either does not occur, or if it does, it is inefficient and results in poor ventilation of the lungs. Thus, pain from a thoracic wound prevents full inspiration, or pain from an abdominal wound prevents full descent of the diaphragm. The same result can be caused by strapping the chest or allowing the patient to lie completely flat so that full descent of the diaphragm is prevented by the pressure of the abdominal contents. Full expansion of the lung may also be prevented by the presence of air, pus or blood in the pleural cavity, and occasionally persistence of relaxant drugs causes weakness in the muscles of respiration. The respiratory centre in the brain is sometimes depressed by drugs or changes in the blood gases. This can occur when one drug interacts with another, following too heavy premedication or when there is an excessive change in the level of carbon dioxide in the blood.

The principles of treatment of respiratory insufficiency are to remove the cause, where this is possible, aspirate the air or drain the pus or blood from the pleural cavity, relieve the pain of a chest wound with analgesics and prevent splinting of the diaphragm by proper positioning of the patient. In those patients in whom there is persistent action of relaxant drugs, adequate amounts of reversal agents must be given, and when there is central depression of respiration this must be supported until the body has excreted the excess drugs. This support entails either manual or mechanical ventilation.

Cardiovascular system

While the patient is in the recovery room the nurse must record the pulse rate and the blood pressure, which are the two most important indices of the state of the cardiovascular system. The pulse rate may be increased by surgical shock, haemorrhage, lack of oxygen, and pain, and decreased by drugs or cerebral compression. The blood pressure may be elevated by drug interaction or a return to its high preoperative level in a hypertensive patient, or it may be depressed by pain, bleeding or bad positioning. The pulse and blood pressure should serve as important early warning signs to the nurse who may otherwise be lulled into a sense of security by the apparent quietness of the patient.

General management

The wound

It is important that the nurse should look at the area of the wound at the earliest opportunity. The site of any drainage tubes and the extent of any loss of blood on the dressings should be noted. In this way a baseline is established by which any further blood loss can be gauged; thereafter intermittent inspection of the wound should be carried out. Severe blood loss can occur into dressings beneath clothes without it being immediately apparent. When a leg or arm is the site of the operation an inspection should be carried out; tourniquets can be left on and bandages may become too tight.

Position of the patient

Most patients are better nursed on their side in the immediate postoperative period, especially those who have undergone a bronchoscopy with the subsequent production of much mucus, or an operation on the nose or throat attended by bleeding. In this position the tongue does not readily obstruct the airway, and blood, mucus and vomitus can drain away. Some patients have to be nursed in a supine position by the very nature of their operations and, therefore, particular attention should be paid to them.

Once consciousness has been regained some elderly patients with poor circulation and bronchitis find respiration easier if they are slightly propped up. Care must be taken in this procedure, especially if the blood pressure is low.

Drains and tubes

Chest drains are employed in most thoracic operations, and their management requires meticulous care. Their function is to drain fluid from the chest without allowing air from the outside to enter the pleural cavity. This is ensured with the aid of a water-sealed bottle. The bottle should never be elevated above the level of the patient; otherwise siphoning occurs and water followed by air enters the chest. If raising the bottle is unavoidable, then before it is done the tubing must be doubly clamped with forceps. Peritoneal drainage is often employed following leakage of infected or otherwise harmful material into the peritoneal cavity. It is not only useful for drainage but also for diagnostic purposes. For example, a drain placed in the area of the gall bladder ducts after cholecystectomy will not only drain blood and debris but also bile on occasions when there has been damage to the biliary ducts. Early diagnosis of a biliary **peritonitis** may be of the greatest importance.

Nasogastric tubes are also often used, inserted via the nose or the mouth. The tip of the tube is designed to rest in the most dependent part of the stomach where the fluid collects. If the stomach is kept free of fluid, the patient cannot vomit gastric contents which might then be inhaled; also, keeping the stomach free of fluid and air prevents it dilating. Bladder catheters are of many different types and are inserted for drainage purposes. In certain operations on the bladder, such as **prostatectomy**, the flow of blood-stained urine must be kept running to avoid clot formation. Some form of bladder irrigation is employed and the recovery room nurse must be conversant with it and thus able to prevent clot formation in the bladder.

Intravenous fluids

On receiving the patient into the recovery room the nurse must satisfy herself that the intravenous fluid is running at the correct rate into the circulation. It is as well to check the solution being used, the tubing for leaks and the needle site to see whether the fluid being administered is passing satisfactorily into the vein or outside it into the tissues of the arm. Enquiry should be made of the anaesthetist as to what further fluid is required and instructions should be given, preferably in writing, for further infusion in the ensuing few hours.

Peritonitis Inflammation of the peritoneum.

Prostatectomy Excision of the whole or part of the prostate gland.

THE RETURN TO CONSCIOUSNESS

Modern anaesthetic techniques have now reached the point where the patient becomes conscious while in the recovery room. He may be restless and not fully in touch with his surroundings. Firm reassurance and reiteration that he has had his operation and is alright does much to quieten him and return him to a normal state.

When the patient is awake and talking, can obey simple commands, maintain his own airway and has a stable pulse and blood pressure, he may, after permission from the anaesthetist, be returned to the ward. The first phase of his postoperative management is now over.

MANAGEMENT IN THE WARD

The patient's transfer from the recovery room to his bed in the ward should be as comfortable and as smooth as possible. Rough handling can result in severe shock. It is important that enough personnel are present to lift him from the trolley to the bed without strain and place him in the correct position. As was the case in the recovery room, most patients are safer resting on their side, particularly those who have undergone operations on the mouth or nose, when blood, mucus or vomitus can drain away. Some patients, however, have to be nursed on their backs, a position dictated by the site or type of operation.

The patient should also be kept warm. Overheating, however, is to be avoided since this causes vasodilatation and a further fall in blood pressure in an already shocked patient. Hot-water bottles and electric blankets must not be used as their use may lead to severe skin burns in the unconscious patient.

It is very important that an adequate record of the patient's pulse and blood pressure be kept in the immediate postoperative period. The pulse particularly will give the earliest warning of the commencement of postoperative bleeding as well as provide an index of the patient's continuing progress in many other respects.

From the moment of his arrival on the ward, the patient must be encouraged to move. If he is unable to do this for himself, then he must be turned frequently by others. Immobility can only lead to the development of a pressure sore which is to be regarded as a preventable condition. A patient, particularly an older one, often resents mobilization immediately following an operation. A combination of tact, cajolery, exhortation and bullying may be necessary before he will move. A nurse who has had the foresight to get to know her patient and befriend him before the operation is most likely to succeed in this, and will markedly reduce his time in hospital and the likelihood of his developing postoperative complications. The term 'mobilization' does not just apply to the patient's limbs, but also to the chest and abdomen.

Every patient who undergoes a major operation should be instructed in breathing exercises preoperatively so that after the operation he knows what is required of him and his nurse and physiotherapist can see that it is done. Immediately following his return to consciousness he is told to breathe deeply several times every 15 minutes. If there is any mucus in the chest, this must be coughed up and he should be shown how to press on the wound as he does so in order to reduce the pain caused by the expulsive effort. These respiratory activities tend to frighten some patients who do not understand their necessity and who fear that they may 'burst their stitches'. These patients require frequent reassurance and analgesia.

On their return to the ward some patients are very restless and disturbed, which may be due to pain. Today a wide variety of analgesics is available and one drug must be selected which will effectively suppress pain without giving rise to respiratory depression. In this respect the dosage and frequency of administration is of vital importance. For example, an intramuscular injection of 75 mg of pethidine hydrochloride may relieve the patient's pain but may also cause respiratory depression. The same amount of pethidine given in three divided doses of 25 mg at intervals during the same time also relieves pain but without causing respiratory depression.

Restlessness is not always due to pain. Another frequent cause is **hypoxia**, the blood leaving the lungs being insufficiently oxygenated due to airway obstruction or respiratory insufficiency. Obviously the cause of the condition should be corrected, and for a time oxygen will have to be administered by nasal catheter or face mask.

A patient returning to the ward will often have a nasogastric tube and intravenous infusion attached to him. It is therefore obligatory that those who nurse him understand the fundamentals of fluid balance. There is an enormous amount of mystique surrounding the subject which causes much confusion, and yet the basic concept is simple. In a healthy person the amount of water in the body remains relatively constant. That is to say there is a balance existing between fluid intake and loss. This body water has a number of inorganic chemical substances dissolved in it which in solution dissociate into positively or negatively charged particles called anions and cations respectively. The total number of anions in the body at any one time is exactly matched by an equal number of cations and a state of electrical neutrality therefore exists. In disease this delicate ionic balance may be

Hypoxia The condition of inadequate oxygenation.

disturbed, and in its efforts to maintain it the body may lose or retain water. Health can only be regained when the former water and electrolyte balance has been restored. In order to do this not only the amount, but also the electrolyte content of the fluid gain or loss must be known. With these principles in mind, seriously ill patients or those who have undergone major surgery have their fluid intake and output from all sources separately charted. A specimen of this chart is shown in *Figure 4.1.* At the end of each 24-hour period the total

DAILY FLUID BALANCE CHART

S. 299

| Name | | | | | | Ward | Date | Sheet No. |

| Time | INTAKE | | Blood (B) Plasma (P) Dextran (D) | OUTPUT | | | Remarks |
	By mouth	Intravenous		Urine	Vomit (V) or Aspiration (A)	Other	
9 am							
10 am							
11 am							
noon							
1 pm							
2 pm							
3 pm							
4 pm							
5 pm							
6 pm							
7 pm							
8 pm							
9 pm							
10 pm							
11 pm							
mid-night							
1 am							
2 am							
3 am							
4 am							
5 am							
6 am							
7 am							
8 am							
Totals							

Total intake .... c.c.   Total output .... cc.

Figure 4.1. An example of a fluid balance chart

intake is compared with the total output and it will be seen whether the patient has retained or lost fluid, and its approximate electrolyte content can be estimated from a knowledge of its source. Thus a correction can be made to the amount of fluids and their type to be infused during the next 24 hours. The keeping of an accurate balance chart is of paramount importance.

The daily fluid requirement of a patient in balance is approximately 2.5 litres, and the amount lost or gained during the previous period must be added to or subtracted from this figure. Of the amount to be infused in the ensuing 24 hours no more than 0.5 litre should be in the form of isotonic saline solution ('normal' saline) unless there has been an excessive loss of salt. In patients who have undergone abdominal surgery normal peristaltic motility of the intestine is suspended, that is, the waves of contraction which move the gut contents onward cease for one or two days. With the return of bowel activity the gastric aspirates fall in amount and at this stage small amounts of water may be given by mouth at regular intervals. Gastric aspiration is continued, but the interval between aspiration is lengthened; once again the fluid balance chart indicates whether the oral fluid is being absorbed. If this is so, then larger amounts of fluid are given and the use of the nasogastric tube and intravenous infusion abandoned. As soon as possible, part of the patient's fluid requirement is given in the form of thin soups and from this point onwards the diet is progressively built up until he is once more taking solid foods.

The management of the patient's drains in the postoperative period is the subject of much confusion. Wound drains are placed superficially and are inserted with the object of preventing haematoma formation. These may be safely removed in 2 to 3 days. Peritoneal drains are employed to remove pus, blood or other fluid from the abdominal cavity. In the main these are removed when they cease to function. Bile duct drains, however, must be left *in situ* for at least 10 days. Unfortunately there are a number of exceptions and wide variations in the personal preferences of surgeons. The wisest course the nurse can adopt is to ask the doctor before taking the drain out.

Most operation wounds heal satisfactorily without infection and the skin stitches can be removed 6 to 10 days postoperatively. The exact time depends on the type of incision and the speed of wound healing in each individual patient. Following stitch removal the patient is sent home having enjoyed a smooth postoperative course. A few patients are unfortunate enough to develop complications of a local or general nature.

Local complications

Haematoma

Sometimes a haematoma, which is a collection of blood, develops in the wound. This is usually due to ineffective haemostasis or arrest of bleeding at the time of operation and therefore must be regarded as a preventable condition.

Once the haematoma has become established it delays healing of the wound and acts as a site where bacteria may flourish and infection can develop.

Wound infection

The first sign of a wound infection occurs with the development of a fever on the fourth or fifth postoperative day, the wound becomes red and inflamed and some part is found to be tender. Treatment consists of establishing drainage by probing the wound, or removing stitches and allowing the pus to escape. At the same time some pus may be taken for culture and the patient given a course of the appropriate antibiotic. Once the wound abscess has been drained the patient's **pyrexia** rapidly subsides and complete healing occurs.

Wound dehiscence

Approximately 3 to 4 patients in every 100 suffer from the condition known as an abdominal wound **dehiscence** or 'burst abdomen' (which is a more accurate and graphic term of description). This condition may occur on about the tenth day, sometimes about 1 to 2 days earlier and sometimes as late as the third or fourth week postoperatively. It is due essentially to poor healing of the tissues, aggravated by bad surgical technique, coughing, vomiting, old age of the patient and malnutrition. The wound suddenly begins to leak rather watery, blood-stained fluid, the stitches give way and sometimes loops of bowel may extrude from the wound. This happening, naturally enough, causes the patient great alarm, but it is not nearly such a grave occurrence as he may imagine. The wound and any extruded gut should be covered with an abdominal pack which has been moistened with sterile saline solution, and the whole abdomen then wrapped in an abdominal binder. It is vital that the patient is reassured and that at the earliest opportunity a secondary suture of the wound is carried out in theatre under general anaesthesia.

Haemorrhage

Arterial haemorrhage occurring in the postoperative period may either be of reactionary or secondary type. Reactionary haemorrhage occurs within 24 hours of the operation when the blood pressure returns to normal. A ligature may slip or a piece of blood clot becomes dislodged and a brisk bleed results. Secondary haemorrhage occurs much later in the postoperative period and is due to the presence of infection. When bleeding is visible diagnosis usually presents no problem and it is only when it is internal or concealed that difficulties and danger arise. A large haemorrhage should be suspected when the patient suddenly becomes pale, anxious, restless

Pyrexia Fever.

Dehiscence Gaping, usually applied to an operational wound that has come apart.

and sweaty, his pulse rate begins to rise and the blood pressure begins to fall. Eventually a sighing type of respiration, known as 'air hunger', develops and the patient may faint or lose consciousness entirely. On occasions early recognition and prompt interpretation of these symptoms and signs may be life-saving. The nurse's first duty is to stop the bleeding if it is possible, and this can usually be done by applying pressure to the site of the haemorrhage, or in the case of a limb, by putting on an emergency tourniquet. The patient should be laid flat and the foot of the bed elevated slightly. Medical aid should then be summoned.

General complications

Atelectasis

Of all the possible postoperative complications by far the commonest are those affecting the lungs. The anaesthetized patient, breathing mixtures of mildly irritant gases, produces large quantities of mucus in the lungs. This mucus frequently blocks the smaller and sometimes the larger air passages; thus an area of lung ceases to function, the air trapped within it is absorbed, and it collapses. Not only is this collapsed lung useless from the point of view of gaseous exchange, but it inevitably becomes a site where infection develops. The condition of lung collapse or **atelectasis** is more prone to occur in those with pre-existing lung disease, such as asthma, bronchitis or bronchiectasis, in the elderly and in those who smoke. It is also more likely to occur in patients who are allowed to be immobile after an operation, breathing inadequately and failing to cough up the secretions present in the lungs. Atelectasis occurs in the first 2 to 3 postoperative days and shows itself initially by a slight rise in the pulse rate which is rapidly followed by fever; the patient is slightly cyanotic and **dyspnoeic**. It is important to diagnose the condition early because with vigorous treatment it is correctable at an early stage. Deep breathing, coughing and postural drainage should be instituted immediately and any infection already established controlled with antibiotics. Humidification of the inspired air helps, and bronchodilators are also of value if there is an element of bronchospasm present.

Pneumonia

Pneumonia and bronchopneumonia occur postoperatively and are almost always a consequence of previous complete or partial collapse of the lung. The infection commences in the collapsed segment and extends from there throughout the lobes and bronchi of the lung. The success of treatment depends on the choice and early use of the correct antibiotic.

Atelectasis Local collapse of a segment of lung.

Dyspnoea Shortness of breath.

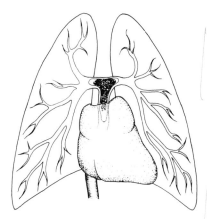

Figure 4.2. Diagram showing embolic occlusion of the main pulmonary arterial trunk

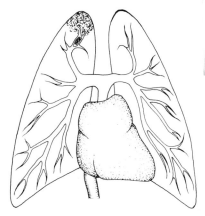

Figure 4.3. Diagram showing occlusion of one of the smaller branches of the pulmonary artery with devitalization of a wedge-shaped peripheral segment of the lung

Pleurisy Inflammation of the pleural covering of the lungs.

Pulmonary embolism

Pulmonary embolism is unfortunately common and frequently follows operations on the abdomen and pelvis in the middle-aged, obese woman. Both sexes and all ages, however, can be affected. The condition usually commences as a thrombosis or blood clot in the deep veins of the calf which become painful, swollen and tender. These clots lie within the veins but unattached to them and are very liable to move onwards in the bloodstream via larger and larger veins until, by passing through the right side of the heart, they lodge in the pulmonary artery or its ramifications in the lung. If the main pulmonary trunk is occluded the patient usually collapses and dies as a result of the sudden arrest of the circulation (*see Figure 4.2*). If one of the smaller branches of the pulmonary artery is affected, the area of lung that it supplies becomes starved of blood and necrotic. This area of dead tissue is usually in the more peripheral parts of the lung which are furthest from its blood supply (*see Figure 4.3*). Occlusion of the main pulmonary artery manifests itself by sudden collapse, cyanosis and hypotension, whereas a small embolism results in an area of **pleurisy**, cough production of small amounts of blood-stained sputum and inspiratory difficulty due to pain. A radiograph of the chest does not immediately show any lesion, but after 1 to 2 days a small triangular area of peripheral consolidation, showing as an opacity, can be seen in the lung. These signs may be accompanied by a change in the electro-cardiograph tracing.

If a pulmonary embolus is suspected, treatment should immediately be instigated. The patient is given anticoagulants, pleuritic pain is relieved by analgesics and cyanosis prevented by giving oxygen. Not only should anticoagulants be given in established cases, but also if the patient develops a deep vein thrombosis. Occasionally when a patient has multiple emboli it is necessary to ligate the long saphenous vein or plicate the inferior vena cava; that is to say, to stitch it so that the single lumen is converted into a number of channels, each small enough to prevent the onward passage of a large embolus.

Paralytic ileus

After abdominal operations the peristaltic activity of the gut is normally inhibited for one or two days. Thereafter there is a slow return to spontaneous bowel movements. This condition is known as paralytic ileus and is a natural response and not of any serious significance unless the gut continues to be inactive, distended with gas, and silent. If it persists, it may be due to the development of peritonitis due to infection or a leakage bowel anastomosis. Paralytic ileus, in that the bowel fails to propel its contents onwards, constitutes a type of obstruction and its conservative treatment in no way differs from that of other types of obstruction. The bowel is decompressed by intermittent suction through a nasogastric tube and the patient's fluid and electrolyte balance maintained by an intravenous drip infusion until normal bowel function returns.

Retention of urine

Retention of urine is a very common sequel to abdominal, perineal and rectal operations, particularly in the male. Pain, mental stress or certain drugs may cause spasm of the urinary sphincter muscles and the patient finds he is unable to pass urine despite an intense desire to do so. Failure to pass water postoperatively must not be confused with acute renal failure when the bladder is found to be empty on catheterization. In acute retention the distended bladder can be felt and sometimes seen rising above the pubic symphysis. Initial treatment should be directed towards encouraging the patient to pass urine. He is helped to stand, pain is relieved with analgesics, and a water tap is turned on. Sometimes the drug carbachol

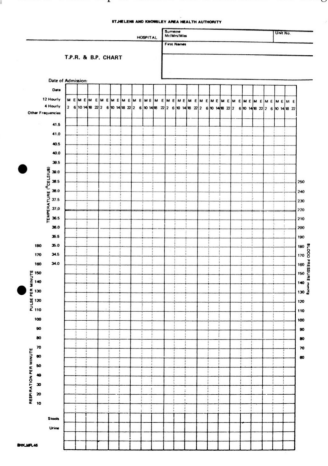

Figure 4.4. An example of a standard temperature chart

is given which stimulates the bladder muscle and causes relaxation of the sphincter. If these simple measures fail, the patient will require catheterization before over-distension of the bladder occurs.

Postoperative pyrexia

Many patients following surgery exhibit a temporary pyrexia, and this is a natural response to injury (*Figure 4.4* shows a standard type of a temperature chart). However, its persistence for more than 24 hours warrants further investigation. The first step is to examine the wound, part of which may be inflamed, swollen or excessively tender — signs indicative of the presence of a **haematoma** or focal abscess. In the absence of such a discovery the search for a cause must be widened. Tenderness in the calf may disclose a venous thrombosis; a chest radiograph following the advent of a cough may demonstrate lung collapse, bronchopneumonia, an **infarct**; a rectal examination may reveal a pelvic abscess. Examination of the urine may show infection in any part of the genito-urinary tract. Lastly, if no cause is found, the presence of a subdiaphragmatic abscess should be suspected.

Bedsores

Sores are caused by persistent pressure on areas of skin situated over bony prominences, such as the heels or the buttocks. The skin becomes devitalized and necrotic and breaks down with the formation of an ulcer. Sores are preventable, but malnutrition, anaemia, old age and the presence of moisture are predisposing factors; patients with diseases of the nervous or cardiovascular systems are particularly vulnerable.

Haematoma A collection of blood in the tissues.

Infarct Death of tissue resulting from interruption of blood supply.

5

The intensive therapy unit

A. A. Gilbertson

INTRODUCTION

An intensive therapy unit (ITU) is defined in a report by the Royal College of Nursing and National Council of Nurses of the United Kingdom (Intensive Therapy Units, 1969) as a unit where care is taken 'of patients who are deemed recoverable but who need continuous supervision and need or are likely to need prompt use of specialized techniques by skilled personnel'.

In an ITU there is more space, staff and equipment available for the care of a patient than can be provided in the ordinary wards. This allows for continuous observation of the patient's vital functions and prompt treatment of complications, should they arise.

In some units treatment of a wide variety of patients is undertaken; others may have very specialized functions, such as the treatment of coronary thrombosis, chest injuries, respiratory failure or the management of renal failure by **dialysis**.

Surgical patients are likely to be admitted to an intensive therapy unit when:

(1) extensive resuscitation will be necessary before sugery;
(2) the magnitude or type of operation has been such that there is a risk of failure of vital functions in the post-operative period (for example, following 'open heart' surgery);
(3) respiratory, cardiac or renal failures are anticipated because of the patient's poor general health; and when
(4) major complications have arisen during the operation or postoperatively (for example, pulmonary embolus).

This chapter will be concerned with the main procedures which will apply particularly to such patients.

RESTORATION OF FLUID BALANCE

There are two types of fluids which may be given intravenously to restore fluid balance:

Dialysis A procedure to remove the (unwanted) soluble substances from the body; used in renal failure when either the blood is passed through a machine (haemodialysis q.v.) or fluid is passed through the peritoneal cavity (peritoneal dialysis).

(1) fluids which stay in the circulation for a long time after transfusion because they contain large molecules (for example, blood, plasma and dextran solutions);

(2) solutions which rapidly diffuse out of the circulation and add water, or water and electrolytes, to the fluid bathing the cells ('electrolytes' in this context are mainly sodium (Na^+), potassium (K^+) and chloride (Cl^-) ions).

Patients who are not critically ill will usually be able to have their fluid and electrolyte imbalance or blood loss restored in the surgical ward. However, more severe fluid depletion will need very rapid treatment, necessitating continuous monitoring of the electrocardiogram and central venous pressure. It may well be best to transfer these patients to the ITU.

In severe fluid loss the most important consideration is to restore the blood volume to an acceptable level. When this has been done, the fluid in the tissues both inside and outside the cells can be restored to normal volume and content. Only then will the various organs be able to function normally. During this second stage of resuscitation the function of the heart and kidneys will improve and it will be found that as this proceeds, the circulating blood volume will need to be adjusted continually for some time.

Stage 1 — Restoration of blood volume

A reduction of the amount of blood circulating in the blood vessels is called oligaemia. In some cases **oligaemia** may be due to the loss of whole blood, for example in haemorrhage or burns. Treatment of such cases will be by whole blood transfusion. In other cases, for example in vomiting due to intestinal obstruction, only water and electrolytes may be lost; the cells and proteins remain and the blood is more concentrated than usual. The packed cell volume (PCV) and haemoglobin will be raised above normal values. In those patients blood volume will be restored to normal by transfusion of electrolyte solutions, usually 0.9 per cent sodium chloride and carefully calculated amounts of added potassium chloride.

Patients with severe oligaemia may need very large volumes of fluid before the circulation improves but there is a danger of overloading the circulation and causing heart failure if too much fluid is given. This is particularly important if the heart is weakened by pre-existing disease. A typical case would be a patient who has had a coronary thrombosis and who is bleeding profusely from a gastric ulcer. If a little too much blood is

Oligaemia A circulating blood volume below normal.

transfused in treating his **haematemesis**, he may pass into cardiac failure due to overloading of his weak left ventricle.

By measuring the pressure in the great veins near the heart (the central venous pressure, or CVP) it is easy to restore blood volume safely and to avoid raising it to a level which might overload the heart.

Measurement of central venous pressure

The measurement of central venous pressure is a procedure which takes only a few seconds once the CVP catheter has been introduced. The CVP catheter is a long flexible plastic tube which is passed into a vein either through a needle,

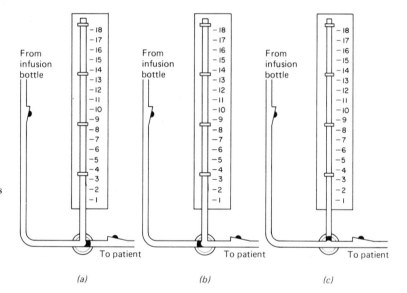

Figure 5.1. Measurement of central venous pressure. (*a*) The three-way tap is turned off to patient so that manometer chamber may be filled with solution. (*b*) The three-way tap is turned off to infusion bottle and on towards patient. (*c*) The three-way tap is turned to open line between bottle and patient and clamp off manometer

From infusion bottle — To patient (a)

From infusion bottle — To patient (b)

From infusion bottle — To patient (c)

Haematemesis Vomiting blood.

Cannula A tube to be inserted into a body cavity, duct or blood vessel to effect a communication with the exterior.

through a special **cannula** or directly into the vein which has been exposed by an incision under local anaesthetic. It is threaded into the vein until the tip reaches the vena cava, or even the right atrium. The other end is joined to a three-way tap so that the catheter may be connected to either the tube from the infusion bottle, or to a pressure-measuring tube (a manometer) (*Figure 5.1*). The manometer is simply a tube which is filled with fluid and placed vertically with its base at the level of the patient's heart. It is filled with solution by turning the three-way tap to position *a* and opening the clamp on the tubing until the manometer tube is full. The tap is then turned to position *b* and the fluid runs from the manometer, through the catheter into the vena cava. When the pressure of the column of fluid in the manometer equals the pressure in the vena cava, the fluid in the manometer will fall no further. The height of the column of fluid in the

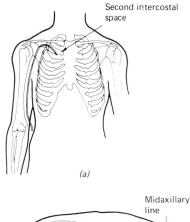

Second intercostal space

(a)

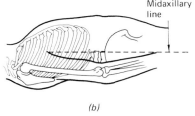

Midaxillary line

(b)

Figure 5.2. Points on the body surface accepted as indicating the position of the heart: (*a*) the anterior surface of the chest in the midline at the level of the second intercostal space; (*b*) the mid-axillary line

manometer is then the central venous pressure and it is expressed in cm of water (or saline or dextrose). When the height of the column has been observed and noted, the tap is turned so that the drip is routed through the catheter (position *c*) and the rate of transfusion is regulated in the usual way with the clamp.

It is important that the height of the column of fluid in the manometer is measured from the level of the patient's heart. Two different points on the body surface are accepted as indicating the position of the heart (*Figure 5.2*): (1) the anterior surface of the chest in the midline at the level of the second intercostal space, and (2) the midaxillary line.

The normal central venous pressure is 0 to 3 cm water measured with zero at the first point or 7 to 10 cm water measured from the midaxillary line.

Sometimes it is important to have a continuous recording of the CVP or of the arterial blood pressure. One way of doing this is to connect the central venous catheter, or an arterial cannula to a pressure-measuring device called a transducer. The transducer alters an electrical current as the pressure changes, and so enables the pressure to be read off on a meter. The transducer and recorder may need to be calibrated at regular intervals and the cannula must be flushed with saline to prevent it blocking. In some systems these operations are performed automatically.

Stage 2 — Tissue rehydration

After the volume of fluid in the blood vessels (intravascular volume) has been restored to a safe level (stage 1), attention is directed to restoring the water and electrolyte content of the tissues (stage 2). To do this a large volume of water containing sodium, chloride and potassium must be transfused. Overloading of the circulation is prevented by monitoring CVP. If potassium is given too quickly, cardiac irregularities or even cardiac arrest may occur. The electrocardiogram is therefore monitored carefully. An increase in the size of the T-wave (*see Figure 5.10*) is the sign of too rapid an infusion of potassium.

During this rehydration phase of resuscitation the fluid intake and output must be accurately recorded. It is necessary to measure the output of urine at frequent intervals and to be able to relate this to the amount of fluid transfused in the same period. Fluid lost from sources other than urine must also be recorded. As each entry is made on the chart, the total intake or loss since the day began (or the patient was admitted) should be calculated, i.e. a running or cumulative total must be kept. Special intake/output charts make this necessary chore very simple. The specific gravity of each urine sample should be measured and in many cases the urine will be sent for analysis of its electrolyte content so that losses can be accurately replaced.

RESPIRATORY FAILURE IN SURGICAL PATIENTS

Some common causes of respiratory inadequacy in surgical patients are:

(1) inhalation of blood in patients with injuries in the upper respiratory tract, or haematemesis or of vomit, particularly in intestinal obstruction;

(2) trauma to the chest wall or lungs; and

(3) in the postoperative period — depression of the respiratory centre by analgesics or anaesthetic agents, weakness of respiratory muscles due to residual effects of relaxant drugs, sputum retention when coughing is ineffective due to pain or weakness, and pulmonary oedema due to heart failure or overtransfusion.

Respiratory embarrassment may be caused by **pneumothorax**, which may follow abdominal operations (for example, **nephrectomy**) as well as thoracic operations, or by **haemothorax** or a pleural effusion.

TREATMENT OF RESPIRATORY FAILURE

The management of respiratory distress is described in Chapter 15. In some cases, however, the measures used to help patients to breathe satisfactorily will fail and, to a variable degree, the lungs will not succeed in absorbing enough oxygen or in excreting enough carbon dioxide. Emphasis is usually placed on the elimination of carbon dioxide rather than on the absorption of oxygen because, to a certain extent, failure of the lungs to oxygenate the blood can be countered by giving a higher proportion of oxygen in the inspired air but, if respiration is not adequate to remove the carbon dioxide produced in the tissues, the only possible remedy is the artificial ventilation of the lungs. A dangerously high carbon dioxide level in the arterial blood is the best indication of the need for artificial ventilation.

The function of the lungs is to remove carbon dioxide from the venous blood as it passes through the pulmonary circulation. How well the lungs have succeeded in performing this function can only be discovered by analysing arterial blood, that is, blood which has just passed through the lung.

Pneumothorax Air within the pleural cavity.

Nephrectomy Removal of a kidney.

Haemothorax Blood in the pleural cavity.

The results are expressed in terms of the partial pressure of carbon dioxide in the blood, usually abbreviated to P_{CO_2}. The normal P_{CO_2} is 36 to 44 mm of mercury. A P_{CO_2} higher than 44 mm Hg indicates that the lungs are not adequately removing carbon dioxide from the venous blood and that the level in the arterial blood is therefore rising. Many patients with chronic bronchitis have impaired elimination of carbon dioxide but manage to live with a P_{CO_2} level of 50 to 60 mm Hg. They are thus permanently in a state of at least partial respiratory failure. An episode of pneumonia may cause complete respiratory failure. The P_{CO_2} may rise to over 100 mm Hg and unless treatment is quickly successful the patient will pass into 'carbon dioxide coma' and die.

Such patients will of course also suffer from the inability of their lungs to provide adequate oxygen for the tissues. In the early stages, administration of oxygen will help them, but later this procedure may actually be dangerous because oxygen therapy does nothing to help carbon dioxide elimination — indeed, it may actually depress respiration by removing the stimulation of the respiratory centre in the brain. The normal tension of oxygen in arterial blood (P_{O_2}) is about 100 mm Hg, or rather less in older people. As long as the P_{CO_2} is reasonably normal, a low P_{O_2} (hypoxaemia) can be treated by administering oxygen. If the P_{CO_2} is rising to dangerous levels, however, and other measures have failed to restore a normal P_{CO_2}, artificial ventilation of the lungs will be required. In some cases, the P_{CO_2} can be kept perhaps just within safe limits but the effort of doing so will so exhaust the patient that it will be safer (and kinder) to relieve him of this effort by instituting artifical ventilation.

Artificial ventilation

It should be understood that artificial ventilation of the lungs will always be seen as a temporary measure to save the patient's life while his lungs recover their ability to function adequately without such help. Thus, the decision to commence artificial ventilation should only be made by a doctor with sufficient knowledge of the patient's history and prospects to enable him to assess the likelihood of the patient regaining, sooner or later, adequate lung function. Remember, the definition of intensive therapy is 'the care of patients who are deemed recoverable ...'. This means that the patient must have a good chance of being restored to a normal, reasonably enjoyable, quality of life. Although individual cases may present very difficult decisions, one should strive to avoid committing patients with irreversible respiratory failure to a life of permanent artificial ventilation.

Mouth-to-mouth or mouth-to-nose ventilation

Mouth-to-mouth or mouth-to-nose ventilation is the only effective method of ventilating a patient's lungs without any equipment. It will rarely be necessary in an intensive therapy unit because convenient equipment for more elegant methods will be available, but such equipment may fail and in such case the inflation of the patient's lungs with one's own expired air may save his life.

Manual methods of ventilation

In manual methods of artificial ventilation of the lungs self-inflating bags (for example, Ambu, Air Viva), or anaesthetic reservoir bags are used.

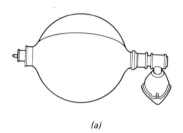

Self-inflating bags Self-inflating bags (*see Figure 5.3*) regain their oval shape following compression. They are attached to a mask or endotracheal tube. When the bag is squeezed, air is forced into the patient's lungs. When the pressure is released it recovers its expanded shape and refills with air through a one-way valve, and the patient exhales through a non-rebreathing valve. If oxygen is available, it may be added to the bag via the inlet tap which is usually provided.

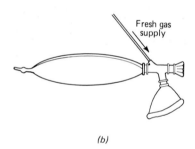

Anaesthetic circuits By squeezing the reservoir bag in the breathing circuit of an anaesthetic machine, oxygen or oxygen-containing mixtures can be forced into the patient's lungs. The closed circuit is particularly suitable for this and is frequently used to ventilate the lungs of anaesthetized patients who are unable to breathe after the administration of relaxant drugs. The 'Waters' circuit is a type of anaesthetic circuit frequently used to inflate a patient's lungs in an emergency, such as in cardiac arrest or in a respiratory failure. It can be, of course, used with an oxygen cylinder or pipeline outlet instead of an anaesthetic machine. The expiratory valve must be opened just enough to prevent the bag overinflating. If it is wide open, all the gas will escape and the lungs will not be inflated.

Figure 5.3. Self-inflating anaesthetic bags: (*a*) Ambu Compact resuscitator; (*b*) 'Waters' circuit used for resuscitation

Mechanical ventilation of the lungs

Machines which automatically ventilate the lungs often look frighteningly complicated, but in fact the majority of them are not difficult to control.

It is very helpful to think of each breath which the machine provides, or assists, in two separate parts.

(1) Inspiration — the chest expands as the machine inflates the lungs with gas.

(2) Expiration — the machine allows the lungs to contract by their own elasticity. The gas in the lungs escapes either to the atmosphere or back into the ventilator to be used again after oxygen has been added and carbon dioxide removed. Expiration ceases when the machine starts to inflate the lungs again for the next inspiration.

As the lungs are inflated by filling them with gas under increased pressure, the phrase 'intermittent positive pressure ventilation' (IPPV) is often used to distinguish this type of ventilation from that produced by an 'iron lung' in which the thorax is enclosed in a case in which the pressure is lowered to suck air into the lungs during inspiration (i.e. intermittent negative pressure).

Various types of ventilators inflate the lungs in different ways.

Constant volume ventilators In constant volume ventilators (for example, Cape ventilators) the volume of gas to be delivered to the lungs is selected on a dial. This volume is then delivered during each inspiration (tidal volume). The respiratory rate (the number of times per minute the patient's lungs are inflated) is set by a separate control. The volume of gas delivered each minute (minute volume) can easily be calculated by multiplying the tidal volume by the respiratory rate. These constant volume machines usually work by a bellows

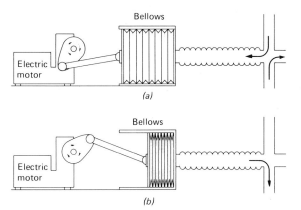

Figure 5.4. Bellows mechanism of a constant volume ventilator; (*a*) during expiratory phase, and (*b*) during inspiratory phase

mechanism which can be set to deliver the volume required at each inflation (*Figure 5.4*). As the bellows force gas into the lungs the pressure of the gas in the lungs rises. If the lungs are 'stiff' or the amount of gas is large, the pressure will rise more, say to 40 cm of water gauge (cm H_2O). If the lungs are compliant or only a small volume of gas is selected, the pressure needed for the inflation will be lower, perhaps 10 cm H_2O. This pressure is always shown on a gauge so that changes in the stiffness or compliance of the lungs can be appreciated, and so that volumes of gas which would require dangerously high inflation pressures can be avoided. The tidal volume, respiratory rate, and inflation pressure are recorded, usually every 15 minutes, on specially prepared charts, so that changes in ventilation and compliance of the lungs can be detected. Conditions in which the compliance ('stiffness') of the lung may alter are pleural effusions, pulmonary oedema, pneumonia, or collapse of all or part of a lung. Variation in the amount of pressure needed to inflate the lungs with a given volume of gas may be an indication of improvement or deterioration in these conditions.

Constant pressure ventilators This type of ventilator (for example, East Radcliffe, Manley) is very frequently used. It does not deliver a set volume of gas to the patient; instead it fills the lungs by inflating them at a certain pressure, which can be varied by the attendant who will move the pressure control until the pressure is found to be sufficient to 'blow up' the lungs to the required amount at each inspiration. This is shown by the reading on an instrument called a 'spirometer' which measures the volume of air which flows at each breath (tidal volume) or each minute (minute volume).

It is important to remember that it is the inflation pressure which is fixed in these ventilators. If the stiffness or compliance of the lungs changes, the volume of air introduced into the lungs by the selected inflation pressure will also vary. For example, a pressure of 15 cm H_2O may be selected and the spirometer may show that this pressure is sufficient to inflate the patient's lungs with 500 ml of gas at each breath. If the stiffness of the lungs increases, however, as a result perhaps of an attack of pulmonary oedema, then the pressure set (15 cm H_2O) may be only enough to blow 300 ml of gas into the lungs. This may not be enough to maintain the patient's respiration, therefore a higher inflation pressure will now have to be selected to restore satisfactory ventilation. In this situation a constant volume ventilator would have continued to pump 500 ml of gas per inflation into the lungs, but the pressure in the lungs would have risen. There is usually a safety valve to prevent the pressure rising high enough to burst the lung.

The principal control regulating inspiration in a constant pressure ventilator is the inflation pressure control. This may be perhaps a knob or a dial which is set to the pressure required or, as in the East Radcliffe and Manley machines, a set of weights which are moved along a lever arm until they exert the desired pressure on the bellows to inflate the patient's lungs (*Figure 5.5*). The weights are lifted off the bellows during the expiratory phase either by an electric motor or by the pressure of gas from a cylinder or pipeline. During inspiration the weights drop onto the bellows and exert the necessary inflation pressure.

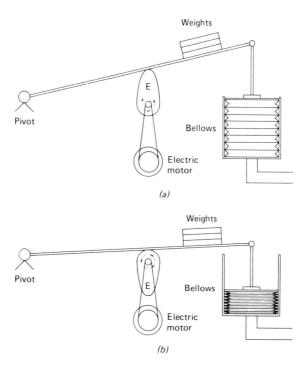

Figure 5.5. Bellows mechanism of a constant pressure ventilator during (*a*) expiratory phase and (*b*) inspiratory phase. The pivot is fixed and the lever arm raised by rotation of the eccentric cam (E)

As with constant volume machines, charting of the tidal or minute volumes, the inflation pressure, and the respiration rate will be necessary. With these machines the inflation pressure, having been set, will not be expected to alter, but the tidal or minute volume will vary with the lung compliance. Accurate charting will allow attention to be drawn to any major change in ventilatory volumes.

Respiratory rate or time Most ventilators have a control by which the number of breaths provided per minute may be regulated. In some machines the ratio of inspiratory to expiratory time is fixed; in others it is variable. An example of a fixed ratio machine is the East Radcliffe machine, in which the expiratory time is always twice as long as the inspiratory (inflation) period. For example, if a rate of 20 breaths per minute is selected on the rate control, then each breath must take 3 seconds. This period will be divided into 1 second for inflation and 2 seconds for expiration. In contrast, the Bennett ventilator has separate controls for inspiratory and expiratory times and a rate of 20 breaths per

E

minute could be achieved by setting expiratory and inspiratory times of 1.5 second each or any other combination of times which totals 3 seconds. Some patients are better ventilated by slow inflation, others by faster rates, and the doctor will select the pattern of respiration best suited to the individual patient.

Expiration In most respirators the only control regulating expiration is one which selects the time between inspirations. Indeed, even this is not always necessary as in many machines expiration is simply fixed as, for example, twice the length of inspiration. Occasionally, however, instead of merely allowing the patient to breathe out by removing the inflation pressure and opening an expiratory valve, a suction (or negative) pressure is applied to the lungs during expiration. This is done primarily to aid circulation. In ventilators with this facility there will be a negative pressure control for regulating this expiratory assistance. More commonly, when ventilating diseased lungs, it is helpful to maintain the pressure in the airways a little above atmospheric pressure during the expiratory period. This improves the transfer of oxygen through the lungs and is called 'positive end-expiratory pressure' usually referred to by its initials as 'PEEP'.

Triggered ventilators Whereas it is usually convenient to ventilate the lungs at a rate set by the medical attendant, there are cases in which it may be possible for the patient to select the rate at which he needs to start inspiration. Certain ventilators, for example, Bird, Bennett and Harlow machines, can 'sense' the suction exerted by the patient starting to breathe in, and they then immediately inflate his lungs until, usually, a pre-set pressure is reached. They then allow the patient to breathe out, and they wait patiently until the patient 'triggers' the machine by starting his next inspiration. These machines in fact assist the patient's own inspiration rather than completely take over his ventilation. There is an expiratory time control on triggered machines but it is inactivated when the patient is triggering, because expiration must then last until the patient's inspiratory effort starts inflation. Only if the patient ceases to make adequate inspiratory efforts to trigger the machine is this control set so that the machine does not wait a dangerously long time between breaths.

Triggered ventilators have a 'sensitivity' control which sets the amount of suction which the patient has to exert to cause the machine to start to inflate his lungs. If the patient is very weak, the machine will have to be very sensitive to detect his feeble inspirations and assist them. In other cases (for example, in a patient with hiccough or a very large heaving heart) such sensitivity could lead the machine to inflate the lungs at too high a rate and so the control is altered to reduce the sensitivity.

Fighting the respirator Most patients who require mechanical ventilation of their lungs are able to make some attempt to breathe, even though their attempts are inadequate. It is surprisingly difficult for a patient to allow himself to breathe at a rate fixed by a ventilator. If he tries to breathe at a rate different from, or out of phase with, the machine (i.e. if the patient tries to breathe out whilst the machine is in the inflation phase), the following may occur:

(1) in many machines, inflation of the lungs may cease prematurely, hopelessly inadequate ventilation of the lungs will result and the patient may asphyxiate; or
(2) dangerously high inflation pressures can build up and may rupture a lung, especially in emphysema.

The observation that the patient's chest and abdomen are not rising and falling regularly, but are jerking and not in time with the machine, and that the pressure gauge on the ventilator is fluctuating wildly, and the tidal volume varying from breath to breath, will indicate to the nurse that the patient is fighting the respirator. These are signs requiring immediate action and the nurse should be constantly watching for them. She should never leave the patient unless she is relieved by a competent deputy.

There are several ways of ensuring that the patient's respiratory efforts do not oppose the action of the mechanical ventilator.

(1) A patient-triggered ventilator (already described) may be used which will inflate the lungs following the inspiratory efforts of the patient.
(2) Intermittent mandatory ventilation (IMV) may be employed. The machine supplies a selected number of breaths each minute (the 'mandated' breaths) but a valve in the breathing circuit enables the patient to breathe freely, if he wishes, between the mandated breaths.
(3) If a fixed rate ventilator is used, (a) the patient's respiratory centre may be depressed, or (b) the respiratory muscles may be paralysed.

Depression of the respiratory centre

The respiratory centre is composed of groups of cells just under the surface of the ventral part of the medulla oblongata in the hind-brain. These cells are stimulated by increasing acidity (for example, when there is a rise in the Pco_2) and impulses then leave the centre to cause an increase in respiration. If this part of the brain is made inactive, the patient will cease to try to breathe, and will allow his lungs to be ventilated at a rate dictated by the ventilator. The respiratory centre can be inactivated by reducing the acidity of the blood by reducing the amount of carbon dioxide in it. This can be done by overventilating the lungs (hyperventilation) so that more carbon dioxide than normal is breathed out. In a short time the blood becomes alkaline and, as the respiratory centre is then not stimulated, no nerve impulses reach the respiratory muscles and the patient's respiratory efforts cease and he will not resist mechanical ventilation. The hyperventilation may be achieved initially by assisting the patient's own ventilation by manually squeezing the reservoir bag of the 'Waters' circuit. When the PCO_2 falls and the patient ceases to breathe, the ventilator can be connected.

Certain drugs are very powerful depressants of the respiratory centre, especially if the PCO_2 is also lowered.

Phenoperidine Phenoperidine is the most useful drug for 'controlling' patients who are being treated by IPPV. Besides depressing the respiratory centre and stopping the patient fighting the ventilator, it is a potent analgesic which makes it the drug of choice in patients with painful chest injuries or surgical incisions.

The intravenous injection of 1 to 3 mg phenoperidine will usually be effective in stopping all spontaneous respiratory activity, and will allow the lungs to be ventilated by the machine without opposition from the patient. Some depression of blood pressure may occur but this is usually of short duration and not dangerous. The main disadvantage of phenoperidine is that its effect only lasts about 30 minutes and will have to be repeated frequently.

Morphine and pethidine Morphine and pethidine, described in Chapter 6, both depress respiration which represents a great disadvantage when they are used to control pain in naturally breathing patients. However, this disadvantage is put to good use when the patient is required to stop breathing and comply with a lung ventilator. The intravenous injection of 50 to 100 mg pethidine or 5 to 10 mg morphine will usually abolish spontaneous ventilation. The effects of these drugs last for about 2 to 4 hours but depress the circulation more than phenoperidine.

Relaxant drugs
Relaxant drugs, also described in Chapter 3, are used to relax the muscles during light anaesthesia. They work at the junction of the nerve and muscle and prevent nerve impulses from

causing muscles to contract. If the impulses are completely prevented from initiating muscle contraction by a large dose of the drug, the patient is paralyzed rather than 'relaxed'. The muscles of respiration (i.e. muscles of the chest wall and the diaphragm) do not escape from this paralysis so that the patient will only survive if lungs are ventilated artificially and he is, of course, quite unable to resist a mechanical ventilator.

Although the relaxants are completely effective in ensuring that the patient will not 'fight' the ventilator, there are some disadvantages to their use.

(1) Relaxants do not make the patient unconscious, or even sedate him. Suitable sedatives are given so that the paralyzed patient will be comfortable and sleep most of the time but, although he cannot move and will appear unconscious, all his senses may be present. That is, he can hear, can feel pain, can see if his eyes are open and so on. Therefore, it is essential that the nurse involved should always talk to the patient whose respiration is being suppressed by relaxants, let him know that she realizes that he is conscious, tell him what she is going to do, and reassure him that he has been weakened by a drug needed to ease his breathing and that this will only be necessary for a short time. She should always try to avoid hurting the patient who looks anaesthetized but, in fact, may be wide awake. The nurse should also avoid shining bright lights directly into the patient's eyes as he may be unable to shut them. Intensive therapy units should therefore have soft, concealed lighting. All these points are very important to the patient's comfort.

(2) A very important disadvantage to the use of relaxants to control ventilation is that they leave the patient completely unable to breathe for himself and entirely dependent upon the ventilator. It is, therefore, vital that the patient should not be left alone for a moment and that, should the ventilator fail, alternative means of ventilating the lungs are available. As a last resort one can always blow into the endotracheal tube or tracheostomy.

The relaxants are not used as much as they once were to control breathing during IPPV. However, analgesics often fail to prevent patients fighting the respirator if hypoxia persists in spite of adequate ventilation as, for example, in severely damaged lungs. Administration of a relaxant drug may be the only effective means of gaining control of pulmonary ventilation in such patients.

Whatever method is used for ensuring that the patient does not 'fight' the respirator, it is essential that it is continuously effective. This means that the senior person in the unit, when he or she observes that the patient's chest is no longer rising and falling rhythmically in time with the ventilator, must be able to take immediate action. There may not be time for a doctor to arrive and drugs (even 'dangerous drugs') may have to be given intravenously via a drip injection site or three-way tap. Delay has led to many ruptured lungs, sometimes with fatal consequences. The administration of drugs into intravenous drips by qualified nurses has now become an accepted fact of life in intensive therapy units.

Tracheostomy

Tracheostomy is the construction of a 'stoma' (an opening) into the trachea through the midline of the neck. Usually the opening is made through the second and third rings of tracheal cartilage, just below the larynx. A hollow tube is inserted into the opening to prevent the tissues closing in over the stoma, and the patient breathes through this tube or, if there is a reasonably airtight fit in the trachea, the lungs may be artificially ventilated through it.

A patient with a tracheostomy should always be nursed in a special respiratory or intensive therapy unit because infection and other complications, which may be fatal, can only be avoided by skilled nursing by experienced staff.

Indications for tracheostomy
Indications for tracheostomy may be summarized as:

(1) obstruction in the upper respiratory tract,
(2) inability to cough,
(3) inability to swallow, and
(4) long-term artificial ventilation of the lungs by IPPV.

Obstruction of the upper respiratory tract Obstruction of the upper respiratory tract occurs, for example, in facial injuries, oedema or damage in the larynx, and can often be temporarily relieved by the passage of an endotracheal tube through the mouth or nose. However, long-term management of such cases may necessitate the construction of a tracheostomy. In a very small number of cases passage of an endotracheal tube may be impossible, and tracheostomy may have to be performed under local analgesia as an emergency. In the vast majority of cases the obstruction is by-passed by an endotracheal tube and then, under general anaesthesia, the tracheostomy may be performed meticulously with good aseptic technique, haemostasis and surgical accuracy.

Inability to cough Many surgical patients suffer from sputum retention because they are unable to cough up their bronchial secretions due to pain from the incision, weakness, or because the secretions are exceptionally profuse or sticky. In most cases physiotherapy or perhaps suction through an endotracheal tube may clear the airway for long enough for the patient to regain his strength but, if the patient does not improve, tracheostomy may be the only way to remove the secretions by frequent suction. The objection to leaving an endotracheal tube in place to enable secretions to be aspirated is that the patient will usually need heavy sedation to enable him to tolerate the tube, and this will depress his cough reflex and respiration still further.

Inability to swallow People who cannot swallow properly tend to aspirate food and secretions into their lungs, especially if the larynx is insensitive. This situation is more common in 'medical' than surgical patients.

Long-term ventilation of the lungs If artificial ventilation is to be maintained for only a few days, the ventilator may be connected to an endotracheal tube, which the patient will tolerate if he is well sedated (or very co-operative). Endotracheal tubes are not usually used for longer than about a week for fear of damage to the larynx, and IPPV via a tracheostomy is needed for longer periods.

Types of tracheostomy tubes

When a tracheostomy is only to maintain a clear airway, or to enable secretions to be sucked out of the bronchi, a plain tube may suffice. These are made of plastic, shaped to fit in the trachea and with a flange to attach tapes which are tied round the neck to hold the tube in position.

When an airtight fit is required in the trachea to enable IPPV to be performed or, if it is necessary to prevent secretions, blood or vomit from the pharynx reaching the lungs, a cuffed tracheostomy tube is used. There are many designs and some commonly used tracheostomy tubes are shown in *Figure 5.6*.

Complications of tracheostomy

Displacement of the tube Care must be taken to fix the tube securely and to prevent heavy equipment dragging on it. A displaced tube can be very difficult to replace as it may pass

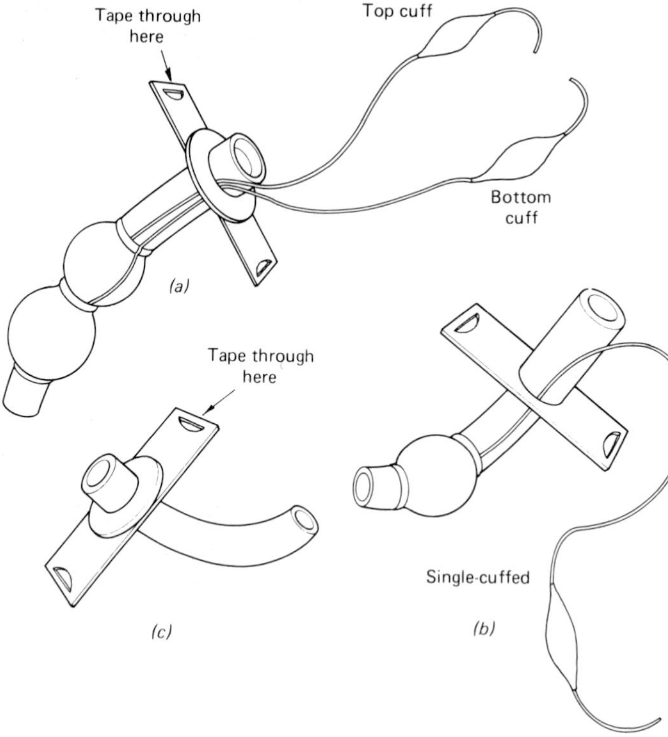

Figure 5.6. Types of tracheostomy tubes. (*a*) Double-cuffed tracheostomy tube; (*b*) single-cuffed plastic tracheostomy tube; (*c*) a non-cuffed tracheostomy tube

through the skin opening into the soft tissues of the neck instead of into the trachea. It is helpful if the lower edge of the tracheal opening is stitched to the skin to facilitate routine changing of the tube and this can be life-saving if the tube is accidentally displaced.

Blockage of the tube If there is bleeding from the lung or bronchi, the tube may be blocked by a clot. Bronchial secretions can become very thick and sticky if the patient is allowed to breathe dry air, or if he is dehydrated. They must be sucked clear or the tube may need to be changed. Occasionally a thick plug of mucus may be displaced from a bronchus and completely block the tracheostomy tube. The patient will asphyxiate unless the tube is immediately cleared or replaced.

Infection The greatest care is needed if infection of the tracheostomy, the trachea and the lungs is to be avoided. A sterile suction catheter is used to remove secretions. The catheter is inserted into the tracheostomy using sterile gloves or forceps. Any catheter which touches a non-sterile area is discarded. The nurse must wear a mask during the suction procedure and in many units all personnel wear masks and gowns routinely. Avoidance of cross infection from other patients is helped by wide separation of beds in units and, where possible, by segregation of vulnerable or particularly infectious patients.

Drying of secretions The air which we breathe is usually warmed and moistened as it passes through the nose. If air enters the lungs directly through a tracheostomy or endotracheal tube, it will dry up secretions and form crusts in the bronchi. Inspired gases must therefore be warmed and humidified for these patients. Several different types of humidifier are used for this purpose.

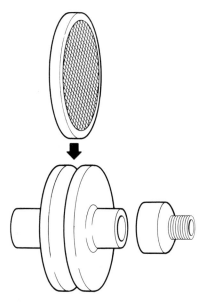

Figure 5.7. Condenser humidifier (artificial nose)

(1) The artificial nose (condenser humidifier). A short wide tube containing a replaceable metal mesh element is attached to the tracheostomy tube. Exhaled water vapour condenses on the mesh and then moistens the inspired air (*Figure 5.7*). This simple humidifier will usually prevent excessive drying but will not be enough to moisten secretions which are already sticky. It is therefore used for maintenance rather than for treatment.

(2) Heated water baths. The inspired air is passed through a container in which water is maintained at 45 to 55°C. By the time the air has passed through tubing to the tracheostomy it should be cooled to 36°C and be comfortable to breathe. A fan may blow the humidified air through the delivery tubing which is usually attached to a Gilston 'T-piece' which fits into the tracheostomy tube and directs the moist air across its open end. The temperature of the humidifier is controlled thermostatically but the nurse should check and record it frequently.

(3) Nebulizers add a fine mist to the air. They may be cold or heated. Most form the mist by directing a jet of air or oxygen past the end of a capillary tube. Water is sucked through the capillary and forms a fine spray. Ultrasonic nebulizers form the mist by dropping water on to a plate which vibrates at very high speed. Although most of these nebulizers are very efficient they may carry bacteria into the lungs on the small water particles.

Damage to the trachea The presence of a tracheostomy tube in the trachea may cause ulceration of the mucosa, scarring and narrowing of the trachea or erosion of blood vessels and haemorrhage.

These serious complications may be minimized by gentle and careful handling of the tracheostomy, and by avoiding infection.

Nursing care of tracheostomized patients

Tracheostomy is a valuable life-saving procedure and skilled nursing is a major factor in reducing complications to a minimum. As no air passes through the larynx, tracheostomy patients cannot usually talk so that nurses have to be particularly considerate and sympathetic in interpreting their needs and allaying their fears.

The operation of tracheostomy is performed with full sterile technique under general anaesthesia and should, if at all possible, be performed in a fully equipped operating theatre. When the patient returns to the unit he should be observed for excessive blood loss. The dry dressing should at first be changed as soon as it is soaked with either blood or secretions, or later, every 8 to 12 hours. Failure to keep the skin dry will lead to excoriation and infection. When changing the dressing the skin should be cleaned with 3 per cent aqueous Savlon, then after the area has been dried with sterile swabs it is sprayed with povidone-iodine powder and covered with a dry dressing.

The introduction of large low pressure ('floppy cuffs') has reduced the incidence of complications due to pressure of the cuff on the tracheal wall. The cuff should be inflated with the smallest amount of air which will produce an airtight seal in the trachea. Periodic deflation of the cuff is not now recommended. The tracheostomy tube should be changed weekly to allow more thorough cleaning of the wound, or more often if the lumen is becoming blocked by inspissated secretions, although with adequate humidification this should rarely happen.

As patients with tracheostomies cannot cough up bronchial secretions, the trachea must be sucked out frequently, or else pulmonary collapse and pneumonia will occur.

Aspiration of secretions must be a meticulously aseptic procedure, but the technique must be simple so that the standard is invariably maintained. The essentials are:

(1) The sterile suction catheter is attached to the suction tubing and the sucker is turned on, but the part of the catheter which will enter the tracheotomy is not withdrawn from its sterile wrapping. The connector between the suction tube and catheter should have a side hole so that no suction occurs until the hole is blocked by the nurse's finger.

(2) The nurse dons a mask and one sterile glove. With the ungloved hand the ventilator or humidifier is disconnected from the tracheostomy tube, then the catheter is pulled clear of its wrapping. With the gloved

hand the catheter is introduced as far into the tracheostomy as it will go. It must only touch the inside of the tracheostomy tube. It is withdrawn slightly, the side hole in the suction connector is covered with a finger on the non-sterile hand and secretions are sucked out as the catheter is fully withdrawn. The patient must be reconnected to the breathing circuit before he becomes **hypoxic**. It is wise to increase the oxygen concentration to 100 per cent for a few minutes before tracheal aspiration in patients with marginal pulmonary function.

NUTRITION IN THE ITU

Patients who are severely ill need more food than healthy patients, not less. If they do not get it they suffer from gross protein loss, increase in total body water and anaemia. This 'syndrome of depletion' is seen after major surgery and is made much worse if any **sepsis** occurs. As patients are frequently not able to eat well, they must often be nourished by other means. The only methods of practical importance are tube feeding and intravenous feeding (also called parenteral nutrition).

Tube feeding

Tube feeding is the method of choice whenever normal oral feeding is impossible or inadequate. A nourishing thick liquid diet is introduced into the stomach by a nasogastric tube. 'Meals' of about 300 to 500 ml of the mixture may be injected down the tube with a syringe in small portions of about 50 ml each. Meals should be 2 to 3 hourly. In many cases it is wise to **aspirate** the stomach before each meal. The contents of the mixture may be either 'homogenized' normal diet made in a food mixer, or various 'concoctions' designed to supply a large number of calories and nutrients in a small volume of fluid, and in well-balanced proportions, and cause minimal initiation of the intestine.

It is important to check that the tube is in the stomach before feeding. This can be done by withdrawing stomach contents, or by injecting a little air and listening for bubbling noises in the stomach with a stethoscope. The feed must be fresh and uncontaminated by bacteria. If it has been refrigerated, it should be warmed to body temperature. Careful oral hygiene is also extremely important.

Hypoxia The condition of inadequate oxygenation.

Sepsis A non-specific term for infection, usually local and with the production of pus.

Aspiration (1) Removal of fluid or air from a body cavity by needle and syringe or suction apparatus. (2) The breathing in of fluid into small air passages (leading to, for example, aspiration pneumonia).

Complications of tube feeding

Diarrhoea is a very common complication of tube feeding. It may be due to:

(1) food poisoning, i.e. contamination of the diet;
(2) intolerance to fat or sugar in the mixture. In this case the formulation should be changed or the volume reduced. 3 g/litre Celevac (methylcellulose) may be included in the mixture routinely to help prevent diarrhoea; finally
(3) broad spectrum antibiotics may cause severe diarrhoea.

Another complication of tube feeding may be ulceration of the oesophagus or larynx caused by the tube. This is less common when plastic tubes are used. It is recommended that they should be changed once a week.

These highly concentrated feeds can remove water from the tissues and dangerous fluid and electrolyte imbalance (hypertonic dehydration) may result unless consideration is given to this possibility.

Tube feeding is of course impossible if the alimentary tract is not functioning, for example in postoperative ileus. If it is expected that normal feeding will not be possible within 2 to 3 days at the most, nutrition should be maintained by the intravenous route.

Intravenous feeding

The main constituents of a normal diet may be supplied by an intravenous infusion which must contain, in the correct proportions:

(1) water;
(2) electrolytes — mainly sodium and potassium chloride;
(3) carbohydrates, proteins and fats; and
(4) vitamins.

Water and electrolyte requirements are discussed elsewhere in the book.

Carbohydrate is supplied usually as concentrated glucose or laevulose (fructose) solutions. Glucose requires insulin for its metabolism, whereas laevulose does not.

The gross protein loss from the body which occurs after major trauma, particularly if sepsis is present, causes poor healing, liability to infection, clotting defects and oedema. These ill-effects may be mitigated by ensuring an adequate supply of protein-building substances called amino acids. Proprietary solutions of amino acids are available for intravenous infusion (Aminosol, Vitrum, Trophysan).

By using soya bean emulsions (for example, Intralipid), it is now possible to give fat intravenously without causing the adverse reactions which complicated the administration of earlier preparations. Fat represents a source of concentrated energy (1 g fat provides 9 calories, whereas carbohydrate and protein each provide about 4 calories per g). It is difficult to provide enough calories intravenously without using fat, and also protein is utilized more effectively if given at the same time as fat (using a double infusion through a T-connector). Heparin 2500 units per litre is added to increase the rate of uptake of fat from the blood. In general, addition of other medication to fat emulsions should be avoided.

Multivitamin preparations are available for intravenous use and they are added daily to the infusion.

Intravenous feeding is now safe and it is possible to maintain most patients in a reasonable metabolic balance. As many of the solutions used are very irritating to veins, they are usually given through a cannula passed into the vena cavae, where the rapid flow of blood dilutes the solution and minimizes damage. The number of veins available is often very limited; it is of the utmost importance that the nurse is careful to avoid causing displacement, kinking or blocking of the cannula, or sepsis at the site of **venepuncture**. If such care is exercised, the same vein may be used for several weeks.

MONITORING

In the treatment of seriously ill patients it is often important that the attendants should know immediately that a significant change has occurred in any vital function. It is possible to attach apparatus to the patient which will give a continuous reading or pictorial display of many functions of the body. These machines will even energize warning devices if the particular function should vary outside desirable limits. They are very appropriately called monitors (Latin *moneo* — I advise, or I warn). A good and common monitor is a pulse monitor, which will give a continuous display of the pulse rate on a meter, and which may be set to buzz or flash if the pulse is faster than, for example, 100 beats per minute or slower than 60 beats per minute. The machine receives information about the pulse from a 'pick-up' which may be attached to a finger. It shines a light through the finger and as the finger fills with blood at each **systole**, less light falls on the light detector in the pick-up, and a beat is registered on the monitor. Thus, the machine not only counts the number of times per minute the finger fills with blood (that is, the heart rate) but also it indicates that the heartbeats are strong

Venepuncture Puncture of a vein to extract blood or to inject a fluid.

Systole The period during which the heart contracts.

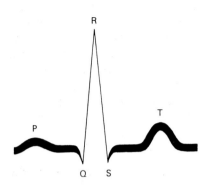

Figure 5.8. The normal components of the ECG during one heartbeat

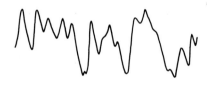

Figure 5.9. An ECG of ventricular fibrillation

Fibrillation A quivering, unco-ordinated movement of muscle, usually the heart.

enough to fill the finger with blood, that is, it is an indicator of the adequacy of peripheral perfusion. Unfortunately, movement of the finger or constriction of peripheral blood vessels make this type of pulse monitor unreliable. Pulse monitors which count the heart rate from the electrocardiograph give a more reliable indication of the heart rate, but no indication of the strength of the heartbeats.

The electrocardiogram (ECG) is frequently displayed continuously on a cardioscope. The following are the normal components of the electrocardiogram during one heartbeat (*Figure 5.8*).

(1) The P-wave — a small wave due to the spread of the electrical impulse through the atria.
(2) The QRS complex — point Q is the bottom of the first downward wave, R is the apex of the upward deflection, and S the bottom of the second downward wave. The QRS complex is due to the spread of electrical activity through the ventricles.
(3) The T-wave — normally an upward deflection of small size and rounded. It follows the QRS complex and represents recovery of the ventricle after contraction.

The normal progression of P-, QRS and T-waves may be seen continuously crossing the screen of the cardioscope. The most important abnormalities to be recognized are asystole (that is, complete cessation of the heart's action) and ventricular **fibrillation**, which is a completely ineffective rippling movement of the ventricular muscle.

Asystole shows as a flat line on the ECG and ventricular fibrillation (*Figure 5.9*) is revealed in the ECG as a completely chaotic pattern of irregular peaks and valleys changing in size, shape and frequency. Both asystole and ventricular fibrillation stop the heart pumping blood, i.e. they are causes of cardiac arrest. On seeing either of these patterns on the ECG screen the nurse should immediately feel the carotid pulse (because loose ECG electrodes can cause a similar appearance) and, if the pulse is not palpable, the cardiac arrest alarm must be raised.

Apart from these ECG indications of cardiac arrest, the nurse may recognize extra beats or more correctly 'premature beats' (PB). An occasional premature beat is of no significance but frequent ones, particularly if the beat is abnormal, may warn of impending ventricular fibrillation.

Changes in the shape of the electrocardiogram may be significant. For example, during potassium therapy an increase in the size of the T-wave (*Figure 5.10*) may be a sign that the rate of infusion is too fast. Changes in the segment between the QRS complex and the T-wave (S—T segment) may indicate

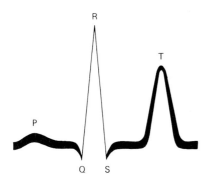

Figure 5.10. The 'tented' T-wave seen in hyperkalaemia (potassium intoxication)

damage to the heart or digoxin overdosage. However, these minutiae will be of more interest to the medical staff. The nurse will be more concerned with the presence and regularity of the electrocardiogram.

Nurses may be required to familiarize themselves with pressure transducers which provide a continuous record of the pressure with the heart or great vessels, temperature monitors, and respirator alarms and other monitors of various types. Consideration of all of these in detail is beyond the scope of this chapter but, by means of the information they afford, surgical patients may be treated with greater precision and abnormalities corrected before they become irreparable.

There are two 'golden rules' to be observed at all times when nursing patients who are being 'monitored'.

(1) When an alarm condition is indicated, never check the monitor first; always check the patient first. The alarm is to draw the nurse's attention to the patient.
(2) Monitors exist to provide staff with more information. They cannot replace the presence of an experienced nurse by the bedside.

In this chapter some aspects of nursing have been described which are particularly relevant to the care of surgical patients in an intensive therapy unit. It must not, however, be thought that general nursing care is unimportant in these very ill patients. The more traditional nursing skills are merely supplemented by modern technology; they must never be replaced. No machine yet devised can encourage a despondent patient by a smile.

REFERENCES

Feldman, S. A. and Crawley, B. E. (1977). *Tracheostomy and Artifical Ventilation in the Treatment of Respiratory Failure,* 3rd Edn. London: Edward Arnold

Clarke, D. B. and Barnes, A. D. (1975). *Intensive Care for Nurses,* 2nd Edn. London: Blackwell

Intensive Therapy Units. (1969). The Function and Staffing of Intensive Therapy Units and the Preparation of Nurses to Work in the Units. London: Royal College of Nursing and National Council of Nurses of the United Kingdom

6 The management of pain

J.E.Utting

The control of pain is one of the most important functions of medical practice, but the ability to do so is still very incomplete. The main method of combating pain remains the use of powerful analgesic drugs, such as morphine and, for more trivial pain, such drugs as aspirin. Other methods are used less often. Local analgesic solutions may be injected into the subarachnoid or epidural space or round nerve trunks or nerve endings. When pain is of great severity and of long duration, especially when associated with cancer, nerves carrying painful impulses can be deliberately damaged by such agents as phenol, or pathways in the spinal cord which are responsible for carrying pain impulses to the brain can be surgically interrupted. In some situations analgesic agents are administered by inhalation; for example, the anaesthetic agent trichloroethylene can be given in subanaesthetic concentrations in labour and during painful dressings.

Severe pain is one of the most compelling of bodily sensations, and it is impossible for the patient who feels severe pain to ignore it. Drugs are the main defence against pain but this is not to say that good general management is unimportant, for simple measures may sometimes go far to provide relief.

Pain is an abstract and subjective phenomenon and cannot be quantified, but it does seem that there is great individual variation in response to pain — as though, indeed, one man's agony may be another man's discomfort. Not infrequently a patient with an upper abdominal incision may be found to be in great distress, and another say that he is only mildly uncomfortable.

There is also great individual variation in response to pain-killing drugs. Some patients have unusually severe side-effects when a normal dose of drug is given. Morphine, for example, frequently causes nausea and vomiting; some patients vomit continually after the administration of morphine and may be said to show 'intolerance' to the drug.

GENERAL MANAGEMENT

The suffering which is associated with severe injury is not only due to pain but also to fear and anxiety. For example, the victim of a traffic accident lying in the road with a broken leg is not suffering merely because he is feeling pain, indeed he may not be feeling pain at all, but he is afraid of the pain he knows he may feel in the near future and of mutilation and death. In these circumstances a quiet air of confidence and optimism on the part of those at the scene of the accident may be of great value to the patient. It is unwise to tell a patient before an operation that he will suffer neither pain nor discomfort, because when he finds that this is not true he may think that something is amiss. Even when a patient is suffering from severe and intractable pain, as may occur in some types of cancer, general management is of great importance; indeed a sympathetic ear alone may have a therapeutic effect.

It is sometimes important that one is sure what pain one is trying to treat. In the postoperative period, for example, the primary pain may be related not to the operation site but to the patient's back. Not infrequently in these circumstances simple attention to the patient's position in bed can help alleviate pain. A full bladder, too, is a common cause of discomfort in the postoperative period and may be easily overlooked.

Two general points may be made about the use of drugs to relieve pain. First, the use of repeated small doses of drug may be more effective in relieving pain than larger doses at less frequent intervals. Secondly, it is usually easier to stop severe pain from occurring than it is to get rid of it once it has appeared.

PHARMACOLOGICAL MANAGEMENT

Powerful analgesics

Human beings have used the opium poppy (*Papaver somniferum*) since before history began. Opium, a mixture of alkaloids, is made from the seed capsules of this poppy whilst the pure alkaloid morphine (from Greek Morpheus — god of dreams) is extracted from opium. Examples of other powerful analgesic drugs are heroin (made from morphine), and pethidine and methadone, both of which are synthetic.

An important feature of these agents is their ability to produce, to a greater or lesser degree, drowsiness, tranquillity, indifference to surroundings and, in some patients, euphoria. These properties are well exemplified by morphine and can be valuable. In the postoperative period, for example, there is no need for the patient to be mentally alert and a period of tranquil somnolence will do good rather than harm. In these circumstances morphine is very valuable. In many situations, however, analgesia is required but the patient wants to be wide awake. A housewife who has an incurable carcinoma of the cervix wants pain relief but does not want sedation and hypnosis. Her main desire may be to look after the housework and her husband and children. Here some of the newer synthetic analgesics may be of greater value.

Unfortunately all the narcotic drugs have important side-effects such as addiction, respiratory depression, nausea and vomiting, and constipation. These are rightly given prominence, but it must be remembered that though it is important to know and appreciate these side-effects their existence must not be allowed to detract from the fact that the powerful analgesics are among the most valuable drugs in medical practice.

Addiction

The powerful analgesic drugs are all drugs of addiction. That is to say repeated administration can produce a state of physical and psychological dependence characterized by an overpowering desire to continue taking the drug. The dose required gradually increases, and the addict will go to any length to obtain the drug. If he is unable to do so, the withdrawal of the drug leads not only to psychological prostration but also to adverse physical effects such as convulsions.

Many drug addicts complain that their addiction was initiated by inappropriate medical treatment. In some cases this may be true, but it must be remembered that these unfortunate patients show a tendency to blame other people for their condition. The possibility of addicting a patient to narcotics must always be kept in mind when these drugs are used. It is, however, all too easy to take an unrealistic view of the dangers. Those in severe pain need the powerful analgesics, and in these circumstances the risk of addiction is small.

Respiratory depression

Extreme respiratory depression can, of course, kill the patient. But even a moderate degree of respiratory depression can lead to pulmonary complications and this is especially likely in the postoperative period. The powerful analgesics, in addition to causing respiratory depression, depress the cough reflex; morphine, for example, is very active in this respect, and heroin is the most powerful cough suppressant known. Depression of the cough reflex leads to sputum accumulation. Sputum accumulation is vitally important. If obstruction by sputum takes place in the lungs, the air distal to the obstruction will be absorbed and pulmonary collapse will follow. Sputum accumulation is likely if the cough reflex is depressed. It is because there is a greatly increased secretion of sputum in patients who smoke that they have an increased tendency to such postoperative respiratory complications as pulmonary collapse and pneumonia.

Another point of cardinal importance should be stressed here; pulmonary infections follow hypoventilation and retention of sputum as night follows day and consequently pulmonary infection leads to increased sputum production — a vicious circle which has usually to be broken with antibiotics and physiotherapy.

But all this is only one side of the coin. It is true that the administration of excessive amounts of analgesic drugs will result in postoperative respiratory depression and retention of sputum; but it is also true that inadequate analgesia can contribute to postoperative respiratory complications. This apparent paradox is explained by the fact that a patient with, for example, an upper abdominal incision who is not given an analgesic will tend to hypoventilate because it is too painful to breathe deeply, and he will also be afraid to cough. He, too, will be in danger of developing postoperative pulmonary complications.

Finally, it should be noted that morphine may cause a bronchospasm, particularly if it is administered to asthmatics. This factor combined with its tendency to produce respiratory depression makes its use particularly dangerous in bronchial asthma. If an analgesic is needed by an asthmatic, pethidine is usually the drug of choice.

Nausea, vomiting and constipation

Nausea and vomiting are both important side-effects of the administration of analgesic drugs, women being somewhat more susceptible than men. For several reasons this is a difficult problem to investigate. Thus, for example, a patient may complain of nausea one day and have completely forgotten about it the next day.

There is no doubt that nausea and vomiting are both peculiarly unpleasant. In some circumstances as, for example, after cataract extraction, vomiting can have disastrous consequences. To some extent the incidence of these complications can be reduced by combining the powerful analgesic with an **antemetic**. The proprietary preparation Cyclimorph, for example, is a mixture of morphine and cyclizine, the latter being an antemetic well known by its proprietary name as a remedy for travel sickness (Marzine). It must be remembered, however, that the addition of the antemetics adds to the depressant effect of the analgesic drug.

Constipation is another important side-effect of the analgesic drugs but is mainly of concern when long-term therapy is being considered.

Antemetic A remedy to arrest or prevent vomiting.

Individual drugs

The narcotic agents are metabolized into inactive forms in the liver. Patients with severe liver dysfunction, therefore, may be markedly sensitive to the drug. In these cases caution is obviously required.

Almost all the analgesic agents can be administered orally or parenterally (intramuscularly, subcutaneously or intravenously). In many cases the oral use of the drugs makes for considerably less consistency in action than when they are given parenterally. Morphine, for example, is not as satisfactory as an oral analgesic as is methadone.

The relative dosage of some of the analgesic drugs is given in Table 6.1. Below, a few notes on some of the salient features of the more important individual drugs are appended.

Table 6.1   Relative dosage of some of the analgesic drugs

Analgesic	Dosage, mg	Duration of effect, h
Codeine phosphate**	10–60	4–6
Dihydrocodeine (DF 118)**	60	4–5
Diamorphine (heroin)*	3	3–4
Methadone (Physeptone)*	7.5–10	3–5
Morphine*	10	3–5
Papaveretum (Omnopon)*	10–20	4–5
Pentazocine (Fortral)**	30–60	2–4
Pethidine*	50–100	2–4

*Controlled by the Misuse of Drugs Act (1971). These drugs, used orally or parenterally, are under very stringent control (Abuse of Drugs Regulations, 1973).

**Controlled by the Misuse of Drugs Act (1971). These drugs are controlled, when given by injection, under the Misuse of Drugs Regulations, (1973).

Morphine Morphine is still the most widely used of the powerful analgesic drugs and this despite the fact that over the years many drugs have been hailed as being much better, only to fall into disuse or to be used solely by a few enthusiasts. Its marked sedative and tranquillizing action makes it very useful in surgical practice, though it is a powerful drug of addiction and the incidence of nausea and vomiting is high. Its use is associated with a pin-point pupil — a useful diagnostic sign. Papaveretum (Omnopon) is a mixture of some of the opium alkaloids and contains 50 per cent morphine. It is said to cause less vomiting than morphine but there is little evidence for this. Diamorphine (heroin) is manufactured from morphine and is, therefore, described as semi-synthetic. It is the most powerful of all drugs of addiction.

Pethidine Pethidine is a synthetic drug introduced in 1939. It has less sedative, hypnotic and tranquillizing effects than has morphine and therefore is less useful if fear and apprehension are present; it is of no use as a cough suppressant. On the credit side it causes less nausea and vomiting than morphine and does not constipate. Like morphine it is a powerful respiratory depressant but it does not cause pinpoint pupil. Pethidine poisoning may be associated with signs of central nervous excitation including convulsions.

Methadone Methadone is another synthetic drug similar to morphine but with less marked tranquillizing and sedative properties. It is given as an example of a powerful analgesic which is widely used by mouth; pethidine and dextromoramide (Palfium) are others.

Dihydrocodeine Dihydrocodeine is a derivative of codeine, an opium drug (opiate) which is a poor analgesic but a good cough suppressant. Dihydrocodeine is said to be virtually non-addicting. It is a useful analgesic for minor pains and is usually given orally.

Pentazocine Pentazocine is technically an opiate antagonist like nalorphine and levallorphan (*see below*) but has marked analgesic properties. It is almost free of addicting properties and has achieved considerable popularity, being usually administered orally (it is somewhat irritant if given parenterally). Clinically, however, it is not as effective as morphine in cases of severe pain. Toxic effects include hypertension, tachycardia, respiratory depression and, occasionally, nightmare-like states and hallucination.

The analgesic antagonists

The action of the powerful analgesic drugs is opposed by certain antagonists, for example nalorphine and levallorphan. These drugs are of value in cases of poisoning by analgesics or in situations in which a slight overdose of analgesic has been given therapeutically and the patient has become more depressed than might reasonably have been expected.

Levallorphan has also been used mixed with an analgesic, the whole injection being considered to contain, as it were, its own built-in antidote. The hope is that there will be less respiratory depression than there would be if no antidote were included. The preparation Pethilorfan consists of a mixture of pethidine hydrochloride and levallorphan tartrate in the ratio of 100 mg to 1.25 mg, respectively.

These mixtures, however, have not achieved wide popularity, though Pethilorfan is still commonly used in obstetric practice.

The reason for this may be that the diminution of the respiratory depressant effect obtained by using the antidote may be associated with a diminished analgesic potency.

Non-narcotic analgesics

The non-narcotic analgesics are very useful drugs but are not suitable for the treatment of severe pain against which they are relatively ineffective. They are often, however, quite effective against postoperative pain after the first period of 48 hours.

Such drugs are numerous and the list of analgesics given below is, of course, very far from exhaustive. In addition there should be mentioned a group of drugs used for their analgesic as well as other actions in such diseases as rheumatoid arthritis; this includes indomethacin, ibuprofen and others.

Salicylates Salicylates have a mild analgesic effect, but are also very important in the treatment of acute rheumatism. The commonly used salicylate is aspirin (dose 0.3—1 g orally). Soluble aspirin containing citric acid and calcium carbonate in addition to aspirin (acetylsalicylic acid) is less of a gastric irritant, being more soluble. Until recently this was commonly combined with phenacetin in such formulations as 'APC' (aspirin, phenacetin and caffeine. It is now realized, however, that phenacetin is dangerous because it produces renal damage and it is, therefore, no longer used.

Aspirin is a constituent of many preparations besides being frequently used by itself. Thus there are preparations containing aspirin with codeine, paracetamol and several others.

Aspirin is far from being non-toxic. The symptoms and signs of poisoning are nausea and vomiting, ringing in the ears (tinnitus), deafness, headache, confusion and hyperventilation. Failure of blood clotting due to **hypoprothrombinaemia** may also occur. Aspirin itself is a powerful gastric irritant and haematemesis following its use (or following overdosage) is an important and not infrequent side-effect. Finally, urticarial rashes, itching, bronchospasm and even anaphylactic reactions may occur in people who are sensitive to the drug.

Paracetamol Paracetamol (Panadol) is an aniline derivative. It appears to be an effective minor analgesic. Overdosage (which has been seen with increasing frequency in recent years) can cause hepatic necrosis. Paracetamol is a constituent of many proprietary preparations: Sonalgin, for example, contains paracetamol with codeine and butobarbitone.

Hypoprothrombinaemia A decrease in the amount of prothrombin in the blood giving rise to a defect in clotting.

Dextropropoxyphene Dextropropoxyphene is related to amidone, but is not subject to Controlled Drugs regulations. With paracetamol it is the active component of Distalgesic. The drug has slight, though real, abuse potential and long-term consumption of large doses can cause psychosis.

Tranquillizing agents

As pain is usually associated with fear, anxiety and apprehension, drugs whose main therapeutic use is in relieving anxiety have a considerable place in the treatment of pain. Two facts, however, must be kept in mind. First, such treatment is not likely to be successful unless an analgesic is used as well as the tranquillizing agent. Secondly, the use of these drugs together can be associated with a greater degree of central nervous depression than would be found with either of them separately.

Some of the phenothiazines are used in this way and can also help the patient by their antemetic action. Chlorpromazine, for example, is used in conjunction with pethidine or morphine and will increase the efficacy of these drugs. More recently the so-called minor tranquillizing agents like diazepam (Valium) have been increasingly used.

Other drugs

Inhalational agents

Some of the anaesthetic agents can be inhaled in subanaesthetic concentrations to produce analgesia. Three agents in common use in midwifery are trichloroethylene, methoxyflurane and nitrous oxide. The first two agents will lead to stupor and unconsciousness if inhaled, even intermittently, for long periods. This is because they accumulate in the tissues of the body. Nitrous oxide, too, can rapidly give rise to unconsciousness if used in 50 per cent concentration though once administration ceases it is relatively rapidly eliminated. Self-administration is possible with all three agents and the apparatus for this may be arranged so that should unconsciousness supervene the hand drops and the mask falls away from the patient's face. Nevertheless effective supervision is required.

Preoperative and postoperative pain is usually continuous and the inhalational methods are clearly not ideal in this case, and their main use will continue to be in midwifery. Nevertheless they may be of wider value in surgical practice than is now realized in such relatively short-lived but severe pains as those associated with changing burns dressings and passing a catheter. Nitrous oxide is now sometimes used in ambulances to relieve the severe pain in road accidents and in myocardial infarction. Given continuously in concentrations as low as 20 per cent it has also been used to provide postoperative analgesia as in this concentration it does not give rise to unconsciousness. Unfortunately, however, these methods give rise to pollution and, as it is difficult to duct away the inhalate, their use is unlikely to increase.

MANAGEMENT BASED ON KNOWLEDGE OF THE NERVOUS SYSTEM

Pathways for transmission of pain

Before considering spinal and epidural analgesia and local blocks as methods of pain relief it is necessary to outline briefly the pathways by which pain is perceived (*Figures 6.1, 6.2 and 6.3*).

Pain from skin and muscle arises by stimulation of nerve endings. Impulses are carried along the axon of the nerve fibres which run in the nerve itself. For example, in the case of an upper abdominal incision the nerves supplying the area are the intercostal (thoracic) nerves (about T5–T10). Each nerve splits into motor and sensory roots before entering the spinal cord; the nerve cells of the sensory nerves are situated in the dorsal root ganglia (*Figure 6.1*). After the nervous impulses denoting pain arrive in the spinal cord other nerve cells take impulses up to the brain in the lateral and anterior spinothalamic tracts of the 'opposite' side of the body, the axons of these second neurones crossing over in the spinal cord (*Figure 6.3*). Painful impulses from the head and neck are conducted mainly in the fifth cranial nerve (trigeminal), but the seventh (facial), ninth (glossopharyngeal), tenth (vagus) and upper cervical nerves are also involved.

Painful stimuli from the viscera travel by a different path, that is by the sympathetic nervous system mainly (and to a lesser extent in the parasympathetic system). The impulses denoting pain are carried to the sympathetic chain where the fibres may travel up and down before they enter the spinal cord via the somatic nerves (*Figures 6.1 and 6.2*). Before entering the sympathetic chain some of the sympathetic fibres form networks — the plexuses. The whole arrangement is much more complicated and this is only a very simplified account.

The spinal cord, like the brain, is covered by membranes known as the meninges. The innermost layer, closely investing the spinal cord, is known as the pia mater, and the outermost as the dura mater. Applied to the inside of the dura

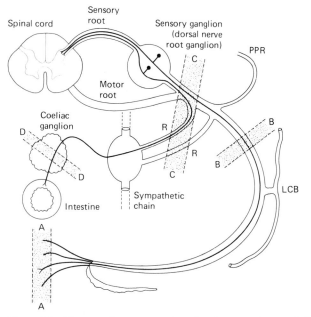

Figure 6.1. Diagramatic representation of an intercostal nerve. Pain fibres from, for example, the mesentery of the intestine travel by the coeliac ganglion through the sympathetic chain and into the intercostal nerve by a ramus communicans (R). The somatic sensory fibre ending in the midline skin incision travels in the main branch of the nerve. In both cases the nerve cells are situated in the dorsal nerve root ganglion. PPR, posterior primary ramus, a minor branch of the nerve; LCB, lateral cutaneous branch. The blocks represented by letters A, B, C and D are explained in the text. (Redrawn after Macintosh and Bryce-Smith, 1953)

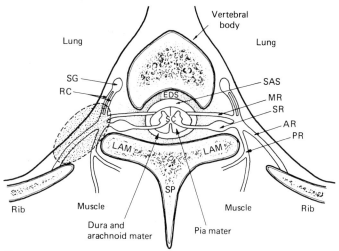

Figure 6.2. The extradural and subaracharoid spaces (EDS and SAS respectively); a detail of the transverse section in *Figure 6.1.* The approximate position of the paravertebral space is indicated by the dotted line on the left side of the diagram. The sympathetic ganglion (SG) is connected to the spinal nerve by the rami communicantes (RC). LAM, lamina of vertebrae; SP, spinous process of vertebrae; MR, motor root of nerve; SR, sensory root (with ganglion); AR, anterior ramus of nerve (the main 'intercostal' nerve); PR, posterior ramus. (Redrawn after Macintosh and Bryce-Smith, 1953)

mater is the third membrane — the arachnoid mater. The arrangement of these three membranes is shown in the diagram (*see Figure 6.2*). It is in the subarachnoid space that the cerebrospinal fluid is located.

Local analgesic agents

There are a number of local analgesic drugs. The first local analgesic was cocaine, but this is not now used except on mucous membranes; lignocaine is the local analgesic which is probably the most popular one — it is a most versatile drug and can be used as a surface analgesic on mucous membranes, for nerve block and to provide extradural and spinal analgesia.

It is all too frequently forgotten that the local analgesics are, to a greater or lesser extent, very toxic drugs and can give rise to convulsions and depression of the heart. Doubling the strength of an analgesic solution more than doubles its toxicity. The toxic dose is less in well vascularized areas than it is in relatively avascular areas as it is more rapidly absorbed from the former, which will result in a higher concentration in the blood before the drug is broken down. Conversely, if

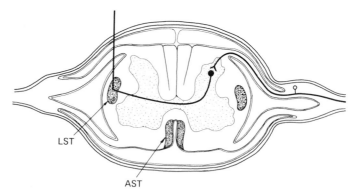

Figure 6.3. Section of spinal cord showing the anterior and lateral spinothalamic tract (AST and LST respectively). In these tracts fibres subserving the modality of pain ascend to the brain. Notice that pain fibres cross the midline before ascending. It is the anterior and lateral tracts which are interrupted in anterolateral **chordotomy**

Chordotomy Surgical division of a nerve tract or tracts of the spinal chord.

Vasoconstriction Diminution of the calibre of blood vessels associated with diminished flow of blood.

Hyaluronidase An enzyme which, by decomposing a constituent of the intercellular spaces, allows a more rapid spread of solutions through tissues.

adrenaline be added to the analgesic solution, the toxic dose is increased as absorption will be less rapid due to the **vasoconstriction**; if, on the other hand, **hyaluronidase** is added to the solution (to help it to spread through tissue planes and to widen the area of action), then the toxic dose will be smaller because absorption will be faster. The effects of local anaesthetic agents last at greatest only a few hours.

An expert can use local anaesthetic agents with great precision. He is able, for example, to insert a needle in the back of a patient and through it inject local analgesic solutions into such apparently inaccessible structures as the coeliac plexus. Some of these techniques will be described in barest outline below. There are many complications of these blocks (sepsis or haemorrhage) which are not described here.

Nerve blocks

Nerve endings

Painful impulses can be blocked by infiltrating local analgesic solution round nerve endings (for example position A — *Figure 6.1*), a technique frequently used in operations under local analgesia (infiltrating the line of incision). It is also used in some forms of intractable pain, though as the local analgesic agents only last for a short time it is surprising that this should be so. Solutions of long-acting local analgesic used to be employed in the treatment of postoperative pain, particularly proctological, oily solutions being frequently used for this purpose. Unfortunately these methods were found to be unsatisfactory because, for example, sloughing of tissues sometimes occurred.

Infiltration of local analgesic into the wound is also used from time to time.

Nerve trunks

Nerve blocks are used to provide analgesia in surgical operations, occasionally for postoperative pain relief and in intractable pain. The local analgesic solution is deposited round the nerve (position B in *Figure 6.1*). Blocking the intercostal and abdominal nerves in this way can be used to provide pain relief for abdominal operations though the sympathetic nerves are not blocked and visceral pain will be unaffected. Blocking intercostal nerves has also been used to provide postoperative analgesia, but the procedure is difficult because several blocks are required and several injections will be needed in the postoperative period. Nevertheless intercostal block is popular in the USA and there is some indication that its use is increasing in the UK. Some believe that even blocking of several intercostal nerves on only one occasion provides useful pain relief.

Another type of block, paravertebral block (position C in *Figure 6.1*), blocks the sympathetic fibres as local analgesic solution diffuses through the space round the vertebra — the paravertebral space — and comes into contact with the rami communicantes which connect the sympathetic chain to the somatic nerve. This procedure, too, has been used in the postoperative period as well as for operation, but is a tedious method.

There are, of course, many other individual nerve blocks available for other somatic nerves, such as the trigeminal nerve or some of its branches in the head, the cervical plexus, and so on. Methods also exist for blocking part of the sympathetic nervous system, coeliac plexus block (position D in *Figure 6.1*) and stellate ganglion block are examples.

Spinal analgesia

Two other methods of pain relief using local analgesic drugs require mention — spinal and epidural analgesia. Both can be used to provide pain relief for surgical operations with the patient conscious (though a light general anaesthetic may be given as well), both are used in the treatment of intractable pain and, in addition, epidural analgesia can be used to provide postoperative analgesia.

In spinal analgesia the local analgesic solution is placed in the cerebrospinal fluid in the subarachnoid space after a lumbar puncture has been performed (*Figure 6.2*). The sensory nerves are blocked as they leave the spinal cord and there is a degree of motor block present as well, though motor nerves are more resistant to the action of local analgesic drugs than are sensory nerves. The sympathetic nerves, on the other hand, are the most sensitive of all to a block by local analgesic drugs. The sympathetic motor fibres, supplying the blood vessels, are partly responsible for the maintenance of blood pressure as they cause vasoconstriction. When this vasoconstriction is abolished there is a tendency for blood pressure to fall. Hypotension is thus a side-effect of spinal analgesia.

Spinal analgesia as a method of providing pain relief for surgical operations is not popular in this country because permanent neurological damage may occur, though this is very uncommon.

Epidural analgesia

In epidural analgesia the local analgesic solution is deposited in the space outside the dura mater, the extradural (epidural, peridural) space (*Figure 6.2*). This space is sometimes approached from below through the sacral **hiatus** (a caudal epidural). Exactly how this epidural injection of analgesic solution causes analgesia is not known for certain. Possibly the local analgesic drug may diffuse across the dura into the cerebrospinal fluid and thus cause a subarachnoid block, or alternatively the solution may spread out into the paravertebral space and affect the nerves there.

Hiatus A gap or opening in a structure (especially of the diaphragm where penetrated by the aorta, inferior vena cava and the oesophagus).

A much larger dose of analgesic drug is required for epidural than for spinal block, and the risk of toxic reaction is, therefore, somewhat greater. The injection is made using a special needle, and the lumbar region is usually chosen for the block, but an epidural injection can even be made in the neck. As with spinal analgesia, a fall in blood pressure will take place with an extensive epidural block though this fall is less than in the case of spinal analgesia. Loss of consciousness, hypotension and failure of respiration will also occur if the relatively large amount of analgesic solution used in epidural analgesia is injected accidentally into the subarachnoid space (total spinal analgesia). This situation requires treatment with artificial ventilation of the lungs and with drugs which will raise the blood pressure. On the other hand, permanent neurological sequelae are rare after epidural block.

Epidural analgesia is more difficult to establish than is spinal because it is more difficult to find the epidural space. The pressure in the epidural space is below that of the atmosphere, and there are various techniques for localizing the space which depend on that fact. For example, if a drop of fluid is left hanging in the needle as it is advanced, it should be sucked into the needle when the space is reached.

The duration of pain relief after a single epidural injection is relatively brief, but an advantage of epidural analgesia is that it can be made into a long-lasting method by inserting a polythene cannula into the epidural space. Through this small doses of local analgesic solution can be given as required and the cannula can be left in for many hours.

Unfortunately, continuous epidural analgesia is not without risks and is very consuming of time and of skilled personnel; for this reason it is not as popular as it might otherwise be.

PREOPERATIVE PAIN

The problem of premedication is dealt with in Chapter 2. Here only the problem of pain before operation will be dealt with.

The useful function of pain is that it draws attention to the diseases or injured part of the body and facilitates diagnosis. The administration of an analgesic to a patient in pain before a diagnosis has been made may make it more difficult to tell what is wrong. For example, it may be unwise to administer morphine to a patient with acute abdominal pain before the surgeon has had an opportunity of seeing the patient. However, once the diagnosis has been made there is usually no reason why an analgesic should not be administered preoperatively to a patient in severe pain.

The route of administration in these circumstances may sometimes be important. Analgesic drugs are usually given subcutaneously or intramuscularly as premedication. If, however, the patient is severely shocked, as after a bad road traffic accident, then there will be a considerable degree of peripheral vascular shutdown, and because the circulation in the skin and muscle is impaired, the drug will not be absorbed. In these circumstances a larger amount of a drug is sometimes given because previous doses have been ineffective, but when resuscitation with adequate blood replacement has taken place and perhaps after anaesthesia has been induced all the drug is absorbed and the patient's vital functions can become severely depressed.

POSTOPERATIVE PAIN

The agents used in general anaesthesia are probably all analgesics and, as they are not got rid of immediately, they provide a source of analgesia in the immediate postoperative period. Until relatively recent years deep anaesthesia was the rule for surgical operations. After 2 hours of deep anaesthesia induced with an agent such as ether, the patient was asleep in the ward for some time and had a good degree of analgesia when he woke up. With the advent of light anaesthesia combined with the use of muscle relaxants and with the increased use of halothane (which is a poor analgesic agent) patients are more likely to need analgesic drugs immediately after their return to the ward from the operating theatre.

Drugs

Postoperative pain is probably most severe in association with upper abdominal and thoracic incisions; it is less severe in operations on the limbs and head and neck. Pain in the postoperative period consists of a dull, constant ache but a sharp pain is produced by moving or by coughing. Powerful analgesics are effective with the former but they do not remove completely the exacerbations felt on coughing and moving. Nevertheless, the powerful analgesic drugs still remain the mainstays of attack against postoperative pain, and of these morphine and pethidine are the most widely used. As has been mentioned these may be combined with other drugs such as the phenothiazines. Increasing the dose of drug does not necessarily increase the analgesia provided. After 48 hours have passed since operation the need for powerful analgesics usually disappears and simpler remedies like dihydrocodeine, and even aspirin can be used instead.

Drug therapy of severe postoperative pain is usually inadequate. This is partly because of deficiencies in the drugs used but is also partly due to failure of general management. In the immediate postoperative period, for example, patients often only receive a small fraction of the powerful analgesic drugs which have been prescribed for them, and this despite the fact that they will say later that the pain was indescribably severe.

There are many reasons for this unfortunate state of affairs. Pain does not directly kill the patient and there is, therefore, a temptation for nursing staff to give a low priority to the administration of the analgesic drugs. Patients, too, are often reticent about asking for pain relief (thinking that they may be regarded as cowardly or addicted). Nursing staff often do not observe patients for the signs of pain, – the screwed up face, irregular respiration, characteristic phonation and muscular rigidity.

There is, of course, a need for nursing staff to watch carefully for side-effects of drugs: deep unconsciousness, decreased frequency of respiration, hypotension, etc. Unfortunately, though, the impression is not infrequently given that side-effects (such, for example, as respiratory depression and hypotension) are so common as to make it dangerous ever to give a powerful analgesic drug. This attitude, too, is unhelpful.

Other techniques

The use of local techniques such as intercostal and paravertebral block is effective but time consuming, as is epidural analgesia which has been mentioned above. They are more widely used in the USA and a good case can be made for extending their use in the UK as well.

Inhalational techniques are unlikely to assume greater importance as there is now a greater consciousness of the dangers of pollution.

INTRACTABLE PAIN

Intractable pain can be defined as pain which is not easily managed by medical or surgical treatment. Pain of this sort is best dealt with by someone who has a special interest in the subject, and pain clinics to which patients with intractable pain can be referred can contribute a great deal. Nevertheless treatment is unsatisfactory.

The most common, but by no means the only, cause of intractable pain, is cancer, and because it is the commonest it will be dealt with first and other forms of intractable pain will be briefly mentioned later.

Cancer pain

Intractable pain due to cancer is most commonly associated with pelvic growths, with carcinomata of the lung and colon, and with various types of new growths in the head and neck. There are several mechanisms by which cancer may cause pain; for example a nerve may be infiltrated or compressed by growth, primary or secondary, or a hollow organ (such as the bladder) may be obstructed and pain result from this.

It is very important to know if a pain is due to cancer because treatment is affected by the diagnosis, and diagnosis can sometimes be very difficult. If pain is due to incurable cancer, there will be little fear of causing drug addiction since the duration of the patient's life will be limited, nor will the physician be as afraid of nerve injury as he would be if the pain were not due to cancer.

Cancer pain has several characteristics which may be important in diagnosis. The pain is frequently described as aching or boring, it wakens the patient up at night, and frequently there are severe attacks of it; indeed there are often no periods of complete relief though analgesic drugs usually help. The site of cancer pain is typically constant but it gradually spreads and increases in severity as the weeks pass. When severe the pain becomes the most important feature of the patient's life, not infrequently to the detriment of his personal appearance and his relationship with his friends and family.

Drugs

Nerve blocks and chordotomy sometimes provide complete relief but often these methods cannot be used; even when they can be used relief is often only partial and analgesic drugs have to be used to supplement the effects of the procedure.

The mild analgesics such as aspirin may be surprisingly effective in the treatment of cancer pain and may be particularly helpful if used in conjunction with the powerful narcotic drugs; they are, of course, all administered orally. All too often it is forgotten that the powerful analgesics can also be given orally, and there is a tendency to turn too early to parenteral drugs when oral drugs would still be adequate.

Not infrequently when dealing with intractable pain it is found that a patient may find one drug virtually useless and another, closely related, will give considerable relief.

The antemetics have frequently to be combined with the powerful analgesics as nausea and vomiting may be the crippling features of treatment. The tranquillizing drugs and sedatives, too, can play a useful part; not only may they make life more acceptable to the patient but they also tend to slow down the development of tolerance to the analgesic drugs.

Subarachnoid block

The basic idea behind the use of subarachnoid block in the treatment of intractable pain due to cancer is to injure the posterior (sensory) nerve roots by injecting toxic substances (alcohol or phenol) into the subarachnoid space. It is usually possible to avoid affecting the motor nerve roots. Quite clearly this is a manoeuvre which is far from being devoid of risk and the patient must be gently made aware of the possibilities before treatment is commenced. Some degree of loss of sensation is usual, but urinary and faecal incontinence and a degree of motor **paresis** are also far from rare. It might be noted that the blocks have often to be repeated.

Epidural block is also used for the treatment of intractable pain but it does not seem to be popular, at least not in the United Kingdom.

Anterolateral chordotomy

Anterolateral chordotomy consists of the destruction of the fibres carrying painful stimuli as they ascend in the spinal cord (*Figure 6.3*); it must be remembered that these fibres are crossed, and come from the opposite side of the body. Anterolateral chordotomy can be carried out as an operative procedure, but recently methods have been developed for accomplishing the same effect without a formal operation when probes are inserted under radiographic control. This percutaneous chordotomy has, it is claimed, the virtue of being more suitable for very ill patients.

Nerve blocks

Blocking of nerves is another method of importance in the treatment of intractable pain and again alcohol or aqueous injections of phenol are used. The intercostal nerves may be blocked in some cases of carcinoma of the lung and the superior laryngeal nerves in carcinoma of the larynx. Sympathetic nerve block is also sometimes performed. Thus the coeliac plexus in the upper abdomen can be blocked using alcohol in patients with carcinoma of the pancreas, liver or gall bladder.

Paresis Incomplete paralysis.

Radiotherapy

The use of radiotherapy for the management of pain is dealt with in Chapter 10.

Other forms of intractable pain

It would be quite wrong to give the impression that intractable pain is only associated with cancer. In pain clinics a wide variety of patients will be found: patients with the so-called 'phantom limb' syndrome after amputation, patients with vascular disease of the lower limb, patients with **postherpetic neuralgia** and many more.

Treatment of these unfortunate people is often difficult and unsatisfactory, and the physician is frequently (though not always) compelled to avoid using methods which would be acceptable in cancer pain, but which might cause sequelae unacceptable to those who have not got malignant disease.

REFERENCE

Postherpetic neuralgia A painful condition occurring after an attack of herpes zoster (shingles).

Macintosh, R. and Bryce-Smith, R. (1953). *Local Analgesia: Abdominal Surgery*. London, Edinburgh: E. and S. Livingstone

7 Congenital defects

N. V. Freeman

The diagnosis of congenital abnormalities may be delayed; 43 per cent are found at birth and 80 per cent by the first 6 months of life and therefore the surgery of congenital malformations is not confined to the neonatal age group.

The incidence varies in different parts of the world, but about 2 per cent of all infants born have congenital malformations, many of which are lethal if left untreated. The incidence of the various anomalies in Liverpool is summarized in Table 7.1. A similar incidence was seen in

Table 7.1 The incidence of congenital abnormalities (Liverpool and Bootle population survey 1960–66)

Malformation	Incidence, per 1000 total births
Congenital heart disease	6.3
Total CNS malformations	6.98
Spina bifida	3.35
Total cleft lip and palate	1.57
Total genito-urinary defects	2.73
Total skeletal defects	8.15
Total alimentary defects	1.78
Total defects	31.84

England and Wales from 1969–1976 (Registrar General Statistics).

Each year, as the infant and perinatal mortality decreases, the numbers of babies surviving with congenital abnormalities increases (*see Figure 7.1*). The care of these babies is best undertaken in a neonatal surgical unit by a team of nurses, anaesthetists, paediatricians and paediatric surgeons who, together with the paramedical staff, specialize in this field.

AETIOLOGY AND GENERAL CONSIDERATIONS

Cause of congenital abnormalities

Research and epidemiological evidence suggests that a large proportion of common anomalies i.e. (anencephalus, spina bifida and cleft lip and palate) may be the result of

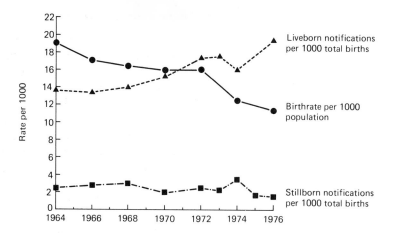

Figure 7.1. Notifications of congenital abnormalities in England and Wales. Abstract of statistics 1977

environmental factors acting on genetically vulnerable individuals.

Every cell in the body contains a nucleus which contains 46 chromosomes (23 pairs). The genetic code of the cell is contained in the double 'helix' DNA molecule which, in combination with nucleoprotein, forms the chromosome. The gametes (sperm or ovum) undergo a reduction during division (meiosis) and contain 23 chromosomes. When conception occurs the zygote is formed, containing 22 pairs (autosomes) and one pair of sex chromosomes either XX (female) or XY (male).

Chromosome anomalies

During division of the gametes extra chromosome material either from unequal division (non disjunction) or translocation may be transmitted to the daughter cells. This results in autosomal trisomy, such as mongolism — Trisomy 21 (incidence 1.45–1.8 per 1000 births). Maternal age is an important factor, the frequency of mongolism (Down's syndrome) rising rapidly between 30 and 44 years of age.

Sex chromosome

Lymphoedema Retention of fluid in the tissues because of lymphatic malfunction.

Sex chromosome anomalies are more common, about 1 in 500 of the population having a sex chromosome defect. Loss of a whole autosome is incompatible with life, and absence of a small fragment is associated with severe mental retardation and physical malformation. Loss of a complete X or Y chromosome may lead to nothing more than severe sexual failure or dwarfism. The Turner's syndrome (XO) may be seen in early life because of troublesome **lymphoedema** of the legs.

Single gene abnormalities

The different patterns of Mendelian inheritance are, autosomal dominant, autosomal recessive and sex-linked recessive disorders. The autosomal dominant is rare and not likely to be seen by the paediatric surgeon. Autosomal recessive disorders, such as fibrocystic disease of the pancreas, adrenogenital and testicular feminization syndrome, occur when the gene for this disorder is located on an autosome, and is expressed when present in the homozygous state. The risk for each conception is 25 per cent (1 in 4). Chromosome abnormalities occur in 1 in 200 live born babies and in 36 per cent of spontaneous abortions.

Babies weighing less than 2500 g at birth have a higher incidence of malformations, often multiple. Hydramnios during pregnancy is associated with a higher incidence of abnormalities, often of the gastrointestinal tract.

Other agents responsible for congenital defects are:

(1) Infection — most maternal infections apparently have no effect on the fetus, but the following protozoal, bacterial or viral infections cause significant birth defects (Table 7.2).

Table 7.2

Protozoal	Bacterial	Viral
Toxoplasmosis	Syphilis	Rubella
(Malaria)	Listerosis	Cytomegalic
	E. coli	Variola-vaccinia
	Proteus	Herpes simplex
	Klebsiella	Varicella-Zoster
	Streptococci	Hepatitis B
	Staphylococci	Poliomyelitis
	Streptococcus faecalis	Influenza
	Mycoplasma	Mumps
		Coxsackie B Echo

It is estimated that the risk for an affected birth is 50 per cent if the illness occurs in the first month, and decreases to 20 per cent in the 2nd month and to 7—8 per cent in the third month.

(2) Drugs — any drug is potentially harmful during the first 3 months of pregnancy and this includes alcohol and tobacco, antihistamines, antibiotics, thalidomide, anti-

convulsants and cytotoxic agents and endocrine preparations, especially hormone pregnancy tests, have been known to have harmful effects.

(3) X-rays — x-rays in early pregnancy can cause congenital abnormalities, hence the '10 Day Rule' in x-ray departments. No female from 12 to 50 years of age should have an abdominal or pelvic x-ray until 10 days after the first day of the last menstrual period.

(4) Mechanical factors — abnormal pressures exerted on the developing fetus *in utero* may be responsible for such anomalies as **talipes** and 'pressure dimples';

(5) Intrauterine vascular accidents — a **volvulus** or intussusception to the developing gut are responsible for **atresia** and **stenosis** of the bowel. The mechanism is shown in *Figure 7.2.*

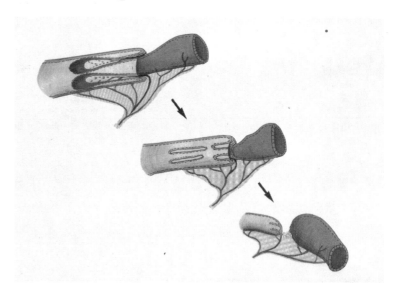

Figure 7.2. Diagram showing possible causes of intestinal atresia (From *Embryology for Surgeons* by S. W. Gray and J. E. Skandalakis, published by W. B. Saunders & Co. Reproduced with permission of Authors and Publishers)

Talipes Club foot.

Volvulus Twisting of a part of the gut.

Atresia Failure of development, for example, of an organ.

Stenosis Narrowing.

Hydrocephalus An abnormal increase of cerebrospinal fluid within the skull.

(6) Mother's health during pregnancy — abnormalities are seen with vitamin deficient diets and with folic acid deficiency during pregnancy. Women working in such places as operating theatres with poor venting of anaesthetic waste gases are shown to have a higher risk of infertility, spontaneous abortions and birth of infants with congenital malformations.

Geographical differences are seen. Anencephalus and spina bifida are 40 times more common in Belfast than in Ljubljana in Yugoslavia.

Ethnic differences are noted, for example, in the relative incidence of **hydrocephalus** and spina bifida in the white and negro population of New York.

Embryology

Once the fertilized egg has been implanted on the uterine mucosa, the period of embryonic development starts, extending to the eighth week after fertilization. This is the period in which all differentiation of the fetal organs takes place. By the end of the second week after conception the fetus consists of an embryonic disc comprising **endo-** and **ectoderm**; a primitive streak appears and the formation of the intra-embryonic **mesoderm** starts. During the third week the neural groove is formed and the cardiogenic plate appears. After this, development takes place very rapidly and simultaneously in many organs. Around the eighth to tenth week after

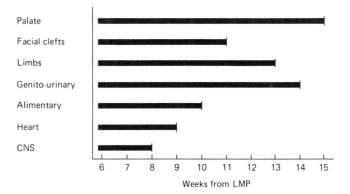

Figure 7.3. Critical periods of fetal development

conception the most important differentiation in the fetal organs is terminated, signifying the end of the embryonic period. The continued development is above all characterized by further growth and differentiation of tissue. During this period the fetus is relatively insensitive to influences so that actual malformations rarely occur (*Figure 7.3*), apart from the late intrauterine vascular accidents which are responsible for many of the intestinal atresias seen.

Prenatal diagnosis

Rapid advances are being made in the prenatal diagnosis of congenital abnormalities. Therapeutic abortion is being offered at about 18 to 20 weeks of pregnancy when an affected fetus is discovered.

Screening programmes for raised alpha feto protein in the maternal serum, followed by **amniocentesis** to confirm the raised level, and abortion if necessary are now available.

Via amniocentesis, fetal cells can be obtained and cultured. The sex of the child, chromosome abnormalities and many inborn errors of metabolism can be diagnosed by this technique.

Endoderm (entoderm) The innermost of the three germinal layers in the embryo; gives rise to the lining of the respiratory and alimentary systems.

Ectoderm The outermost of the three germinal layers in the embryo, from which is derived the skin and its related structures and the nervous system.

Mesoderm The middle germinal layer of the embryo, the origin of connective tissue and the locomotor and genito-urinary systems.

Amniocentesis Puncture of the amniotic sac, which contains the fetus, to remove amniotic fluid.

The ultrasound scan is totally non-invasive. The size of the baby, multiple pregnancies and various external anomalies, such as **anencephaly**, **spina bifida** and **exomphalos** can be visualized by this means (*see* Chapter 33).

Plain radiography in late pregnancy or enhanced with the injection of water-soluble contrast in the 2nd and 3rd trimester (amniography), may outline many congenital anomalies.

Recently the development of **fibre-optic endoscopy** (fetoscopy) has been used to view the fetus either via the cervix or through the uterus.

SOME DIFFERENCES BETWEEN PAEDIATRIC AND ADULT SURGERY

The newborn infant cannot be considered as a 'miniature adult'. Rapid and dramatic alterations occur in his circulatory and respiratory systems at birth which allow him to adapt from his intrauterine to his extrauterine existence.

Not only are the surgical conditions which are seen and treated unique in this age group, as will be discussed later, but there are fundamental differences in respiratory function, cardiovascular function, metabolism, fluid and electrolyte regulation and immune response.

Table 7.3 **Differences in respiratory function between the neonate and adult**

	Neonate	*Adult*
Respiratory centre	Immature	Mature
Trachea	6 mm	20 mm
Vital capacity	140 ml	1500 ml
Breathing	Diaphragmatic	Both
Surfactant	Lack	Present
O_2 toxicity	Eyes, lungs	Lungs

Anencephalic Characterized by having no brain.

Spina bifida A congenital failure of fusion of the lamina of the vertebra. Usually several vertebrae are affected. There may be nerve damage and thus serious interference with bladder function, locomotion, etc.

Exomphalos A condition in which part of the abdominal viscera protrudes into the umbilical cord.

Fibre-optic endoscopy Endoscopy is a general term for internal inspection of a part of the body with an instrument; fibre optic means that light, usually for illumination as well as to carry the image, is conducted by numerous very fine glass fibres.

The fundamental changes in the cardiovascular system which will occur following birth from a placental to neonatal circulation are dependent on the establishment of an adequate pulmonary expansion. Some of the differences are shown in Tables 7.3 and 7.4.

Not many people appreciate that a baby weighing 3 kg has a total blood volume of something in the order of 250 ml. Blood loss in the order of 30 to 40 ml would probably cause severe shock in such a child. Therefore, in every operation blood loss is monitored very carefully from an early stage. There are two main methods of measuring blood loss, either by weighing swabs or by a colorimetric method measuring the haemoglobin extracted from the swabs.

Table 7.4   **Differences in cardiovascular function between the neonate and adult**

	Neonate	*Adult*
Blood volume/kg body wt	108 ml (premature) 85 ml (full-term)	70 ml
Haematocrit	50–70%	30–40%
Shunting of venous blood	Ductus arteriosus Ductus venosus Foramen ovale	Mature

Frequent **apnoeic** attacks — the exact mechanism of these attacks being uncertain — easy blockage of the small diameter trachea and bronchi and the fact that the respiration is primarily diaphragmatic are major problems. Conditions such as exomphalos, which necessitate the return to a small abdominal cavity of grossly distended or thickened gut, cause subsequent embarrassment of the breathing by pushing up the diaphragms. This problem can now be overcome by positive pressure ventilation or by increasing the size of the abdominal cavity by sewing in a Silastic patch to the abdominal wall.

Table 7.5   **Differences in renal function between the neonate and adult**

	Neonate	*Adult*
GFR	2/3	3/3
Excretion of water load in 4 hours	50%	100%
Sodium load	Retention	Excretion
Concentration ability (urine water/kg urine)	600 m Osm	1200 m Osm

The renal function differs from an adult (*see* Table 7.5) by a reduced glomerular filtration rate, inability to excrete a water or a sodium load and relatively poor concentrating ability.

The composition of the body water not only differs quantitatively from the adult but there is a distribution difference in the various compartments and one of the major factors of great importance in managing these babies is to

Apnoea Temporary cessation of breathing.

FLUID REGULATION

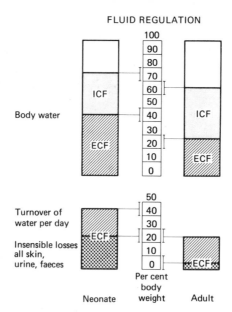

Figure 7.4. Diagram comparing relative composition of body water between neonate and adult, and showing relative daily turnover

note that something like 50 per cent of the extracellular water is turned over each day compared to 10 per cent turn-over in the adult (*Figure 7.4*). This has serious implications when managing these small infants with problems such as vomiting and diarrhoea in that they are able to deplete their body fluid very much more rapidly than an adult.

Table 7.6   Daily intravenous fluid requirements of a neonate

Neonatal		Children and adults
Day 1 — 10 ml 2 — 20 ml 4 — 40 ml 6 — 60 ml 8 — 80 ml 10 — 100 ml	per kg body weight	100 ml per kg body weight for the first 10 kg 50 ml per kg body weight for the next 10 kg then 20 ml per kg body weight

The average fluid requirements of the baby are shown in Table 7.6. It will be seen that a baby weighing 3 kg at birth will require something in the order of 2 ml per hour of intravenous fluid for maintenance. For these slow infusion rates the use of an infusion pump (such as the Ivac 501) and a giving set with a graduated burette chamber is essential.

The baby has special metabolic problems one of which is hypoglycaemia. Detection of hypoglycaemia, using a Dextrostix on a heel prick every 4 hours from birth, is standard practice and if present should be corrected by intravenous glucose infusions.

Thermal control of the infant's temperature may be difficult. This is due to a large surface area, minimal sub-cutaneous fat, inability to shiver and to use muscle energy. With cold there is a decrease of carbon dioxide in the extra-cellular fluid causing acidosis (*Figure 7.5*).

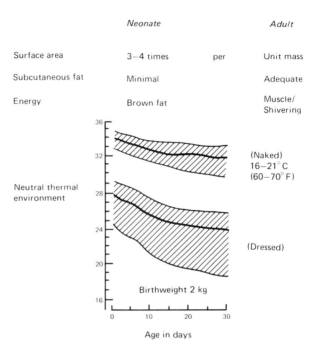

	Neonate		Adult
Surface area	3—4 times	per	Unit mass
Subcutaneous fat	Minimal		Adequate
Energy	Brown fat		Muscle/ Shivering

(Naked)
16—21°C
(60—70°F)

(Dressed)

Birthweight 2 kg

Neutral thermal environment

Age in days

Figure 7.5. Differences in thermal control between a neonate and adult

Table 7.7   **Drugs to be used with caution in neonates**

Unusual drug reactions

Caution: Vitamin K
            Chloromycetin
            Tetracycline
            Muscle relaxants — curare
            Atropine
            Morphine

The baby should be nursed in an incubator or infra-red heater to facilitate monitoring and handling of drainage tubes, infusions, etc. The infant should be nursed in 'an optimum thermal environment'. Within this temperature range the baby can be expected to maintain a normal body temperature without increasing heat production or evaporative water loss by more than 25 per cent. There is evidence that oxygen consumption is at a minimum when the skin (rather than the core temperature) is between 36 and 37°C (*Figure 7.5*).

Certain drugs have unusual reactions in neonates and should be used with caution (Table 7.7).

Furthermore the newborn is at special risk with infection due to low immunoglobulins, poor phagocytosis and the difficulty in establishing a diagnosis.

Hypoglycaemia The blood sugar can be measured simply by the Dextrostix method (Ames) on a drop of blood obtained from a heel prick. The acute symptoms of hypoglycaemia are apnoea, cyanosis, limpness, twitching and convulsions, and the long-term effects of untreated or undiagnosed hypoglycaemia may be permanent brain damage and subsequent low intelligence. Hypoglycaemia is prevented by early feeding or by giving intravenous glucose solutions. All babies should be tested at birth, and this repeated regularly if the blood sugar is low.

NEONATAL HYPOCALCAEMIA

Neonatal hypocalcaemia is a common cause of clonic convulsions in the first two weeks, in mature full time infants. Convulsing neonates have been traditionally treated with calcium supplements (10 ml of 10 per cent calcium gluconate with each feed) or phenobarbitone (7.5 mg 6-hourly orally). Magnesium sulphate (0.2 ml of 50 per cent solution, intramuscularly on 2 occasions at 12-hourly intervals) was found to be more effective, because of the essential role of magnesium in neonatal calcium metabolism.

General care

Transport

As neonatal surgical units are few in number these sick infants will need to be moved to a suitable centre soon after birth. Vomiting and inhalation of vomitus is a major hazard during transportation. This can be prevented by nursing the baby flat on its side, by passing a No. 6 or 8 French gauge nasogastric tube, and keeping the stomach empty by frequent aspirations. Heat loss from the baby must be prevented at all costs. This is ideally achieved by the use of a portable incubator, or by wrapping the baby in plastic or aluminium foil, using a **bassinet** or carry-cot, supplemented by hot-water bottles.

Bassinet A type of cradle for babies.

The incubator

In nursing babies with congenital malformations requiring surgery, it is an advantage to have the baby naked so that the whole body can be seen at a glance. This allows easy supervision of intravenous drips, nasogastric, thoracotomy and gastrostomy tubes, and routine observations on the colour of the baby, the respiration, passage of urine and faeces. The objective of the incubator is to provide warmth, a sterile environment, high humidity, and an oxygen-rich atmosphere. Most modern incubators fulfil these criteria. The temperature of the incubator can be regulated by means of a built-in thermostat, or controlled by means of a servoregulator triggered by a probe on the baby's skin or in the rectum. The temperature in the incubator ranges from 30°C to 33°C (85°F–90°F) and should be adjusted according to the baby's maturity. The humidifier in the incubator may sometimes have to be augmented by the use of an ultrasonic nebulizer. Caution must be observed when using an ultrasonic nebulizer in babies with endotracheal tubes or tracheostomies, as a dangerous amount of water can be absorbed by the lungs. A clean environment is maintained as long as the portholes and doors are shut and the filters are changed regularly. Contamination and cross infection readily occur by inadequate cleaning and sterilizing of the incubators, and by infected hands and gowns of the medical and nursing staff who ignore the basic principles of barrier nursing on handling these babies. The danger of causing retrolental fibroplasia, (a condition in which opacification behind the lens causes blindness) when nursing premature babies in an oxygen-enriched atmosphere (more than 30 per cent) must not be forgotten. Checks should be made using an oxygen analyser.

The room in which the incubator stands must be kept at a constant temperature of 25°C to 27°C to prevent heat loss on opening the doors of the incubator, or heat loss by radiation from the wall of the incubator and from the baby's body. The baby should be moved to a clean sterilized incubator every third day.

General nursing care

The nurse looking after surgical neonates should have experience in handling and feeding premature babies, as a large proportion of these babies with congenital anomalies weigh less than 2500 g. She must also be able to recognize immediately the signs of a sick baby. A slight change in the colour, appearance or activity of the baby, or a subnormal temperature, may be the only clue to a serious infection or septicaemia.

Vomiting or aspiration of vomitus is perhaps the most common cause of death in neonates. Prevention is achieved by means of a nasogastric tube left on open drainage with hourly aspirations. The position of the tube must be repeatedly checked by testing for acid secretion or by listening to the epigastrium with a stethoscope when 5 cc of air is injected down the tube. If the baby does vomit and aspirate, the air passages must be sucked out immediately. For this purpose an emergency trolley containing laryngoscopes, sterile endotracheal tubes of various sizes, syringes, drugs, oxygen and a high pressure suction machine must always be ready for resuscitation. The neonatal nurse should be able to perform closed cardiac massage, and it can be life-saving if she is familiar with the technique of intubation. The nurse is also responsible for aspiration of the pharynx when the secretions are thick and sticky. A careful sterile technique must be used each time. The pharynx must not be aspirated for too long using strong suction as this may collapse the lungs.

Gentle physiotherapy is administered frequently by the nurse using an electric vibrator rather than her fingers or hands to help loosen the tenacious secretions in the small bronchi.

Monitoring

The neonatal nurse is today faced with increasing complexity in the equipment used for monitoring. This is similar in all intensive care units (*see* Chapter 5).

Artificial ventilation may be necessary for several days post operation, and the nurse should be familiar with the various types of ventilator used for neonatal artificial ventilation.

In premature babies, in whom frequent apnoea attacks occur, apnoea alarms convert the breathing movement of the baby via an air-filled mattress or impedance electrodes to an audible signal. This allows the nurse to listen for apnoeic attacks rather than watching the baby.

Oxygen tension in the arterial blood is measured via an indwelling umbilical artery probe or surface membrane electrode. Further developments are rapidly taking place such as indwelling pH tissue probes, giving a constant reading of the tissue fluid pH. These probes can give continuous readings over several days.

Cross infection

Stringent precautions about admitting babies with suspected infection, isolation and barrier nursing must be observed to prevent gastroenteritis and other infections spreading from one baby to the next. The nurse should change into a short-sleeved dress and change her shoes before entering the unit. During feeding or handling the baby a specific plastic apron should be allocated to each baby, and should be used by the nurse to prevent her dress from becoming soiled. The hands and forearms should be washed with 3 per cent pHisohex each time the baby is handled. The temperature is taken rectally with a low reading thermometer 29.4°C (85°F), or continuously by using an indwelling rectal probe. The baby's position is changed from side to side in 2-hour periods and the disposable nappy changed when soiled, but the infant should not be disturbed unnecessarily.

On admission to the ward or when the condition has improved after surgery, cleaning of the skin with olive oil or Cidal soap, dusting the skin with hexachlorophane powder (Ster-Zac powder) and treating the umbilical stump with methylated spirit helps to reduce the incidence of pathogenic organisms and skin sepsis.

Feeding

Oral Early feeding in small or premature babies is essential to avoid the dangers of hypoglycaemia. In mature babies with good sucking and swallowing reflexes, a bottle with a suitably-sized teat may be used. Babies too weak to suck should be fed by a plastic gastric tube (No. 3 French gauge) to prevent aspiration. In premature babies, 2 ml of feed 2-hourly and increasing to 20 ml 2-hourly at 7 days, and 30 ml 2-hourly at 14 days would be a suitable regimen for a baby weighing 2 kg (4.4 lb). Diluted half-cream powdered milk, which is gradually increased to full strength, is a suitable feed if breast milk is not available.

Intravenous If the baby is unable to tolerate oral fluids the intravenous route is used for water, electrolyte and calorie requirements. The scalp veins are most often used, the needle being secured by means of plaster of Paris. Very occasionally, for prolonged intravenous feeding, a cannula introduced at the ankle or arm is used and the limb secured by means of a lead splint to prevent movement. When all the peripheral veins have been used, a central venous Silastic catheter passed from the scalp via the jugular vein into the atrium (heart) can be used. A paediatric administration set (Soluset 100 (*Abbott*) with a 100 ml burette calibrated to give 60 drops to 1 ml) is essential to avoid the risks of overinfusion of large amounts of fluid. An infusion pump (Ivac 501) which automatically controls the rate of flow is helpful in maintaining the drip at a very slow rate, 2 to 3 ml per hour, which is sometimes required.

Subcutaneous infusions should be regarded as obsolete as the intravenous route is always possible.

Gastrostomy

A gastrostomy (i.e. a Malécot catheter fixed into the stomach and brought out through the abdominal wall) is an operation frequently performed in neonatal surgical practice. This is used for decompression of the intestines or for feeding. The catheter is fixed to the abdominal wall by means of sutures, kept at right angles to the abdominal wall by means of two pieces of sponge rubber fixed to the catheter and secured further by strapping to the abdominal wall. The baby's hands must be restrained by using 'mitts' made of stockinet* (*see Figure 7.6*). The end of the catheter is fixed to a barrel of a syringe which is left open to allow escape of air from the stomach.

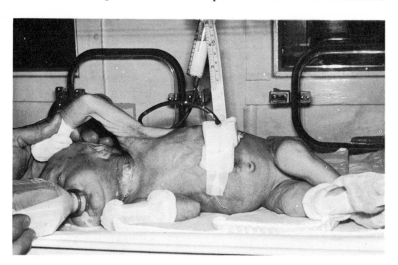

Figure 7.6. Baby feeding with cervical **oesophagostomy** and **gastrostomy**. Note the method of fixation of the catheter, keeping the tube at right-angles to the abdominal wall, and the height above the stomach of the milk level in the reservoir

For feeding, milk is placed into the syringe barrel. The upper level of milk in the reservoir, which is suspended above the baby, must not exceed 10 cm (4 in) above the level of the stomach, as this increases the pressure in the stomach and may rupture an oesophageal anastomosis by reflux up the oesophagus (*Figure 7.7*). The baby should be given a dummy to suck while the gastrostomy feed is given. This allows the pylorus to relax and milk to be expelled into the duodenum. A serious complication arises if the Malécot catheter is pulled out inadvertently within the first 4 weeks after operation. It should be replaced by the surgeon, often under general anaesthesia, because of the risks of replacing it in the peritoneal cavity instead of the stomach.

Oesophagostomy Surgical opening through the neck into the oesophagus.

Gastrostomy Surgical opening through the abdominal wall into the stomach, usually for feeding through a tube.

---

*The mitts should be checked 4-hourly as gangrene of the fingers has occurred by constrictions caused by threads from the stockinet.

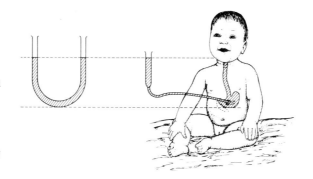

Figure 7.7. In a U-tube the level of fluid is equal in both open limbs. This principle applies in gastrostomy feeding as gastro-oesophageal reflux is common and spill-over into the trachea and lungs will occur if the level of milk in the barrel of the syringe is above the level of the pharynx

Rectal wash-outs

Rectal wash-outs are used both diagnostically and therapeutically in the treatment of Hirschsprung's disease, meconium ileus, and the meconium plug syndrome to remove sticky meconium or hard faeces. A lubricated soft rubber No. 8–10 French gauge Jacques catheter is passed for 5 to 10 cm into the rectum stopping the moment any resistance is felt, and 10 ml of isotonic saline (because of the danger of water intoxication) is slowly injected, moving the catheter gently up and down. The baby usually passes the fluid around the catheter, or it may be removed by aspiration. Further aliquots of 10 ml at a time may be injected up to a 50 ml total. If any blood is noted, the procedure must be abandoned at once.

Nursing position

As has been pointed out, nursing on the side, flat or slightly head down is the safest to prevent aspiration of vomitus. Occasionally the baby with free gastro-oesophageal regurgitation (i.e. lax oesophagus or hiatus hernia) needs to be propped up 45 degrees in a special baby chair. Where obstruction of the airway by the tongue presents a problem, for example **retrognathia** (Pierre Robin syndrome), nursing face down on a special frame (Burston) can be life-saving. Babies with oesophageal atresia should not be nursed prone until the tracheo-oesophageal fistula has been ligated, as this forces gastric contents into the bronchial tree.

INDIVIDUAL CONDITIONS AND THEIR MANAGEMENT

DISEASES OF THE NERVOUS SYSTEM

Spina bifida

Retrognathia Congenital recession of the jaws.

Spina bifida (meningocele, myelomeningocele) is the commonest condition treated in the neonatal period (incidence 3.35 per 1000 births). It is estimated that 20 per

G

cent of severely handicapped children suffer from the condition. The spinal cord develops by an infolding of the ectoderm to form the neural groove. Fusion starts in the mid-dorsal region and proceeds simultaneously headwards and tailwards. The primitive mesoderm now starts to organize to form the vertebrae, skull and meninges enclosing the neural tube (future spinal cord). The spinous process of the vertebrae are formed by the mesoderm uniting around the neural tube. Failure of this process leaves the neural tube exposed, and the spinous process of the vertebra split in two, hence the term 'spina bifida'. Spina bifida varies in degree. Sometimes skin, or abnormal skin, containing a hairy patch or haemangioma, may overlie the abnormal spine. This is called spina bifida occulta. If only the meninges protrude onto the back, the lesion is called a meningocele. In the most severe form abnormal spinal cord and nervous tissue are exposed on the surface of the back. This is called a myelomeningocele (*Figure 7.8*). The exposed nervous tissue is always abnormal and there is a varying degree of paralysis which affects the muscles to the lower limbs, bladder or anal sphincters.

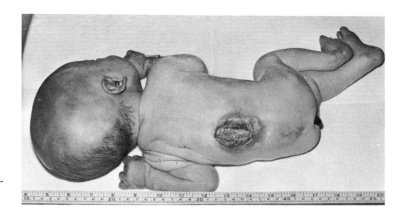

Figure 7.8. Baby with a myelomeningocele, showing paralysed legs and anus, also talipes of feet and hydrocephalus

Herniation of brain tissue is called an encephalocele (*Figure 7.9*).

The diagnosis does not present any difficulty as the condition is usually obvious at birth. Spina bifida may be diagnosed at 16 to 20 weeks by finding a raised alphafeto protein in the maternal blood or amniotic fluid. This can be further confirmed by ultrasound examination or an x-ray in late pregnancy showing the abnormal spine.

Although the abnormality is obvious at birth, it is sometimes necessary to investigate the child further by means of a **ventriculogram**, intravenous **pyelogram** and radiological examination of the spine before undertaking any surgical treatment.

Ventriculogram A radiograph of the cerebral ventricles. Contrast is obtained by filling them with air.

Pyelogram Renal tract radiography (strictly — the renal pelvis).

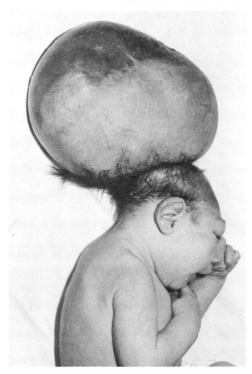

Figure 7.9. Large encephalocele associated with microcephaly

Treatment

When the baby is affected by the most severe degree of spina bifida, that is, complete paralysis from the waist down, paralysis of the bladder and anal sphincters, gross vertebral deformities giving rise to a large hump on the back (**kyphosis**) and gross hydrocephalus at birth, the decision whether or not to operate on the baby can be very difficult. In these circumstances, full discussions should take place between the surgeon, the paediatrician, the general practitioner and the parents before contemplating any surgery. Sometimes it is justifiable in such a case not to embark on a long and complicated series of surgical operations. In England and Wales the number of live and still births with spina bifida and/or hydrocephalus fell from 5380 in 1970 to 3750 in 1974. Surgery was undertaken in 2910 in 1970 and in 1700 in 1974. In most paediatric surgical units about 30 per cent of spina bifida cases are being offered active treatment.

The thin sac of the myelomeningocele may rupture at birth or soon after and leak cerebrospinal fluid. Protection against infection is the most important first-aid treatment. The sac is covered with a wet swab of gauze, (not cotton wool, which adheres and cannot be removed subsequently at operation)soaked in 1 per cent aqueous Hibitane and the baby transferred to a suitable centre for treatment.

Kyphosis Excessive forward spinal curvature

The baby is prepared for a major operation under general anaesthesia. When the myelomeningocele is large, that is, about one-half of the width of the back, the operation can be very difficult and blood loss considerable. A blood transfusion is usually necessary. The principle of the operation is to repair the defect on the back in three layers; the dura mater, a musculofacial layer and the skin are mobilized sufficiently to be brought together in the midline.

Postoperative care

The baby is returned to the ward from the operating theatre in the knee—chest position. The baby is suspended by means of extension strapping to the abdomen from a special frame (*see Figure 7.10*). This position relieves tension on the operative repair and prevents contamination of the wound by

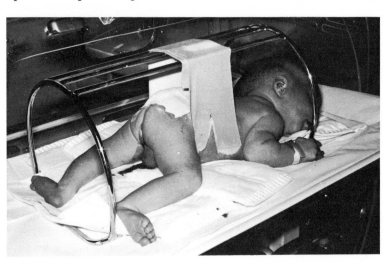

Figure 7.10. Nursing position after myelomeningocele repair

urine and faeces. Feeding may present certain difficulties as the baby is not taken off the frame for feeding. This means that the baby has to suck in this position with the head to one side. Vomiting is quite common, either due to the prone position or due to the pressure on the abdominal contents. Care must be taken of the knees and elbows as ulceration may occur due to abrasion and pressure, especially as the skin overlying the knees may lack sensation.

Retention of urine is a frequent complication seen in myelomeningoceles. The baby's abdomen must be inspected and palpated frequently. If a distended bladder is noted, this can be expressed manually by pressing downwards and backwards. Undue pressure must not be used as rupture of the bladder has occurred. Occasionally forceful dilatation of the urethra is necessary to allow the urine to be expressed more easily and to prevent back-pressure changes on the kidneys.

Rehabilitation and follow-up

The repair of the spinal defect is only the first part of a long and complicated course of treatment in these babies. Over 80 per cent develop hydrocephalus (*see below*) which requires surgical treatment, usually within the first 3 to 4 weeks of life. The paralyzed and deformed legs require orthopaedic attention from an early stage in order to correct any deformity. To achieve this, several procedures, such as manipulation and strapping, tendon transplants and so on, may be necessary. The ultimate aim is to achieve an upright position, with or without the aid of a body caliper, and some degree of independent locomotion.

Over 50 per cent of the survivors suffer from major physical handicaps and attend schools for the physically handicapped. Intellectually about 10 per cent are ineducable; 40 per cent attend normal schools.

Hydrocephalus

Hydrocephalus is a word derived from the Greek, meaning 'water' and 'head'. It is due to the excessive accumulation of cerebrospinal fluid within the skull, usually within the ventricles. This causes the ventricles to become grossly distended, the brain substance to become thinned and the skull bones to separate. About 60 per cent of the cerebrospinal fluid is formed in the ventricles and 40 per cent in the subarachnoid space. The cerebrospinal fluid circulates from the ventricles to the subarachnoid space assisted by the arterial pulse wave. Absorption of the cerebrospinal fluid is mainly via perineural spaces and 10 per cent by the arachnoid villi.

Hydrocephalus is caused by an overproduction of cerebrospinal fluid, such as a tumour of the choroid plexus, or by an anatomical blockage anywhere along the pathway for circulation or absorption of the cerebrospinal fluid. The most common cause of blockage is seen in cases of spina bifida in which the posterior fossa of the skull is small, and the medulla and cerebellar tonsils prolapse, preventing the flow of cerebrospinal fluid (Arnold–Chiari malformation).

Congenital atresia and stenosis of the minute channel between the third and fourth ventricles of the brain (aqueduct of Sylvius) is another common cause of hydrocephalus. Haemorrhage or inflammation (meningitis) around the base of the brain may lead to hydrocephalus by preventing circulation and absorption of the cerebrospinal fluid.

Hydrocephalus is diagnosed by noting a progressive enlargement of the skull (above normal for the age), a large anterior fontanelle which bulges, prominent veins on the scalp and open sutures of the cranial bones. The eyeballs are rotated downwards so that only one-half of the iris appears above the lower eyelid — 'sunset' sign (*Figure 7.11*).

The diagnosis is confirmed by **ventriculostomy** and ventriculogram. Using local anaesthesia and strict aseptic precautions a Tizard brain needle is passed into the brain from the outer angle of the anterior fontanelle. The cerebrospinal

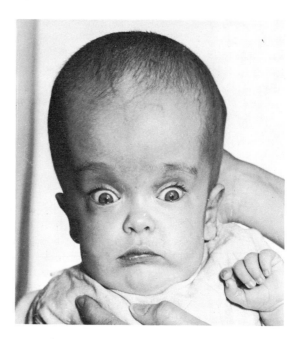

Figure 7.11. Hydrocephalus, showing prominent forehead and 'sunset' sign of eyes

fluid pressure is measured by a manometer, some cerebrospinal fluid is removed (30—50 ml) and replaced with air. A series of radiographs are taken (air ventriculogram). These radiographs will give an indication of the size and shape of the ventricles and the thickness of the cerebral cortex. This invasive technique has been largely replaced by a CAT scan (x-ray computorized tomography) which gives good visualization of the ventricles, but gives no indication of ventricular pressure or whether the blood or infection is present in the CSF. Similarly, ultrasound scans via the open anterior fontanelle can be used to estimate the size of the ventricles.

Treatment

Today, effective treatment for hydrocephalus is available, therefore no longer should one see the baby with a grossly enlarged head, too heavy to lift and covered with pressure ulcers. The hydrocephalus can be controlled by the use of the Spitz—Holter ventriculoatrial shunt, or one of the other types of shunts available, which drains the cerebrospinal fluid from the lateral ventricle back into the bloodstream (*Figure 7.12*).

Ventriculostomy The making of an opening in the ventricles of the brain to allow drainage of cerebrospinal fluid, usually by fitting a tube from the ventricles to the subarachnoid cisternae.

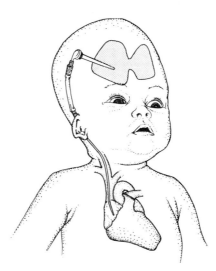

Figure 7.12. Ventriculoatrial Spitz–Holter valve in position. (After Rickham and Johnston, 1969, by courtesy of the Authors)

Postoperatively the baby should not lie on the valve as the overlying scalp is thin and pressure necrosis may develop with extrusion of the valve. Occasionally the valve causes rapid overdrainage with collapse and overlapping of the skull bones with depression of the fontanelle. If this occurs, the baby should be placed in a head-down position. Nurses and parents should be familiar with the form of the Spitz–Holter valve beneath the scalp and know how to test whether or not the valve is working by pumping it.

DISORDERS OF THE ALIMENTARY TRACT

Oesophageal atresia and tracheo-oesophageal fistula

In oesophageal atresia the baby is born without continuity of the oesophagus. The condition may be suspected in a mother who has **hydramnios**. There are several varieties (*Figure 7.13*), the most common one being associated with a tracheo-oesophageal fistula in which the upper third of the oesophagus ends as a blind pouch and the lower segment joins the trachea just above the carina (bifurcation). The baby is unable to swallow saliva and, therefore, regurgitates a frothy mucus, chokes and has cyanotic attacks. During respiration air enters the stomach and abdomen. Vomiting back into the trachea along the fistula is a lethal hazard. The surgical treatment of these babies can be difficult and complicated, and the overall mortality is still about 50 per cent. An attempt is made to join the two ends (primary anastomosis) together with division of the tracheo-oesophageal fistula via a right lateral **thoracotomy**.

Hydramnios Excessive amniotic fluid which surrounds the fetus *in utero*.

Thoracotomy The operation of incising the wall of the thorax.

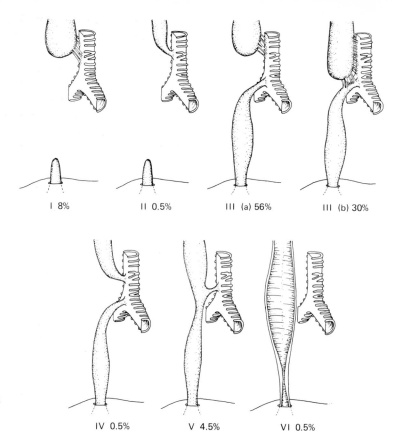

I 8%   II 0.5%   III (a) 56%   III (b) 30%

IV 0.5%   V 4.5%   VI 0.5%

Figure 7.13. Diagram showing types of oesophageal atresia and tracheo-oesophageal fistula. (After Rickham and Johnston, 1969, by courtesy of the Authors)

A gastrostomy is made for decompression of the intestines and for subsequent feeding. If joining of the oesophagus (primary anastomosis) is not possible, the upper blind pouch is brought out above the clavicle (cervical oesophagostomy). The baby is fed via his gastrostomy and also by mouth, so that the suck-swallow reflex can develop. When the baby is thriving and able to take solids by mouth a second operation is necessary to bridge the gap between the cervical oesophagus and the stomach. This operation is performed via a left thoracotomy, opening the diaphragm and mobilizing the transverse colon on a vascular pedicle (*see Figure 7.14*).

Postoperatively, following a primary repair of the oesophagus, the baby is nursed on his side and in a slightly head-down position to allow the mucus and saliva to drain from his mouth. Gentle pharyngeal suction to a measured distance, usually about 7 cm, is necessary for the first 3 or 4 days. Although the operation is performed retropleurally, the chest (retropleural space) is drained via an underwater seal. The nature and amount of fluid draining (either serum or blood) should be noted. Any air bubbles or saliva in the tube should be reported immediately as this is suggestive of disruption of the anastomosis. Intravenous feeding is continued for 36 to 48 hours until gastrostomy feeds are established. Oral feeding is started when it is seen that the child is coping well with his saliva — usually in about 5 to 6 days. Dilute gentian violet is given by mouth to test the patency and continuity of the oesophagus by seeing whether dye appears in the chest drain or gastrostomy tube.

Intestinal obstruction

There are many causes of intestinal obstruction in the newborn baby. This condition should be suspected in any baby who fails to pass meconium within 24 hours of birth, who vomits bile and whose abdomen becomes distended. A single erect radiograph of the abdomen and chest will often show fluid levels in various characteristic patterns, which confirm the diagnosis. Once the diagnosis is made or suspected a No. 6 FG stomach tube is passed and continuous nasogastric suction started. Fluids are given intravenously. Occasionally, in a low large bowel obstruction due to Hirschsprung's disease,

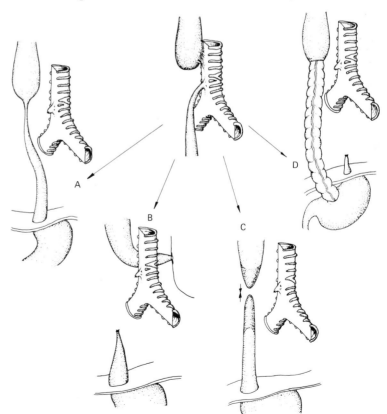

Figure 7.14. Diagram showing various methods of dealing with oesophageal atresia and tracheo-oesophageal fistula. (A) Primary anastomosis. (B) Ligation of fistula with cervical oesophagostomy. (C) Lengthening of upper and lower segments by regular stretching. (D) Bridging the gap by means of colonic interposition

or a sticky meconium plug, a gentle rectal wash-out will relieve the obstruction. Recently, Gastrografin enemas have been used to relieve the obstruction in meconium ileus. However, a **laparotomy** is usually necessary to deal with the specific intestinal pathology found. This may include stenosis (narrowing), atresia (absence of canalization), malrotation, meconium ileus or Hirschsprung's disease.

CONGENITAL MALFORMATION OF SMALL AND LARGE INTESTINES

Atresia and stenosis

Atresia means 'absence of' and stenosis means 'narrowing' of the normal lumen of the intestine. Atresia can occur in any part of the intestinal tract from the oesophagus to the anus.

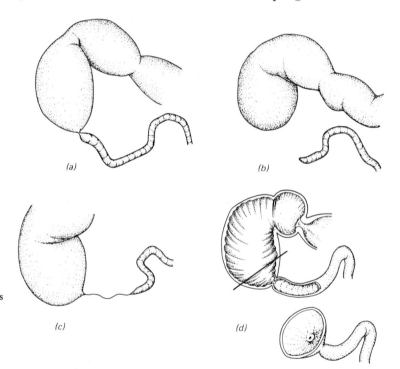

Figure 7.15. Types of duodenal obstruction. Atresia is shown in (a) and (b). In (c) the ends are joined by a fibrous cord. In (d) the stenosis is due to a diaphragm with a central hole. (After Rickham and Johnston, 1969, by courtesy of Professor Rickham)

Laparotomy An incision made through the abdominal wall to explore the abdominal cavity.

The types of atresia and stenosis of the duodenum are shown in *Figure 7.15;* similar examples can be seen anywhere in the small or large bowel. In most cases except in the oesophagus, duodenum and rectum the cause is due to an intrauterine vascular accident occurring late in pregnancy such as volvulus, intussusception or strangulation of the bowel at the umbilical ring. Because, unlike the child, the fetus is germ-free and the gangrenous portion of the bowel is absorbed and disappears almost without trace.

Because the atresia causes a complete obstruction of the lumen, the proximal bowel **hypertrophies** and dilates and fills with bile-stained fluid. Bile-stained (green, not yellow coloured) vomiting is the most important sign, which should alert one to the presence of an obstruction. The diagnosis of the site and probably the cause of the obstruction can be made by a single good quality erect x-ray film of the abdomen.

Operation is reasonably urgent, after resuscition and re-hydration of the baby. Laparotomy, using a transverse, muscle-cutting, supra-umbilical incision is sufficient in most instances to explore any part of the abdomen. The grossly dilated proximal bowel is resected and joined to a small distal bowel by means of a single-layer anastomosis using 4/0 black silk sutures, in an end-to-end or end-to-back fashion.

Meconium ileus

A mature (40 weeks' gestation) baby should pass meconium within 24 hours after birth. Meconium, is the first black tarry stool which is passed and consists of bile (secreted from four months' gestation), mucus and cells which have been desquamated from the superficial epithelial surfaces of the stomach and intestines, along with squamous cells and hairs from the vernix caseosa swallowed in the **amniotic fluid**. Meconium is kept fluid by the action of pancreatic enzymes. If, however, pancreatic function and mucus gland secretion is deficient, for example in fibrocystic disease of the pancreas, the meconium becomes thick and putty-like which may obstruct the terminal ileum by small pellets of inspissated meconium. Twisting (volvulus) of the grossly distended proximal bowel may lead to atresia and perforation.

Gross abdominal distension and bile-stained vomiting, with no passage of meconium are the main presenting features. Large coils filled with the rubbery meconium may be palpated through the abdominal wall, and a straight abdominal x-ray shows the typical mottled granular appearance due to fat granules trapped in the sticky meconium.

As the condition is due to a genetic defect (autosomal recessive) a family history of affected siblings may give a clue. Laboratory investigations may show absence of the pancreatic enzyme, trypsin, from the stool, or the amount of sodium chloride in the sweat can be measured. Values above 80 mmol per litre are diagnostic of cystic fibrosis.

The obstructed bowel may be deflated by the use of a 'gastrografin' enema. This substance has a very high osmolarity and detergent action which attracts fluid into the lumen of the bowel thereby softening the stool. In more severe cases, laparotomy, **enterotomy** or resection of the dilated bowel

Amniotic fluid The fluid which surrounds the fetus.

Enterotomy Incision, division or dissection of the intestine.

Hypertrophy Increase in the size or number of cells in a tissue.

with an end-to-side (Bishop—Koop) anastomosis is performed. This leaves a 'chimney' opening on the abdomen through which pancreatic enzymes can be instilled. Once the bowel has been cleared of the sticky meconium, oral supplementary pancreatic enzymes are given with each meal throughout life.

Anomalies of intestinal rotation

Up to the tenth week of gestation the gut lies outside the abdominal cavity in a physiological hernia at the umbilicus. The gut returns in an orderly fashion to form the typical 'C' loop of the duodenum, the oblique attachment of the small bowel mesentary, and the attachment of the ascending, transverse and descending colon.

The process of rotation of the mid-gut (extending from the area of the bile duct papilla to the middle of the transverse colon) may be arrested at any stage and several abnormalities develop. The main effects of these abnormalities are:

(1) that the intestine remains free on a narrow-based mesentery and is therefore very liable to undergo twisting, or volvulus;
(2) that tight bands of peritoneum or fibrous tissue cross and obstruct the second part of the duodenum and stretch from below the liver to the caecum, which is situated in the epigastrium, close to the origin of the superior mesenteric artery.

Volvulus may lead to partial obstruction of the blood vessels of the intestine, which may ultimately become gangrenous. More frequently, the symptoms that result are due to obstruction of the duodenum immediately below the entry of the bile duct into the duodenum. Vomiting usually begins very early in life and the vomitus may contain bile. Radiological examination will demonstrate that the first part of the duodenum and the stomach are distended by swallowed air. A valuable investigation is the injection of 20 to 30 ml air through a nasogastric tube to distend the stomach and duodenum before the abdominal x-ray.

Treatment is by operation. Any volvulus is corrected by derotation in an anti-clockwise direction, with division of the obstructing bands from the caecum across the duodenum. The small and large bowel cannot be returned to a normal anatomical position, therefore the duodenum is freed and made to lie in the right paracolic gutter, the narrow mesentery is opened up as much as possible as an apron, and the colon placed on the left side of the abdomen with the caecum and appendix in the left hypochondrium. No anchoring is necessary.

Congenital megacolon — Hirschsprung's disease

The ganglion cells of the small and large bowel migrate from above downwards in intrauterine life, and should reach the anus by birth. Failure of this migration to reach the anus will cause an aganglionic zone, which extends upwards, for a varying distance from the anus. The segment of bowel, without ganglion cells and proper innervation by the autonomic nervous system is unable to conduct a co-ordinated peristaltic wave, and acts as a physiological obstruction to the onward passage of bowel contents. This results in obstruction with gross dilatation and hypertrophy of the proximal colon. Eighty per cent present as acute large bowel obstructions in the neonatal period, with failure to pass meconium, abdominal distension and bile-stained vomiting. About 20 per cent present less acutely, with failure to thrive or severe constipation from early infancy. They require laxatives, suppositories and enemas to evacuate their colons. The diagnosis is made by showing the characteristic narrow segment, 'cone' area and dilatation of the colon on barium enema, or by examining histologically a strip of rectal mucosa removed through the anus (rectal biopsy) showing the absence of ganglion cells.

Treatment consists of a **loop colostomy** to relieve the obstruction, followed 6 to 12 months later by a definitive operation to remove most of the aganglionic segment, restore continuity and preserve faecal continence.

Imperforate anus

Imperforate anus is a term used to describe a number of congenital anomalies, some of which may be complex, which affect the anus, rectum, urinary and genital tracts of both sexes (*Figure 7.16*).

During the early stage of embryological development (4—6 weeks' gestation) the hind-gut (rectum) communicates with the future bladder in a common cavity — the cloaca. Division into two separate chambers occurs. The female genital tract (vagina and uterus) develops from further differentiation of tissue between these cavities. Arrested development at an early stage leaves the colon (rectum) communicating with the vagina in females and with the urethra in males. No development of the rectum or sphincteric muscles occurs. Only the anus is affected by arrested development at a later stage, and may be ectopic or stenosed. Two major problems arise, one of intestinal obstruction in the neonatal period, which is usually relieved by a colostomy; secondly, without a normal rectum or anal sphincteric muscles

Loop colostomy A temporary artificial opening made between the skin and the colon which is brought out as a loop.

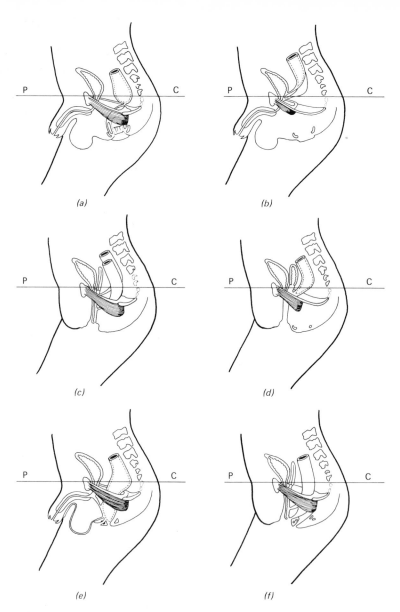

Figure 7.16. Diagram showing various types of anorectal anomalies. (*a*) Rectal atresia in a male infant. (*b*) Anorectal agenesis with rectovesical and recto-urethral fistula. (*c*) Anorectal agenesis and high and low rectovaginal fistula in a female infant. (*d*) Anorectal agenesis with rectocloacal fistula. (*e*) Anobulbar, anocutaneous, anoperineal, anoscrotal and anopenile fistulae. (*f*) Anovulvar fistula. (After Rickham and Johnston, 1969, by courtesy of the Authors)

it is very difficult to achieve normal faecal continence. The anus must always be inspected at birth and a thermometer passed to determine its patency. The diagnosis is usually obvious on inspection. A radiograph taken with the baby held upside down for 2 to 3 minutes will allow the air bubble to rise in the lowermost portion of the bowel and the distance between the blind pouch and perineum can be measured. In the 'low' varieties the anal canal ends blindly just above the perineal skin. In these cases operative treatment is via a perineal **anoplasty** to widen the opening of the anus. If the abnormality is 'high', intestinal obstruction is usually present, although there may be a fistula between the bladder, urethra or vagina and the rectum. A transverse colostomy relieves the obstruction.

At a later stage, when the baby is thriving, and 6 to 12 months of age a 'pull-through' operation is performed usually via an abdominal sacroperineal approach. Great care is necessary to preserve the delicate pelvic muscle fibres forming a sling around the colon, in order to achieve any degree of continence.

Postoperative care

The buttocks are left exposed, any soiling is immediately removed by gentle mopping or irrigations and the area dried and sprayed with an antibiotic aerosol. Dilatation of the new anus with Hegar dilators starts on about the tenth day.

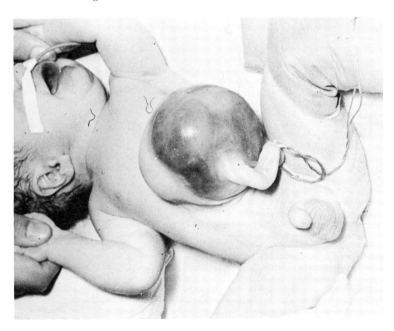

Figure 7.17. Showing exomphalos with intact sac

Anoplasty Plastic repair of the anus.

Exomphalos

Exomphalos is a special type of umbilical hernia. The size varies from small, in which only a knuckle of bowel appears, to very large, in which most of the abdominal contents lie within the sac (*Figure 7.17*). The sac consists of a thin, translucent, avascular membrane which is usually intact but may be ruptured. To prevent infection and heat loss the sac should be covered by placing the contents in a sterile plastic bag such as the Aldon intestinal bag (*Aldington Laboratories*). Continuous nasogastric suction should be started immediately to prevent distension of the gut.

Operative repair is easy in the small defect. In the large protrusions, return of the abdominal contents to a small abdominal cavity may markedly interfere with respiration and the venous returns to the heart. In these cases a staged procedure, using a sheet of silicone rubber to close and enlarge the abdominal cavity and then serially reducing the size of the hernia, can be used. Alternatively, by painting the sac with mercurochrome 1 per cent, granulation and epithelialization of the defect of the abdominal wall can occur.

Duplication of the alimentary tract

Any part of the alimentary tract from the mouth to the anus may be duplicated. The duplications take three forms — a localized cyst, a tubular structure intimately related to some part of the gut or two complete organs lying close together. The duplication may be asymptomatic throughout life or cause intestinal obstruction by pressure on the adjacent bowel. As the duplications are frequently lined by ectopic gastric mucosa, peptic ulceration causing haemorrhage or perforation may occur (*Figure 7.18*). Treatment consists of excision of

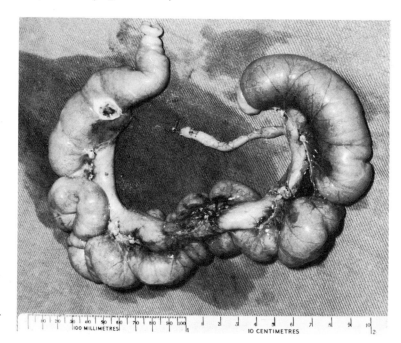

Figure 7.18. Duplication of ileum showing perforated peptic ulcer

the duplicated structure, together with the adjacent bowel as the blood supply is shared. In the extensive duplications a laparotomy and a thoracotomy may be necessary to remove the portion in the chest related to the oesophagus and the prolongation through the diaphragm into the abdomen.

Meckel's diverticulum

This is the commonest manifestation of the persistence of portion of the vitello-intestinal duct which in the very young embryo connects the mid-gut to the yolk sac (*see Figure 7.19d*). The other possibilities of non-obliteration of the duct are shown in *Figure 7.19a, b, c*.

A similar sequence of embryological events is seen elsewhere in the body, i.e. the processus vaginalis causing a hernia, hydrocele or encysted hydrocele of the cord, the thyroglossal duct causing a fistula, cyst or sinus or the formation of a branchial fistula, cyst or sinus in the neck.

The Meckel's diverticulum projects from the antimesenteric side of the ileum about 2 ft (60 cm) from the ileocaecal valve. If the diverticulum forms a very short wide-mouthed

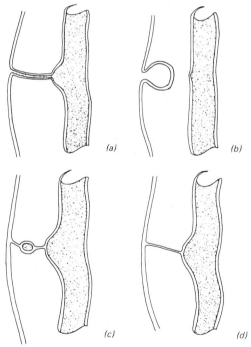

(a)   *(b)*

(c)   *(d)*

Figure 7.19. The various abnormalities associated with a persistent vitello-intestinal duct. In (*a*) there is a patent fistula between the Meckel's diverticulum and skin at the umbilicus. In (*b*) there is a sinus at the umbilicus. In (*c*) there is a closed cyst suspended in a fibrous cord between the Meckel's diverticulum and the umbilicus. In (*d*) there is a Meckel's diverticulum which may be attached to the abdominal wall by a fibrous band

pouch lined by intestinal epithelium there is usually no problem. The diverticulum may be elongated, with the mucosa containing ectopic gastric mucosal cells including oxyntic cells which secrete acid. A peptic ulcer forms at the junction between gastric and small bowel mucosa, which may

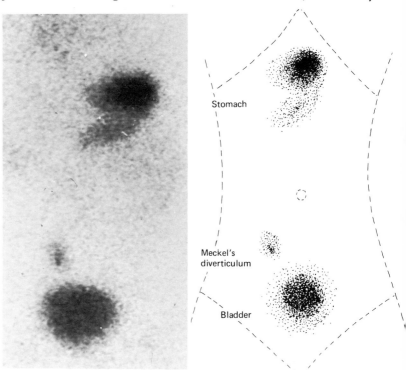

Figure 7.20. Technetium pertechnetate (^{99m}Tc) scan showing ectopic gastric mucosa in Meckel's diverticulum just above the bladder

cause serious haemorrhage. This usually occurs in the first two years of life, is copious, painless and symptomless, with exsanguination of the child. A radio-isotope scan using technetium pertechnetate ^{99m}Tc may confirm the presence of ectopic gastric mucosa within the abdomen (*see Figure 7.20*). Emergency operation with resection of the diverticulum may be required. Other complications of a persistent vitello-intestinal duct include cyst formation, volvulus of the small bowel and invagination of the diverticulum causing intussusception.

Congenital pyloric stenosis

Congenital pyloric stenosis affects infants between a narrow age range of 3 to 8 weeks and it is rarely seen in children outside this age limit. Pyloric stenosis is a common condition affecting one in every 150 male children and one in every 600 girls (ratio 4:1). It is genetically determined. Babies with affected parents have a 1 in 5 chance of having pyloric stenosis.

Pathology

Thickening and hypertrophy of the pyloric muscle occurs gradually in the first few weeks of life. The exact cause of this is still unknown. The thickening of the muscle causes narrowing of the pyloric canal and prevents the emptying of the stomach. This in turn causes dilatation of the stomach and hypertrophy of the stomach wall in an attempt to overcome the partial obstruction. Stagnation of the food in the stomach causes gastritis (bleeding from the mucosa).

Clinical presentation

The baby is usually considered to be perfectly normal during the first 3 to 4 weeks of life. Vomiting then occurs. This is the main symptom and certain features are important. At first the vomiting is only small in amount. As the stomach hypertrophies and dilates, the vomiting becomes more forceful (projectile) and larger in volume. The vomiting occurs during or soon after a feed and consists of curdled milk and mucus. If gastritis is present, blood in the form of coffee grounds may be noted but bile is never seen and this negative finding should always be recorded.

With the persistent vomiting and the inability to retain feed the secondary signs and symptoms are noted, dehydration being of great importance. If this is severe, the baby appears wizened, the eyes large and anxious and the lips and mouth red and dry. His weight may be below his birth weight. Due to the loss of gastric secretions containing water, hydrochloric acid, sodium and potassium ions, the baby develops a biochemical alkalosis.

Two physical signs are looked for to confirm the diagnosis. In a warm quiet room the baby is given a milk test-feed by the nurse. The abdomen is exposed and inspected for visible **peristalsis** which represents contractions of the dilated hypertrophied stomach. Waves are seen starting from under the left costal margin and moving towards the umbilicus like golf balls under the skin. The examiner palpates with the middle finger of his left hand in the area of the duodenum. The enlarged and thickened pylorus is felt like a small peanut and is called the pyloric tumour. The baby frequently demonstrates a projectile vomit during the examination. Doubt may exist in about 5 per cent of cases, when it may be necessary to resort to a barium meal to confirm the diagnosis.

Treatment

Once the diagnosis has been confirmed, preparations are made for treatment. Although 'medical' treatment, consisting of carefully graduated feeds, gastric lavage and giving an antispasmodic (Eumydrin Drops — 0.6 per cent solution of

Peristalsis The process by which solids are carried along any of the hollow tubes of the body — the oesophagus, intestines and so on. The muscles of the tube in front of the solid relax, while those behind it contract, and hence push the mass along.

atropine methonitrate in alcohol) 15 minutes before feeds is described, in practice it is not often used. Preparation for surgery should not be regarded as an emergency. It is important that fluid and electrolyte imbalance is corrected by intravenous therapy and the stomach washed out several times, especially if there is evidence of gastritis. This preparation may take 24 to 36 hours.

The baby is sent to theatre with a stomach tube (No. 8 FG Jacques catheter) in position. The operation is performed under general anaesthesia as local anaesthesia is rarely used today. A small transverse muscle-cutting incision over the upper right rectus muscle is made to expose and deliver the stomach and pylorus. The peritoneum and thickened muscle are split longitudinally along the whole length of the elongated pyloric canal down to the mucosa. This allows the mucosa to pout and releases the constriction and obstruction of the canal (Ramstedt's operation, first performed in 1912). The abdomen is closed in layers with a subcuticular catgut suture to skin.

Postoperatively the child's temperature is checked by a low reading thermometer. The stomach tube is aspirated hourly and a stomach wash-out given at 4 hours. Feeding is then started with 5 per cent glucose feeds, 2-hourly, gradually increasing the volume from 5 ml. After 6 hours, dilute milk is introduced and if this is tolerated, the strength of the milk is increased. The aim should be to have the baby on 2-hourly full strength feeds by 48 hours. Thirty years ago the mortality for pyloric stenosis was 25 per cent, today it should be less than 0.5 per cent.

Diaphragmatic hernia

In babies with diaphragmatic hernia there is a congenital defect, usually in the posterolateral aspect of the left dome of the diaphragm. This allows the abdominal contents to enter the chest, compressing the lungs and pushing the heart over to the right side. The baby may have great difficulty in breathing immediately after birth; nearly one-half of them are stillborn. Any air which distends the stomach and intestines will aggravate the position and therefore a stomach tube must be passed immediately, to which constant low grade suction is applied. Due to the extreme respiratory embarrassment which may occur at any moment, the baby may require intubation and positive pressure ventilation as an emergency. A resuscitation trolley should, therefore, always be on hand. If transfer is arranged, an experienced paediatric anaesthetist should accompany the baby. Tension pneumothorax on the unaffected side is not uncommon and should be watched for and treated by an underwater seal. An emergency abdominal operation is needed to return the chest contents to the abdomen and to close the defect in the diaphragm. The chest is drained via an underwater seal until the lung expands. A chest drain is usually placed into the contralateral chest prophylactically.

OTHER CONDITIONS

Genito-urinary anomalies

Two important problems, *ectopia vesicae* and *posterior urethral valves*, are discussed in Chapter 30.

Adrenogenital syndrome

The adrenogenital syndrome is due to an inborn error of adrenocortical metabolism caused by an abnormal autosomal recessive gene. There is a biochemical block in the production of hydrocortisone. The pituitary responds by producing more **adrenocorticotrophic hormone** (ACTH), which causes an excess production of adrenal androgens and masculinization of the external genitalia. Mistakes regarding the sex of the infant can be made. One-quarter of the infants also lose excess salt and may die of hydrocortisone deficiency if the vomiting, dehydration, constipation and peripheral circulatory failure are not diagnosed early. Treatment is by hydrocortisone replacement therapy and later by surgery for the enlarged clitoris.

Hare-lip and cleft palate

Clefts of the lip and palate may occur separately or together. Clefts of the lip may be unilateral or bilateral and vary in severity from a small notch of the red margin (vermilion) of the lip, or extend backwards as a complete gap of the alveolar margin. Likewise, the cleft in the palate may start as a bifid uvula in its mildest form or extend forwards to the alveolus as a large gap of the hard and soft palate. The deformity affects the skeleton of the whole middle third of the face. In planning treatment, attention must be directed towards correction of the twisted nose, the malaligned alveolar margin and the gap in the upper lip. The best cosmetic results are obtained when treatment is carried out by the combined efforts of orthodontic and plastic surgeons. If only the lip or the palate is affected, surgical repair is usually straightforward and is usually carried out, if the baby is thriving, at the age of 3 months for the lip, and at 18 to 24 months for the palate.

Adrenocorticotrophic hormone (ACTH)
A hormone which stimulates the cortex of the adrenal gland.

When the premaxilla is deformed, early orthodontic treatment is necessary. To realign the premaxilla, a pressure pad is carefully strapped onto the face and renewed daily (*see Figure 7.21*). A cast is made of the alveolus and a plastic splint worn as soon as possible. This allows early bottle feeding and the suck-swallow reflex to develop.

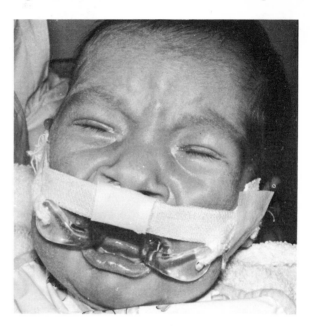

Figure 7.21. Bilateral cleft lip and palate showing pressure pad and obturator in position

The incidence of cleft lip and palate is 1.56 per 1000 live births. In 50 per cent both lip and palate are affected, and in 25 per cent the lip, and in 25 per cent the palate is affected. Mental subnormality is 10 times more common in this group than in normal children. The disorder is genetically determined. If one child is affected with a hare-lip, the risk to subsequent children is about 1 in 20, and 1 in 50 if he has a cleft palate. If one parent is affected, the risk is about 1 in 5.

The shock to the mother of seeing her baby with an ugly deformity can be lessened by showing her photographs of similar children before and after surgical treatment.

Feeding

Handling and feeding the baby may present problems. Breast-feeding is not usually possible in severe cases of cleft lip and palate, but breast milk can be expressed and utilized.

Feeding does not present any difficulties with suitably trained staff (*Figure 7.22*). Lying the baby across one's knee and using a special lamb's teat is not necessary. With the obturator in position the baby is held as normal and a teat (Griptight—Maws) with a larger hole is used.

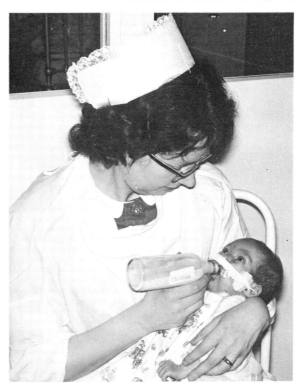

Figure 7.22. Baby with cleft lip and palate feeding with pressure pad and obturator in position

Preoperatively the baby should be isolated to prevent infection, photographed, haemoglobin estimated and any anaemia treated and swabs taken of the nose and throat to exclude the presence of haemolytic streptococci or other pathogenic organisms. If these are present, operation is postponed and the appropriate antibiotics given.

Operation

Operation is performed under general anaesthesia. There are many methods by which the local tissue can be used to repair the deformity, and specialized books on the subject should be consulted. When these babies are managed by a team of specialists in the manner outlined above the cosmetic results achieved are truly excellent.

Postoperatively, apart from the routine surgical care, special care must be directed towards preventing any strain on the suture line. The baby is kept clean, warm and dry and well supplied with fluids. Elbow splints are needed for 4 to 5 days to prevent interference with the suture line. A Logan's bow is applied to further reduce the tension on the suture line, and crying is prevented at all costs. Cleaning of the suture line should be achieved by means of gentle swabbing with hydrogen peroxide and suction should be avoided if at all possible.

Feeding can start at 4 hours after repair of the cleft lip following return to the ward. This is by means of a spoon until sutures are removed on the fourth or fifth day.

The aim of surgical treatment is that the child should look well, feed well and speak well. Staged operations over several years, together with the help of a speech therapist, may be necessary to achieve this aim.

REFERENCES

Craig, W. S. (1969). *Care of the Newly Born Infant*. 4th Edn. Edinburgh: Churchill Livingstone

Duncombe, M. and Weller, B. F. (1969). *Paediatric Nursing*. London: Bailliére Tindall

Farrow, R. and Forrest, D. (1968). *The Surgery of Childhood for Nurses*. 3rd Edn. Edinburgh: Churchill Livingstone

Rickham, P. P. and Johnston, J. H. (1969). *Neonatal Surgery*. London: Butterworths

Young, D. G. and Weller, B. F. (1971). *Baby Surgery: Nursing Management and Care*. London: Harvey, Miller and Medcalf

Inflammation

A. H. Cruickshank

INTRODUCTION

Inflammation is the reaction of living tissue to irritation or damage. Only living tissues are capable of reacting and if an injury is overwhelming, there will be no reaction, only death. But an injury may cause death of only a part of an organ and then the surviving tissues at the edge of the dead area respond by becoming inflamed and the inflammation is followed by the formation of new cells to replace those that have been killed. A certain amount of inflammation is probably necessary to initiate healing but excessive inflammation impairs healing. Thus, even in a sterile wound, minor inflammatory changes precede repair, but in a septic wound severe inflammation may delay healing indefinitely.

Nature of the inflammatory reaction

The inflammatory response consists of the changes that occur at the site of the injury — the local effects, and the responses of the body as a whole — the general effects. The two groups of reactions are closely associated. The responses may develop very rapidly in acute inflammation or build up gradually in chronic inflammation. It is quite common for an inflammation to begin acutely and then pass into a chronic phase. The diagram in *Figure 8.1* contains the main components and stages of the inflammatory reaction, and the various ways in which it may end.

AETIOLOGY

Types of injury that cause inflammation

The injuries that will be followed by an inflammatory reaction may be, for example, wounds due to mechanical violence; the burns caused by heat, sunlight, artificial ultraviolet light, x-rays, many caustic and irritant chemicals; the damage caused by harmful immunological responses; and several types of living agent. The living causes of inflammation differ from the inanimate causes in that they reproduce themselves

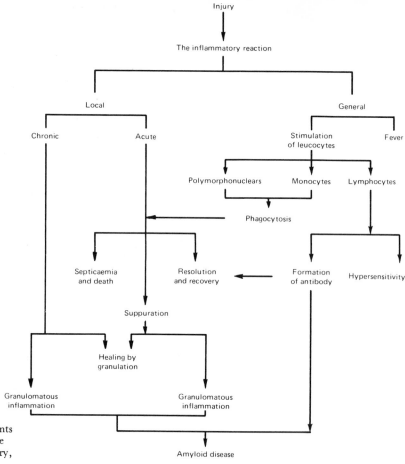

Figure 8.1. Diagram of the components of the inflammatory reaction with the main courses that may lead to recovery, death or chronicity

after their entry into the host and thus may cause progressive damage. Such agents of disease are microbes, which include viruses, bacteria, fungi, and protozoa. Inflammation may also be caused by certain larger animal parasites. Because living agents are such important causes of inflammation, it is necessary to say a little more about the main types.

Living causes of inflammation

Viruses

Viruses are the smallest of all micro-organisms and cannot be seen with the ordinary microscope but the electron microscope has provided much information about their size and shape. Their size is measured in units called nanometres (nm).

In trying to imagine such small units it may help to remember that a small object that can be seen easily with the naked eye is probably about 1 millimetre (mm) in diameter. One-thousandth of a millimetre is a micrometre (μm) and a nanometre is one-thousandth of a micrometre. The largest viruses are 200 to 300 nm in diameter — the viruses that cause chickenpox and smallpox are about this size. The smallest viruses, for example the virus of foot-and-mouth disease, measure 20 to 25 nm in diameter. The chemical structure of viruses is distinctive. They contain only one of the two nucleic acids that are present in all the higher forms of living things. The two nucleic acids are deoxyribonucleic acid (DNA) and ribonucleic acid (RNA). The viruses that cause inflammation in man may contain one or the other of these nucleic acids but not both. Viruses have to enter the bodies of living cells in their hosts before they can multiply and cause damage. Their infectivity is very great.

Bacteria

Bacteria are microbes that differ from the animal cells that are classified as protozoa by having no recognizable nucleus although, unlike viruses, they contain both DNA and RNA. The vast majority of bacteria cause no disease in man or animals and live in the soil, water or on plants. Certain other bacteria live in great numbers in the intestines of all healthy people and, at least as long as they remain in the intestines, do not harm; but there are some bacteria that are pathogenic, that is, they cause disease. Bacteria can never be trusted to be harmless and all operations, and all dressing of wounds, must be carried out aseptically, especially as hospitals tend to harbour bacteria that have become resistant to antibiotics.

Bacteria can be seen with the microscope, and various ways of staining them with dyes make them much more easily seen. Some, the cocci, are spherical and are about 1 μm in diameter while many others, the bacilli, are rod-shaped being from 2 to 10 μm long and about 1 μm in diameter. Certain cocci cause acute inflammation in wounds and certain types of rod-shaped bacteria cause diseases such as diphtheria, gas **gangrene** and **anthrax**. The ordinary bacteria that live in the intestines are rod-shaped; in the intestines they are harmless, but if they escape into the peritoneal cavity or the urinary tract or contaminate a wound, they can cause severe inflammation. Most disease-producing bacteria can be grown artificially in the laboratory and their precise identification and the determination of their sensitivity to antibiotics is carried out on cultures prepared from the material sent to the laboratory.

Gas gangrene An infection with tissue necrosis and gas formation due to an organism of the Clostridia group.

Anthrax A very serious pustular, or more widespread, infection derived from cattle and sheep.

Fungi

Fungi form a large group of organisms and their appearance and size vary greatly; for example, yeasts, moulds, mushrooms and toadstools are all fungi. Tiny single-cell fragments of the network (the mycelium) that makes up the substance of most fungi, can survive when separated from the original colony of fungus and give rise to a new colony. Yeasts are fungi that do not form mycelium, and each cell is unattached to its neighbour. Yeasts reproduce by budding new cells that separate from the parent cells.

The dispersal of many types of fungi is facilitated by the formation of single-cell forms (spores) that are capable of reproducing the fungus and act rather as seed do for plants.

The chemical activities of fungi have many valuable uses, for example, yeasts are used in baking, wine-making and brewing, and the fungus *Penicillium notatum* is the source of the antibiotic penicillin. Certain fungi, however, are pathogenic and cause inflammatory disease in man and animals. Ringworm is a fungous infection of the skin, and actinomycosis is a serious chronic inflammatory fungous disease of the subcutaneous tissues and of internal organs.

Protozoa

The protozoa form a group of animals whose whole body consists of a single cell that contains everything necessary for the life of the animal. The word protozoa is a Greek word for primitive animals. Many of the creatures in this group live in water or the soil and are completely independent of man and other animals, but some cause human disease. They are all too small to be seen without a microscope, being for example about 20 to 30 μm in diameter, and, like the cells that make up the bodies of the more complex animals, have a nucleus and cytoplasm. The amoeba is an animal of this type. Its shape is always changing because it puts out extensions of itself, called pseudopodia, into which the rest of the body then flows, so that the whole cell moves gradually along. This type of amoeboid movement is seen also in the case of the white cells of the blood of man and animals when they migrate from the blood vessels into the more solid tissues of the body as part of the inflammatory reaction. One type of amoeba, the *Entamoeba histolytica,* is of medical importance for it invades human tissues to cause amoebic dysentery, a type of severe ulcerative inflammation of the colon. The microbes that cause the various types of malaria are also protozoa and they have a complicated life cycle that includes a stage when they live in the bodies of mosquitoes until they are ready to invade the blood cells of the next victim that is bitten by the infected mosquito.

Larger animal parasites

Animal parasites often have complicated life cycles that involve an adult stage in one type of animal and immature stages in some other species of animals. The adults are usually large enough to be seen with the naked eye but their eggs and the larvae that hatch from the eggs are microscopic. The adult parasite, for example a tapeworm several yards long in the small intestine of a man, provokes almost no inflammatory reaction but when the microscopic larval stages invade the body and migrate from place to place they provoke inflammation. The microscopic eggs of parasitic worms also provoke an inflammatory reaction which almost certainly assists in their discharge into the urine or faeces to contaminate soil or water and allow the larvae that hatch from the eggs to find new hosts in whom they can complete the next phase of their life cycle.

PATHOLOGY AND MANAGEMENT

Local signs of inflammation

The local signs of inflammation have been recognized since ancient times. They are redness, heat, swelling, pain and a change in the way that the affected organ or part works. Of these, pain is the most important and the least well understood. The redness, the heat, and the swelling all depend on changes in the walls of the blood vessels in the affected area and experimental studies have provided much information about these changes, but exact knowledge about the mechanism by which inflammation stimulates the nerves to cause pain is scanty. Movement increases pain, and total rest, with immobilization of the affected part, assists recovery.

Altered function

The altered way in which an inflamed organ functions varies from organ to organ, but a good example is provided by the behaviour of the mucous glands in inflamed mucous membranes. Normally such glands provide only the appropriate amount of mucus required to lubricate and protect the surface of the mucous membrane. But when the membrane becomes inflamed there is usually excessive secretion of watery fluid by the glands. The thin watery mucus that pours from the nose in the early stages of the common cold and the watery diarrhoea that accompanies inflammation of the mucous membrane of the colon are familiar examples.

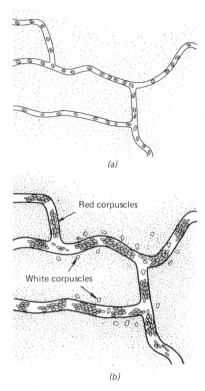

Figure 8.2. (*a*) Normal capillary blood vessels containing red blood corpuscles. (*b*) The same vessels as in (*a*) after the inflammatory response has caused dilatation, congestion and migration of white blood corpuscles

Reactions in the walls of vessels

The changes in the walls of small blood vessels that cause the redness, the heat and the swelling have been observed in great detail. The vessels that react are too small to be seen individually with the naked eye, they are capillaries and venules, but they can be watched in the living state with the microscope by various experimental techniques. Their reactions have been filmed, and the electron microscope has been used to study the minutest changes that occur in their walls. Such studies have shown that the very first reaction is momentary contraction of the arterioles causing transient pallor in the affected part, visible to the naked eye. This is followed by dilatation of the arterioles (*Figure 8.2*) so that the capillaries contain more blood which, at first, flows more rapidly and more strongly. This lasts for less than a minute and then the flow becomes sluggish and may stop completely; the whole area looks red. Spaces between the endothelial cells of the venules enlarge to allow protein molecules larger than those that normally pass through the vessel wall to escape, and the part becomes swollen because of the accumulation of protein-rich plasma that has passed through the walls of the vessels into the tissue spaces outside the vessels. This is inflammatory oedema, which combined with the increase in the amount of blood in the innumerable tiny vessels, causes the swelling. The increased blood in the vessels and the opening up of previously unfilled capillaries produce the redness.

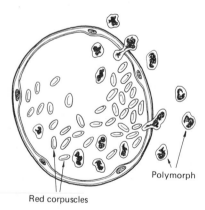

Figure 8.3. Migration of polymorphonuclear leucocytes through the walls of a capillary in inflammation

Migration of leucocytes

When the flow of blood in the capillaries in an area of inflammation has become sluggish the leucocytes of the blood, especially the polymorphonuclears, become much more conspicuous. They stick to the walls of the capillaries and venules and then migrate through them (*Figure 8.3*). The stimulus that makes the leucocytes migrate is a chemical one and, once the polymorphonuclear leucocytes have escaped from the vessels, the same stimulus makes them travel by a kind of liquid crawl, in which the cells enclosed by their membranes direct themselves through the tissues to reach the area that has been damaged where they become phagocytic. Phagocytosis means that the leucocytes take into their own cell bodies (their cytoplasm) the bacteria or other organisms that caused the damage, which then become surrounded by lysosomes, little packets of digestive enzymes, and are gradually dissolved.

Resolution

If inflammation does not progress to cause death of tissue, it is possible for a rapid return to normal, the cause of the inflammation having been eliminated by the natural defences of the body or by antibiotics. The flow of blood in the vessels returns to normal and the abnormal redness disappears. Fluid that has escaped from the vessels into the tissue spaces is drained away by the lymphatics and the swelling subsides. If the fluid in the tissues has coagulated to form a mesh of fibrin, there is liquefaction of the fibrin by the digestive action of leucocytes and by the activation of fibrinolysin, an enzyme derived from the plasma of the blood. The liquefied fibrin, like the other fluid in the tissue spaces, is removed by the lymphatics. Leucocytes in the tissue spaces, with the material that they have phagocytosed, also leave by the lymphatics and further digestion may be carried out by the cells lining the sinuses of the lymph nodes through which the lymph is carried on its way back to the circulation by way of the thoracic duct.

Suppuration and abscess formation

In severe inflammation the injury or infection kills a substantial amount of tissue and many of the phagocytic polymorphonuclear leucocytes die from the effects of their contact with the microbes. Their bodies are added to the accumulation of dead material in the area of most intense inflammation. Digestive enzymes from the dead leucocytes continue to act and the remains of the leucocytes and the dead tissue remnants are liquefied to form pus. The process has now reached the stage of suppuration. The most dangerous type of suppuration is diffuse and without a definite margin; if suppuration is limited by a defensive reaction at its margins, it forms an abscess.

An abscess is a collection of pus in a circumscribed cavity formed by the destruction or displacement of tissue. Pus is a turbid yellowish or green liquid, sometimes thin and very fluid, sometimes thick and viscid. If it is allowed to stand, it may separate into a layer of almost clear fluid similar to serum and a deposit of solid material. The solid material is made up of living and dead polymorphonuclear leucocytes, degenerate remains of the original tissue, and, usually, an abundance of the bacteria or other microbes that caused the inflammation. The colour of pus varies from creamy white to reddish yellow or bluish green. The colour depends upon the presence or absence of red blood cells and upon the presence or otherwise of the pigments that are produced by certain types of infecting microbes. During the acute stage of an inflammation it is quite common for red blood cells to escape from the vessels, a phenomenon named diapedesis. Red cells have no defensive function and their escape is incidental to the reactions of the vessel walls but in some inflammations red cells may escape in such numbers that the exudate may be almost as red as blood, a haemorrhagic type of inflammation. If pus formation follows such an inflammation, the pus may be reddish or rusty looking. If the inflammation has been caused by the *Staphylococcus aureus,* a common bacterial cause of inflammation, the golden pigment produced by the organism may colour the pus, while in infection by *Pseudomonas pyocyanea,* the bacteria produce a pigment that makes the pus look blue or greenish.

As has been mentioned earlier an inflamed part becomes swollen because of the escape of fluid from small blood vessels. As a rule the extravasated fluid coagulates on contact with the extravascular tissues to form a network of fibrin threads that form a pale yellowish layer on surfaces such as the outer coat of an inflamed appendix or the surface of a lung affected by pneumonia. In the subcutaneous tissues there is less marked coagulation of the fluid and it can be moved by pressure. The condition is one of inflammatory oedema and gentle firm pressure with a finger on the overlying skin leaves a depression that persists for some time after the pressure has been removed. This clinical sign of oedema is called 'pitting'.

If the inflammatory process has formed an abscess, the important clinical sign of fluctuation may be elicited. This is the transmission of a wave-like motion from one side to the other in a cavity with flexible walls filled with fluid; this can be felt clinically on gentle palpation.

By the time that pus has developed in the centre of an abscess, blood monocytes have begun to migrate from the blood vessels. They are even more effective at phagocytosis (*Figure 8.4*) than the polymorphonuclears and, unlike the polymorphonuclears, they remain phagocytic under the conditions of increasing acidity that accompany the development of an abscess. The monocytes phagocytose dead polymorphonuclears, bacteria, the red cells that have escaped from vessels and the fat droplets that are commonly left after damage to fatty tissue. An abscess may progress by further necrosis of its walls with increase in its purulent contents until some part of its walls gives way and allows the pus to escape. The escape may be to the surface of the skin, or, in the case of deep abscesses, into one of the body cavities or into some hollow organ. The release of pus through the skin usually causes marked improvement in the patient's general condition but rupture of an abscess into a body

Figure 8.4. Phagocytosis of bacteria by monocytes

cavity may spread the inflammation. Thus peritonitis may be produced if rupture occurs into the abdominal cavity, or **empyema**, in the case of rupture into the pleural cavity.

Repair and healing

If death of tissue has occurred, the damage stimulates the adjacent tissues to make good the loss to the best of their ability but the capacity for repair varies greatly in different tissues. Epithelial surfaces and fibrous connective tissue can regenerate very effectively. The nerve cells of the brain and spinal cord cannot regenerate at all and muscle, voluntary, smooth and cardiac, has such a limited capacity for regeneration that damage is usually made good by a fibrous scar instead of muscle. Bone, on the other hand, can replace large amounts of lost bone in a truly remarkable way.

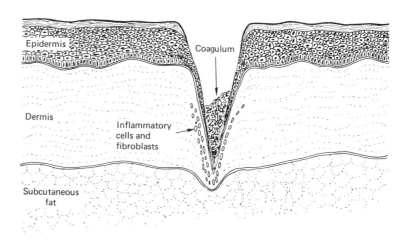

Figure 8.5. The migration of epidermal cells to the deepest parts of an incision through the skin at about 5 days after wounding

An incised wound without infection, in which the edges are kept together, heals by 'first intention'. Almost at once the deepest parts of the wound become filled by a coagulum formed by the fibrinogen of blood from the divided vessels which is converted to fibrin by contact with the injured tissues. The more superficial parts of the wound remain free from coagulum and during the 24 to 48 hours following the injury, epidermal cells, that is the epithelial cells that cover the skin, have been mobilized from the epidermis at the margins of the wound and begin to spread down the raw walls of the wound. They reach the deepest parts of the skin after 5 to 8 days (*Figure 8.5*). The migration of the epidermal

Empyema Pus in the pleural cavity.

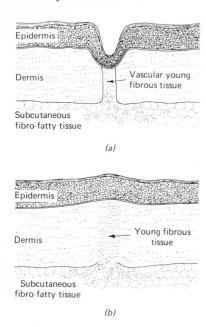

(a)

(b)

Figure 8.6. (*a*) Healed incised wound of the skin at about 14 days. (*b*) Healed incised wound of the skin after a month

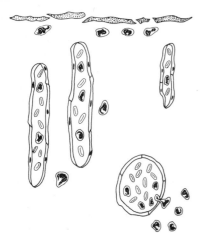

Figure 8.7. A microscopic section through granulation tissue, new capillary vessels are present in the background of fibrin and ground substance. Polymorphonuclear leucocytes are migrating from the vessels

cells is produced by amoeboid movement but the moving cells never lose contact with their neighbours and a membrane, one cell thick, spreads over the raw surfaces. The supply of cells to form the membrane is mainly by a sliding effect in which the stratified epithelial cells at the margins move from being piled one upon the other in many layers into a single cell layer in which each flattened cell lies alongside its neighbours, the cells being attached only at their edges. The effect is similar to that of spreading a pack of cards from the stacked position to an arrangement with each card upon the table with its edges in contact with adjacent cards. When the membrane of migrating cells meets a similar membrane from the other edge of the wound, the two membranes unite and the cells of both membranes travel no farther. Once the epithelial cells have ceased their migration they divide to form new cells that gradually pile up into layers. In the meantime, immature connective tissue cells in the subcutaneous tissue have begun to multiply and during the 10 to 15 days following the damage newly formed cellular fibrous tissue begins to grow into the space that the wound has created and in doing so pushes the epithelium that has spread down to cover the lips of the wound back to the surface (*Figure 8.6a*), often leaving residual clumps of epithelial cells in the depths of the wound or in the tracts left by stitches. After about a month the wound has been filled by vascular fibrous tissue and the epidermis has been lifted slightly above the level of the original skin surface (*Figure 8.6b*). During the months that follow, the immature connective tissue cells (the fibroblasts) in the young scar lay down collagen fibres that become bound together and contract to obliterate the vessels and leave, eventually, a white avascular scar of mature collagenous fibrous tissue.

When an injury, either suppurative or traumatic, has left a large defect, healing is much slower because much more reparative tissue has to be produced. In areas of mobile skin, however, the size of the injury is sometimes much reduced by contraction. The phenomenon of contraction is due to the migration of fibroblastic cells within the skin that surrounds the wound, the so-called picture-frame area, and contraction is sometimes so effective that a defect may be reduced by 80 per cent of its size. The remaining gap has to be filled by granulation tissue. Granulation tissue is the precursor of fibrous scar tissue. It consists of fibroblasts, primitive connective tissue cells produced by undifferentiated connective tissue cells in the subcutaneous tissues, and new blood vessels (*Figure 8.7*). The new blood vessels appear as buds or sprouts from undamaged capillary vessels at the margins of the wound. Fibroblasts and capillaries accompany

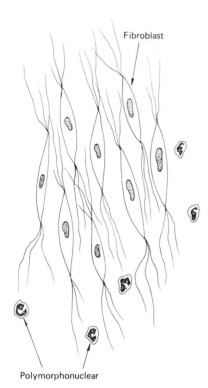

Fibroblast

Polymorphonuclear

Figure 8.8. Fibroblasts and polymorpho-nuclear leucocytes

each other as they grow into the coagulated blood on the floor of the wound. The tips of the new vessels unite with the tips of adjacent new vessels to produce loops through which blood can flow, and from which blood monocytes migrate to phagocytose damaged cells and digest the coagulum of blood that is being penetrated by the granulation tissue. The cells of the new capillary loops multiply so that the loops lengthen until, along with their accompanying fibroblasts, they have filled the cavity of the wound. The fibroblasts (*Figure 8.8*) between the capillary vessels align themselves in the direction of the fibrous tissue cells of the original skin and lay down collagen fibres that become bound together by mucinous material.

When the defect in the deeper tissues has been reduced as much as possible by contraction and the remaining space has been filled by granulation tissue, the epithelial cells at the margins, which have been spreading themselves from their layered arrangement into a much larger single cell layer from the edges towards the centre of the defect, usually succeed in covering the raw surface. As soon as they meet the layer of cells spreading from other parts of the edges of the defect, their migration ceases. Simultaneously, the growing granulation tissue, having been covered by a layer of epithelium, ceases to grow and gradually matures into avascular scar tissue similar to that of an incised wound.

When the raw surface is very large the spreading out of the layered epithelial cells at the margins may not be sufficient to provide a covering. Healing may then be delayed, for epithelial cells that are migrating cannot reproduce themselves and if no more marginal cells are available, it may take a very long time for new epithelial cells to be produced. In such cases grafts of epithelium will often supply much needed new epithelial cells. In the case of the large raw areas caused by burning, it often happens that sweat glands, which are relatively deeply situated in the subcutaneous fat, escape destruction by the heat and provide sources from which epithelial cells can spread. It is usual for granulation tissue to be mixed with cells that are the aftermath of the inflammatory process and, if the inflammatory process has passed into a stage of chronicity, active inflammation and the formation of granulation tissue may go on simultaneously so that there is destruction of the leading margin of the zone of granulation tissue by the still active inflammatory process. A balance between the two processes can sometimes exist for years as in a chronic peptic ulcer in which the healing process and the destructive process exist simultaneously with destruction dominating at times of active ulceration, and the healing process dominating during phases of remission of the disease.

The cells of chronic inflammation

When inflammation has lasted for more than a few days, new cells appear among the polymorphonuclears and monocytes on the scene. Lymphocytes migrate from the blood vessels and, after having migrated, certain lymphocytes become transformed into plasma cells, so called because of their pear-like shape which suggests that their form must have been squeezed or moulded. Plasma cells are concerned with the formation of antibody, a most important type of immune response. Eosinophil leucocytes, so called because they contain granules that stain vividly with the red stain eosin, migrate from the blood vessels. The function of the eosinophils is not clear. Giant cells may be formed by the coalescence of monocytes to produce a single cell with a much enlarged cytoplasm in which the nuclei of the original cells persist. The function of the multinucleated giant cells is to engulf particles that are too large to be tackled by a single phagocyte. Multinucleated giant cells are found when foreign material, a suture for example, is present, or when the area has been contaminated by insoluble particles of vegetable, mineral or lipoidal material, and, for this reason, they are called foreign body giant cells.

The chemical mediators of inflammation

In spite of the many diverse and unrelated injuries that initiate the inflammatory reaction the changes that follow the onset are, nevertheless, stereotyped. The probable explanation is that the injury, whatever its nature, acts as no more than a trigger and that the actual vascular and cellular responses depend upon the liberation, from the injured cells and tissues, of chemical substances that are the actual causes of the inflammation. A number of substances that will cause some of the changes of inflammation have already been identified and there is a strong suspicion that the earliest changes are in the jelly-like material in which most tissue cells are embedded. Changes in the degree of its acidity and an increase in its fluidity have been noted among the earliest responses to injury. The chemical mediators already recognized include histamine, serotonin (5-hydroxytryptamine) bradykinin and prostaglandins, but other mediators, as yet unrecognized, undoubtedly exist.

Failure of the local inflammatory reaction

The inflammatory response may be delayed or fail completely in shock. In shock there is failure of the peripheral circulation with paralysis of the small vessels that are responsible for the inflammatory reaction and, if bacterial infection occurs during a period of shock, the bacteria can proliferate in the tissues without hindrance from the leucocytes that would ordinarily migrate to prevent their survival or delay their multiplication.

The adrenal cortical hormones have a direct suppressive effect upon most of the cells concerned in inflammation and when patients are receiving large doses of such hormones (the **steroid** drugs) they are quite abnormally vulnerable to infections that they would normally overcome with little in the way of symptoms. Also in Cushing's syndrome, in which there is excessive secretion of cortisol (hydrocortisone) by the adrenal cortex, there is also abnormal vulnerability to infections that would ordinarily be trivial.

Diseases that cause abnormalities in the number and maturity of the leucocytes of the blood also make patients liable to infections by organisms that would be incapable of producing disease in a person with normal leucocytes. Thus patients with leukaemia, Hodgkin's disease, lymphosarcoma, agranulocytosis, aplastic anaemia and myelofibrosis may all have inadequate defence against infection and may, moreover, be receiving steroid drugs that further reduce their capacity to produce an effective inflammatory response.

Certain virus infections, especially in the respiratory tract, reduce the capacity of the mucous membranes to resist bacterial infection and there is an inherited abnormality of the immunological reactions, the condition of **hypogammaglobulinaemia**, that causes abnormal susceptibility to infections.

Granulomatous inflammations

In addition to the type of inflammation that begins acutely and then passes into a chronic phase, there is an important group of inflammatory diseases that are chronic from the outset. Pain may not be a feature, at least in the early stages, and the presence of a lump may be the first abnormality to be noticed. The name granuloma, meaning a tumour of granulation tissue, is given to such a swelling. Most of the granulomas are due to infections but chemical irritants, beryllium for example, may also produce granulomatous disease.

Tuberculosis is one of the most important of the granulomatous diseases. In this disease the characteristic cellular reaction takes about a month to develop. The mycobacteria that cause tuberculosis have a covering of wax-like material that provokes the most characteristic parts of the reaction. When the bacteria that cause tuberculosis enter the tissues of the body, the first reaction in patients that have

Steroid A class of chemical compound including sex hormones, adrenal cortical hormones, cholesterol and cholic acid. They all have a nucleus of joined carbon rings.

Hypogammaglobulinaemia Low level of a serum protein fraction, the gamma globulins, and usually, therefore, a low antibody level.

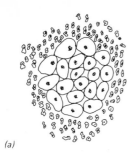

(a)

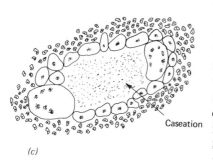

Langhans'
giant cell

(b)

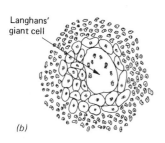

Caseation

(c)

Figure 8.9. (*a*) A tubercle with central epithelioid cells surrounded by lymphocytes. (*b*) Epithelioid cells have coalesced to form Langhans' giant cell. (*c*) The central part of the tubercle is undergoing caseous necrosis

Actinomycosis A chronic inflammatory disease due to infection with a fungus, *Actinomyces israelii.*

Amoebic dysentery An inflammatory disease of the bowel due to infection with the organism, *Entamoeba histolytica.*

had no previous contact with the organisms, is a migration of polymorphonuclear leucocytes from the vessels without escape of fluid or dilatation of the vessels to cause redness. The polymorphonuclears phagocytose the bacteria but fail to kill them and, in fact, die themselves leaving the still surviving bacteria to be dealt with by monocytes. The monocytes are more durable but their contact with the bacteria alters their appearance in a characteristic way to produce cells described as 'epithelioid cells' that accumulate in clumps. The clumps of epithelioid cells enlarge until the clumps, though not of course the individual cells, can be seen with the naked eye as greyish pin-head-sized tubercles that give the name tuberculosis to the disease. Some of the cells in the tubercles coalesce to form giant cells that have multiple nuclei arranged in a crescent just inside the boundary of the cytoplasm. A giant cell with this appearance is a Langhans' giant cell because a Swiss pathologist called Langhans first described that type of cell. As monocytes are clumping and changing their appearance to form tubercles, lymphocytes accumulate around the edges of the tubercles and at this stage the central parts of the tubercles undergo 'caseation' (*Figure 8.9*). Caseation is necrosis of a type that produces a soft cream-cheese-like white material that looks, even with the naked eye, quite different from the pus that forms in suppuration. The onset of caseation in tuberculosis coincides with the development of the delayed type of hypersensitivity and depends upon the presence of sensitized lymphocytes. If caseation involves the skin over an area of tuberculous infection, a tuberculous sinus to the surface may develop. Such sinuses were common when tuberculosis of lymph nodes in the neck was commonly caused by milk from tuberculous cows. The discharge from such sinuses is infective and the mycobacteria of tuberculosis can usually be identified bacteriologically in the discharge. If, however, as sometimes happens, the organisms of tuberculosis cannot be identified in the discharge, the finding of the characteristic microscopic changes in a sample of tissue may be an important diagnostic clue.

Tuberculosis is still probably the most important of the granulomatous diseases but granulomatous inflammation may be produced by viruses, which cause, for example, lymphogranuloma inguinale and cat scratch disease; or bacteria, which cause, for example, syphilis, yaws and leprosy; or fungi which cause **actinomycosis**; and protozoa, which cause **amoebic dysentery**. Non-infective irritants can also cause granulomatous disease, for example when they are inhaled, or contaminate wounds as may happen when somebody is cut by fragments of a radio valve that contains beryllium.

The general responses in inflammation

The general reactions in inflammation are complex and include elevation of the body temperature (fever), leucocytosis (an increase in the number of white corpuscles circulating in the blood), and the development of immunity.

Fever

An increase in body temperature is usual in inflammation. This response to inflammation is most marked in the young and is inconstant in the aged. Certain types of infection cause characteristic fluctuations in the patient's temperature and in such cases the temperature chart may be almost diagnostic. One type of malaria is an example of such an infection. The minor variations in body temperature that occur at different times of the day and at the time of ovulation in women are much less than the response to infection and are unlikely to be confused with it. When there has been extensive necrosis of tissue, however, such as occurs in **coronary thrombosis** with infarction of the myocardium, fever similar to that of infection may occur.

The temperature of the body is regulated by groups of nerve cells in the hypothalamic region of the brain that are sensitive to chemical substances that circulate in the blood. Such substances are called pyrogens and when blood carrying pyrogens reaches the sensitive hypothalamic nerve cells these send messages by the motor nerves of the blood vessels of the skin. The result is constriction of the skin vessels with reduction of heat loss by the skin, and a corresponding rise in temperature. The circulating pyrogens are derived from two sources: one 'exogenous', that is from a source other than the patient's own tissues, and one 'endogenous', that is from the patient's own tissues.

In most cases of bacterial inflammation, the febrile response is due to the combined effects of exogenous and endogenous pyrogens but endogenous pyrogen can also be liberated without the action of exogenous pyrogen from muscle and accounts for the fever that may accompany cardiac infarction.

Leucocytosis

Certain infective inflammations may cause a marked increase in the number of circulating leucocytes, with white cell counts of 15 000 to 30 000 per mm^3 blood, instead of the normal number which is between 5000 and 10 000 per mm^3. The increase is nearly always due to an increase in the polymorphonuclear leucocytes (the granulocytes) and because of the circulation of the blood, more polymorphonuclear cells reach the site of the inflammation to combat the infection.

Coronary thrombosis The obstruction of a coronary artery by a thrombus; this may cause death of the area of heart muscle that becomes deprived of blood (a myocardial infarct).

The increased number of white cells in the blood, at least in its early stages, is due to the liberation of mature polymorphonuclears from the bone marrow in which there is normally a large reserve of mature polymorphs. If the inflammation lasts more than a few days, the bone marrow increases its production of polymorphs and recognizably young leucocytes appear in the circulation. Certain special infections do not stimulate a leucocytosis although they may cause severe inflammation at the seat of the disease; they may even depress the number of circulating leucocytes. These special infections include typhoid fever, measles, infective hepatitis, chickenpox, and some types of tuberculosis.

An increase of lymphocytes above the normal maximum of 4500 per mm³ blood is rare except in glandular fever.

The development of immunity

There are two types of immune response: humoral immunity and cell-mediated immunity.

In humoral immunity the penetration of the body by bacteria, or their toxins, the entry of viruses, and of various proteins, and sometimes other chemical substances, leads to the appearance of neutralizing substances in the blood plasma. These are antibodies and, although an infinite number of significantly different varieties can be produced in response to the entry of different substances, all antibodies are closely related chemically and form the group of immunoglobulins. Each immunoglobulin antibody will combine absolutely specifically with the substance, the antigen, that stimulated its formation. In the case of a toxin, the union makes the toxin harmless. In the case of bacteria whose previous entry has stimulated the formation of antibody, the combination of antibody with subsequently invading bacteria of the same type makes them ineffective, and easy prey for the leucocytes.

The formation of antibody is one of the functions of the lymphocytes. Lymphocytes are not formed in the bone marrow, as are the polymorphonuclears, but develop in masses of lymphocyte-forming tissue situated in the lymph nodes, the thymus gland and in the submucosa of the alimentary and respiratory tracts. They migrate from these areas of lymphoid tissue into the bloodstream in which they circulate for a few hours before leaving it again to return to the lymphoid tissue, while other lymphocytes take their places in the bloodstream so that the number of lymphocytes circulating in the blood remains fairly constant. The capacity to form antibody as a result of contact with a foreign antigen is not present in all lymphocytes but only in those that have been derived embryologically from the submucosal lymphoid tissues of the fetal alimentary canal. Moreover, the formation of antibody coincides with changes in the microscopic appearances of these lymphocytes. They take up their position near the site of the inflammation and in the lymph nodes adjacent to it and, as they form antibody, they change their appearance and become transformed into plasma cells (*Figure 8.10*).

Lymphocytes

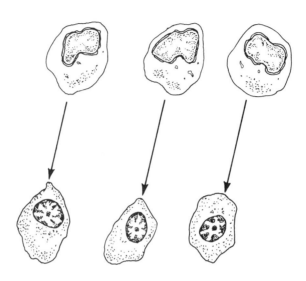

Plasma cells

Figure 8.10. The transformation of lymphocytes into plasma cells that takes place when lymphocytes are stimulated to produce antibody

Because of an inherited abnormality, certain individuals fail to form antibody to the normal extent. This condition is called hypogammaglobulinaemia and people with this condition are abnormally liable to infections.

The cell-mediated immune response does not depend upon the presence of antibody in the plasma but upon the presence of sensitized lymphocytes. Such lymphocytes cause a state of hypersensitivity to an originally harmless substance that has acted as an antigen. When such a substance enters the tissues of somebody whose lymphocytes have been sensitized by previous contact with that substance there will be a marked inflammatory reaction. The lymphocytes concerned with this type of immune reaction differ in their embryological origin from the lymphocytes concerned with the formation of circulating antibody and are derived from the fetal thymus gland. Hypersensitive inflammatory reactions of the cell-mediated type are of importance in granulomatous disease, especially in tuberculosis, in the rejection of grafted organs, and in the auto-immune group of diseases — diseases in which the patient develops an immune type of inflammatory reaction against his own tissues.

Amyloid disease

When inflammatory disease has lasted for many years amyloid disease may develop. The inflammation may be of the suppurative type as in chronic osteomyelitis or bronchiectasis or it may be non-suppurative as in rheumatoid arthritis. In amyloid disease an abnormal substance coated with immuno-globulins is laid down in the walls of blood vessels and in the supporting tissues of many organs. In certain organs amyloid is very damaging. In the kidneys, for example, it may cause the nephrotic syndrome, or lead to renal failure.

There is also an inherited metabolic abnormality in certain people that makes them liable to develop amyloid disease without preceding chronic inflammation. This is the so-called primary type of amyloid disease.

9 Tumours

A. H. Cruickshank

INTRODUCTION

Cells in many parts of the body reproduce themselves by division throughout life, and in tissues from which there is a continuous loss of cells active proliferation is necessary to make good the losses. Such cellular proliferation occurs, for example, in the skin, the bone marrow and in the mucous membranes not only while a young person is growing but also throughout adult life. Normally such proliferation is controlled and does not exceed what is required for maintenance; the loss of control gives rise to tumours. Living growing cells are also the essential units of a tumour. Such cells are descendants of normal ones but have undergone modification that usually makes them continue to divide and reproduce themselves in excess of the needs for cellular replacement to such an extent that sooner or later a mass develops and causes symptoms. Because tumour cells are the descendants of normal cells they resemble their ancestors and therefore the classification of tumours depends upon the recognition of the type of normal cell from which the tumour originated. If the resemblance to the normal cells of origin is close, the tumour is said to be well differentiated and, in general, such tumours are benign. If the tumour cells have lost much of their resemblance to the cells from which they had their origin, the tumour is said to be poorly differentiated, or anaplastic. In general, anaplastic tumours behave malignantly.

The change from a normal cell into a tumour cell is irreversible and the tumour cells reproduce themselves to form a colony of permanently altered cells. It is rare for such cells to lie dormant and as a rule they proliferate more or less rapidly. Because the essential change in a cell or cells can sometimes take place without immediate proliferation and enlargement of the affected area, it is perhaps more accurate to refer to the irreversible change as neoplasia, which does not necessarily imply enlargement. The ordinary behaviour of a tumour, however, is to enlarge progressively without the establishment of any equilibrium with the other tissues of the host and with no limit to its progress. A tumour is thus autonomous and independent of the influences that control the replacement of cells in normal tissues and it can continue to increase in size even when the host is suffering from starvation. According to Berenblum (1962), a tumour is thus 'a cellular tissue in which the normal growth-controlling mechanism is permanently impaired, permitting progressive growth'. Although it is difficult to provide a definition that takes into account all the academic information that is available about tumours, most tumours are easily recognized clinically and pathologically. It is of far greater practical importance to differentiate between simple (benign) and malignant tumours.

While it is true that there is a spectrum of tumours with all intermediate grades between simplicity and malignancy, most tumours can be classified, more or less satisfactorily, as being either simple or malignant and the outstanding difference is that simple tumours remain at their site of origin while malignant tumours disseminate the cells of which they are composed to sites distant from the original tumour. This is the process of metastasis by which new colonies of tumour cells form secondary tumours in organs and tissues quite remote from the site of the original tumour. The outstanding task in the surgical treatment of cancer is to eradicate the tumour before metastatic spread has occurred. The extent of the excision that may be necessary should follow the most accurate possible identification of the tumour and consideration of the known behaviour of tumours of that type.

Terminology

The names of most tumours, both simple and malignant, have the ending '-oma'. The first part of the name usually indicates the tissue of origin of the tumour or gives some kind of description of the tumour. The suffix '-oma' is Greek for a tumour and many of the first parts of the names of tumours are also Greek, but Latin and other names have also been linked to the ending '-oma'. 'Cancer' is not a precise term. It was originally the Latin equivalent of the Greek 'carcinoma' but it is now commonly used to include all the malignant tumours. Carcinoma, from Greek words meaning crab and tumour, perhaps because of the crab-like shape of one of the common types of carcinoma (*Figure 9.1*), is used for all the malignant tumours that arise from the epithelial cells covering the skin, the lining of the air passages and the alimentary canal, and forming the glands that secrete into the ducts opening on to these surfaces. The malignant tumours that originate from the cells of fibrous connective tissue, muscle, bone, cartilage and the cells of the lymphoid organs are sarcomas.

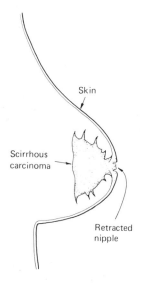

Skin

Scirrhous carcinoma

Retracted nipple

Figure 9.1. A drawing of the naked eye appearance of a slice through a cancer of the breast to show the shape that may have suggested a crab and given rise to the name 'cancer'

SIMPLE (BENIGN) TUMOURS

No simple tumour gives rise to metastatic (secondary) deposits of tumour at a distance from the site of the primary tumour. The danger of simple tumours depends upon effects such as, pressure, obstruction or the abnormal amounts of secretion that a glandular tumour may produce. In many sites, too, simple tumours project enough to become injured, with the formation of bleeding ulcers on their surface. They nearly all have a strong resemblance microscopically to the tissue from which they originated. A lipoma, for example, is indistinguishable histologically from the normal fat in which it arose, and can be recognized only by its having formed a lump of fat where no lump should be. It is of no diagnostic importance, but of great interest, that a lipoma does not shrink if its host becomes emaciated and the histologically similar normal fat almost disappears. Because simple tumours nearly always resemble their tissue of origin microscopically they can usually be classified according to their origin. The following are some of the well recognized types of simple tumour.

Tumours of epithelium

If the epithelium covering a surface such as the urinary, alimentary or respiratory tracts, produces a benign tumour, the tumour usually projects on the surface and is called a papilloma because it has a certain resemblance to a nipple (*papilla* in Latin) (*Figure 9.2*). In fact, not all papillomas

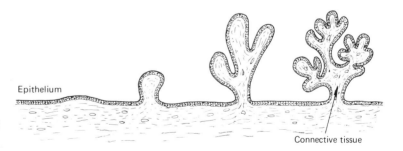

Epithelium

Connective tissue

Figure 9.2. Stages in the development of a papilloma

resemble a nipple and several different types of shape may occur. A broad-based papilloma is said to be sessile (Latin *sessilis*, sitting), while one with a narrow stalk is said to have a pedicle (in Latin, a little foot). If a papilloma is made up of a number of projecting processes each of which has a central delicate core of fibrous tissue and blood vessels covered by epithelium the papilloma is said to be villous (Latin *villi*, shaggy hairs). The name epithelioma is not used for simple epithelial tumours, for epithelioma has come to mean a type of a malignant epithelial tumour of the skin for which a more precise name is squamous cell carcinoma.

Adenoma

Adenoma is the name for a simple tumour of glandular tissue. Such a tumour develops as a lump in glandular organs or may project on a surface that is lubricated by the secretions of glands. Adenomas develop in endocrine glands such as the thyroid, where they appear as a lump or nodule in the substance of the gland or in the secreting glandular epithelium lining an organ like the uterus or colon where they tend to project into the cavity of the organ, sometimes on quite a well developed stalk (*Figure 9.3*). Any tumour with a stalk

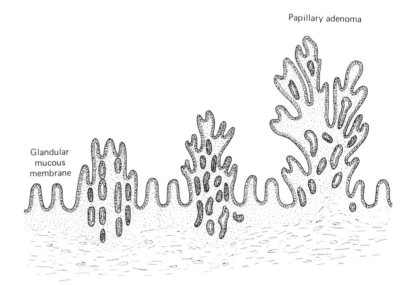

Papillary adenoma

Glandular mucous membrane

Figure 9.3. Diagram of the microscopic stages in the development of a papillary adenoma of a mucous membrane

may be described as a polyp and the name polyp does not indicate what microscopic structure the tumour may have. Adenomas resemble the normal glandular tissue from which they arise and, like the parent tissue, they secrete (*Figure 9.4*). On a surface the secretion may be discharged and escape but in a deep situation secretion may accumulate within the adenoma forming fluid-filled cavities and making the adenoma into a cystadenoma. If there are marked projections of the secreting tumour cells into the cystic spaces, the tumour may be described as a papillary cystadenoma. Mucus is the secretion most likely to accumulate in a cystadenoma and the presence of much retained mucus may provoke quite a marked inflammatory reaction. In the case of endocrine glands, whose secretions (hormones) pass into the blood, a secreting

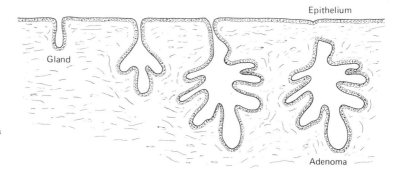

Figure 9.4. Diagrammatic representation of the stages in the development of an adenoma that does not project to form a polyp. Low magnification

adenoma can cause dramatic changes in the general health and illnesses, such as, **Cushing's syndrome**, thyrotoxicosis, and **acromegaly** are often due to secreting adenomas: of the adrenal cortex in the case of Cushing's syndrome, the thyroid in thyrotoxicosis, and the pituitary in acromegaly. An adenoma of the tiny parathyroid glands may, through its secretions, cause widespread disease of the skeleton, with weakening of the bones, or, because an excess of calcium is excreted in the urine, form **calculi** in the urinary passages.

Non-epithelial tumours

Simple tumours develop also in non-epithelial tissues of the body. Thus the supporting tissues give rise to tumours such as a fibroma, from fibrous connective tissue, chondroma, from cartilage, and osteoma, from bone. The common lipoma of fatty tissue has already been mentioned. Some tumours may contain an epithelial and a connective tissue component as, for example, in fibroadenoma of the breast, a common benign tumour in young women.

Muscle, especially smooth muscle, commonly gives rise to simple tumours. A tumour of muscle is a myoma and if the tissue of origin is smooth muscle, then the name leiomyoma, meaning smooth muscle tumour, is given. Leiomyomas are common in the smooth muscle of the uterus; they are less common in that of the alimentary canal and turn up only occasionally in other sites where smooth muscle is normally found. Rhabdomyoma, or striped muscle tumour, is very rare indeed which is perhaps surprising in view of the large amount of striped (voluntary) muscle present in the body. Nerve cells usually in the ganglia of the sympathetic nervous system may give rise to a tumour of well differentiated nerve cells, a ganglioneuroma, and the supporting cells of the central nervous system, the glial cells, can give rise to a whole group of tumours, the gliomas, some of which are well differentiated and histologically benign, and others of which are histologically malignant, while the fibrous sheaths of nerves give rise

Cushing's syndrome A disease produced by excess production of steroids from the adrenal cortex characterized by obesity of the face and trunk, abdominal striae, hypertension and the presence of glucose in urine.

Acromegaly A disease characterized by progressive enlargement of the bones of the head, chest, hands and feet.

Calculus A stone.

to neurofibromas. Tumours of blood vessels (haemangiomas) and of lymphatic vessels (lymphangiomas) also occur but most of these are not true neoplasms although they form lumps clinically and have names that are similar to those of tumours. Many of the angiomas are really malformations of blood or lymph vessels and do not have the quality of autonomy that is the characteristic of a true neoplasm. The name hamartoma, from a Greek word meaning an error, is sometimes given to malformations that cause tumour-like lumps.

MALIGNANT TUMOURS

Most malignant tumours except those of the nervous system, can be classified as carcinomas (arising from epithelial cells) or sarcomas (arising from tissues other than epithelium). Carcinomas are much commoner than sarcomas.

Carcinoma

Carcinomas arise in the type of epithelium that also gives rise to the simple epithelial tumours and the various types of simple tumours usually have a malignant counterpart.

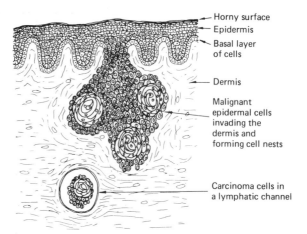

Horny surface
Epidermis
Basal layer of cells

Dermis

Malignant epidermal cells invading the dermis and forming cell nests

Carcinoma cells in a lymphatic channel

Figure 9.5. Drawing of the microscopic appearances of a squamous carcinoma of the skin

Carcinomas are classified according to the microscopic characters of the epithelium from which they have arisen. Thus the carcinomas that arise from surfaces covered by flattened layers of epithelial cells, such as, the epithelium of the skin, lips, mouth, tongue, lower pharynx, and oesophagus, are of cells that retain some at least of the characters of the parent epithelial cells. Such carcinomas are squamous carcinomas (*Figure 9.5*). Other sites covered by squamous epithelium that are liable to develop squamous carcinoma are the anal canal and the vaginal part of the cervix uteri. The

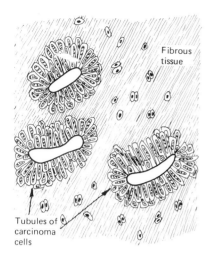

Figure 9.6. Microscopic appearances of an adenocarcinoma. The carcinoma cells are arranged in tubules with a central channel

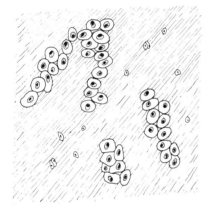

Figure 9.7. Microscopic appearances of an undifferentiated scirrhous carcinoma with irregular rows of carcinoma cells embedded in fibrous tissue

Figure 9.8. In this photomicrograph of a carcinoma the dark groups of cells are poorly differentiated cancer cells and the brighter areas are the fibrous reaction which has been provoked. (Stained by haematoxylin and eosin and magnified X 150)

vagina itself, though lined by stratified squamous epithelium, is a rare site for squamous carcinoma. In addition to the sites where squamous epithelium is normally present, certain sites lined by columnar or transitional epithelium sometimes also develop squamous carcinoma. Such a change of cellular character is called metaplasia; it can occur without being associated with the development of a tumour but is relatively common in malignant tumours. Carcinoma of the bronchial epithelium, normally columnar ciliated epithelium, is commonly a squamous carcinoma and a similar squamous metaplasia is not infrequent in carcinomas of the urinary tract. Carcinomas of the epithelium lining the stomach and colon and of many glandular organs such as the breast or the pancreas, are of columnar cells and tend to produce a type of tubular or acinar (berry-like) structure that resembles that of a normal gland (*Figure 9.6*). Carcinomas with this structure are adenocarcinomas, and quite commonly they secrete mucus. Carcinomas on a surface sometimes project and have a papillary arrangement. Such a pattern may be present in either a squamous carcinoma or a carcinoma of columnar cells, but in addition to projecting they also invade the base to which they are attached. Quite commonly there is little projection on the surface and much invasion with death of the central parts that leads to ulceration. The carcinoma then appears as an ulcer with edges that are thickened, rounded and firm or even very hard because the infiltrating carcinoma cells provoke an inflammatory reaction of the chronic type with lymphocytes and fibroblasts that mature and lay down collagenous fibrous tissue. The fibrous reaction around invading clumps of carcinoma cells is illustrated in *Figures 9.7* and *9.8*. It is this reaction against the invasion of the

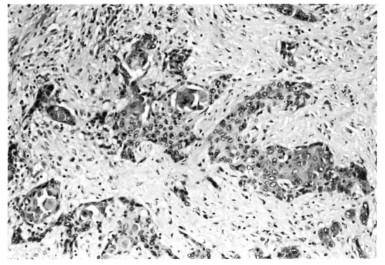

I

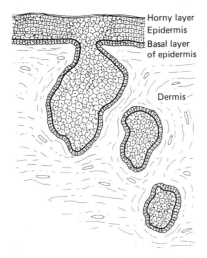

Horny layer
Epidermis
Basal layer
of epidermis

Dermis

Figure 9.9. Diagrammatic drawing of the microscopic appearances of a basal cell carcinoma of the skin with invasion of the dermis by groups of epithelial cells from the basal layers of the epidermis. Later the tumour would ulcerate to form a rodent ulcer

tumour that is responsible for the sensation of hardness that is felt on handling a carcinoma. But carcinomas are not invariably hard; some of the most malignant ones seem to cause little fibrous reaction. Hardness is important however in suggesting that an ulcer or a lump, especially a lump in the breast, is malignant. The hardness is often so marked that it suggests stone and the carcinoma is said to be scirrhous or stone-like. Carcinomas that have not provoked a scirrhous reaction may be so soft as to suggest brain tissue and these are said to be encephaloid or brain-like. Another name used to describe a soft carcinoma is 'medullary' because of a resemblance to bone marrow or spinal cord.

Rodent ulcer

A rodent ulcer, is a special type of carcinoma of the skin in which the malignant cells seem to be related to the cells of the basal layer of the epidermis (*Figure 9.9*). The cells of a rodent ulcer show some tendency to form structures with a resemblance to hair follicles, but never form hairs, and are less dangerous than an ordinary carcinoma (squamous epithelioma) of the skin for although they form a malignant ulcer, hence the name rodent or gnawing ulcer, and may be very destructive, they do not spread to distant organs to form metastatic colonies.

Metastatic spread of carcinomas

All truly malignant tumours invade and infiltrate the anatomical structures that are close by and in doing so, almost inevitably, lymphatic channels and blood vessels are penetrated by the tumour. Sometimes the vessels become obliterated by thrombosis of the lymph or blood that they contain but even this does not prevent the spread of the tumour along the channels. Carcinoma has a special tendency to penetrate lymphatic vessels. It seems that sometimes the carcinoma cells, having entered the lymphatic vessel, are carried by the flow of fluid lymph to the nearest lymph node through which the lymph is filtered and there is another, slower, way in which spread of carcinoma by the lymphatics can occur. In this the lymphatic vessel becomes filled with thrombosed lymph in which the carcinoma cells survive and grow as a solid cord along the thrombus; this is spread by lymphatic permeation. In most carcinomas, spread by the lymphatics happens earlier than spread by the blood vessels, and sometimes the carcinoma may kill by, for example, its obstructive effects without spread other than to the lymph nodes that receive the drainage from the site of the tumour.

Although carcinoma seems to have a special tendency to spread by lymphatics it spreads also by the blood vessels.

Because carcinoma invades locally it penetrates the walls of the veins in its vicinity and carcinoma cells that have penetrated a vein may be carried as single cells or small clumps of cells, usually with some fibrin thrombus around them, to the next capillary bed through which the blood must pass. Here the clumps become jammed in the capillaries and remain to reproduce themselves and give rise to a metastasis or secondary carcinomatous colony. Carcinoma cells travelling singly, however, may pass through the capillaries of the liver or the lungs, reach the arterial circulation and be carried to any organ of the body. It is rare for carcinoma cells to penetrate the relatively thick wall of arteries and most of the dissemination of carcinoma by the bloodstream is believed to follow the penetration of the walls of veins. Thrombosis of blood within a vein that has been penetrated by carcinoma sometimes occurs and then there may be permeation of the thrombus by carcinoma cells sometimes for a distance of several centimeters, as may happen when a carcinoma of the kidney permeates thrombus in the renal vein. Later portions of the mixture of thrombus and carcinoma cells break off to form emboli containing enough carcinomatous cells to form large secondary tumours very quickly in the lungs.

It is almost certain that a number of the cells that escape from a carcinoma to be spread by the lymphatics or by the blood are destroyed when they lodge in a new site. The host develops a certain amount of immunity with circulating antibody against the tumour cells and activated lymphocytes may form a barrier against the invading cells. It is rare for such resistance to be completely successful and lymph nodes in spite of all their immunological capabilities are a common site for secondary carcinoma. The spleen, however, seems to have a high resistance to the development of secondary carcinoma and it is unusual to find deposits of secondary carcinoma in the spleen even in cases where most of the other major organs contain blood-borne deposits of secondary carcinoma.

Certain organs are particularly liable to be involved by blood dissemination of carcinoma; the liver and the lungs are such organs. Carcinoma is common in the stomach and in the colon. The veins from both these organs drain to the portal vein which carries blood to the sinusoidal system of vessels within the liver. It is thus not surprising that the liver is a common site for blood-borne secondary carcinoma in cases of carcinoma of the stomach or colon. It is also common, however, for the liver to be a site for secondary carcinoma by blood dissemination from sites whose veins do not drain into the portal system and secondary carcinoma of the liver is common, for example, in carcinoma of the lung and of the breast. The lungs of course provide the first capillary system through which blood carried by veins other than those of the portal system has to pass and blood-borne deposits of secondary carcinoma are common in the lungs in, for example, carcinoma of the kidney. In addition to spreading by lymphatics and by the bloodstream, carcinoma in organs within serous cavities such as the pleural or peritoneal cavities may liberate living carcinomatous cells into the serous fluid, that is normally present in small amounts in these cavities, to be carried by the movement of that fluid to new sites on the surface of organs within the serous cavities or on the wall of the cavity. Such spread often provokes an inflammatory response with an effusion of fluid into the body cavity — malignant ascites in the case of the peritoneal cavity, and malignant pleural effusion (malignant hydrothorax) in the chest cavity. The pericardial cavity is sometimes similarly affected if it is invaded by carcinoma in one of the adjacent bronchi. Dissemination across serous body cavities is known as transcoelomic spread. When transcoelomic spread occurs within the peritoneal cavity certain organs are specially liable to be involved, partly at least, because of the effects of gravity. In a woman the ovaries seem to be particularly vulnerable and large secondary carcinomas in each ovary may be found before the presence of a symptomless primary carcinoma in the stomach or colon is recognized. Such secondary carcinomas of the ovary form the so-called Krukenberg tumours of the ovary. Primary carcinoma of the ovary is also very liable to spread itself by transcoelomic spread.

Cancer and age

The 'cancer age' refers to the age at which people may develop carcinoma. Sarcomas may develop in children or young adults but carcinoma is a disease of adult life and of old age. Carcinoma in any organ is quite unusual in childhood and in the decade between the age of 20 and 30 years. Between the age of 30 and 40 years it is still uncommon, though by no means rare, and after the age of 40 years carcinoma becomes quite common in all the usual sites. The relatively late age at which carcinoma becomes common has suggested that a long preliminary or precancerous stage may exist before fully developed carcinoma becomes apparent. It is in the skin, and on the vaginal aspect of the cervix uteri that precancerous changes can be recognized by microscopic examination of samples from the surface. The examination of smear preparations from the cervices of apparently healthy women may detect carcinoma of the cervix in the pre-invasive stage when successful treatment is far simpler than when the disease has reached the invasive stage.

Sarcoma

Unlike carcinoma, sarcoma tends to occur in much younger people and certain types of sarcoma are almost limited to children and young adults. Fortunately sarcoma is much less common than carcinoma. Certain sarcomas seem to be related to normal growth and proliferation of cells. Sarcoma of bone, for example, tends to occur near the growing ends of long bones in adolescents and young adults whose bones have only recently ceased to grow. When sarcoma of bone occurs in older people it is usually a complication of the condition of Paget's disease of bone in which abnormal growth-like activity develops in the bones of old people. Certain types of cellular connective tissues continue to produce cells throughout life. The blood-forming cells of the bone marrow and of the lymph nodes are of this type and it is in these tissues that sarcoma, and tumours akin to sarcoma, are most common.

In lymph nodes a sarcoma may develop from, and consist of, cells almost indistinguishable from normal lymphocytes; such a tumour is called a lymphosarcoma. Sarcoma in lymphoid tissues, however, may not consist of lymphocytes but of more primitive cells, more akin to embryonic cells than to any type of adult cells. Such a sarcoma is called a reticulosarcoma or reticulum cell sarcoma. Lymphatic leukaemia is somewhat akin to lymphosarcoma and the microscopic changes in the lymph nodes are very similar indeed but, in addition to enlargement of the lymph nodes and spleen, the patient's blood contains a great excess of lymphocytes. Myeloid leukaemia is a similar malignant proliferation of the cells of the bone marrow that produce the polymorphonuclear leucocytes. There is replacement of all the bone marrow and spleen by the precursors of polymorphonuclear leucocytes along with flooding of the blood by similar cells.

Myeloma

Myeloid leukaemia is one type of malignant overproduction of cells in the bone marrow in which the abnormal cells are liberated into the circulation but there is also a solid type of malignant tumour arising from cells in the bone marrow; that tumour is a myeloma. The name myeloma simply means 'marrow tumour'. There is nothing in the name itself to indicate malignancy but myeloma is malignant and by the time the tumour is discovered multiple areas of tumour may be present throughout the skeleton, a condition of myelomatosis. Fracture of bone may occur under stresses that are no more than those that are caused in bone by ordinary movements. Such a fracture is called a pathological fracture. In becoming malignant, the cells forming a myeloma undergo a type of differentiation which does not normally occur to any extent in the bone marrow. They become plasma cells with the appearances, staining properties and the capacity to form immunoglobulin of normal plasma cells. This immunoglobulin (usually IgM) is not produced in response to any antigen and is present in such large amounts that the total protein content of the blood plasma may be raised by 20 to 30 g per litre. There are important secondary effects upon the kidney. A special type of protein, the Bence-Jones protein, may appear in the urine and the patient may die of renal failure.

Behaviour of sarcomas

Most sarcomas are highly malignant and the sarcoma of bone (osteosarcoma) that occurs in young people is among the most malignant. The blood vessels that form within the tumour have walls of tumour cells and it is thus not surprising that dissemination of the tumour by the bloodstream occurs with the greatest of ease to produce secondary tumours in the lungs. Pathological fracture may occur in the bone at the site of the tumour and the injuries to vessels that this involves also favour blood-borne metastatic spread of the tumour. In general, sarcomas have only a slight tendency to spread by lymphatics but are even more likely than carcinomas to spread by the bloodstream. The exception is, of course, the sarcomas of the lymphoid tissues, such as, lymphosarcoma, reticulosarcoma, and the tumour-like condition, Hodgkin's disease. These conditions tend to involve one group of lymph nodes after another and, unlike carcinoma, may involve the lymphoid tissue in the spleen, causing an enlargement of the spleen which can be felt clinically.

Special types of tumour

A large number of tumours have special names and special characters; some are benign, some behave like carcinomas, some like sarcomas, and the exact nature of some is still uncertain. A few of special interest and importance will be mentioned here.

Hydatidiform mole and chorion carcinoma (choriocarcinoma)

These tumours are of special interest for the cells of which they are composed are really those of another individual. They follow conception and are tumours of the placenta, in which the cells are those of the fetus and not of the mother. Normally, chorionic villi, projections of the placenta with a covering of epithelial cells, penetrate blood vessels in the endometrium and obtain oxygen and nourishment for the fetus.

The relatively benign tumour of the placenta is the hydatidiform (so called because of its grape-like cysts) mole; and the malignant counterpart is the chorion carcinoma in which the tumour cells, being derived from cells that normally invade blood vessels, spread rapidly by the bloodstream.

Teratoma

In chorion carcinoma the tumour cells are those of an individual whose genetic material differs from that of the host and in at least a certain number of teratomas it has been shown that the chromosomes of the tumour cells differ from those of the host. Teratomas seem to develop from a cell with at least some of the developmental potentialities of a fertilized ovum and can give rise to a mixture of embryonic and mature tissues that occurs in no other type of tumour. One of the suggestions made in the various attempts to explain the structure of a teratoma is that the tumour is a much malformed and slowly developing twin of the host. Teratomas may be benign or malignant and the site of growth is the ovary in a woman or the testis in a man. If they develop elsewhere the site is somewhere in the midline of the body. Most ovarian teratomas are benign and tend to form cysts lined by skin in which sebaceous glands are numerous and which normally grow some hair. Remarkably well formed teeth are not uncommon in such cystic tumours, or dermoid cysts, of the ovary. A solid thickening in part of the wall of a dermoid cyst usually contains a jumbled mixture of tissues including smooth or striped muscle, nervous tissue, glandular tissue of various types, cartilage and bone. Such tumours enlarge to produce a cystic mass in the pelvic cavity without causing acute symptoms unless, through twisting, one becomes strangulated.

In the testis a teratoma is more solid with only small cysts lined by epithelium of various types. The solid areas between the small cysts often contain cartilage. A testicular teratoma is a dangerous tumour whose epithelial elements may behave as a carcinoma. These elements may include malignant placental epithelial cells that give rise to chorion carcinoma of the testis.

Melanoma

The name means black tumour and sometimes these tumours may be very black indeed but occasionally the pigment may be so scanty that an amelanotic or non-pigmented variant is recognized. The pigment that makes these tumours black is melanin. This pigment is produced in the epidermis of normal skin and most people have a number of tiny malformations in the skin that consist of clumps of misplaced melanin-producing cells in the dermis, a site from which melanin-producing cells are normally absent. These are pigmented naevi and it is thought that malignant melanoma of the skin arises in a pre-existing pigmented naevus. The other site in which malignant melanoma occurs is in the choroid, the malanin-containing layer of the retina of the eye. Malignant melanoma behaves like a carcinoma with a marked tendency to spread by the lymphatics as well as by the bloodstream.

Seminoma and dysgerminoma

Teratoma of the testis has been mentioned but there is another well-known tumour of the testis, the seminoma. In general, seminoma occurs in older men and teratoma in younger ones but the age groups overlap and it is by no means exceptional for the two types of tumour to occur simultaneously in the same testis. Seminoma is a tumour of the spermatogenic cells of the testis, it is malignant, and its behaviour is that of a carcinoma. Rather surprisingly a tumour that is histologically identical occurs in the ovary and it seems that under the stimulus of neoplasia the gonads of both sexes may produce an identical, poorly differentiated, tumour from their reproductive cells. The ovarian tumour is named dysgerminoma.

Hypernephroma

The name hypernephroma, which literally means 'tumour above the kidney', is still used quite commonly for a carcinoma of the tubules of the kidney. The cells of the tumour contain so much golden-yellow lipoid that the mass in the kidney resembles adrenal glandular tissue and it was suggested at one time that the tumour actually arose from displaced adrenal cortical cells within the kidney, hence the name hyper-nephroma or suprarenal tumour. It is no longer believed that the tumour is derived from suprarenal glandular tissue but the term hypernephroma has persisted.

Hepatoma

The name hepatoma simply means liver tumour. Both simple and malignant types occur; a benign adenoma of liver cells is a rare tumour, that is, a benign hepatoma; a malignant hepatoma is a primary carcinoma of liver cells. Such a carcinoma is by no means a rare complication of cirrhosis of the liver. It is also the commonest type of all the cancers in certain parts of the world, and is particularly well known as a very common cause of death in men of the Bantu people of South Africa.

AETIOLOGY

In man the cause of most tumours is not known but simple and malignant tumours of various types can be produced experimentally in animals by a number of apparently quite unrelated methods. It is probable that a combination of factors contributes to the development of natural tumours. The circumstances that are known to be carcinogenic, that is, to be capable of inducing tumours, fall into certain groups. Thus there are certain things that are hereditary, there are the influences of hormones, there are physical agents and chemical substances that people may encounter at work, or in their recreation, or in habits such as smoking, and there are living agents, especially viruses that may be important in causing tumours. Combinations of factors of these types associated with variations in the immunological and other responses that the host may be capable of developing to prevent the growth of a tumour all contribute to the complexity of the aetiology of tumours. It may be that additional carcinogenic factors remain to be discovered but it may also be that it is only the interaction of the known carcinogenic influences which remains to be learned to discover the cause or causes of natural tumours.

Hereditary factors

Ordinarily no significant family history of cancer or other tumours can be obtained from a patient with any of the commoner cancers but in the case of certain rare tumours there is a clear history of the disease in the family. Examples of such tumours are familial **polyposis** of the colon, **retinoblastoma** of the eye, von Recklinghausen's neurofibromatosis, skin cancer in **xeroderma pigmentosum**, and carcinoma of the oesophagus in tylosis palmarum. In the case of at least some of these conditions it is not the actual tumours that are inherited but an abnormality of the metabolism of the cells concerned that leads in time to the development of tumours.

Polyposis A condition in which a large number of polyps (mucosal outgrowths, usually with a stalk) cover the mucosa.

Retinoblastoma A malignant tumour of the retina which occurs in infants and is congenital in origin.

Xeroderma pigmentosum A condition characterized by reddening of the skin with blistering and pigmentation, on even very slight exposure to sunlight.

Hormonal effects

In clinical studies there are also some striking effects that are almost certainly hormonal. For example the type of primary carcinoma of the liver that is so common in the Bantu tribe of South Africa is almost entirely a disease of males. In established cases of carcinoma of the prostate, even when secondary deposits are present, the progress of the disease is often reduced very much if oestrogenic hormone is administered. In advanced carcinoma of the breast, the course of the disease can sometimes be slowed down by the removal of the ovaries and adrenal glands, the patient being given artificial cortisone to replace the natural adrenal cortical secretions. Even the removal of the pituitary gland is sometimes undertaken to palliate advanced carcinoma.

Physical agents

Excessive exposure to sunlight, especially in fair-skinned people, greatly increases the incidence of skin cancers and the effects of x-rays are even more liable to produce carcinoma of the skin and, because of their penetrating effects, may also induce sarcomas in the deeply situated connective tissues or bone. Many of the early workers with x-rays developed carcinomas of their skin before the risk was recognized and suitable protection provided and sometimes the successful treatment of one type of malignant tumour may be complicated years later by the development of a post-irradiation sarcoma. Also the introduction of radioactive chemicals into the body carries a risk of causing either carcinoma or sarcoma, depending upon the type of tissue in which the radioactive material accumulates. Only substances with long-lasting radioactivity have this effect and radioactive isotopes with a half-life of a few days or hours can safely be administered for diagnostic or therapeutic purposes.

Chemical carcinogens

Many substances that are capable of inducing tumours when they are applied to the skin, or swallowed, or inhaled, have been discovered. Some of these substances are related chemically to each other and some are not. The chemical nature of a substance may arouse suspicion that it is carcinogenic, but testing on animals is the only reliable method at present by which carcinogenic power can be judged. Substances with entirely different chemical structures may also induce cancers. Such carcinogens include certain dye substances, arsenic, asbestos, and the products of some fungi. Some of these substances do not cause cancers where they first come in contact with the body but are absorbed and may undergo chemical modifications in the body before causing tumours in some of the organs in which they accumulate, such as the liver, or in organs like the kidneys or urinary passages, by which they are excreted.

Tumour-inducing viruses

The fact that tumour-inducing viruses can cause certain simple and malignant tumours in animals has been known since the early years of this century but until recently there was no evidence that such viruses played any part in the cause of human tumours. However, the discovery that a virus is at least one of the factors that induces a type of lymphosarcoma, the Burkitt lymphoma, affecting African children has renewed interest throughout the world in the possibility that virus infection may play some part in the cause of leukaemia and sarcomas of lymphoid tissues.

REFERENCE

Berenblum, I. (1962). The nature of tumour growth. In *General Pathology*, p. 538. Ed. H. Florey. London: Lloyd-Luke

10

The patient with advanced cancer

J. E. Dalby

INTRODUCTION

Cancer is the second commonest cause of death in the western world and more than 120 000 people now die of the disease each year. In spite of this unhappy state of affairs — and perhaps paradoxically in a chapter discussing management of advanced disease — it is well worth stressing that many more patients are cured of their cancer than is generally appreciated even by doctors and nurses. For example, over 80 per cent of early cancer of the vocal cord is cured by radiotherapy, over 80 per cent of early seminoma of the testis is cured by a combination of surgery and radiotherapy and it is fair to estimate that about one-third of all patients suffering from cancer (both early and late) are cured.

However, the problem of the management of the patient with advanced cancer remains, and it is well to begin by stating the magnitude of the problem. In 1968, 10 416 new cases of cancer were recorded by the Liverpool Clinical Registry from an estimated population of just over 2.8 million.

Analysis of treatment policy for these 10 416 patients shows that 43 per cent received curative treatment, 25 per cent were given palliative treatment, that is treatment aimed only at relief of symptoms for a time, not cure, and 32 per cent were not treated at all because their disease was too advanced. Table 10.1 shows in rather more detail the proportion of patients receiving curative and non-curative therapy for six important types of cancer.

It is seen that the outlook, or prognosis as it is called, varies considerably. Nevertheless, no cancer has a 100 per cent cure rate and the problem remains how to manage those patients who because their disease is too advanced are not to be treated curatively.

It is a difficult situation and one where personality, sympathy and understanding are much more vital than mere

Table 10.1   Treatment policy in cases of cancer in 1968

Site of cancer	Total number of cases	Treatment policy, % of total	
		Curative	Non-curative
Uterine cervix	494	86	14
Breast	1069	68	32
Throat	180	65	35
Ovary	236	28	72
Stomach	958	21	79
Lung	2010	14	86

technical expertise. It is a situation in which the nurse has an immensely important — and also rewarding — part to play.

Management of patients with incurable disease may be discussed under three main headings: management of the patient as an individual; active treatment of the disease; and terminal care of the patient.

MANAGEMENT OF PATIENTS AS INDIVIDUALS

The individual approach to the patient is of paramount importance; it is of little use to relieve a patient's physical symptoms if he remains worried because no one has spoken to him about his disease, his treatment, his future prospects or any other of the many problems he may have. The nurse can, and should, be the link between the patient and the doctor, and can often pass on to the doctor questions from the patient which he himself may be reluctant to ask.

What to tell the patient suffering from advanced cancer is one of the most difficult problems that the doctors and nurses have to face. It would be much easier, of course, were it possible to lay down hard and fast rules, if one could say, perhaps, that all patients should be told of their prognosis, or that no patients should be told that they have malignant disease, or again that they have a malignant disorder which is curable, whether or not this is, in fact, the truth.

It does not work out like this, of course. Each patient must be treated individually, but what is certain is that it is very important indeed that the nurse knows the view of the doctor in charge in each case and thus avoids the possibility that she and the doctor may tell the patient a different story.

In my experience, it is not very common for a patient genuinely to want to be told that he has an advanced malignant disease, even though he may say that he wishes to be told the truth. I can think of cases where I have bitterly regretted being entirely open with the patient as regards his prognosis. Occasionally, of course, there are situations when, for example, financial and family affairs must be settled and when one feels that the patient really must be given more than just an inkling of the true position in his case. But it should be said that it is seldom, if ever, justifiable to take away all hope from any patient.

Often, of course, the patient knows that he is dying, knows that the nurse and the doctor know, and yet the subject is never broached in exactly these terms. The pretence, as it were, is kept up by both sides and this, in my view, is far better than a blunt statement of the true position by the doctor.

It is said by some experienced doctors that if a patient asks the question 'Have I got cancer?' or, alternatively, 'Is the cancer from which I am suffering incurable?', he must be told the absolute truth as, if he subsequently discovers that the doctor has not been completely honest with him, he will immediately lose all confidence in the doctor. It is, of course, a perfectly valid point of view, but I personally feel very strongly that when these questions are asked, in the majority of cases the patient is really asking for reassurance and will often be very upset if he is told the whole truth. There is a difference here, of course, between 'early' and 'advanced' cancer. I find myself more and more inclined — if asked — to tell a patient suffering from an early cancer that he or she has a growth which is curable and, on the whole, I have not regretted this 'honesty'. The situation is different however, when the disease presents in an already advanced state. I very, very seldom, if ever, tell such a patient that his disease is incurable and I do not think that I shall ever alter this view. It is advisable, though, to inform at least one member of his family, usually the husband or the wife, often after prior consultation with the general practitioner, who knows the family so much better, of the prognosis and prospects for the patient's future.

Here again the ward sister and nurse have vital roles to play because it is to them that near relatives will turn for information and for reassurance. It is, therefore, worth repeating that there must be the closest possible collaboration between doctor and nurse, for nothing is more disturbing to relatives than to receive differing opinions and statements about the patient. Often the cancer is spoken of as an 'ulcer', a 'gland', or a 'growth which may spread if it is not treated straightaway', and the nurse will clearly need to know the exact details of what has been said.

ACTIVE TREATMENT

It is worth repeating that treatment in these circumstances, though active, is not radical, that is, with intent to cure. It is palliative, which implies treatment aimed at relief of symptoms with the minimum of upset to the patient.

Principle of treatment

The principles on which palliative treatment should be based have been admirably defined by Professor Ralston Paterson (1957): (1) there must be reasonable expectation of relief; (2) treatment should be as short as possible with minimal discomfort; (3) beyond a certain stage of decline, no palliative treatment is possible; (4) avoid rescue from 'the frying pan into the fire'. It is worth considering these four points in a little more detail.

Expectation of relief

It has been well said that the duty of the doctor is to prolong life, but not to prolong the act of dying. There must be something quite real to palliate and the patient must become aware that he has benefited from the treatment that has been given to him. An example of where it would be unwise, and indeed unkind, to give definitive treatment, even of a palliative nature, would be when an aged and incurable patient has developed bronchopneumonia — antibiotics should not be given. On the other hand, a patient who is suffering from swelling of the neck due to engorgement of the veins caused by the pressure of malignant glands in his chest, can very often be significantly helped for a period of time by radiotherapy and he will certainly be aware that he has benefited from it.

Minimal discomfort

It is clearly quite unjustifiable to give a prolonged course of treatment, either surgical, radiotherapeutic or medical, involving perhaps weeks in hospital, for a patient with incurable malignant disease. It is also quite unjustifiable to subject the patient to a treatment which produces, in the case of radiotherapy, unpleasant reaction which lasts for some considerable length of time or, in the case of surgery, a long and perhaps difficult operation with a period of discomfort afterwards. It would however, be quite justifiable to give a short course of treatment to the patient perhaps not even involving him in in-patient therapy.

Treatment not possible beyond a certain stage

To decide whether a patient is beyond a certain stage of decline when no palliative treatment is possible, can be exceedingly difficult. It is never easy to withhold or refuse treatment. Nevertheless, there is no doubt that some patients have malignant disease which has already developed to such an extent that one knows from experience that no form of treatment has really the slightest chance of relieving him significantly. An example of this type of case would be a patient suffering from advanced cancer of the stomach with liver metastases.

Treatment in patient's interest

One must attempt to avoid the more distressing kinds of death in favour of the most merciful ones. It is, for example, not advisable to give a blood transfusion to a woman with very advanced cancer of the uterus who has either severe anaemia or who has had a brisk haemorrhage: what happens then is that although she is relieved of the immediate risk to her life, the chances are that the growth as it extends will, as it so often does, involve nerves in the pelvis and she will suffer very severe pain which is extremely difficult to relieve. She may also develop a rectal or bladder fistula. This is not a good palliative treatment as it is not in the patient's interest.

The treatment for the relief of symptoms should now be considered in more detail. Results can be achieved by medical treatment (for example, administration of pain-killing drugs and hormones), surgical treatment (**chordotomy**, **colostomy**) or by radiotherapy (for example, healing of ulceration, relief of bone pain).

Medical and surgical treatment will be more familiar to nurses than radiotherapeutic treatment and it is, therefore, necessary to deal with the latter in a little more detail at this stage.

Radiotherapy is the treatment of disease, almost always malignant disease, by radiation.

Radiation used in radiotherapy are x-rays produced by high-voltage machines or γ-rays produced either by naturally radioactive substances like radium, or by elements such as cobalt and caesium which it is possible to make radioactive artificially. If a beam of x- or γ-rays is shone on to a part of the human body, there is damage to tissue, that is to the cells making up that part of the body on which the beam was directed. Normal or abnormal cells of the body can be affected adversely by radiation, and indeed destroyed if the amount of radiation given to that part of the body is great enough.

Chordotomy Surgical division of a nerve tract, or tracts, of the spinal cord.

Colostomy An opening made through the abdominal wall into the colon (*see* Glossary).

Fortunately, many malignant tumours are more liable to damage by irradiation than the normal cells surrounding them. If this were not so, of course, radiotherapy would not be possible. Indeed, there are some tumours whose sensitivity to radiation is such that the normal tissue in which they are growing is damaged to the same extent as the tumour cells and radiotherapy has no part to play in tumours of this type. Not only do malignant tumours vary in their response to radiation, normal cells of the body also vary. For example, the bone marrow cells and the epithelial cells of the alimentary tract are very sensitive to radiation and, therefore, special care has to be taken when large beams of radiation are directed on to this part of the patient's body.

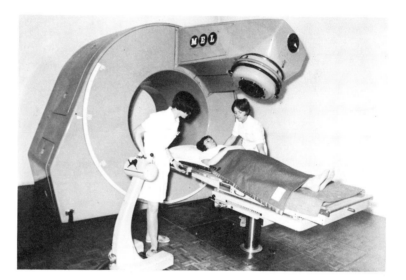

Figure 10.1. Linear accelerator (6 million V)

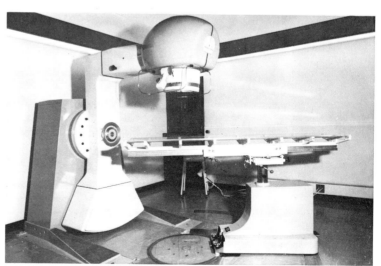

Figure 10.2. Radioactive cobalt therapy machine

The most usual x-ray unit now available for treatment is the linear accelerator. *Figure 10.1* shows the 6-million volt machine installed at the Liverpool Regional Radiotherapy Centre in Clatterbridge Hospital. The higher the voltage of these x-ray units, the greater the penetration of their x-ray beams. There is now no part of the body, however deeply situated, which cannot be adequately 'reached' by these beams.

The commonest γ-ray beam unit in use at the present time utilizes radioactive cobalt (*Figure 10.2*). However, it is not as powerful as the linear accelerator and treatment takes rather longer, but it is considerably cheaper and its beam has precisely the same effect on cancer cells as has the x-ray beam.

Radioactive substances such as radium — a naturally occurring radioactive element discovered by Madame Curie in 1898 — cobalt produced artificially by subjecting the element

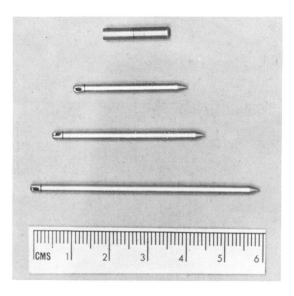

Figure 10.3. Radium tube and needles

cobalt to bombardment in a nuclear reactor, and iridium, are also used in the treatment of malignant disease. They are used in the form of needles, tubes or wires (*Figures 10.3* and *10.4*) which can be inserted or 'implanted', as it is termed, into tissues or organs invaded by cancer. Examples of their use in palliative treatment will be discussed later.

While a course of radiotherapy given with curative intent — as it often is — may take some 3, 4, 5 or even 6 weeks, it is desirable, and almost always possible, to drastically reduce this time when symptomatic relief only is the aim; in fact, a single treatment by x-rays is quite often effective and may not even necessitate admission to hospital. This, of course, has obvious advantages to the patient and his relatives.

There are occasions when a single application of x-rays achieves excellent pain relief. One of these is when cancer has spread to bone; this occurs relatively frequently in breast cancer, in lung cancer and also in cancer of the thyroid gland. Such treatment causes the minimum of disturbance to the patient and is very worthwhile.

Inoperable lung cancer often produces severe pain; in my experience the prospects for relief are not as good as in the case of deposits in bone, but palliative irradiation, often given over a course of 1 to 2 weeks, offers the best hope.

Relief of symptoms

The relief of symptoms will now be discussed in more detail. The problem of management of pain has been discussed in Chapter 6. Nevertheless, it is mentioned again briefly because pain is a rather frequent accompaniment of advanced malignant disease and is also the most important symptom for which relief must be sought. It is very nearly always possible to achieve this.

The mainstay of the management of pain is regular medication, be it 8-hourly, 6-hourly or less, for in the terminal stages, pain is often unremitting and unless adequately relieved is infinitely distressing.

There is a great variety of available drugs. The following list is based on practice in wards at the Liverpool Regional Radiotherapy Centre and on the experience of the senior nursing staff. It is not possible to be dogmatic as the choice of drugs will often depend on personal preference.

Analgesics, hypnotics and sedatives

Analgesics for the management of mild, moderate and severe pain caused by cancerous growth are summarized in Table 10.2. Hypnotics and sedatives used for the same purpose are listed in Table 10.3.

Surgical methods

Surgical methods used to relieve pain include: injection of nerves (for example, the fifth cranial nerve which supplies the face) by substances such as phenol; phenol injections into the subarachnoid space (a complication of this treatment may be paralysis of the sphincter of the bladder, usually of short duration); and electric chordotomy when the fibres of part of the spinal cord are destroyed by an electrode inserted under local anaesthetic.

These surgical methods, although merely mentioned here, are, as has already been stressed in Chapter 6, valuable tools

Table 10.2   Analgesics used for the management of mild, moderate and sever pain

Analgesic	Dose	Remarks
Mild and moderate pain		
Paracetamol (Panadol)	1 g 6 hourly	
Acetylsalicylic acid (Soluble Aspirin)	600 mg 4—6 hourly	
Soluble aspirin, codeine; (Codis) tablets	2 tablets 4—6 hourly	Tendency to constipate; useful for relief of **tenesmus** and diarrhoea
Dextropropoxyphene hydrochloride 32.5 mg, paracetamol 325 mg; (Distalgesic) tablets	2 tablets 6—8 hourly	Effectiveness equal to Codis but does not constipate
Dihydrocodeine tartrate (DF 118)	30—60 mg 6 hourly	More effective than Codis; considerable individual variation of preference
Severe pain		
Pentazocine (Fortral)	Oral 25—50 mg 4—6 hourly; intramuscular injection 30—60 mg 4—6 hourly	Frequently no more effective than Distalgesic, aspirin or codeine; more effective by intramuscular injection
Pethidine*	Oral or intramuscular injection 50—100 mg 4—6 hourly	
Dextromoramide (Palfium*)	10 mg 6—8 hourly	
Dipipanone hydrochloride 10 mg, cyclizine hydrochloride 30 mg (Diconal*) tablets	1 tablet 6—8 hourly	The author finds it more effective than oral pethidine; not advised in the presence of hepatic or renal disease
Oxycodone pectinate 30 mg (Proladone*) suppositories	1 suppository 8 hourly	Very effective for relief of severe pain
Morphine*	Intramuscular injection 10—30 mg 4—6 hourly	Used in terminal stages of malignant disease; causes depression of respiration, drowsiness and vomiting; to minimize vomiting Largactil (chlorpromazine 25—50 mg) is given orally or by intramuscular injection
Diamorphine (heroin*)	Intramuscular injection 1—3 mg	Has fewer side effects than morphine
Mist. Euphoria*. Various mixtures of morphine, cocaine, gin, honey and chloroform water	As prescribed by physician	The proportion of morphine can be increased without varying the quantity of mixture the patient is to take

*Controlled by the Dangerous Drugs Act (DDA)

Table 10.3   List of the more popular hypnotics and sedatives used for management of pain

Hypnotic or sedative	Dose	Remarks
Butobarbitone (Soneryl)	100—200 mg at night	
Quinalbarbitone (Seconal Sodium)	50—100 mg at night	
Dichloralphenazone (Welldorm)	650 mg—1.25 g at night	Particularly suitable for the elderly patient
Nitrazepam (Mogadon)	5—10 mg at night	

Tenesmus Continual and painful feeling of wanting to open the bowel.

in the endeavour to relieve intolerable pain; an example of their application is in advanced uterine cancer where the pain of nerve invasion can often be significantly relieved.

Although pain is the commonest problem and often the overriding consideration of the patient with incurable disease, there are many other symptoms, some even more distressing for the patient such as bleeding, discharge, dyspnoea and obstruction, to mention but a few.

Space does not allow detailed discussion of the ways of relieving symptoms produced by cancer in every site of the body. It is, though, important to realize that surgery, radiotherapy, hormones and chemotherapy all have their part to play.

Examples of the use of surgery

Bleeding or discharging masses

A surgical procedure is used to remove unsightly, bleeding or discharging masses. This is probably most often necessary in advanced carcinoma of the breast when a toilet mastectomy is performed to remove an ulcerating tumour. Rarely, metastatic glands, for example in neck or axilla, are excised as a palliative procedure.

Obstructions

Surgery is also used to relieve obstruction. Probably the most satisfactory method of palliation for advanced oesophageal cancer (other than morphia) is intubation with a Celestin tube. **Gastrostomy** should seldom, if ever, be performed, as it does not relieve the distressing symptom of the inability to swallow saliva.

Colostomy for inoperable bowel cancer is also a valuable procedure.

In late pharyngeal and laryngeal cancer, **tracheostomy** is sometimes necessary and relieves the patient's symptoms most dramatically.

Fistulas

Gastrostomy Surgical opening through the abdominal wall into the stomach, usually for feeding through a tube.

Tracheostomy Artificial opening made in the trachea.

Surgery can also be used to relieve symptoms due to fistulas. One of the most distressing terminal events in advanced pelvic malignancy in women, later cancer of the uterus, is a vesicovaginal or rectovaginal fistula. If prognosis in the individual case is estimated to be months, rather than days or a few weeks, ureteric transplant or colostomy may be justified.

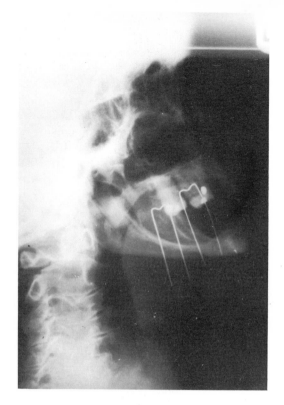

Figure 10.4. Radioactive iridium wires in the side of a tongue containing a carcinoma

Endocrine operations

In addition, surgery is used in endocrine malignant disease. In certain cases of advanced breast cancer, the operations of **oöphorectomy**, adrenalectomy and **hypophysectomy** are performed. A response in between 20 and 40 per cent of cases is achieved.

Examples of the use of radiotherapy

Ulcerations

Radiotherapy is used to heal ulceration. A perfectly acceptable alternative to toilet mastectomy in breast cancer (and indeed the treatment of choice for fixed lesions) is a short course of x-ray therapy (*Figures 10.5* and *10.6*).

Advanced skin cancer, e.g. a rodent ulcer on the face, can show remarkable improvement following palliative irradiation.

One of the sites where implantation of radium needles or iridium wire (*Figure 10.4*) is indicated is the tongue. Even though the tumour is considered to be incurable, such therapy can relieve symptoms of pain, discharge and bleeding and even temporarily heal ulceration; in the meantime, dissemination of the disease may take place together with an

Oöphorectomy Surgical removal of an ovary or ovaries.

Hypophysectomy Removal of the pituitary gland.

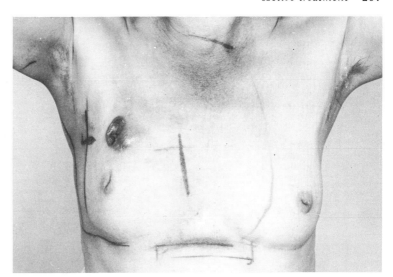

Figure 10.5. Ulcerated breast cancer before irradiation treatment

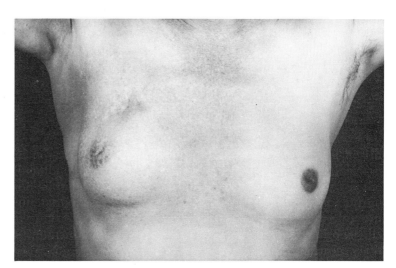

Figure 10.6. Ulcerated breast cancer after irradiation

easier death for the patient. This concept of bringing about a 'more comfortable death' for the patient is perhaps, on first thought, somewhat macabre: reflection, however, will bring realization that it is, in fact, a most merciful one, though not by any means easy of fulfilment.

Haemorrhage

Radiotherapy may also be used to stop haemorrhage. The relief of **haemoptysis** — often an alarming symptom to the patient and his relatives in the now increasingly common disease of lung cancer — is often achieved by modest doses of x-ray therapy.

Haemoptysis The coughing up of blood.

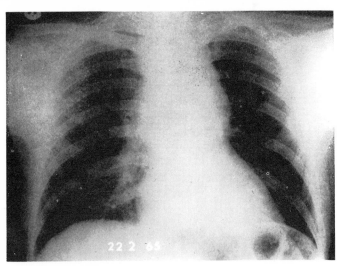

Figure 10.7. Lung cancer; mediastinal glands before irradiation

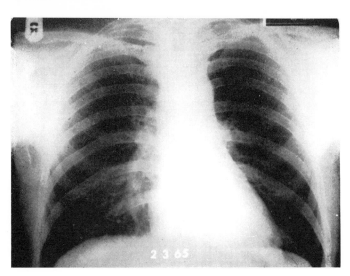

Figure 10.8. Lung cancer; mediastinal glands after irradiation

Similarly, **haematuria** from advanced bladder cancer is usefully relieved in many cases, if only for a period of weeks or months, by irradiation.

Bleeding from uterine cancer (even though too advanced for curative therapy) is often treated by insertion of radium tubes into the uterine cavity and vagina. This procedure does, of course, require a short anaesthetic. The radium need remain *in situ* for only some 72 to 96 hours. The patient, therefore, needs to be hospitalized for only a few days.

Obstruction

Very often radiotherapy is used to relieve obstruction. Superior mediastinal obstruction, due to metastatic glandular

Haematuria The presence of blood in the urine.

spread of lung cancer, is all too common nowadays (*Figure 10.7*). The swollen neck and face with eyelid oedema, dilated veins and dyspnoea is quite typical. There is also an equally typical response to irradiation, especially when the tumour is an undifferentiated one (*Figure 10.8*); often within a few days, symptoms are significantly alleviated. There are few results in the palliation of malignant disease more pleasing to both doctor and patient.

Again, in lung cancer, a blocked bronchus can be opened up by a short course of irradiation with re-expansion of lung and relief of dyspnoea.

When pharyngeal or laryngeal cancer threatens to obstruct breathing and/or produce dysphagia, irradiation is indicated, with or without preliminary tracheostomy. If the tumour is sensitive to irradiation, relief for many months, even years, can be the result of this type of treatment.

Neurological symptoms
Radiotherapy can be very successful in relieving neurological symptoms. It is not particularly uncommon for breast and lung cancer to metastasize to the brain with ensuing symptoms of headache and vomiting, **ataxia**, personality changes and so on.

In a worthwhile percentage of cases, temporary relief can be achieved by irradiation of the whole brain.

The majority of primary malignant cerebral tumours are, of course, incurable. Although a radical course of irradiation is often given, the fact that so few patients are cured means that the treatment given — and the symptomatic relief achieved — is essentially of a palliative order.

Paraplegia, sometimes of sudden onset, is an urgent situation demanding urgent treatment. If the source of the metastasis (as such it often is) is known, for example breast cancer or **Hodgkin's disease**, it is possible to make an immediate choice between surgery and radiotherapy. **Laminectomy** will often bring about the quickest relief, but if the primary malignancy is reticulo-endothelial or some other **anaplastic** (and, therefore, often radiosensitive) tumour, radiotherapy will be preferred and is clearly easier for the patient.

It is usually necessary to institute treatment within 1 or 2 days at the most if recovery of function is to be hoped for, though there are cases when recovery from paraplegia has occurred after a delay of as long as a week.

Reduction of malignant masses
Radiotherapy can also be used with considerable success to reduce the size of malignant masses. The glandular deposits

Ataxia Loss of control over movements and balance.

Paraplegia Paralysis of both legs and the lower part of the body.

Hodgkin's disease A malignant disease of the reticuloendothelial system (lymph nodes, spleen, bone marrow).

Laminectomy An operation to remove the laminae of a vertebral arch. Done to expose the spinal cord.

Anaplastic Characterized by imperfect development or a change back to a more primitive form of cell.

K

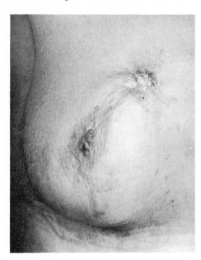

Figure 10.9. Recurrent breast cancer before oestrogen treatment

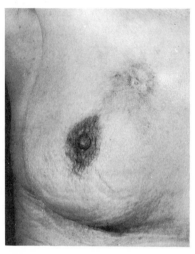

Figure 10.10. Recurrent breast cancer 3 months after oestrogen treatment started (note pigmentation of nipple)

Androgen A general name for the male sex hormones.

Oestrogen General name for certain types of female sex hormones.

Anti-oestrogen Will usually act by blocking the effect of an oestrogen at the site of its action.

Progestogen Substance possessing the activity of the corpus luteum hormone of the ovary.

of late reticulo-endothelial disease, for example Hodgkin's disease, are very responsive to irradiation and resolve after modest doses of x-ray therapy.

Occasionally, secondary carcinoma in glands responds to radiotherapy but, where operable, surgical treatment is to be preferred.

Examples of the use of hormone therapy

In incurable breast cancer, both **androgens** (for example, Ultandren 10 mg t.d.s.) **oestrogens** (for example, ethinyl-oestradiol 0.1 mg t.d.s.) **anti-oestrogens** (for example, tamoxifen 20 mg b.d.) and **progestogens** (for example, norethisterone acetate 10 mg t.d.s.) are often used and can help to relieve symptoms in some 30 per cent of patients (*Figures 10.9* and *10.10*).

Oestrogens are used in the management of advanced prostatic cancer and symptomatic relief can be expected in a high percentage of patients.

Examples of the use of chemotherapy

More and more chemical agents are being developed and used to treat patients with incurable malignant disease.

Such drugs as cyclophosphamide (Endoxana) methotrexate, bleomycin, vinblastine and 5-fluorouracil (to mention only a few) are increasingly used, usually in combination rather than singly and striking remissions have been achieved in such diseases as advanced Hodgkin's disease. This form of therapy is likely to be increasingly useful in the management of advanced cancer.

TERMINAL CARE

In the management of patients with incurable disease, there must inevitably come a time when no further active treatment is indicated.

Such palliation as can be expected has been achieved and it becomes a question of caring for the patient throughout the terminal phase of the illness.

When the patient can be cared for adequately at home, this is by far the best; it is clearly more pleasant for the patient to be in familiar surroundings during this time (whether or not he appreciates the true position) and to have his family near at hand. It is in these circumstances that the services of a home help and district nurse can be so valuable. The former is able to relieve relatives of daily chores so that more time may be spent with the patient and the sympathetic district nurse is of immense importance, not only in the giving of injections and the dressing of ulcers and so on but also in keeping up the patient's morale.

Sometimes, of course, ward care is necessary (probably about 15 per cent of cancer patients are in hospital during their terminal illness) and it is then that nursing staff can do so much to ease the burden during this time.

It is always desirable — though often not possible — for such a patient to be nursed in a side ward as the death of a patient in a crowded general ward, particularly when for some days the outcome has been obvious, is discouraging, to say the least. It is easier, also, to relax ward routine if the patient is nursed in a side ward — and this is very often desirable. The patient should be able, within fairly broad limits, to sleep when he wishes, eat the sort of food he fancies and drink when he wishes and should certainly not be pressed in any way to conform to standard ward practices, essential though these are in general.

This, of course, means extra work for the nurse but a minute's reflection will show how desirable it is, from the patient's point of view. More time, and infinitely more patience, is also required of the nurse; patients often want just a few minutes, to discuss their problems and voice their worries and it is the nurse rather than the doctor to whom they turn. It is admittedly often very difficult indeed to find the time, but no emphasis can be too great for this aspect of care of the patient in the terminal phase of a malignant disease. What might be called the more 'practical' nursing problems, for example, the prevention and care of pressure-sores, which so quickly develop, must, of course, be dealt with, but when all is said and done, the skills of nurse and doctor count for relatively little, if care, understanding and compassion are lacking.

It would not be right to conclude this chapter without referring to the splendid work of Dr. Cicely Saunders in focussing attention on the problem of patients with terminal disease. An account of the approach adopted at St. Christopher's Hospice, London, may be found in an excellent book *The Management of Terminal Disease*, edited by her.

REFERENCE

Paterson, R. (1957). The use and misuse of palliative radiotherapy. *J. Fac. Radiol.* **8** (No. 4), 235

Saunders, C. (Ed.) (1978). *The Management of Terminal Disease.* London: Edward Arnold

11 Transplantation surgery

Robert Sells

INTRODUCTION

The objective of organ transplantation is to restore to normal life a patient suffering from fatal disease of some organ or system. As such, this objective is in no way different from that of general physicians and surgeons who attempt to restore to normal the function of the diseased organ before it is irretrievably damaged by a pathological process. The practical difference is that in patients who are considered for transplantation, an organ or system has been totally destroyed or removed. Without some form of replacement therapy, the patient would die.

Of course, not all such conditions demand the replacement of a complete organ for the restoration of health; the revolutionary advances in physiology during the last century have enabled the identification of organ function, clarification of the biochemical mechanisms involved, and in many cases, the purification or artificial synthesis of agents which can be administered to the patient in the event of a breakdown in function of a simple organ or gland. There are several obvious examples which immediately come to mind: insulin in the treatment of diabetes, cortisone therapy in adrenal failure, and thyroxine in patients with hypothyroidism. These conditions are all treated fairly simply by the substitution of a single missing hormone or gland extract.

Where the function of an organ is more complex, for instance the clearance of metabolites from the circulation by the kidney, then failure of the organ demands replacement of the blood filtering system to prevent the lethal build-up of toxic metabolites and electrolytes in the blood. A kidney transplant can save a patient's life and give him an independent existence. It is possible to treat patients successfully using haemodialysis machines designed to rid the blood of excessive water, salt and urea. However, the number of young patients who develop renal failure each year far exceeds the number of machines available, even in the world's richest countries; it is, therefore, essential to provide a method of treatment which offers the patient a normal existence, not only for his own good, but to enable the most efficient use of the dialysis machinery available. It is because of this need that renal transplantation is at present the most widely practised form of transplant surgery. This chapter describes the development and technique of kidney transplantation and attempts to present outstanding problems as well as the results.

GENERAL ASPECTS OF TRANSPLANTATION

Immunological factors

Allograft rejection

Using modern techniques of vascular surgery, it is now possible to transplant almost any organ from one individual to another. The basic method of sewing blood vessels together forming a secure joint was developed in 1906 by Alexis Carrel; this far-sighted man was quick to see the potential of the method in the field of transplantation and he performed many kidney transplants in experimental animals. He was the first man to observe that if a kidney was transplanted to an unrelated recipient whose own kidneys had been removed, the animal enjoyed normal renal function for a few days, and behaved like any other healthy animal. After a week the signs of renal failure set in, with eventual coma and death; postmortem examination revealed a dark, swollen kidney which, on microscopic examination, was seen to be largely destroyed. The characteristic histological appearance was leucocyte infiltration and thrombosis of the small vessels within the kidney substance with consequent necrosis of the renal tissue. Carrel was describing the process known as 'rejection', and his account of this remarkably consistent immunological phenomenon has not been bettered. Since Carrel there have been many accounts describing identical processes occurring in transplanted livers, hearts, pancreases and skin grafts. It is a sober thought that the basic technique for transplanting organs had been available for nearly 50 years before significantly successful therapy to combat rejection was discovered.

A lot is known about the mechanisms of rejection even though it cannot be completely prevented. The process is an immunological one; it is the response on the part of the immune apparatus as a whole to foreign **antigen** present in the graft.

Immune reactions may be rapid (for example, **anaphylaxis**) or slow (for example, tuberculous lesions); rejection falls into the latter category, and like other 'delayed hypersensitivity' responses, the principal immune effector agent appears to be the lymphocyte.

Antigen A substance which, under suitable circumstances, can stimulate a specific immune response.

Anaphylaxis A violent reaction usually to a foreign protein to which the subject is sensitive.

The mechanism of graft rejection

When foreign tissue in the form of a graft is implanted in one individual from a different animal, the blood of the host circulates through it and supplies it with all its metabolic needs so that it may function adequately. Skin grafts grow hair, kidney grafts produce urine, and heart grafts pump blood. But despite this satisfactory state of affairs subtle changes occur in the blood supplying the graft soon after

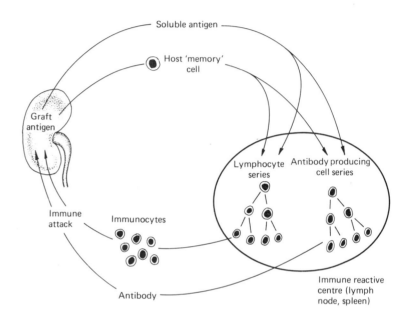

Figure 11.1. Schematic representation of **allograft** rejection

grafting, which lead to the damaging effects of rejection. It appears that some lymphocytes in the bloodstream are altered by their encounter with foreign grafted material, and are capable of initiating rapid growth of other lymphocytes in the spleen, lymph nodes, and other parts of the immunological factory. (Interestingly, the spleen very often enlarges after transplantation in man, as do the local lymph nodes draining the area of a skin graft applied to a mouse: these changes reflect the lymphoid hyperplasia which is a natural immune response to foreign antigen, and are seen also of course in many types of infection).

The lymphocytes from these immune reactive centres spill into the bloodstream, and when they encounter the graft they stick to the vascular lining, creep through it and attack the cells of the graft (*Figure 11.1*). It is also possible that lymphocytes set up small colonies of rapidly dividing progeny within the graft; the focal distribution of white cells in rejection certainly favours this theory (*Figure 11.2a*).

Allograft (homograft) A tissue graft between two unrelated members of the same species.

In addition to this cellular attack, the host also produces antibody against the organ tissue antigens in exactly the same way as in a bacterial infection. The consequent injury affects mainly the blood vessels, which become blocked up with cellular and thrombus-like material (*Figure 11.2b*). The organ supplied by such diseased arteries will quickly die due to impairment of blood flow, ischaemia and necrosis.

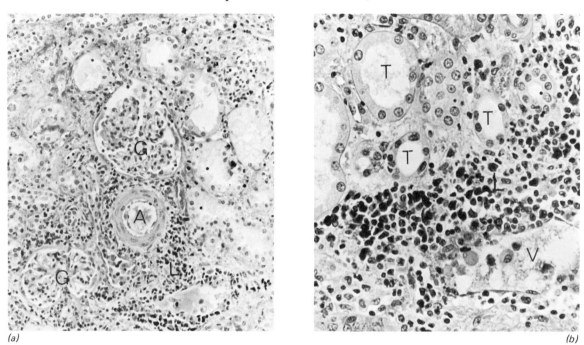

(a) *(b)*

Figure 11.2 Histological appearance of human kidney graft rejection. (*a*) Dark-staining lymphocytes (L) infiltrating around an artery (A) and two glomeruli (G). The high-power photograph (*b*) shows lymphocytes apparently emerging from a blood vessel (V) and infiltrating the adjacent tubules (T)

Sometimes the recipient may have antibodies to human tissue in the bloodstream prior to transplantation, and if they are active against the grafted tissue, then hyperacute rejection takes place. This consists of thrombosis of all the vessels, and death of the graft within hours or 1 to 2 days of grafting. Such antibodies may be present as a result of previous blood transfusion or pregnancy — in which case the host's immune system produces antibodies against the white cells present in the blood of the blood donor or the fetus. Fortunately they may be identified preoperatively, and hyperacute rejection can be prevented in renal transplantation.

Immunosuppression

From the above description of the rejection reaction it can be seen that in theory rejection may be depressed by interfering with the response at any of its three stages.

Antigen recognition and cell killing may be prevented experimentally by biological means and such an approach may form the basis of immunosuppression in the future. However, the most successful immunosuppressive agents used in human transplantation aim at suppressing the reactive phase, the proliferation of immunocytes in the regional reactive centres. These agents are listed below.

Imuran

Imuran (azathioprine) is chemically related to the anti-leukaemia agent 6-mercaptopurine. It may be given by mouth in doses of up to 4 mg per kg body weight per day. Its main action is to depress cellular proliferation, and since the demonstration in 1961 by Calne that dog kidney allograft survival could be considerably prolonged by giving Imuran after transplantation, it has been universally used in clinical transplantation. Its action is unselective, in that reticulo-endothelial elements other than lymphocytes are also suppressed; thus patients on this drug are prone to develop a low white cell count (leucopenia) and platelet deficiency (thrombocytopenia). These complications may, of course, lead to infection and bleeding, so daily white cell and platelet counts have to be performed on the blood of transplant recipients until the doctors supervising therapy are sure that the patient can tolerate the drug and that the maintenance dose is not too high. Transplant recipients are given this drug indefinitely while their graft remains functional, to prevent rejection.

Steroids

In addition to Imuran, the mainstays of immunosuppression are prednisone and hydrocortisone. Prednisone is the more powerful preparation and exerts an anti-inflammatory effect as well as a toxic action on lymph node cells (this action explains its successful use in disorders of excessive lymphoid proliferation). Large doses are required for immunosuppression (up to 200 mg/day) and so steroid-induced complications are regrettably frequent in transplant recipients. As well as the classic manifestations, such as Cushing's syndrome, peptic ulcers and diabetes, resistance to infection is lowered (a particularly unfavourable complication when Imuran is being administered simultaneously), and hypertension and fluid retention may also develop.

Antilymphocyte serum

Antilymphocyte serum, antilymphocyte globulin, and anti-lymphoblast globulin comprise a group of agents which theoretically should provide a specific form of immuno-suppression without the unwanted complications mentioned above. They are preparations of antibody (raised in another species) against human lymphocytes, prepared by injecting an animal (for example, the horse) with a pure human lymphocyte preparation and injecting the horse serum containing antilymphocyte antibody into a human transplant recipient. The use of the crude serum may lead to unwanted and dangerous complications, the most important of which is unselective killing of other blood cells. A purer preparation may be made by extracting the globulin from the serum, although the selectivity of action against lymphocytes cannot be obtained simply by purification. This is because the lympho-cyte suspension injected into the horse usually contains minute quantities of other blood constituents which promote antiplatelet and antineutrophil antibodies.

A recent substantial development in this field has been the injection of horses with pure lymphoblasts derived from cultures of human lymphatic tissue. The resultant antibody is not dangerous, but its efficiency in antirejection therapy has yet to be demonstrated. Although antilymphocyte prepar-ations are now used routinely in some centres, uncertainty regarding their efficiency, toxicity and mode of action prevents their universal use in immunosuppressive regimens.

Tissue typing

It has been demonstrated that the rejection reaction is triggered by the presence of foreign antigen on the surface of the grafted cells. It is known that blood group (ABO) com-patibility is necessary for allograft survival. There are other antigens (HLA = Human Leukocyte Antigens) present on the cell surface which also play a part in rejection. Techniques have been developed which allow these antigens to be defined and detected.

By studying the distribution of tissue antigens within families, it has been possible to show that histocompatibility antigens are inherited from both father and mother. Further-more, each parental chromosome bears a group of antigens which are conveyed to the offspring intact. The possible patterns of inheritance are illustrated in *Figure 11.3*. One can see from this illustration that although antigen patterns inherited by the four siblings are all different, there is a 1 in 4 chance that the inherited antigens will be identical to that of another sibling. It has been established that kidney transplants from sibling donors survive longer than grafts between unrelated individuals. When the sibling donor and recipient

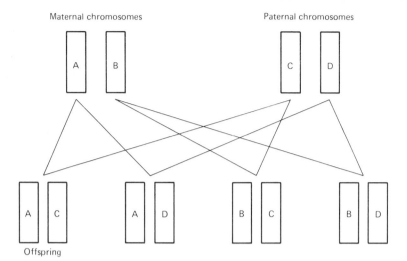

Figure 11.3. The four possible patterns of inheritance of histocompatibility antigen by the offspring of the two unrelated individuals

are exactly matched (the 1 in 4 chance), then the survival figures are significantly better than for any other group.

Clearly it is of great importance to know whether tissue matching (that is, obtaining the closest fitting donor and recipient) will improve the longevity of a cadaveric unrelated graft. The early results of two European surveys are encouraging enough to warrant the tissue typing of all cadaveric donors and the selection of the best recipients on a tissue-matching basis.

When the tissue type of a donor is known, a rapid comparison is made with the tissue types of all the recipients in the country (using a computer), and the destination of the kidney is decided. Thus it is important that kidneys can be preserved for up to 12 hours to allow tissue typing and transport to take place.

This simplified account of tissue typing is intended as a guide to the principles involved and not as a final vindication of the technique. There are many examples of unexpectedly successful transplants between grossly mismatched recipients: the explanation of this will have to await further knowledge on the chemistry and immunology of histocompatibility antigens.

The legal aspect of transplantation

Dissection of dead bodies for the purpose of removing organs for transplantation is allowed in Great Britain by the Human Tissue Act of 1961. This Act was passed at a time when transplantation was in its youth and was mainly directed at loosening the restrictions on the procurement of bodies for anatomical dissection. (These restrictions were introduced by a Victorian parliament following the scandalous grave-robbing activities of Burke and Hare). It is an unwieldy Act from the point of view of the transplant surgeon, since there is a necessity for speed in the removal of organs for transplantation which is not anticipated in the Act. The Law (as it affects transplantation) may be summarized as follows:

(1) If a person gives permission for his organs to be removed after his death, then it is lawful for a doctor to proceed with removal after death has been declared.

(2) If no such permission has been granted, the 'person in charge of the body' must ensure that every reasonable effort has been made to contact the relatives, to ascertain whether they object to the removal of organs. If there is no objection then it is lawful for a doctor to proceed with removal after death has been declared.

(3) When death is due to unnatural, violent, or unknown cause, the act of organ removal must be sanctioned by the Coroner (or Procurator Fiscal in Scotland).

Although these legal restrictions appear at first sight to limit substantially the freedom of transplant surgeons, and therefore the supply of donor kidneys, a policy has evolved in the United Kingdom which adequately maintains ethical and legal standards whilst allowing successful cadaver **nephrectomy**. The main points of this policy are now described.

(a) The donor

Patients who are suitable as donors are people who suffer severe brain damage and who during their admission are found to have brain death. They fall into the following categories:

(1) Major brain trauma: such patients often have musculoskeletal and visceral injury in addition to brain damage, and are suitable as donors if resuscitation has been successfully carried out and there is no evidence of serious renal injury.

(2) Brain haemorrhage: the commonest condition resulting in brain death and subsequent kidney donation is found in young patients following a massive haemorrhage beneath the arachnoid membrane (a layer of the meninges lining the skull). In these cases the subarachnoid haemorrhage bursts through into the brain substance, causing coma and eventual destruction of the vital centres controlling respiration and cardiovascular activity.

(3) Anoxic brain death: occasionally patients may be resuscitated following a temporary cardiac arrest when

Nephrectomy Excision of a kidney.

the circulation has ceased for more than four minutes (the longest ischaemic period which the brain can tolerate) and on restoring the circulation the patient is found to have total brain death.

(4) Cerebral tumours: people suffering from inoperable brain tumours often are admitted to hospital where they develop progressively deepening coma and destruction of vital centres.

Patients who are not suitable are those suffering from infection of lungs, urine, or bloodstream, and also those who have cancer anywhere in the body other than primary tumours of the nervous system, which do not spread to the rest of the body: pathogenic organisms and cancer cells can cause disease in the recipient if transplanted with a cadaver kidney graft.

(b) Brain death

Although artificial respiration techniques have existed for many years it is only recently that efforts have been made in the U.K. to prepare formally a list of criteria by which a patient may be diagnosed as having brain death. The advent of transplantation has certainly brought home the need for a clarification of this contentious subject, and a valuable report was issued in 1976 by a committee of the combined colleges of Surgeons and Physicians. The main recommendations of this report are summarized below.

The following conditions may simulate brain death and should be excluded: **hypothermia**, metabolic disorders (e.g. diabetic coma, hepatic coma), overdose with depressive drugs such as barbiturates, the administration of relaxants. If none of these have occurred the following neurological characteristics should be looked for:

(1) Coma: the patient with brain death is unresponsive to noise, and facial movements in response to pain should be absent. There should be no spontaneous movement.

(2) Cranial nerve reflexes: the following reflexes should be absent:

(a) the conjunctival reflex (no lid movement on touching the cornea).

(b) the oculovestibular reflex (no eye movement on filling the external auditory **meatus** with icy water).

(c) the response of the pupils to light.

(d) the gag and cough reflex.

(3) Spontaneous breathing should be absent. (After making sure that the level of CO_2 in the arterial blood is high enough to stimulate an intact respiratory centre, the patient is disconnected from the ventilator for 5

Hypothermia Low temperature for the given species. In the human, in current clinical usage, temperatures down to 28°C are called moderate hypothermia. Below that, profound hypothermia — a temperature of 15°C is the lowest that has been occasionally induced for operations on the blood vessels of the brain.

Meatus A passage or opening.

minutes and a catheter is left in the trachea delivering pure oxygen to the lungs. In cases of brain death no respiratory movements occur.)

(c) Compliance with the law

If a patient dies in hospital and a signed kidney donor card is found in the possession of the patient then it is lawful to remove the kidneys without asking whether relatives object. However since at the time of writing the Department of Health donor card scheme is still in its infancy, the number of people who carry such cards is negligible. In the majority of cases, efforts have to be made to find the relatives. In practice this does not usually pose a problem since nearly all kidney donors are respirator cases who spend at least 12 hours in an intensive care unit after their admission, and there is ample time to get the relatives to hospital and interview them. The interview is conducted by the doctor looking after the case, or the transplant surgeon, and although it is not always necessary for a consent form to be signed, a witness (usually a nurse or ward sister) should sign the doctor's statement in the patient's notes so that a true record of the relatives' decision exists for legal purposes.

Fortunately most relatives have no objection to the removal of organs, even when they are faced with the decision at a time of profound emotional trauma; it speaks well for human nature that they can recognize the good which may be achieved by their decision, that from the death of their loved one, two other lives may be saved. But crucial to that decision is complete confidence that the doctors in charge are convinced as to the diagnosis of brain death and that they will maintain the highest ethical standards during the management of the patient.

Finally if the patient is a Coroner's case, permission must be obtained from his office before organs may be removed. Permission will normally be witheld in cases of homicide or where forensic evidence will be interfered with by the removal of the organs.

(d) Renal function in the kidney donor

Patients whose renal function has deteriorated, or who suffer from chronic renal disease, are also unsuitable as donors. The former category can be recognized by a fall off in urine output and a rise in the blood urea and creatinine levels; if these changes are preceded by hypotension and are detected early, it is often possible to resuscitate the renal function by administration of blood or Hartmann's solution in combination with a diuretic such as Mannitol or Lasix, given intravenously. Such resuscitated kidneys may be perfectly satisfactory for transplantation provided blood volume, fluid and electrolyte balance, and a diuresis are all maintained. Experiments in kidney preservation have demonstrated the usefulness of certain drugs in improving the tolerance of kidneys to ischaemic injury: heparin, Largactil, frusemide and phenoxybenzamine are given routinely to the donor by intravenous injection before removal of organs.

(e) Other ethical considerations

It is of the utmost importance that the doctors in the transplant team should not be involved with any aspect of the donor's management until brain death has been certified by two doctors independent of the transplant team. After this has been done, then it is ethically correct that the transplant surgeon, having satisfied himself also that death has occurred, should arrange for resuscitation of renal function if necessary, take blood for tissue typing, and, if he receives approval from the relatives of the deceased, the Coroner and the person in charge of the body, he should arrange for the body to be taken to the operating theatre. Ventilation and circulation should be maintained and operation of nephrectomy may be carried out while the blood is still circulating or very soon after it has stopped. The kidneys are removed using a normal sterile operative technique, they are flushed with an ice-cold salt solution, and are stored in sterile bags in ice. A postmortem should be carried out on the donor soon after nephrectomy to check for the presence of an occult neoplasm which might jeopardize the safety of the recipient.

By paying strict attention to these rules and by developing good relationships with busy district hospitals, organs for transplantation may be removed successfully and decorously with the minimum amount of fuss and publicity. Yet the supply is still very small compared with demand, and constant efforts are needed to maintain a high degree of awareness in the minds of doctors and nurses that many people die each year for lack of a kidney transplant, and that the solution to this problem lies in their hands.

KIDNEY TRANSPLANTATION

Transplantation of the kidney has been carried out in well over 25 000 cases in the world, to date. There are many good reasons why the kidney has enjoyed such popularity in transplant surgery and these are summarized below.

The kidney is a paired organ; this means that one kidney can be removed from a living related donor with a very small risk of the donor suffering more than the temporary discomfort of a nephrectomy. In some countries (for example, in the United States of America) more than half of the kidney transplants have been performed using live related donors.

Patients who develop terminal renal failure display the familiar pattern of **uraemia**, hypertension, fluid retention with oedema, subsequent heart failure and gross electrolyte imbalance. In addition, they usually suffer from cerebral impairment and muscle weakness. Patients in this condition are not fit for surgery, and reversal of these changes must be effected before anaesthesia, transplantation and immuno-suppression can be carried out. Any patient who is considered for a kidney transplant must therefore be given a course of **haemodialysis** therapy to restore electrolyte balance, reduce hypertension, and allow full physical rehabilitation.

Transplantation cannot be carried out without the expert knowledge of renal physicians in attendance on the transplant unit together with adequate dialysis facilities. In addition, the patient will usually require dialysis temporarily following the operation until renal function has recovered to a level which allows the patient to live an independent existence.

Patient selection

The patient's ability to cope with the psychological and physical trauma of transplantation must be carefully assessed beforehand. A successful renal transplant recipient must have a reasonable degree of intelligence and stability and willingness to co-operate.

Before any patient can be considered for a renal transplant it must also be shown that there is no intercurrent disease, for example, tuberculosis, diabetes or collagen disease.

Preoperative management

When terminal renal failure has been diagnosed the patient is admitted as soon as possible to hospital and a shunt is inserted into the radial artery and cephalic vein of the arm. This allows twice- or thrice-weekly access to the bloodstream for dialysis. An alternative method of access to the bloodstream may be afforded by creating an arteriovenous fistula in the arm which causes the superficial veins to become dilated, which may be cannulated with wide bore needles. During the period when the patient's health is being restored to near normal by dialysis (a process which may take 3 months or more), a careful search is made for established infection in the lungs, kidneys and bloodstream, and any infection is eradicated by suitable means.

In some patients, for example, those with **pyelonephritis**, there is persistent infection in the kidneys and lower urinary

Uraemia Excessively high blood level of urea usually resulting from renal failure when other metabolic products are also retained in the body and cause a type of poisoning.

Haemodialysis A procedure to remove (unwanted) soluble substances from the body; used in renal failure when the blood is passed through a machine.

Pyelonephritis Inflammation of the kidney.

tract. In immunosuppressed patients there is obviously a danger that such infection may spread throughout the body due to impaired immune defence mechanisms. Infection must therefore be eradicated whenever it is detected; thus bilateral nephrectomy may be necessary prior to transplantation. This operation may also prove useful in controlling hypertension of renal origin which cannot be controlled by haemodialysis.

If possible, the patient is put on a full diet and encouraged to become ambulant and redevelop the muscle mass which is usually wasted during uraemia. Because the patient will be given steroids following the operation, radiological tests are performed for presence of peptic ulceration, and surgical treatment performed if necessary. Patients with renal disease may develop disturbances of calcium metabolism, and hyperparathyroidism does occur in about 20 per cent of cases. This may be reversed by dialysis or may require parathyroidectomy.

Anaemia is common in patients with renal failure and should be corrected by oral iron therapy or blood transfusion.

When the patient is thought to be fit for the operation then he is either maintained on dialysis in the hospital, or a machine is supplied for him to dialyse himself at home. It is important that a potential recipient should be within easy reach of a telephone so that he can come to the hospital at short notice when a cadaveric kidney becomes available.

The operation

When the donor kidney (*Figure 11.4*) has reached the operating theatre the patient is anaesthetized and an endotracheal tube passed. An incision is made above the left or the right groin about 12.5 to 15 cm (5–6 in) long. The muscles are divided down to the peritoneum. This is not divided but is reflected off the pelvic wall until the iliac vessels are exposed. The peritoneum is carefully retracted to allow the surgeon to dissect the internal iliac artery from the surrounding tissue. This artery supplies the pelvic contents and may safely be **ligated** on the side of the operation without causing necrosis of the pelvic organs because the opposite internal iliac artery has free anastomotic branches across the midline. The distal vessel is ligated and divided, the proximal end having been clamped, and the end of the artery is prepared to receive the renal artery of the donor kidney. The external iliac vein is also mobilized. When all is ready, the kidney is removed from ice and transferred to the recipient's pelvis. The renal vein is cleaned and any small tributaries are ligated securely. The end of the vein is anastomosed to the side of the external iliac vein using a conventional running silk

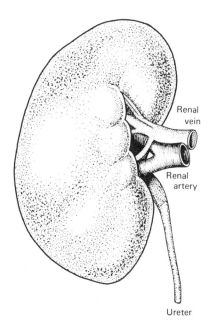

Renal vein

Renal artery

Ureter

Figure 11.4. The donor kidney

Hyperparathyroidism Oversecretion of parathormone which is produced by the parathyroid glands and is concerned with the regulation of calcium and phosphorus metabolism.

Parathyroidectomy Removal of a parathyroid gland.

Ligation The tying off (with a ligature) of a blood vessel or other hollow structure.

vascular suture. The clamps are released to allow blood to return up the external iliac vein and a small clamp is applied to the renal vein to prevent blood from passing into the kidney in a retrograde fashion. The renal artery is then anastomosed end-to-end to the internal iliac artery. The venous clamp and then the arterial clamp are removed and the blood is allowed to flow into the organ. If preservation has been successful then the kidney usually rapidly becomes

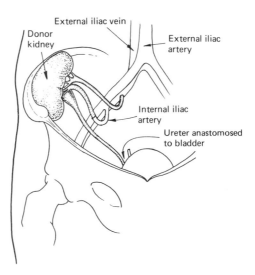

Figure 11.5. The operation of renal transplantation

red and swells visibly. Within a few minutes a normal consistency and colour should have been achieved. The suture lines are checked carefully for bleeding and additional sutures placed if necessary.

The donor ureter is then brought down to the bladder and carefully anastomosed through a muscular tunnel to the mucosa of the bladder, just above the trigone. A small **biopsy** is taken of the kidney for histological examination. A repeated check is made for bleeding and when the surgeon is satisfied that haemostasis has been secured, the layers are sewn together over the kidney, a drain being left *in situ*. A catheter may be left in the donor ureter if the kidney does not pass urine visibly during the operation. A self-retaining catheter is left within the bladder for 4 days after the operation. *Figure 11.5* illustrates the basic technique of the operation.

Postoperative management

Nursing care
The patient is returned to a clean cubicle environment which is air-conditioned with filtered air. Routine precautions against cross-infection should be rigorously employed. If the

Biopsy Inspection during life (from the Greek *bios* = life, *opsis* = view; c.f. necropsy = inspection after death), usually relating to small pieces removed from the body for a tissue diagnosis.

donor kidney function returns to normal rapidly after the operation, and if there is no evidence of haemorrhage or infection, then the nursing care of these patients is not at all difficult. As the peritoneal cavity has not been involved in the operative field, there is usually little disturbance of gastrointestinal function, for example, ileus. The patient should be mobile within 24 hours of the operation and is encouraged to sit out of bed on the following day. A soft diet may be commenced as soon as return of bowel function has been noted. After wound healing has occurred the patient is allowed up in the general ward and is discharged home as soon as renal function is satisfactory. With good renal function a patient may enjoy a normal diet and a full degree of physical activity.

Immunosuppression

Immunosuppressive drugs are started immediately after the operation. Initially prednisone 150 mg per day is given orally, and the dose reduced over a two-month period to 20 mg per day.

As Imuran is excreted by the kidneys, extreme caution must be used in its administration while the donor kidney is recovering its function. Initially 50 mg per day are given by mouth, and when the patient is passing more than 1 litre of urine per 24 hours the dose is gradually raised to 150 to 200 mg per day. A careful watch is kept on the white cell count and platelet count. These investigations plus routine blood tests of renal function (blood urea, creatinine, urine volume, electrolyte estimations) are carried out daily during the patient's stay in hospital. Should the white count or platelet count fall, the dose of Imuran is omitted for the next 2 to 3 days and recommenced at a reduced level when the total white cell count starts to rise. Careful checks are made for the onset of infection during the early postoperative phase and nose, throat, shunt and urine exit sites are swabbed every 3 to 4 days and cultured. If a respiratory infection occurs, then sputum cultures and routine chest radiographs should be performed. Suitable antibiotic therapy is instituted if such an infection occurs.

Haemodialysis

Postoperative **oliguria** is common after renal transplantation and dialysis treatment may be necessary. Ideally this should be carried out in the patient's own cubicle to prevent cross-infection. Post-transplantation oliguria rarely lasts for more than 30 days; following the onset of good renal function, dialysis may be discontinued.

Oliguria Urine output below the normal level.

Rejection

Some degree of rejection can be expected after transplantation of a kidney allograft and in most cases rejection can be controlled by the appropriate therapy, although a number of cases are resistant, resulting in the loss of the kidney.

Clinical signs
The clinical signs of the rejection reaction are as follows.

(1) The patient develops a fever and complains of symptoms of malaise not unlike those of influenza. He may also develop hypertension, and on physical examination there is enlargement and tenderness of the graft.
(2) There is a fall in urinary output and **proteinuria** occurs.
(3) There is a decrease in the glomerular filtration rate with a commensurate rise in the blood urea, creatinine and potassium levels.

The identification of rejection in the early postoperative phase may be difficult, particularly if the kidney is still recovering from ischaemic damage incurred at the time of grafting. In some cases other investigations may be of help, for example, isotope renography, arteriography and laboratory studies on the peripheral blood lymphocyte activity. If, after these tests have been performed there is still doubt, then a definite diagnosis can be made by performing needle biopsy of the graft and histological examination of the kidney tissue.

Treatment of rejection
As soon as rejection is diagnosed 1G. methylprednisolone is given intravenously and is repeated daily up to 4 grams. Imuran therapy is continued and other immunosuppressive agents (for example, actinomycin C) may be added to the regimen for a short period. As the renal function improves, the dose of prednisone is brought down to less toxic levels. Failure to resuscitate the graft after rejection is treated by graft nephrectomy and return to dialysis.

Long-term therapy
It is essential that these patients are followed up regularly for the rest of their lives while on immunosuppressive drugs. Quarterly or twice-yearly examinations may be carried out at the local hospital with the co-operation of the physicians or general practitioners in the area. Regular white cell counts and haemoglobin estimations should be performed. If there is any sign of rejection, the immunosuppressive dose must be adjusted during a period of close observation in hospital. It is

Proteinuria The presence of protein in the urine.

important to emphasize that these patients require immuno-suppressive drugs for the rest of their lives, albeit in very small doses in patients with prolonged graft survival.

Chronic rejection

In addition to acute rejection mediated mainly by host lymphocytes, the kidney may also incur chronic damage to its blood vessels by antibodies. This causes sclerotic changes in the renal vessels and subsequent atrophy of the kidney tissue and impairment of renal function. This type of rejection usually appears several months after the transplantation and is resistant to any form of treatment. Ultimately the patient will have to be returned to haemodialysis and the kidney removed.

Second and subsequent kidney transplants

If a patient rejects a graft and it has to be removed, a further graft may be considered. Before performing the second operation, however, it is important to test for the presence of antibody in the host's circulation which is active against the donor tissue. The second renal graft may be placed in the pelvis on the opposite side to the previous graft, or inserted into the abdomen. It is interesting that patients who receive a second graft fare as well, or better than, the primary allo-graft group.

The results of renal transplantation

The results of patient and graft survival are given in Table 11.1. Grafts between identical twins (isografts) are not rejected as there is no difference between donor and host histo-compatibility antigens, so in this group no immunosuppression is necessary: the 2-year patient and graft survival rate is 100 per cent. The 2-year graft survival figures of 67 per cent and

Table 11.1   One and 2-year patient and graft survival following renal transplantation. (From the Ninth Report of the Human Transplant Registry)*

			Donor		
Identical twin (isograft)			*Non-identical sibling*	*Parent*	*Cadaver*
Patient survival	1 year	100%	84%	78%	67%
	2 years	100%	76%	77%	61%
Graft survival	1 year	100%	75%	70%	56%
	2 years	100%	71%	67%	45%

*The disparity between patient survival and graft survival occurs because when a kidney stops functioning it may be removed and the patient returned to a haemodialysis programme.

77 per cent in the live related donor groups are very significantly better than the 45 per cent cadaver donor graft survivals.

Examination of the world results of kidney transplantation during the last 10 years shows that yearly the future is becoming brighter for renal transplant recipients. Many factors may explain this, but improvement in preservation techniques, further knowledge of immunosuppression, and the emergence of tissue typing as a means of improving donor-recipient matching are, no doubt, all significant. There is reason to suppose that with the utilization of new biological techniques, mortality and morbidity will fall even more and thus render renal transplantation a much less hazardous form of treatment of terminal renal failure.

FUTURE DEVELOPMENT

The results of renal transplantation are encouraging: a large proportion of patients treated are restored to a healthy and independent existence when they would otherwise have died. The survival figures compare very favourably with most forms of cancer. The major causes of morbidity and mortality arise from the toxic effect of the drugs which are used to suppress rejection. It is unlikely that any major breakthrough will be achieved until an alternative method of suppressing the rejection of the kidney has been found. In this context antilymphocyte serum (already discussed) provides an exciting alternative form of treatment to Imuran and steroids. However, a thoroughly satisfactory preparation is not yet available.

It is to be hoped that a clinically applicable specific immunosuppressive technique will be available in the foreseeable future for the artificial protection of organ grafts. When this is achieved, it can confidently be expected that the survival figures of renal transplantation will very significantly improve, to the extent that technical problems will represent the major limiting factor. Under these conditions, and using these techniques, it would be justifiable to apply transplant surgery to a very much wider range of human diseases. Tissue transplants which hitherto have been dogged by failure due to inability to suppress rejection, (for example, liver and pancreatic grafts) may well come into their own and be ethically justifiable.

So it seems possible that, like cardiac surgery during the last decade, tissue transplantation will be a routine therapeutic tool in the treatment of human disease.

12

The general management of trauma

Paul Atkins and C. J. E. Monk

The patient who suffers an injury to the body which is both sudden and often violent may subsequently be said to be suffering from trauma. The traumatic incident is usually short-lived and, unlike other factors in disease, it is not a continuing feature of the disease process. Trauma may literally be a short, sharp blow. A series of effects results directly from the injury — the majority being apparent immediately or within a short time. The treatment of the traumatic patient is directed to recognizing and correcting these effects and to preventing infection which may readily occur when body defences are breached (descriptions of specific injuries and their treatment will be found in different sections of this book). As far as the traumatic patient is concerned, the most important place in the hospital is the accident and emergency department (*Figure 12.1*), for it is here that the patient is received, diagnosis made and treatment initiated. It is important to realize that in a large district hospital, the accident and emergency department will be receiving many traumatic cases each day. Consequently, an important factor in dealing with trauma is the organization of this department, an aspect of which the nurse should be aware. It is helpful to consider patients with injuries as being in one of three categories: those with minor injuries, those with major injuries and those with life-threatening injuries.

GENERAL CONSIDERATIONS

Reception of patients suffering from trauma

Some degree of streaming is absolutely essential to the smooth running of a department dealing with traumatic cases.

Life-threatening injuries
The most serious cases will be brought into the department by the ambulance service and accepted immediately to the resuscitation room.

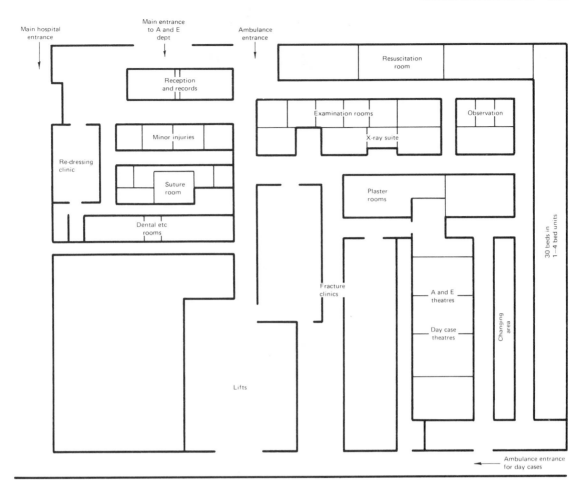

Figure 12.1. A diagram illustrating the layout of an accident and emergency department based on that at the Royal Liverpool Hospital

Major injuries

Most patients brought in by the ambulance service will not need immediate 'on the spot' treatment and these patients are accepted to a consulting room or cubicle, administrative details completed on the department card by the receptionist and the casualty officer informed of the patient's presence. Observations of pulse rate, respiratory rate and temperature should be made and the urine examined for the presence of sugar, **ketones** and protein. Other observations will be noted where appropriate; for example, in a patient with a head injury the level of consciousness will be recorded.

Minor injuries

Many patients attend the accident department with minor injuries. They will be received by the receptionist at the

Ketones Organic compounds (e.g. acetone) produced by an oxidation process.

door. She will issue a department card and the patient will be seen by the doctor as soon as possible. In a busy department it is sometimes inevitable that there will be a delay before the patient's turn to see the doctor comes. In this situation the nurse requires considerable tact to explain and apologize for the delay. The competent nurse will also provide an invaluable service by making sure that there are no patients waiting whose condition demands urgent consideration.

Sorting and disposal

An important function of the accident department is one of sorting. The casualty officer will decide that some injured patients can be managed entirely in the department, but that other patients will require the services of the specialist departments of the hospital. The decision will be made immediately, or after some investigations have been made.

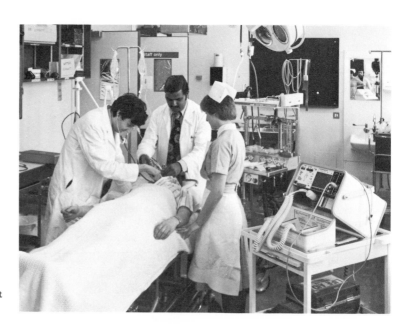

Figure 12.2. The resuscitation room in the Accident and Emergency Department of the Royal Liverpool Hospital

Sometimes the patient will be referred to an out-patient clinic, but more commonly immediate help is required. The appropriate hospital doctor will be contacted and will take charge of the patient's management. When a patient is severely ill, it may be necessary to keep him in the accident department while resuscitation is continued (*Figure 12.2*). Most patients, however, should be moved to a ward as rapidly as possible: either an observation ward within the department, or a ward within the main hospital.

Assessment of injuries

In all but the most minor injuries, the doctor will make a full examination of the patient. It cannot be stressed too strongly that to ensure that injuries are not overlooked, the patient should be fully undressed. In the severely injured it is remarkably easy to miss serious injuries simply through not seeing them. The patient may be unconscious or have all his attention focused on one injury and be completely unaware of another. Diagnosis may, of course, be straightforward, but it should be remembered that patients who sustain injuries often become involved in legal claims for compensation and an accurate record of the injuries is invaluable.

In examining the patient the medical officer makes a very rapid assessment of the condition. The majority of patients will have either major or minor injuries and the medical officer can complete a systematic examination, make a diagnosis and have special investigations, such as radiography, carried out to confirm it. A small proportion of patients with life-threatening injuries will require immediate treatment, and complete diagnosis may have to be deferred until this has been started. The state of a patient seen at the accident department following an injury depends not just on the

Table 12.1   Correlation between the severity of an injury and the anatomical injury

Minor injuries	Major injuries	Life-threatening injuries
Small lacerations	Large lacerations	Head injuries
Bruises	Fractures of long bones	Chest injuries
Fractures of small bones	Spine (fractures)	Abdominal injuries
Dislocations of small joints	Pelvis (fractures)	
Sprains	Multiple injuries	
	Burns	

anatomical extent of the trauma, but on other factors as well: for example, the age of the patient, the time since trauma was inflicted and the first-aid measures taken, are all of importance. Thus the young man with a fractured tibia and fibula, whose leg has been expertly splinted by a 'first-aider', and who has been rapidly transported to hospital, may be in a better state than an old lady who has merely bumped her leg but in doing so has torn a superficial varicose vein. Inadequate attempts at stopping the bleeding and delay in obtaining help have often led to the admission of such patients in a critical

L

condition. Bearing in mind these qualifications, the severity of an injury will probably correlate with the anatomical injury in the way indicated in Table 12.1.

Observation

Many traumatic patients will require careful observation. Most hospitals have charts on which the observations are recorded by the nurse. A medical officer may request the nurse to make observations with one of *three* possibilities in mind. It may be that with a period of observation the diagnosis will be clarified, for example unexpected bleeding in the abdominal or thoracic cavities may be revealed by a rising pulse rate and falling blood pressure. Certain complications are known to be common in particular injuries and careful observation will lead to their recognition at an early stage, for example deterioration in the level of consciousness in a patient who has sustained a head injury may indicate that cerebral compression from an extradural haemorrhage is occurring. Observations may also be made to ensure that treatment is satisfactory, for example adequate transfusion to replace blood loss is accompanied by return of the pulse rate, blood pressure and urinary output to normal. Whatever the reason, the nurse responsible for making the observations must be quite sure that she fully understands the doctor's instructions. Rather than mechanically charting the findings, the nurse should be able to appreciate the significance of them. The doctor or sister will invariably explain this. If this is not done, the nurse should ask about points she does not understand. Invariably the medical staff's written instructions will specify instances when a doctor is to be notified. For example, it may be stated that the casualty officer should be informed if the pulse rate rises above 120 per minute or the systolic blood pressure falls below 100 mm Hg. While obviously such instructions will be followed, it is even more important for the nurse to use her common sense and inform the medical staff promptly if she thinks the patient's condition is deteriorating, whether or not the specific limits have been reached.

COMMON PROBLEMS IN TRAUMA AND THEIR MANAGEMENT

Though trauma can result in many different types of injury, each of which requires a specific line of treatment, there are certain common problems which are very frequently seen. Many patients are frightened and upset by their experience and a kindly word of reassurance should always be given.

Haemorrhage accompanies most injuries. It may be obvious in the patient with multiple lacerations, or it may be concealed in the patient with a fractured pelvis. When a large volume of blood is lost, the patient becomes shocked and if the blood volume is not restored, the patient will die. Respiratory failure is seen in patients with chest injuries, but also in other circumstances, such as head injuries. Wounds and lacerations are the commonest results of trauma and demand skilled attention. The nurse caring for traumatic patients will be intimately concerned with these problems. The time available for starting treatment may often be short. There can hardly be a more serious problem than the traumatic patient who undergoes cardiac arrest, perhaps as the end result of haemorrhagic shock or of failing vital centres, yet it may be the nurse who has to set in motion initial treatment. For these reasons, emphasis is deliberately laid on a practical approach to these problems.

Shock

The clinical picture of shock is rarely difficult to recognize. The patient is pale and cold, has a clammy skin and a rapid, thready pulse with usually a low blood pressure. Shock commonly results from haemorrhage, trauma, burns and loss of gastrointestinal fluid (*Figure 12.3*). In these conditions there is a decrease in blood volume. The kidneys, gut and skin are deprived of blood by selective vasoconstriction thereby maintaining the blood supply of the heart and brain with the blood volume available. Shock also occurs in septicaemia, when there is an increase in circulatory capacity and also when there is a central failure of the heart pump in such conditions as myocardial infarction and **pulmonary** embolism.

Essentially the condition is a failure to perfuse the tissues with blood. As a result the tissues are deprived of oxygen and metabolic processes are disturbed, resulting in the formation of acid products. The presence of acid products causes many more of the small tissue vessels to dilate than usual, thereby increasing the circulatory capacity. The flow in these vessels, however, is so slow that sludging of the red cells takes place in many of them, thereby worsening the perfusion of tissues.

The time scale for developing the features of shock shown in *Figure 12.3* is, of course, variable but usually shock due to a reduction in blood volume develops over a period of hours; in septicaemic shock the features may develop in minutes and, in cardiogenic shock, days. Cardiogenic shock may develop in the patient whose initial problem was hypovolaemic or septic shock. The action of the heart becomes impaired by

Pulmonary embolism Pulmonary artery blockage by a clot carried from elsewhere in the blood until it lodges at this point.

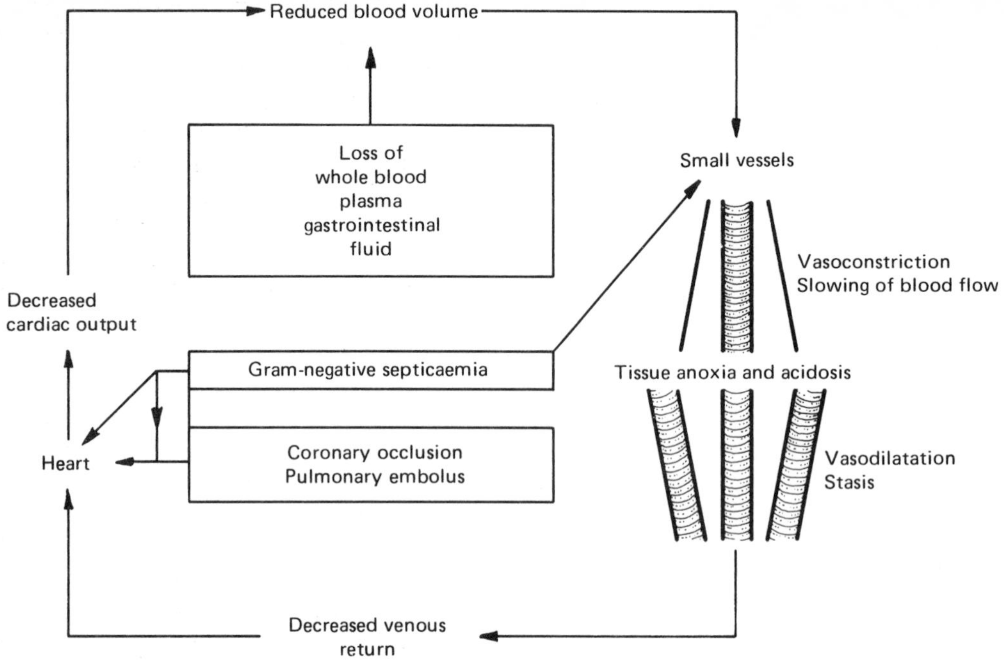

Figure 12.3. Diagram illustrating the cause and effect of shock

acidosis, myocardial ischaemia or the direct action of bacterial toxins.

The patient who is shocked may well have a number of competing requirements. He may need analgesia for pain, an operation to stop bleeding or he may have fractured limbs which require splinting. The priority given to these requirements needs careful judgement in the individual case. Invariably, however, resuscitation is the first step. Concurrently, careful observations are made to monitor the effectiveness of treatment.

Treatment

The treatment of shock depends on the cause. In the traumatic situation shock is invariably due to a reduction in blood volume — so-called hypovolaemic shock. A head-down tilt will help to restore the effective blood volume by emptying blood from the veins of the legs. The next step is to replace the fluid lost; when it is blood from haemorrhage the logical replacement fluid is whole blood. However, a certain amount of time may elapse before blood becomes available, and it is important to realize that the essential requirement is to restore volume rather than red cells, hence the medical officer will often start a transfusion with a solution such as dextran or Ringer lactate fluid. The former is known as a colloid solution and has large molecules. On the other hand, Ringer lactate is a crystalloid solution with small molecules. It should be remembered that the smaller the molecules are the quicker will that fluid escape from the circulation, and large amounts of crystalloid fluids are required if this is the sole replacement fluid. Attempts are often made to lessen tissue anoxia and acidosis by improving small vessel flow. Low molecular weight dextran may be transfused as it reduces red cell sludging. Steroids in large doses are sometimes given to lessen vasoconstriction. The effects of anoxia and acidosis may be mitigated by making the patient breathe oxygen through a mask and by transfusing calculated amounts of an alkaline solution such as 8.4 per cent sodium bicarbonate.

Hypovolaemic shock in patients with burns is mainly due to the escape of plasma through damaged blood vessel walls and in this instance the blood volume should be restored with plasma.

Other forms of shock are less likely to be seen in the traumatic situation but for completeness their treatment is briefly mentioned. Hypovolaemia due to loss of gastrointestinal fluid as in vomiting or diarrhoea is treated by transfusion of crystalloid solutions containing appropriate electrolytes. In septicaemic shock a very large volume of crystalloid fluid is often required but, in addition, large doses of a wide spectrum antibiotic are essential. If a source of infection such as an **empyema of the gall bladder** is found, this will require operative treatment. In cardiogenic shock measures are taken to support the heart.

Monitoring treatment Carefully recorded observations are essential to ensure that treatment is adequate. Recordings of the pulse, blood pressure, respiration and temperature are instituted at 15-minute intervals. In hypovolaemic shock the pulse is rapid but slows with restoration of the blood volume. The blood pressure may be sustained at relatively normal levels until the blood volume deficit is large, but it may then fall rapidly. Air hunger and a temperature below normal may be features of hypovolaemia. Effective treatment is accompanied by a reversal of these signs. Measurements of the central venous pressure and of the urinary output are also extremely important ways of monitoring the effectiveness of treatment.

Intravenous infusions
A trolley is prepared by the nurse and should contain a variety of intravenous catheters for introduction by venepuncture and by the 'cut-down' technique. On the trolley there should

Empyema of the gall bladder Acute cholecystitis with distension of the gall bladder with pus.

also be a giving set and bottles of intravenous fluid, gauze swabs, skin disinfectants, such as Cetavlon and spirit, local anaesthetics (1 per cent procaine or lignocaine), gallipots, sponge-holding forceps, scalpel, dissecting forceps, haemostats, fine pointed scissors, suture materials and needles. Sterile syringes and hypodermic needles as well as skin towels are necessary and gloves and masks must also be available.

The doctor 'scrubs up' and if the 'cut-down' technique is used, he will wear sterile gloves in addition to a mask. The nurse, though not 'scrubbing up', should wear a mask. Whenever possible a vein in the forearm rather than in the leg is selected for the insertion of a catheter (*Figure 12.4*).

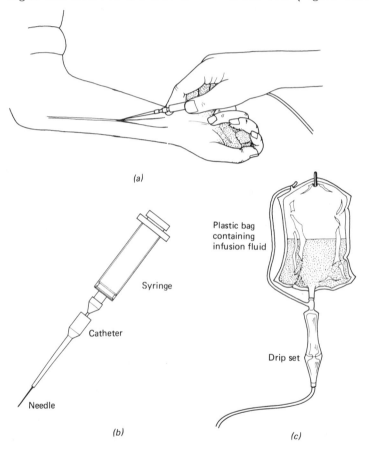

(a)

Plastic bag containing infusion fluid

Syringe

Catheter

Drip set

Needle

Figure 12.4. (*a*) Setting up a transfusion; (*b*) intracatheter; (*c*) transfusion set

(b)   *(c)*

The veins are distended conveniently by inflating a sphygmomanometer cuff on the arm. This should be placed on the arm with the rubber tubing away from the forearm, the opposite way from usual, so that it does not lie over the proposed venepuncture site. The cuff should be inflated to one-half of the systolic blood pressure level. The site is sterilized, towels suitably arranged and local anaesthetic injected to raise a bleb over the vein. The nurse takes a plastic bag or bottle of infusion fluid and places a holder around the latter. If a blood transfusion is being set up, the name and number on the label must be checked against that in the patient's notes. The doctor takes a sterile plastic drip set out of its package and inserts the bevelled end of the set into the outlet of the plastic bag or rubber bung of the infusion bottle. Fluid is then run through the giving set to ensure that it is free of air bubbles and the bottle is hung up on the drip stand in a convenient position.

The doctor will then insert a polythene catheter either by venepuncture or by 'cut-down' technique. If the former method is used, the procedure differs little from a normal venepuncture except that a catheter is left lying in the vein while the needle which acts as a **trocar**, is withdrawn. As the catheter fills with blood the giving set is quickly joined to it.

With a 'cut-down' technique, a small transverse incision is made over the vein (*Figure 12.5*). The vein is dissected out and the distal end ligated with catgut; the ends of the catgut are left long and held in a haemostat. A further length of catgut is placed around the upper end of the vein and the first half of a knot loosely tied — the ends of this are also held in a haemostat. A small cut is made with sharp pointed scissors and a catheter inserted and directed a suitable distance up the vein. The knot on the proximal ligature is completed and the ends of the ligature cut. As blood fills the catheter, the giving set is joined to it and skin sutures are inserted. A small gauze dressing is applied and wide elastoplast is used to fix the drip set in position; the tubing should be placed in the shape of a 'U' on the patient's forearm to prevent a direct pull on the catheter.

The type of fluid and the rate at which it is to be given should be clearly indicated in written, timed instructions. When very rapid infusion of fluid is required, a Martin's pump may be used.

Central venous pressure measurement

In the presence of a low blood volume, the central venous pressure is low; with restoration of blood volume towards normal, the central venous pressure will rise to normal levels. If overtransfusion occurs, or if the pumping action of the heart fails 'damming back' the venous blood, the central venous pressure reading will be higher than normal. Measurement of the central venous pressure is a relatively simple way of monitoring the progress of a patient receiving large transfusions. The procedure for inserting the catheter is as previously described, but the catheter used is longer and it is advanced into the superior vena cava.

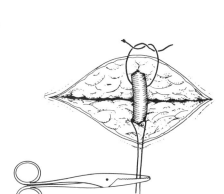

Figure 12.5. 'Cut-down' technique of intravenous infusion

Trocar An instrument which has a sharp point and is placed in the centre of a cannula to allow this to be introduced into a cavity.

This important procedure is described in detail elsewhere (p. 82).

The medical officer will give instructions with regard to the frequency of readings and will indicate the central venous pressure levels at which he should be notified. The way in which three successive readings lead is in many ways more useful than the absolute readings.

Urine excretion

Excretion of urine is decreased in the hypovolaemic state. Rapid restoration and maintenance of the normal blood volume is reflected by a return to normal levels of urinary excretion. In the average adult, this exceeds 50 ml per hour. Urinary output is an extremely useful indication of the circulatory state and it should always be measured in the severely injured. The bladder should be catheterized, using a fully aseptic technique.

Cardiac arrest

Patients may be brought to the resuscitation room with ambulance personnel already performing cardiac massage, or ill patients already in the department may suddenly arrest. In cardiac arrest the vital centres of the body have an inadequate circulation, either because the heart has stopped beating, or because of unco-ordinated contractions of parts of the ventricular muscle. If the heart remains arrested for 4 minutes without resuscitative measures being taken, permanent brain damage occurs. The patient, in losing consciousness, becomes ashen, the pulse impalpable and respiratory movements cease. As soon as this situation is apparent, the diagnosis of cardiac arrest is made and the hospital plan for this emergency is put into operation. In the accident and emergency department, the casualty officer will quickly take charge, but the nurse may well be the first person to recognize the situation. She must detail someone to get in contact with the telephone operator and proceed immediately to inflate the patient's lungs with air; there is no doubt that the rapidity with which mouth-to-mouth respiration may be started is a great advantage in a situation where every second counts. A Brooks airway or an Ambu bag may, of course, be immediately to hand and either can then be used. Once the lungs have been inflated a few times, it is worth trying three sharp blows over the precordium. The main consideration, however, is to continue inflating the lungs. As soon as a second person arrives, effective cardiac massage can begin.

Closed cardiac massage

The patient must be lying on a firm surface. If the trolley does not provide such a surface, a specially designed board should be placed underneath the patient, or failing this, the patient can be transferred to the floor. Closed massage (*Figure 12.6*) is performed by laying the heel of one hand on the sternum with the other placed on top. The sternum is then pushed towards the spine, thereby compressing the

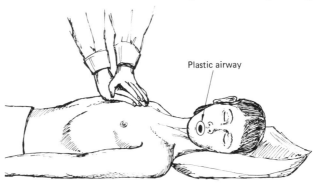

Plastic airway

Figure 12.6. A diagram showing the technique of a closed cardiac massage in a patient in cardiac arrest

heart. By rocking backwards the compression is released allowing the heart to fill. It is advantageous to massage the heart at the rate of 72 per minute at first, but if there is no immediate response, a slower rate with a regular pause to enable inflation of the lungs should be followed. The adequacy of massage can be confirmed by feeling the femoral or carotid pulse, and its effectiveness by noting contraction of previously dilated pupils.

When the telephone operator receives the arrest call, he will inform the designated team and despatch porters with the arrest trolley to the emergency site. The arrival of the team should allow an even more intensive attempt to save life to be made. While cardiac massage is continued, the following changes in procedure are smoothly made by the team. An endotracheal tube is inserted by a doctor which allows the patient's lungs to be inflated more efficiently with oxygen, delivered most conveniently from an oxygen cylinder in a Boyle's machine. It is delivered by way of a 'bag' and valve. An intravenous drip is set up and 100 ml of 8.4 per cent sodium bicarbonate is run in to reverse the inevitable acidosis that results from cardiac arrest. Electrocardiogram (ECG) leads are applied and monitoring established. The ECG will show that either the heart has stopped beating (asystole), or that it is beating in an unco-ordinated fashion (fibrillation). If asystole is present, an injection of intracardiac adrenaline 1 ml of 1/1000 solution should be given. This may result in the restoration of a normal heartbeat, it may induce fibrillation, or the heart may remain in asystole. If normal rhythm is restored, cardiac massage is continued until there can be no doubt about the adequacy of the circulation. If asystole persists, further sodium bicarbonate should be given. Intracardiac adrenaline can be repeated after a 5-minute interval. An injection of 5 ml of 10 per cent calcium chloride may also be administered by the intracardiac route. When ventricular fibrillation is the underlying cause of the arrest, or when it has been induced by adrenaline, an attempt should be made to defibrillate the heart by passing electric shocks through it. An external direct current defibrillator machine should be used. Before using this machine, the ECG monitor should be switched off and metal connections on airways removed. All medical and nursing personnel other than the two people holding the paddle electrodes should stand aside. The two people applying the electrodes will wear rubber gloves and will apply the wide, damp electrodes from opposite sides: one should be placed on the lower part of the sternum and the other on the left anterolateral chest wall. One shock of low voltage is given. If the heart does not respond, three shocks are given in rapid succession. The procedure is repeated at an increased voltage if there is still no response.

Open cardiac massage

Open cardiac massage is less frequently used. It is, however, probably rather more effective and if closed massage fails to establish a satisfactory pulse, it should be utilized if the situation appears to be recoverable. Open massage is desirable in the patient who has arrested in the presence of a chest injury.

Pausing only to ensure that an endotracheal tube is in place, the chest is rapidly cleaned with Cetavlon and opened through the anterior half of the left fourth intercostal space. The ribs are sprung apart and, if necessary, further room is obtained by dividing the costal cartilages of the fourth and fifth rib. The pericardium is opened vertically in front of the phrenic nerve and the heart is compressed between two hands: one placed anteriorly and one posteriorly. The procedure then differs little from closed massage except that, of course, with successful resumption of heartbeat, the chest is closed and an intercostal tube inserted and drained to an underwater seal. Very occasionally, where patients fail to resume a normal beat, the medical staff will decide to use a pacemaker which supplies a continuous electrical stimulus. When the heart has been restarted, the patient must be kept under continuous observation for about 3 days. Arrhythmias and further arrest are most likely to occur during this time. Antibiotics should invariably be prescribed to combat infection.

Arrhythmia Irregular heartbeat.

Respiratory problems

A full description of respiratory problems and their management is given elsewhere. It is pertinent to note here, however, that the first step in looking after the unconscious patient or the patient with a chest injury, is to ensure the presence of an adequate airway. Often this may be accomplished simply by positioning the patient in the lateral position, pulling the tongue forward and introducing an oropharyngeal airway. If, despite these measures, the patient is in respiratory distress, further action will be required to cope with the causative problem.

Wounds and lacerations

The treatment of wounds and lacerations is a recurring problem in the accident department. Many of these are quite simple, such as a cut finger, but if they are not properly treated, they may cause considerable morbidity, with subsequent loss of time from work or school. The type of wound and the circumstances under which it occurs are very important. Two considerations are uppermost in the doctor's mind when he sees a patient with a laceration: (1) the extent of the injury, whether it is merely a wound of skin and subcutaneous tissue, or whether it has involved other anatomical structures, such as tendons and nerves, or even large blood vessels; (2) which applies to all lacerations and wounds, whether infection has occurred or is likely to occur. The risk of infection occurring is relatively small in cleanly incised wounds which are seen in the accident department within the first 6 hours. On the other hand, jagged and particularly penetrating wounds are much more likely to be infected. One infection of great importance is tetanus. The tetanus spores are most commonly found in well manured soil; consequently, the chance of infection with this organism is much greater if the wound has been sustained under dirty conditions. Fortunately, the incidence of the disease of tetanus is low in Great Britain. In countries such as Nigeria, on the other hand, it is still high. The risks of tetanus can be minimized in two ways; one is to give antitetanus serum, which contains antibodies which will directly inhibit tetanus toxin, the other is to give tetanus toxoid which stimulates the production of antibodies to tetanus toxin. Tetanus toxoid can have no immediate effect, but it will boost the production of antibodies to tetanus toxin in a patient who has already been immunized with tetanus toxoid. The side-effects from tetanus toxoid are minimal. On the other hand, with antitetanus serum, allergic reactions are not uncommon.

Since the incidence of tetanus is low in Great Britain, the policy usually adopted is to give patients with dirty wounds and lacerations an antibiotic, such as penicillin, and tetanus toxoid, following this up with a booster dose of toxoid 6 weeks later. This procedure avoids the risk of allergic reactions. In countries where the incidence of tetanus is high, the policy of giving patients antitetanus serum in such circumstances is followed.

Surgical toilet of wounds

Although suturing of a laceration is quite a minor procedure, it should be done under full aseptic precautions, ideally in an operating theatre reserved for clean cases. If the wound is large, a general anaesthetic may be necessary. The vast majority of smaller lacerations and wounds can be dealt with utilizing 1 or 2 per cent lignocaine. It is vital to ensure that where a local anaesthetic is used to anaesthetize a digit, it does not contain adrenaline, since this can readily cause **gangrene** and loss of a finger or toe. The affected area is cleansed with Cetavlon, the area towelled up, a local anaesthetic injected where necessary and the wound explored; obvious bleeding points are caught with haemostats and ligated with fine catgut. On the whole, the doctor dealing with these wounds will insert a minimum of deep sutures. Fine silk sutures are used to close the skin. Where the wound is infected, or treatment has been delayed, it may well be felt wiser by the doctor to excise obviously necrotic tissue and leave the wound open to granulate. Dressings should consist of dry gauze, held in place by a bandage, or where the wound is small, a proprietary plastic spray on dressing may well suffice. Having finished his initial treatment, the patient will invariably be seen at a dressing clinic, where sutures will be removed and an effort made to ensure that the patient is fully rehabilitated from his wound.

MANAGEMENT OF SPECIFIC INJURIES

The casualty officer is concerned with the reception and initial assessment of the injured patient. In a modern hospital accident unit, such as that described earlier, he has the full facilities of the hospital to call on. Experience has shown that no one individual can have sufficient expertise to cover the surgical assessment and treatment of injuries to all parts of the body. The casualty officer therefore assesses the patient in the following order of priority.

Gangrene Tissue necrosis and putrefaction due to cutting off of the blood supply; usually either in the bowel or in a limb, in which case the gangrene may be 'dry' or 'wet'.

(1) Is the airway clear?
(2) Is the patient breathing satisfactorily?
(3) Are there any signs of circulatory failure (shock)?

Any abnormality in these areas must be dealt with immediately. It will be noted that the aforementioned (1), (2) and (3) can conveniently be grouped alphabetically.

(1) — A — Airway
(2) — B — Breathing
(3) — C — Circulation

Having dealt with these 3 assessments the casualty officer then turns his attention to the injuries sustained by the patient conveniently grouped as:—

(a) The body cavities — cranial, thoracic, abdominal.
(b) The rest of the body.

Head injuries

Most injuries to the head cause some damage to the brain and may lead to unconsciousness. This is referred to as concussion and it may last for any period from a few seconds to several days or weeks.

It is important in all head injuries, especially those causing concussion, to make periodic estimations of the patient's level of consciousness and motor activity. This is because there is a possibility that one or more of the blood vessels within the skull has been damaged and there may be bleeding into the cranial cavity. The skull acts as a bony case which cannot be distended and hence any intracranial bleeding must compress the brain substance. Pressure on the brain itself causes a deterioration in the level of consciousness and pressure on the motor centres will cause at first a spastic type of paralysis of the muscles supplied by the particular area of the brain and this is followed, if the intracranial pressure continues to rise, by a flaccid paralysis.

Similar changes are seen in the muscles supplied by the cranial nerves if the intracranial pressure rises. Most sensitive are the muscles of the pupil which constricts first and then dilates. A severe rise of intracranial pressure will cause the pupils on both sides to be dilated thereby not responding to light.

Fractures of the skull may be depressed and the bone fragments themselves may compress the brain substance. Elevation is urgently indicated.

Chest injuries

These are dealt with in detail in Chapter 15. The first priority in the treatment of chest injuries is to keep the patient well oxygenated. This means that the airway (the mouth and larynx) must be checked to ensure that there is no obstruction and the movements of the chest examined to see if there is (a) any paradoxical movement: one segment moving out of step with the rest of the chest wall or (b) any loss of movement which may signify a tension **pneumothorax**.

The ribs are palpated to see if any are tender and if so whether pain is felt at this tender area when the thoracic cage is gently compressed from backwards and from side to side. If there is pain it is possible that there is a fracture of one or more ribs.

Having established that the patient's airway is clear and that he is breathing normally an x-ray of the chest is done to confirm the presence of rib fractures or intrathoracic injury.

Abdominal injuries

Abdominal trauma results in either a penetrating or a closed injury. In civilian practice in Great Britain the majority of injuries are of the closed type. An injury to the abdomen may be the sole injury, but very often it is seen as one of several injuries.

Closed injuries
Closed abdominal injuries may simply give rise to bruising of the abdominal wall or they may cause damage to structures which lie within the abdomen. Most of these structures lie within the peritoneal cavity and others, such as the kidneys and bladder, are only separated from it by a thin layer of peritoneum.

Penetrating injuries
Penetrating injuries may also only damage the abdominal wall, but are much more likely to damage underlying viscera. The problem of abdominal injuries hinges on whether or not there has been damage to the intra-abdominal contents.

The patient may give a clear history of the traumatic incident and complain of abdominal pain or other specific symptoms, such as inability to pass urine or the passage of blood-stained urine. Sometimes, however, the patient does not realize that he has sustained an abdominal injury because his attention is directed to other, more painful injuries. On other occasions, patients with abdominal injuries are unconscious. In the latter instances, the history supplied by bystanders may be extremely useful in judging the likely damage.

The patient is very carefully examined in an attempt to decide whether there is an intra-abdominal injury. His general appearance may suggest that he is shocked and this may be supported by finding a rapid pulse rate and a low blood

Pneumothorax Air within the pleural cavity.

pressure. Penetrating injuries of the abdomen, such as stab wounds, are usually obvious but it must be remembered that an intra-abdominal injury can result from a downward stab in the chest — the knife traversing the diaphragm; hence the importance of having the patient fully exposed for examination. Obvious bruising and tyre marks on the abdomen usually indicate serious mischief.

Injuries to other parts of the trunk may suggest the likelihood of intra-abdominal injury; for example, fractures of the left lower ribs are frequently accompanied by damage to the spleen, and fractures of the pelvis by damage to the bladder and urethra. Tenderness and rigidity may be indicative of peritoneal irritation caused either by blood, or visceral content free in the abdominal cavity. Sometimes it will be possible to palpate a mass due to haematoma in one part of the abdomen and repeated examination may indicate that it is increasing in size.

Investigations

Radiographs of the abdomen are taken. If the alimentary tract has been damaged, gas often escapes into the abdominal cavity, and films taken with the patient sitting up may show this. Sometimes it can be appreciated from the radiographs that there is free fluid in the abdomen. When the possibility of damage to the kidney arises an intravenous pyelogram is performed in an attempt to show up the injury and, even more important, to demonstrate that the other kidney is normal so that, should an operation be necessary, there will be no question of unknowingly removing a solitary functioning kidney.

The haemoglobin level is a useful indication of blood loss and should always be estimated. The white cell count is usually estimated at the same time; it is sometimes found to be increased when the spleen has been ruptured. The urine is routinely examined. When the genito-urinary tract has been damaged, the patient will invariably have haematuria. Aspiration of the abdominal cavity — the so-called four-quadrant tap — may reveal free fluid within the abdomen.

In this way the doctor attempts to decide whether an intra-abdominal injury has occurred. In the majority of patients a firm diagnosis is made. In a small proportion of patients, despite very careful assessment, the medical officer will be in some doubt as to whether or not there is an intra-abdominal injury. It may be a situation where, because of the nature of the injury, the likelihood of intra-abdominal damage is so great that a decision is made to explore the abdomen. On the other hand, it may be decided to observe the patient for a short period of time. When the nurse is requested to make observations on such a patient, it is important that she realizes that her observations will be crucial to the diagnosis.

In instances where intra-abdominal bleeding is occurring, the general appearance of the patient, his pulse rate and blood pressure, may all indicate bleeding. It may become apparent that, despite transfusion sufficient to deal with blood loss from known injuries, the patient is not responding well and that additional bleeding is taking place within the abdomen. Equally, maintenance of a normal pulse and blood pressure may suggest that there is, in fact, no intra-abdominal bleeding in a patient where this was at first suspected. When visceral damage has occurred the signs of peritoneal irritation will increase during the period of observation.

Treatment

In the more severe forms of abdominal injury the first consideration will be to combat hypovolaemic shock with blood or dextran transfusion.

Laparotomy is performed for all penetrating injuries and for closed injuries where there is evidence of blood or free fluid in the peritoneal cavity. Damage to different organs is treated in appropriate ways; thus the spleen is removed, lacerations in the liver are sutured where possible — sometimes a part is excised or at other times a pack may be inserted. Tears in the small gut and mesentery are usually treated by resection of the damaged part and anastomosis of the two ends. Damage to the descending part of the large bowel is treated by bringing the damaged part on to the abdominal wall and forming a colostomy. Damage to the right side of the colon is treated by a right **hemicolectomy**, or where the damage is slight, by suturing the hole. Injury to the rectum is treated by a diverting colostomy and repair of the rectal wall.

Postoperative care is directed towards the prevention of paralytic ileus, the treatment of infection and the relief of pain.

Injuries to the urinary tract

Mention of injuries to the kidneys, bladder and urethra will be found in Chapters 29 and 30; only the salient features are described here.

Renal injuries

A renal injury may be the sole injury or it may accompany other injuries. The patient will usually complain of loin pain and blood may be found in the urine. Examination may show some degree of hypovolaemic shock and tenderness and rigidity of the loin muscles is usually found. If damage is severe, there may be a swelling in the loin caused either by

Hemicolectomy Surgical excision of a portion of the colon.

extensive bleeding or by urine leaking from the kidney. Confirmation of suspected renal damage is obtained by an intravenous pyelogram.

Shock is treated by intravenous fluid and paralytic ileus, which is common in these injuries, is guarded against by inserting a Ryle's tube to allow continuous gastric aspiration.

In most cases the patient with an injured kidney is treated conservatively. He is nursed in bed and very careful observation is made; in particular the pulse and blood pressure are recorded and successive specimens of urine are examined to ensure that the haematuria is decreasing.

Only when there are signs of continuous bleeding or urine leakage as evidenced by the patient's general state, the appearance of a mass in the loin or the radiographic appearance, is a nephrectomy performed.

Damage to the bladder

The bladder lies in the pelvis, but as it fills it rises up into the abdomen. It is separated from the peritoneal cavity only by a thin layer of peritoneum. When the bladder is torn urine may leak either into the extraperitoneal tissues, or into the peritoneal cavity itself. Extraperitoneal rupture is more common than intraperitoneal injury and is usually associated with a fractured pelvis. In this injury a part of the pelvic girdle may be driven into the bladder. An intraperitoneal rupture can occur when a patient with a full bladder receives a blow to the abdomen. When dealing with a drunk who has been in a fight, the possibility of such an injury should always be considered, for these are ideal circumstances under which this injury can occur yet the inebriated man may give little evidence of such damage. The patient will usually be unable to pass urine and suspicion of the injury may be confirmed by finding signs of peritoneal irritation.

As part of the investigation, a catheter is passed under sterile conditions. Radio-opaque dye is injected and radiographs are obtained. In this way and also occasionally by performing a **cystoscopy**, attempts are made to visualize the leak. The presence or absence of urine in the bladder is not diagnostic of a rupture or of its absence, though the presence of heavily blood-stained urine strongly suggests that a tear has occurred.

If a tear in the bladder has occurred, the abdomen is explored. The tear is sewn up and the bladder drained by a catheter in the urethra and usually by one leading through the abdominal wall, a so-called suprapubic catheter. In the case of an intraperitoneal rupture all urine is sucked out of the abdominal cavity. Catheters are removed when the bladder has healed.

Cystoscopy The examining of the interior of the urinary bladder with a cystoscope.

Damage to the male urethra

The urethra may be ruptured at the base of the bladder within the pelvis, or in its perineal course. The former injury may take place when the pelvis is fractured. The urethra, which is rigidly held at the bottom of the pelvis, is acutely distorted and torn across. The perineal urethra is rarely injured, but this can occur when a patient falls astride an object. The clinical features of an intrapelvic rupture of the urethra are similar to those of an extraperitoneal rupture of the bladder. The patient with a ruptured perineal urethra is unable to pass urine, but blood may be seen at the urethral meatus. Considerable swelling and bruising in the perineum may also be apparent.

A urethrogram may be obtained. This is a radiograph taken after dye has been injected into the urethra and this may delineate the tear.

When treating an intrapelvic rupture, a catheter is passed in the operating theatre. If it fails to enter the bladder, but merely drains blood, the presence of a ruptured urethra is almost certain. The bladder is opened, enabling a urethral catheter to be manipulated into the bladder. By drawing down on the catheter the divided ends are closely opposed. Healing then takes place with the catheter acting as a splint.

In the case of perineal rupture, the ends of the urethra are exposed and two or three sutures are inserted to oppose the ends; a catheter is inserted to act as a splint.

Spinal injuries

Fractures and dislocations of the spine are usually relatively easy to diagnose on clinical and radiological examination. The most important aspect of these injuries is that they may be associated with damage to the spinal cord which lies within the bony protection of the vertebrae. Complete cutting of the cord results in complete loss of sensation and voluntary movement below the level of transection. If this occurs at the waist the condition of paralysis of the legs is referred to as paraplegia. If it occurs in the neck the condition of paralysis of all four limbs is referred to as tetraplegia. Both of these conditions require treatment in specialized centres, but it is important for the staff of a Casualty Department to appreciate that the danger to the patient is that he will be left lying on insensitive areas of skin from which the blood will be squeezed and the whole skin and subcutaneous tissue may later necrose and slough. The phenomenon can occur within 2 hours, so that it is essential that the patient be moved often enough and regularly so that his weight is taken on a different area of his body at least every 2 hours.

In tetraplegia and paraplegia the bladder also becomes paralyzed and if the patient is detained in the receiving hospital for more than 12 hours, catheterization may be necessary. This should be done under full aseptic precautions and most authorities accept now that the catheter should be removed at the end of the procedure. The long-term handling of the bladder depends on the current practice in the paraplegic unit to which the patient is transferred.

Pelvic injuries

Since quite a large proportion of the pelvis is easily palpated most of the fractures of the pelvis can be diagnosed on initial assessment. Some of the deeper parts of the pelvis and especially those parts around the hip joint are more difficult to palpate and any suspected injury must be further investigated by x-ray examination.

There are two complications commonly seen in fractures of the pelvis; injury to the genito-urinary tract (*see above*) and haemorrhage.

The large vessels supplying the pelvic organs and the lower limbs are in close contact with the pelvis. Fracture of the pelvis may cause tearing, particularly of the veins, with a large amount of leakage of blood into the tissues in the pelvis and in the extraperitoneal tissues of the back. It is not unusual for a patient to lose 2 to 3 litres of blood into these spaces when a fracture occurs in the pelvis. The difficulty confronting the surgeon is that none of this blood is visible and it is only when the patient develops signs of shock that the degree of haemorrhage becomes apparent. For this reason, it is usual for an intravenous transfusion of plasma or blood to be given to any patient with a severe fracture of the pelvis.

Fractures of limb bones

The emergency treatment of fractured bones is to immobilize the affected limb on a splint until radiographs can be taken and full assessment of the injury can be made. If a limb bone fracture is left unsplinted it can contribute to, or even cause, shock of a severe degree.

In general terms the fractures of the limbs are treated according to the general principles laid down in Chapter 16: reduction, immobilization until union, and protection until consolidation. Normally the reduction and immobilization of fractures are done in the Accident Department before the patient is taken to the ward or allowed home.

Wherever possible the fractures are reduced by the closed methods of reduction (manipulation or traction) and immobilized by external means — (splints, plasters or traction). Those requiring open reduction or internal fixation are admitted to the ward for preparation of the skin preoperatively.

CONCLUSION

At the present time, the individual who suffers an injury has a better chance of surviving it than ever before. Recognition of the major problems associated with trauma and the means by which they may be corrected have led to considerable improvement in the results of therapy. Unfortunately, with this improvement, there has been a parallel increase in the likelihood of an individual suffering a severe injury, largely through road accidents although, even now, the majority of accidents still happen at work and in the home.

During the last decade there have been many attempts to improve the accident services of Great Britain. Perhaps the most important attempts have been concerned with organization. It has been recognized that a more efficient service results when all traumatic cases are sent to a single area accident department, rather than to a number of smaller casualty departments.

In association with the police, fire and ambulance services, all accident centres now have contingency plans to deal with a major disaster, such as a plane or train crash, should it occur in their area. A designated team of doctors and nurses with all the necessary equipment is always available to go to the site of a disaster, while pre-arranged plans to put the hospital into a state of readiness to receive a large number of casualties can be put into effect.

13

Neurosurgery

C. B. Sedzimir and Richard Jeffreys

INTRODUCTION

Organization of neurosurgical services in the United Kingdom

In the United Kingdom, neurosurgical services are organized on a Regional basis, that is to say, a Neurosurgical Department will be responsible for the patients of many District General Hospitals. Some Regions are very large and have several Neurosurgical Departments, others have only one department. All patients needing in-patient investigation and treatment will be transferred to the Neurosurgical Department although out-patients may be seen in the District General Hospital by the Neurosurgeon paying a visit.

It will be seen that many District General Hospitals will not have an in-patient neurosurgical service although the nursing and medical staff will be looking after such patients in the early phase of the illness, and possibly later during the rehabilitation phase after surgery.

Nursing neurosurgical patients

In most general terms neurosurgical patients may be regarded as those suffering from intracranial conditions and those from spinal conditions.

Nursing of both these groups of patients requires the highest standard and understanding of the specialized nature of diseases and trauma of the central nervous system.

In the first group many patients with intracranial conditions may be suffering from an attention defect or clouding of consciousness or may be unconscious. Others may suffer from speech or intellectual defects which may make communication difficult. The onset of symptoms and signs may be sudden as in many vascular conditions, the best example being intracranial haemorrhage. On the other hand there may be a progressive development which may be rapid or slow. These are found in the presence of intracranial neoplasms of the malignant or benign varieties.

After a sudden onset there may be further slow progression. After a gradual development there may be a sudden or rapid deterioration. In patients with head injuries the constant vigilance necessary for evaluation of the trend and fluctuations of the state of consciousness must become a nursing obsession.

Nowadays people are probably more afraid of having something 'wrong' with the brain or heart than any other organ or system in the body.

The emotional fright and shock received by the patient's relatives is frequently tantamount to a state of absolute panic or incredulity or complete rejection of the information given by the nurses and doctors.

Nurses must be aware of the importance of understanding of the mental as well as physical suffering of the patient. The need for sympathy and compassion is even greater than in other branches of surgery. The reason for such a statement is apparent from the knowledge that frequently the acute unexpected, unheralded condition, may be also the terminal. This is most apparent in sufferers from severe head injuries, from intracranial haemorrhage and from some of the intracranial neoplasms and infective processes. The relatives of these patients are particularly subject to mental anguish as they have not been previously conditioned and prepared by a prolonged or recurrent illness.

In the other group, in patients with spinal conditions, paralysis of limbs, loss of sensation and loss of sphincteric control are the most noticeable and terrifying disabilities.

On the one hand the potential for recovery is always there and must be stressed to the patients and the relatives from the very beginning. On the other hand the knowledge of unpredictability, and of the extent of such recovery, is a professional burden. The importance of encouraging and helping the patient to develop and to cultivate persistently the capacity for living is a never-ending task.

The team-work of doctors, nurses, physiotherapists, occupational therapists, social workers and others must give an active support to the patients and relatives at various stages of rehabilitation.

In both groups of patients, to those who survive but whose recovery is restricted and whose disabilities are substantial one can do no more than try to help them to maintain the maximum capacity and the will to live.

Head injuries

INTRODUCTION

Reflection on the present and future

The most frequent source of head injury is the road traffic accident. It accounts for some 30 per cent of traffic victims and for some 60 per cent of fatalities. Next come industrial and other accidents, then domestic accidents, including a proportion of battered babies, and finally, in peace time, a small number of gun-shot wounds and other penetrating wounds of the head, either due to assault or self-inflicted. This 'small' number will vary according to the quality of the 'peace' and to the variable and complex characteristics of communities.

It is rarely wise to be dogmatic, particularly with reference to the future. One feels, however, justifiably certain that the number of victims of severe head injury will rapidly increase. According to recent statistics, 140 000 patients with head injuries of various **aetiologies** were actually admitted to hospital in England and Wales in one year.

The prolonged morbidity resulting in loss of productive work, the high rate of mortality, the cost of hospitalization and of modern treatment will inevitably continue to drain the resources of the National Health Service which in this field as in many others are already grossly inadequate.

The problem of head injuries is not only a nursing and a medical one, but also a managerial, economic and political problem.

Definition of a head injury

When one poses a question 'What is a head injury?' to a young nurse or a doctor in training in a major accident centre, small casualty department, in a general surgical or orthopaedic service, or in a surgical neurology centre, what kind of mental picture would it conjure up in their minds? Very likely anything from a scalp contusion and a black eye to pulped brain oozing amongst fragments of shattered skull; from a child slightly dazed after heading a football to a comatose motor cyclist after a head-on collision with a car. Head injury means many things to many people, all of whom are correct to a degree. For the same reason, confusion and misunderstanding are rife.

Aetiology The science of investigation of the cause of disease.

Structures of the head which can be damaged

Different structures of the head can be damaged, such as, scalp (contusion, laceration, wound, loss of and **avulsion**), skull (closed and compound fractures), meninges and their blood vessels (tears and haemorrhages), and finally also brain and its blood vessels (concussion, contusion, laceration and haemorrhage).

Points to remember

When notifying a patient with 'head injury', specify whether the patient is fully conscious or if not, the level and the trend of the state of responsiveness and the presence of any neurological signs. It is also necessary to observe whether the patient has a compound fracture of the skull, either depressed and comminuted or frankly penetrating. These are potentially more serious than the closed varieties because of the danger of infection.

All other injuries should be specified, such as injuries of the chest, abdomen, limbs, and so on, many of which may be more important with regard to urgent treatment than the head. Particular attention should be directed to examination of the chest and abdomen. Even in 1979 patients are being transferred from a hospital to another hospital with an unrecognized tension pneumothorax.

Determination of the severity of head injury

Primary brain damage

The existence and the degree of damage to the neurones and the white matter of the brain determine the immediate severity of the head injury and are responsible for the early mortality. Such damage may be diffuse throughout the brain, particularly at the junction of the grey and white matter of the frontal lobe, or may be affecting more specifically certain parts of the brain like the hypothalamus and the brainstem (containing the reticular formation, important in the maintenance of consciousness). This damage (and the clinical effects which it produces – unconsciousness, flaccidity, rigidity, hyperthermia) is present from the moment of impact and is therefore called primary.

Should this damage be overwhelming, the patient will succumb. With a somewhat lesser degree of damage, modern treatment may preserve life at a certain level, at least temporarily.

In addition to the wide range of neuronal damage from lethal to fully reversible, the brain may be also contused or lacerated in certain predictable areas, or at random. The latter is caused by penetration, the former by shearing

Avulsion Forcible separation of a part or structure.

movements of the brain throwing the uncinate gyrus of the temporal lobe and the orbital surface of the frontal lobe against the sphenoidal ridge and the roof of the orbit. This is an example of just one of such predictable situations where gross contusion and laceration of the brain may be produced. It is possible, particularly with regard to a shearing injury to the temporal lobe, for the patients to regain consciousness for a variable period. They then deteriorate as a result of a massive swelling of the temporal lobe and die. This is just one example of a patient with brain injury who 'talked' and died.

Secondary brain damage

After the first impact to the head, any further damage to the brain may be inflicted only by virtue of complications of the primary injury. Such complications are referred to as secondary pathological manifestations and are numerous. The most important of these are intracranial haemorrhage, swelling of the brain, increased intracranial pressure and infection. Two major extracranial factors of secondary brain injury are periods of unrecognized or incompetently treated **hypoxia** and circulatory hypotension.

The purpose of treatment of head injuries

The purpose of treatment of patients with a head injury is two-fold: (1) to minimize the effects of primary injury to the brain, meninges, the skull and the scalp; and (2) to prevent the complications and to treat promptly those complications that develop in order to avoid further brain damage.

FRACTURES OF THE SKULL

Closed fractures

Linear fractures of the skull without a scalp wound are in themselves of no consequence. Some of them may, however, point towards the possibility of a complication (for example, extradural haematoma, intracranial infection, and so on).

Depressed fractures

A minor degree of depression, particularly of a large fragment, is not subjected to an operative correction.

A greater degree of depression, more so if the fracture is comminuted as well as depressed (*Figure 13.1*), should be either excised or elevated. The dura mater must be inspected for penetration. Should it be torn, the subdural space and the underlying brain are visualized. Bone fragments and blood clot are removed and any bleeding carefully secured.

Hypoxia The condition of inadequate oxygenation.

M

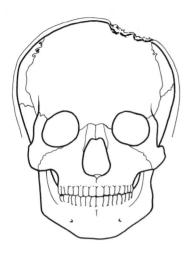

Figure 13.1. Depressed comminuted fracture of the skull. (Reproduced from Jamieson, 1971, by courtesy of the Author)

Meningitis Inflammation of the membranes of the brain or spinal cord.

Internally compound fractures

Any injuries to the frontal area, multiple linear fractures or fractures with displacement, may involve the paranasal sinuses in addition to any fractures of the faciomaxillary bony structure. As a result of these fractures, a communication may be established between the intracranial contents and the paranasal sinuses if the dura mater is torn. For that reason, these fractures are sometimes called 'internally compound'.

As a result of these fractures, the cerebrospinal fluid (CSF) may leak into the nose or nasopharynx (CSF rhinorrhoea), or infection may enter the cranial cavity with the development of **meningitis** or even a frontal lobe abscess, and finally also air may be forced from the paranasal sinuses into the subdural space, subarachnoid space (so-called traumatic pneumo-encephalogram), the brain itself (pneumo-encephalocoele), or even the cerebral ventricles (traumatic ventriculogram). In the case of the leakage of cerebrospinal fluid into the nose and where air is forced into the subdural and subarachnoid space and the brain, prophylactic antibiotic cover is commenced but the nostril is not packed. When the patient improves, the operation of unilateral or bilateral frontal craniotomy is performed. The tear of the dura mater and the fracture are exposed, loose bone fragments are removed and a graft of fascia lata is inserted over the dural defect, either on the outside or on the inside of this membrane.

Diagnostic lumbar puncture

In the case of infection entering the cranial cavity when meningitis is suspected, a lumbar puncture must be performed in order to verify the diagnosis. Suspected meningitis is the only valid indication for the performance of a lumbar puncture in the acute stages of head injury.

Compound fractures

Compound fractures must be operated upon no later than 24 hours and preferably within 6 hours after the injury. This delay is now permissible because of modern antibiotics.

Linear fracture with a wound of the scalp situated directly over it is technically compound. From the point of view of treatment, nothing more elaborate is needed than excision of the scalp wound and scraping of any dirt ingrained in the bone or trapped in the crack.

In depressed, usually also comminuted, fractures the scalp wound is excised and either sutured or suitably enlarged to expose the extent of the comminution. If sutured, an appropriate skin flap is fashioned to expose the fracture. The fracture itself, the dura mater and the brain are dealt with in the same manner as described in the closed variety.

If the dura can be easily sutured this should be done but otherwise time should not be wasted and the exposed area of brain should be simply covered by fibrin foam. Local antibiotic is spread before closing the scalp (no tension).

Recently some surgeons have advocated the replacement of larger fragments of a comminuted fracture, not only in the closed but also in the compound variety. In the latter, this is only carried out if the wound is not grossly contaminated and the operation is not delayed beyond 6 hours after the injury.

Penetrating fractures

Penetrating fractures may be extremely misleading as to the extent and seriousness of the penetration. Delay in their diagnosis may produce dire consequences within hours, days or even weeks. Whenever a penetrating head injury is suspected, the patient (particularly if a child) should be referred to a department of surgical neurology.

TRAUMATIC HAEMORRHAGE

Four types of haemorrhage should be considered in patients with head injury: extradural, subdural, cerebral and haemorrhage into the cerebrospinal fluid. Two, three or all four of them may coexist.

Extradural haematoma (cerebral compression)

The frequency of extradural haematoma is 3 to 7 per cent of the large series of head injuries.

The haemorrhage takes place between the bone of the skull and the dura mater (*Figure 13.2*). The injured vessels are most frequently the middle meningeal arteries or other meningeal arteries and veins. Because of this, about 80 per cent of extradural haematomas are temporal. On more rare occasions, the source of the haemorrhage is an emissary vein or one of the large dural sinuses, usually the superior sagittal or the lateral sinuses.

A linear fracture of the bone overlying the dural sinus or the meningeal bony groove (temporal, occipital, interparietal) may be a corroborative pointer but is not a diagnostic sign of an extradural haematoma. Because the dura mater is in places very adherent to the inner surface of the skull, the blood vessels may be torn even though the injury is not severe and has not produced any or only minimal concussional effect.

The patient may not have have been unconscious, or only briefly so. It follows that the brain itself was either not damaged or only very slightly.

With the enlargement of the haematoma, more dura is gradually stripped away from the bone and more bleeding points are added. The skull, being an unyielding structure, cannot expand to accommodate the additional mass of

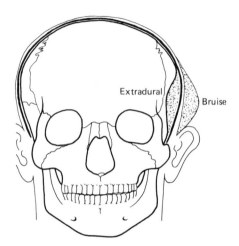

Figure 13.2. Extradural haematoma. See also *Figure 13.3*. (Reproduced from Jamieson, 1971, by courtesy of the Author)

haematoma and the pressure inside the intracranial compartment begins to rise. The bulk of the haematoma competes for space with the normal intracranial contents. Thus, the brain is being displaced medially underneath the falx and the cerebrospinal fluid is expelled from the collapsed lateral ventricle.

Whilst these events are taking place, the patient, who may have become completely lucid after the initial concussion (lucid interval), will begin to deteriorate again. He may become less attentive or frankly drowsy.

This deterioration in the state of consciousness, as judged by the patient's response to verbal or painful stimuli, is the most important and the most sensitive sign of what is called cerebral compression.

In due course, every expanding space-occupying lesion regardless of its nature will produce this syndrome if the responsible lesion is not treated surgically.

With further expansion of the clot, the uncinate gyrus of the temporal lobe begins to herniate between the free border of the tentorium and the lateral aspect of the mid-brain (tentorial herniation). It impinges on the oculomotor nerve (the third cranial nerve) and is instrumental in the production of the dilated fixed pupil, which is a pupil which does not react to light by either direct or consensual stimulation. The pulse rate followed by the respiratory rate may slow down, while the blood pressure rises.

Finally, the brainstem itself becomes compressed and rotated, the perforating blood vessels distorted with the production of ischaemic or haemorrhagic lesions.

By this stage, the patient is deeply unconscious and develops a decerebrate posture and rigidity. There is a rapid pulse and irregular, shallow or periodic respirations. Eventually respiratory failure is followed by a final cardiac arrest.

Diagnosis of cerebral compression

The most important points of diagnosis of cerebral compression in the presence of an extradural haematoma are: history of lucid interval; deterioration of consciousness; dilatation of pupil and loss of light reaction; slowing pulse rate; and rising blood pressure.

Mortality

Ideally and theoretically, there should be no mortality due to the extradural haematoma. In practice, reported mortality varies from 20 to 30 per cent in five large series of head injuries. This percentage includes a number of extradural haematomas, complicated by subdural haematoma and various kinds of injuries to the brain. Naturally the mortality and morbidity rate of these patients is more grave than of the just described cases of simple extradural haematoma.

Influence of state of consciousness In patients operated upon whilst still conscious or drowsy, the mortality is 0 to 9 per cent, while the mortality rises to 55 per cent when the patients are already unconscious at the time of surgery.

Influence of age Children and young people are more resilient to brain compression from extradural haematoma. Average mortality between the ages of 0 to 40 years is about 9 per cent, between the age of 41 to 60 years about 53 per cent, while in some series of head injuries, the mortality of patients over the age of 60 years is 85 to 100 per cent.

In only 5 per cent of all patients with extradural haematomas, mortality is unavoidable because of coexisting brain damage.

Treatment

Urgent operative treatment must be instituted the very moment that cerebral compression due to extradural haematoma is diagnosed in order to prevent the march of events leading to death.

The type of operation employed will vary with the experience of the surgeon and his team and the resources of the hospital.

Because 80 per cent of extradural haematomas are in the temporal region, subtemporal craniectomy or temporal craniotomy is usually performed.

Subtemporal craniectomy For subtemporal craniectomy, a hockey-stick-shaped incision is made in the scalp overlying the temporal fossa and carried down to the zygomatic arch. The temporal fascia and the muscle are split longitudinally and retracted. A hole is made in the exposed temporal bone. The haematoma is immediately noted. The bone is now nibbled away using bone-cutting forceps until most of the blood clot is visible. It is removed by suction, washing and gentle scraping, while all the bleeding points of the dura mater are diathermized. Bleeding from under the edges of the craniectomy can be controlled with insertion of strips of beaten temporal muscle or strips of fibrin foam and the sewing of the dura to the cranial periosteum. When the haemostasis is completed, a drain may be inserted and the muscle and scalp are sutured in separate layers. The bony defect is well protected and hidden by the temporal muscle and in due course, will hardly be noticeable.

Temporal craniotomy A detailed description of a temporal craniotomy or of a craniotomy for a haematoma in other situations is beyond the scope of this book.

Acute subdural haematoma

In acute subdural haematoma (*Figure 13.3*) the bleeding occurs into the space deep to the dura mater and superficial to the arachnoidal membrane. This space varies from a mere slit to a more sizeable cavity in relationship to age, posture and intracranial pressure. The haemorrhage originates as a rule from the veins on the surface of the brain.

The sylvian group of veins is frequently involved and laceration or contusion of the brain is almost invariably associated with the subdural bleeding.

It is true to say that in most instances of acute subdural haematoma, there is a severe general and local brain injury. Therefore, the haematoma is frequently found in lethal cases and its prognosis and mortality is that of the brain injury rather than of the cerebral compression, that is, 40 to 55 per cent.

Any amount of blood in the subdural space, however small, constitutes a subdural haematoma in the pathological

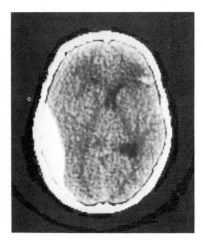

Figure 13.3. CAT scan. Surface clot: extradural or possibly acute subdural haematoma

sense. On the other hand, a surgically significant acute subdural haematoma, i.e. one sufficiently large to produce cerebral compression by itself, is not common. It must be at least 1 cm thick and be large enough to compress and displace the underlying brain.

Clinical diagnosis

Because substantial brain damage and an acute subdural haematoma coexist so frequently, the lucid interval is very rarely encountered. More frequently, the patient is unconscious from the time of injury and the degree of responsiveness when first observed must be thoroughly noted and recorded. It becomes the important baseline with which all subsequent observations are compared. Any improvement in responsiveness is a sign of recovery. Any deterioration may be a sign of developing cerebral compression which may be due to the haematoma. The other signs of cerebral compression, for example, dilated fixed pupil, rise in blood pressure, progressive bradycardia and respiratory dysfunction, may also appear.

The most confusing issue in the diagnosis of the subdural haematoma is that all the signs of cerebral compression will also be present in progressive brain swelling, cerebral haemorrhage and of course for the same mechanical and pathological reasons. Frequently the difficulties of clinical differentiation between those conditions are insurmountable.

The occurrence of an epileptic attack is believed by many surgeons to suggest the presence of an acute subdural haematoma. This is not always so. They appear in only 4.8 per cent of cases and are more likely to be related to the brain contusion or the thrombosis of cortical veins.

Computerized axial tomography (CAT scanning)

Apart from the main neurosurgical and neurological centres, the CAT scanning facilities do not yet exist in this country. The apparatus is extremely expensive and only a small number of the radiologists and neuroclinicians have sufficient experience to interpret the scans reliably. In the course of time and in the case of economic recovery, CAT scanning will be established in every major hospital. This technique revolutionized the diagnosis and radically altered the management of a great number of intracranial lesions.

In the case of head-injured patients the presence of surface, parenchymal or intraventricular haematomas can be demonstrated as soon as they have developed.

When necessary a second or third scan will show an enlargement or contraction and resolution of the clots.

The scan allows for a more accurate assessment of the part played by the haematoma in any given patient. Thus, unnecessary surgical diagnostic and doubtful therapeutic procedures are avoided.

In the meantime it is still not practical to transfer every patient with a major head injury to the neurosurgical centres for CAT scanning.

Surgical diagnosis

Diagnostic burrholes made for the purpose of exploration are the most reliable method available.

Cerebral **angiography** is also helpful when employed in special neurological surgical services.

Surgical treatment

Exploratory burrholes Exploratory burrholes are made first on the side suspected on clinical grounds and then on the opposite side because the acute subdural haematoma is bilateral in about 35 per cent of cases. Three burrholes are usually recommended: frontal, within the hair-line and anterior to the coronal suture, and 3 cm from the midline; temporal, just above the zygomatic arch and 1 cm in front of the ear, over the temporal fossa; and parietal, over the parietal eminence.

These burrholes do not 'decompress' the brain as is so frequently and entirely erroneously believed. If a substantial subdural haematoma is aspirated through the burrholes, then its removal decompresses the compressed brain.

Decompressive craniotomy Some neurological surgeons believe that in the presence of verified and substantial acute subdural haematoma, a craniotomy should be performed to allow its thorough evacuation and to secure a thorough haemostasis. This manoeuvre also provides a large decompression for the oedematous brain but the operation may be very formidable.

Cerebral haemorrhage

Cerebral haemorrhage may be single, large, multiple, small or petechial. These haemorrhages are, as a rule, even more intimately a part and parcel of severe brain injury than the acute subdural haematoma. It would not serve much purpose to discuss these haemorrhages here as a separate entity.

Angiography Radiology of blood vessels by injection of a radio-opaque contrast.

Haemorrhage into the cerebrospinal fluid

Haemorrhage may occur into the cerebral ventricles in lethal brain injuries. In the majority of patients, the bleeding takes place into the subarachnoid space either over the convexity of the brain or into the basal cisterns, usually from an injured arachnoidal vessel or a surface vein of the brain. It may be a minor or a profuse slow bleeding and not necessarily related to the severity of trauma. It may account for headache, stiffness of the neck, **photophobia**, restlessness and irritability and a moderate degree of temperature elevation (37–38°C).

The bleeding process is self-limiting. There is no surgical treatment. The removal of large amounts of blood-stained cerebrospinal fluid as a method of treatment, once recommended in some quarters, is no longer permissible in the face of modern knowledge of intracranial traumatic biomechanics.

Diagnostic and therapeutic lumbar puncture

For reasons mentioned above, 'diagnostic' lumbar puncture is superfluous and may be dangerous, while 'therapeutic' lumbar puncture is condemned.

In this context, it must be remembered that when a spontaneous subarachnoid haemorrhage is suspected, that is, a haemorrhage from an intracranial **aneurysm**, and so on, diagnostic lumbar puncture is indicated.

Raised intracranial pressure; cerebral swelling; cerebral venous congestion

The important minority of surgical patients with raised intracranial pressure and cerebral compression due to an extradural haematoma or an acute and uncomplicated subdural haematoma has already been fully discussed.

The vicious triad of raised intracranial pressure, cerebral swelling and cerebral venous congestion must now be considered. It is through better understanding of the development, perpetuation and mutual interaction of these three that the modern non-surgical management of severe head injuries has been evolved.

After a head injury severe enough to induce unconsciousness for more than a few minutes, there is, one assumes, some generalized brain swelling. It is of no manifest significance.

With a more severe degree of neuronal injury and of scattered contusions, a more serious generalized swelling is bound to develop.

A massive swelling of frontal, or even more characteristically of the temporal, lobe is produced because of the predilection of these parts of the brain to severe contusions and lacerations.

Photophobia Severe dislike of light (for example, in meningitis).

Aneurysm Dilatation of an artery due to disease of its wall or to escape of blood from the artery to beneath its outermost coat.

The veins here are frequently torn and after the production of some subdural bleeding, they thrombose. Large areas of brain around them become infarcted, devitalized and subject to even more serious swelling. The general or regional swelling of the brain, the regional venous congestion and the consequent rise in the intracranial pressure become aggravated and may produce a lethal brain compression in the presence of:

(1) obstruction of respiratory passages (nasopharynx, trachea, bronchi) by blood, secretions, vomitus, collapsed tongue and swelling of faciomaxillary injuries;

(2) chest injury, for example, fractured ribs can prevent adequate respiratory excursion and infection, atelectasis or haemorrhage can reduce the amount of functioning alveolar surface. Tension pneumothorax will displace the mediastinum and cause severe hypoxia of the brain. Chest injury can also result in rise of the central venous pressure;

(3) obstruction of jugular veins in the neck or of the cerebral veins and dural venous sinuses.

In fact, severe injury to the thorax may produce a secondary and terminal brain damage through hypoxia or asphyxiation even if the concomitant brain injury was relatively slight.

TREATMENT

Non-surgical treatment

The instant re-establishment of free respiratory passages and the speedy attention to any significant thoracic injury are, in themselves, the first and the most important steps in the treatment of injury to the brain.

Care of respiratory passages

The care of respiratory passages requires an unremitting watchfulness on the part of the nursing and medical staff. A few minutes of obstruction may ruin the result of hours of care and vigilance. There are several means of achieving this.

The patient should be nursed on the side or in a semiprone position (*Figure 13.4*) with a flat pillow under the head. This prevents the tongue from falling back and allows secretions to run out from the corner of the mouth. A mouth airway should be inserted if it is tolerated. The pillow prevents the head from falling too far below horizontal position, particularly in a broad-shouldered patient, and thus allowing for the veins in the neck to be stretched and obstructed. Such stretching may aggravate intracranial venous congestion which one is trying to reduce.

Atelectasis Local collapse of a segment of lung.

Secretions must be removed at frequent intervals with the help of a suction machine. Should there be any obstruction to the respiratory passages by vomitus and blood clot on admission, intubation and tracheal toilet or even broncho-scopy should be performed immediately. During this, an opportunity should also be taken to pass a Ryle's tube and institute gastric aspiration if required. Alternatively, under such circumstances, an early tracheostomy should be performed, particularly if a concomitant faciomaxillary injury produces profuse nasopharyngeal bleeding or makes repeated laryngoscopy difficult and disturbing.

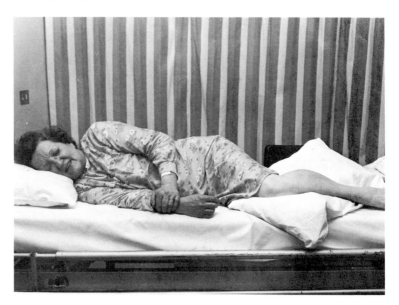

Figure 13.4. Nursing the unconscious patient in a semiprone position

Should the patient still be unconscious after 48 hours and seems liable to remain so for an indefinite period, tracheostomy should always be performed. With the advent of Portex tracheal tubes the necessity to perform tracheostomy may not arise until 7 days or so after the initial intubation. It should be stressed that tracheostomy is not an end in itself, that the tube must be kept free by suction and that the technique of these aspirations, as well as the general management of tracheostomy wounds, must be learned.

The attention of a physiotherapist experienced in chest work is essential at all times.

Maintenance of body temperature
An adequate oxygen supply to the cell is vital for its function and its survival. It is even more vital to the neurone because of its high oxygen requirements and the fact that the neurone does not regenerate. The acceleration/deceleration brain

injury of road traffic accidents impedes in itself neuronal biochemistry. Venous stasis and swelling aggravate it even further. These, together with the underoxygenated arterial blood supply may fail completely to fulfil the basic demands of the neurone, even at normal body temperature.

In a severe head injury, when the brunt of the damage is sustained by central parts of the brain (hypothalamus and brainstem) the temperature-regulating mechanism becomes defective. As the temperature rises, the metabolism of the cells and therefore also their oxygen requirement increases steeply. The breaking-down point is invariably reached when the temperature is elevated to about 40°C. It becomes literally vital that the hyperthermic patients should be rendered **normothermic** or even occasionally hypothermic. In addition to the protection afforded to the neurones by lowering the temperature and therefore the metabolism and the need for oxygen, hypothermia also reduces to some extent the volume of the intracranial contents and therefore also the intracranial pressure. The lowering of the temperature can be relatively easily produced in an unconscious patient by administering chlorpromazine by intramuscular injections to avoid shivering, and then sponging the patient with tepid water, by exposing the patient to air fans or by applying wet sheets. Ice packs may be required and these are placed over the areas of the body overlaying large arteries and also over the heart if there is no injury to the chest.

Dehydration therapy

After initial doubts regarding the rationale and effectiveness of dexamethazone as a rapid brain-dehydrating agent, the use of it became almost universal.

The swelling of the brain associated with injury, abscess, tumour or cerebral haematoma is rapidly reduced as a result of immediate treatment with dexamethazone. The initial dose should be high, e.g. 10 or more milligrams given by intravenous injection. Subsequently 4 to 6 milligrams every 6 hours is given by an intramuscular injection, provided that there is no history of bleeding tendency, i.e. **haematemesis**, melaena, metrorrhagia etc. This medication may be continued for a week or so. It is then gradually reduced during the second week and according to the circumstances it is eventually discontinued.

In the presence of a suspected massive swelling of the brain, an intravenous infusion of 20 per cent mannitol is also recommended. Hypertonic urea is now rarely employed.

The volume of secreted urine after the administration of mannitol is enormous and an indwelling catheter must be inserted into the bladder which is drained continuously.

Normothermic Temperature normal for a given species. In humans: 36–37°C.

Haematemesis Vomiting blood.

In those centres where intracranial pressure is continually monitored by either intra- or extracranial device, one can prevent or at least treat any sudden rise of intracranial pressure by a variety of ways. The controlled judicious use of dehydrating agents just described, is one of them.

Intermittent positive pressure ventilation

In several centres some of these severely brain-injured patients are curarized and artificially ventilated to avoid any possibility of hypoxia. Blood gases and electrolytes are frequently or continuously monitored. The same method may be applied to patients in a post-traumatic or otherwise uncontrollable status epilepticus. An operable intracranial surface clot must be firmly excluded by CT scanning in all such patients.

Intensive care of the patient

In whatever place the treatment of an unconscious patient is undertaken, that place becomes *ipso facto* an intensive care area. It is immaterial whether it is or is not designated as such. This is not a place for an argument between concepts of intensive care units and intensive nursing areas. Facilities available vary from hospital to hospital. Neurosurgical patients require intensive care and intensive nursing.

While referring more specifically to sufferers from severe head injuries, the nursing does not differ from that required by those suffering from a major spontaneous intracranial haemorrhage from an aneurysm. Unconscious patients with an intracranial tumour or a brain abscess or an obstructive hydrocephalus are equally in the same category.

Positioning of the patient (*Figure 13.4*)

The patient should be placed on a bed with a firm mattress and padded cot sides preventing the restless and confused from injuring themselves still further. A bed cage may be required if blankets are used. A sheet is mostly the only covering needed or accepted.

The patient is arranged in a semiprone position. The head is turned to one side so that the nostrils and mouth are not obstructed and the drainage of saliva etc. is free. A pillow placed at the back of the patient prevents him from rolling over. Another pillow is arranged between the legs preventing pressure and rubbing. There must be a free access all around the bed.

The basic requirements of any intensive care area are good lighting, suction apparatus, respirator, humidifier, intubation and bronchoscopy trolley as well as an anaesthetic machine and appropriate gases. Reasons for these requirements have been discussed in the previous text, particularly with reference to the care of respiratory passages.

When available it is helpful to have a continuous monitoring of ECG, blood pressure, pulse and respiration rates, and of blood gases.

In more specialized Units there may be facilities for continuous monitoring of intracranial pressure. Even in the specialized centres caring for patients with neurosurgical conditions this most advanced management is still rarely available.

The intensive care of a patient consists of:—

(1) Conscientious nursing staff — first and foremost.
(2) Nursing and observing the patient for any change in state of consciousness, neurological signs and vital signs (all these observations must be clearly recorded and any changes *reported instantly*). In any patients with an intracranial condition the observation of the state of consciousness and its trend is of the greatest importance. It is stressed that deterioration of consciousness is a better and a more sensitive sign than any other including the size and the reaction of the pupil to light. The reason for this statement, and indeed the reason for the necessity to observe and to note all the enumerated signs have been discussed at length in the section dealing with Secondary Pathological Manifestations. These are the warning signs of the developing brain compression and of other changes of intracranial pressure.
(3) Meticulous attention to complete freedom of respiratory passages and to oxygenation is stressed once again because of the danger of anoxic damage already fully discussed.
(4) Meticulous attention to intake and output fluid (intravenous drips, gastric drips, indwelling catheters and so on) must be maintained. The need for intravenous feeding arises only very infrequently, but the feeding by an intragastric route using a Ryles tube is quite common. One aims at the basic requirements of around 3000 calories per day and vitamins and sodium are added. Standardization of intravenous and intragastric feeding over a prolonged period has been achieved in most hospitals and in this respect the neurosurgical patients do not differ from those in other surgical specialities.
(5) There must be a strict control of electrolyte balance and of level of blood urea, most particularly if dehydration therapy is carried out.
(6) Control of temperature (normothermia and hypothermia) has been already discussed.

(7) Dehydration therapy has been already discussed at some length.

(8) *Sedation* Restless and confused patients must be sedated safely and adequately. All drugs depressing the respiratory centres are ruled out (opiates).

Neuroleptic drugs are suitable. Chlorpromazine 100/50 mg should be given 6-hourly for as long as necessary. If 400 mg or more is administered per 24 hours, one must watch for any signs of jaundice after a week or so. Those neuroleptic drugs which are likely to lower substantially the blood pressure should be used very sparingly while the blood pressure is monitored.

Another drug frequently used is diazepam which was already mentioned in connection with post-traumatic fits. Very restless patients also benefit from IV or i.m. injections of 5 to 10 mg diazepam per dose.

Surgical treatment of head injuries

Excluding minor lacerations of the scalp, surgical intervention in head injuries is called upon in perhaps 5 to 10 per cent of cases.

Surgery is more urgently needed for the relief of cerebral compression due to extradural haematoma. With exceptions, it is somewhat less urgently required for the relief of acute subdural or cerebral haematoma.

Compound depressed and penetrating fractures take precedence over the closed variety and all are excised or elevated.

Finally, major scalp wounds, scalp avulsion and the loss of scalp, may require very urgent surgical attention because of profuse and rapid blood loss. These scalp injuries are treated simultaneously with a vigorous blood replacement.

For the performance of any operation on the head, save for the very minor scalp wounds, it is essential to have the use of good lighting, reliable suction apparatus and diathermy apparatus.

Preparation of scalp

The head should first be shaved to at least 5 cm away from the wound or the proposed line of incision. Local analgesia is used for minor scalp excisions in co-operative or suitable unconscious patients. In all other circumstances, intubation and general anaesthesia are usually preferred in this country.

Scalp wounds

Scalp wounds are excised, inspected, debrided and sutured in two layers (except for the very minor ones). The deep layer, i.e. the galeal layer, approximates the edges of the wound and takes any tension. The superficial layer is haemostatic and must not be under any tension or the scalp will slough. It is well to remember that sensory nerve endings and the blood vessels are situated in the fatty fibrous tissue superficial to the galea.

Burrhole

The basic component of practically every operation on the head is a burrhole.

The scalp is incised down to the bone. The galea is everted over the superficial layer of the scalp or haemostatic scalp clips are used. The periosteum is elevated and a self-retaining retractor is inserted. Using a brace and a perforator, the bone is perforated just through the inner table. The hole is enlarged with a burr. In a case of extradural haematoma, the clot is instantly encountered. Otherwise, the dura is visible. In a case of subdural haematoma, dark plum discolouration is visible deep to the dura mater.

When operating on a comminuted depressed fracture, a burrhole is always made first in the unaffected bone at the edge of the fracture before attempting its excision.

Bone flap (craniotomy)

The scalp is incised in any position and according to any desirable pattern, provided that the blood supply to the area of scalp in question is well preserved. Several burrholes are made. The bone between them is cut by a wire Gigli saw and the bone flap obtained in this way is broken at the base. It remains attached to the rest of the skull by the temporal muscle. In connection with cranial trauma, this operation may be used for extradural, subdural and cerebral haematomas, and certain complicated basal fractures of the skull.

Haemostasis

Digital compression, scalp clips, eversion of the galea over bleeding points, diathermy and closing sutures take care of haemorrhage from the scalp. Bleeding from the bone is arrested by squeezing Horsley's wax into the bleeding surface.

Haemorrhage from the dura mater is dealt with by diathermy, fibrin foam or muscle application, haemostatic sutures, haemostatic clips or gentle packing. Finally, bleeding from the brain is secured by the use of diathermy, haemostatic clips, fibrin foam or muscle. Oozing from tiny blood vessels of the brain may be satisfactorily arrested by application of cotton wool, soaked in hydrogen peroxide. One should not try to ligate or apply Spencer Wells' forceps on bleeding cerebral arteries and veins.

Instruments used

Very few instruments are needed for the performance of a burrhole. Scalpel, Adson's periosteum elevator, self-retaining mastoid or thyroid type of retractor, Spencer Wells' dissecting forceps blunt and toothed, Hudson's brace, perforator and a burr. With the addition of some bone-nibbling forceps, a wire saw and a guide, a No. 11 blade and perhaps a hook and grooved director, a craniotomy can be performed satisfactorily.

For the suturing of the scalp, small spring-eye needles and a larger sized round-bodied needle, together with black silk, are generally preferred for the galeal and superficial layers.

Intracranial neoplasms

INTRODUCTION

Intracranial neoplasms may be primary (that is, they develop from the cells of the brain or its surrounding membrane) or secondary (when they are metastases borne by the bloodstream from malignant tumours outside the central nervous system). They may be extrinsic (they develop outside the brain usually in the surrounding membranes) or intrinsic (arising within the brain itself).

Frequently there is confusion in students' minds when the words benign or malignant are used with respect to intracranial neoplasm. The terms benign or malignant derive from the histological nature of a neoplasm. Elsewhere in the body a benign tumour is usually one that can be removed and the patient cured whereas a malignant tumour may be removed but often the tumour may recur locally or more particularly spread elsewhere in the body either directly or by distant blood-borne metastases. It is very rare for intracranial neoplasms to metastasize outside the central nervous system. Any intracranial neoplasm is potentially lethal and because of this potential could be called malignant. However, here again the terms benign or malignant should be based on the underlying histological pattern. On the whole most extrinsic primary neoplasms are benign whereas most intrinsic primary neoplasms have varying grades of malignancy. It is obvious that a secondary intrinsic tumour is malignant since the original primary was malignant.

It is very rare for neoplasms to arise from the nerve cells of the brain and the vast majority of intracranial neoplasms arise from supporting tissues — for example from the supporting tissue of the brain, glia (gliomas); from the surrounding membranes the meninges (meningiomas); from the linings of the ventricle ependyma (ependymomas); from the sheaths of intracranial nerves (neurofibromas). Tumours, which are nearly always benign, may also arise from the pituitary gland.

Since all intracranial tumours occupy space within a rigid structure of the skull they are often called space-occupying lesions. Benign neoplasms may flatten the brain and cause localized degeneration of the brain (atrophy) and intrinsic tumours may destroy brain as well as acting as space-occupying lesions.

Although individual types of neoplasm may develop particular characteristics (as described later), many of the effects of neoplasm are similar. In describing these general characteristics, it will be easier if the intracranial cavity is thought of as comprising two compartments, namely the supratentorial compartment containing the cerebral hemispheres, thalamus and basal ganglia, and the infratentorial compartment containing the brainstem and cerebellar hemispheres.

Supratentorial tumours

Obviously the site and nature of a given tumour will have some influence on the effect on the brain and thereby the symptomatology, but the common problems of such tumours are listed as follows:

(1) *Epilepsy* Epileptic attacks may take the form of general convulsions affecting all parts of the body in which case the patient usually loses consciousness, or may be focal, in which case the patient may either go on to develop a generalized seizure or remain conscious with only a focal seizure. The nearer to the surface of the cortex that the tumour lies, the more likely it is to produce epilepsy. Epilepsy may take the form of motor involvement, sensory involvement or even temporal lobe involvement in which case there are often attacks involving changes of personality and mood. After some seizures there may be a transient focal neurological deficit (Todd's palsy). The term late-onset epilepsy is used to denote any adult patient who develops epilepsy from no known previous pathology.

(2) *Focal neurological deficit* It does not matter whether a tumour is extrinsic or intrinsic for it to produce a focal neurological deficit due to either pressure (atrophy) on the brain (extrinsic) or focal destruction of the brain (intrinsic). This deficit will depend on the site of the tumour and may take the form of personality change, speech disorder, motor and/or sensory deficit and visual deficit. Since tumours grow this deficit also progresses.

(3) *Brain displacement* Many tumours evoke a reaction from the surrounding brain in that oedema (water in and around the cells) develops and thereby increases the effective size of the tumour. The space occupation of the neoplasm together with the surrounding oedema will lead to displacement of more normal brain away from the site of the tumour. Normal brain may be distorted and pushed against rigid structures such as the falx or the tentorium. When the brain is so distorted, it tends to become ischaemic due to interruption of its normal blood supply and further neurological deficit occurs. Since this is remote from the original focal deficit directly due to the neoplasm, these signs when they develop are called false localizing signs.

(4) *Raised intracranial pressure* Since the skull is approximately a sphere and cannot expand in adult life, any attempt to increase space will inevitably and eventually lead to a rise in intracranial pressure. In the early phases this is manifest by headache which is usually located across the forehead behind the eyes, is worse in the morning, is exacerbated by coughing, sneezing and bending forwards and often not relieved by simple analgesics. There is one infallable sign of raised intracranial pressure at this stage and that is the recognition of oedema of the visual disc in the eye (papilloedema). Later if the pressure is more severely raised, there will be some interruption of blood supply to the brain and eventually this will lead to drowsiness and coma. Tumours of the thalamus and 3rd ventricle may lead to blockage of the passage of CSF from the lateral ventricles and lead to hydrocephalus (*see below*).

Infratentorial neoplasms

These neoplasms develop the following general symptoms and signs.

(1) *Focal neurological deficit* This again depends on the site of the tumour, for example limb ataxia in a cerebellar tumour.

(2) *Displacement phenomena* The brainstem may be either displaced from one side to the other if there is a laterally placed tumour or from behind forwards if there is a midline tumour. In any event this displacement usually causes unsteadiness of gait and standing (truncal ataxia) and disorders of the eye movements, in particular **nystagmus**.

(3) *Raised intracranial pressure* Virtually all infratentorial neoplasms, apart from intrinsic ones of the brainstem, lead to interruption of the flow of CSF by either distorting the passage of CSF into the 4th ventricle at the aqueduct or by stopping the exit of CSF of the 4th ventricle. In either event this inevitably leads to an internal hydrocephalus (hydrocephalus due to an internal block within the brain, with dilatation of the 3rd and lateral ventricles). This will lead to the development of raised intracranial pressure as listed above, but in addition hydrocephalus will lead to thinning of the cortex of both frontal lobes. This leads to another false localizing sign, namely a dementia (a reduction in the higher mental processes and a change in personality).

GENERAL PRINCIPLES OF INVESTIGATION AND MANAGEMENT

Confirmation or exclusion of metastasis

Many patients who are known to have a malignant primary neoplasm outside the central nervous system already diagnosed and treated, develop a metastasis within the brain. However there is a smaller group of patients in whom the first manifestation of a malignant primary neoplasm outside the brain is the development of a metastasis within the brain; that is to say, the primary neoplasm is relatively silent and it is the metastasis which produces symptoms. In such an event neurosurgical treatment is extremely limited (*see later*). It is therefore important to try and diagnose such conditions before proceeding with major neuroradiological investigations. In the absence of any history of primary malignant neoplasm elsewhere in the body, it is usual to look at the more obvious sites that may produce an early metastasis in the brain. These sites include bronchial carcinoma, breast carcinoma in woman, renal carcinoma, tumours of both ovaries and testes, neoplasms of the thyroid, and malignant melanoma of the skin. Occasionally gastrointestinal primary malignant tumours may also present this way and if there is any index of suspicion for these sites they must also be checked.

Assuming that the screen of the rest of the body apart from the brain is negative for such a malignant neoplasm, the

Nystagmus A condition in which there is repetitive rhythmical movement of the eyeballs, usually laterally.

doctor makes a tentative diagnosis of a primary brain tumour and proceeds with further neuroradiological investigation. At the same time it must be pointed out that one can never completely exclude metastasis at this stage, and the possibility must still be kept in mind.

Neuroradiological investigation of intracranial neoplasm

(a) *Skull x-ray* This can show various features that may be helpful in diagnosis such as evidence of raised intracranial pressure or even calcification within the tumour.

(b) *Electroencephalogram (EEG)* As a screening test for a neoplasm an EEG is not as effective as a CAT scan (*see later*) and it is usually reserved for patients presenting with epilepsy and with no real evidence of space occupation.

(c) *Isotope brain scan* Nearly all district general hospitals have facilities for radioactive isotope scanning which produces a two-dimensional image of the brain. The isotope used is Technetium^{99} which is injected into a vein in the arm and the patient has to lie still for a few minutes. This technique will show up large neoplasms as well as other types of pathology but can miss tumours low along the base of the skull, small tumours less than 2 cm in diameter and some intrinsic neoplasms of the brain. It is a very useful starting test although its limitations must be realized.

(d) *Computerized axial tomography (CAT)* This has revolutionized the investigation of intracranial neoplasms. This technique will give a three-dimensional image by building up horizontal slices of the brain and with the enhancement of tumour circulation by iodine injected into the arm vein will nearly always pick up an intracranial neoplasm. It will also delineate the site and size of a neoplasm very accurately although the histological nature of the tumour will have to be inferred from other parameters in addition to the CAT scan. It must be remembered however that the patient may have to lie extremely still for up to 20 minutes. Therefore it is usual to give a general anaesthetic to small children and to confused and demented patients simply in order to obtain an undistorted scan. Apart from on the patients needing general anaesthesia, CAT scans can be performed on an out-patient basis (*Figures 13.5—13.7*).

(e) *Angiography* The historically older technique of angiography is less used now in the diagnosis of tumours but the surgeon may need information on the blood supply to the

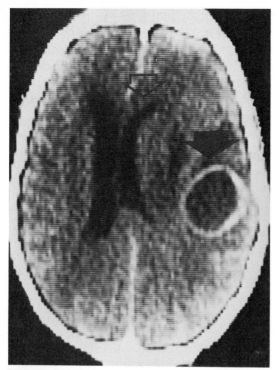

Figure 13.5.

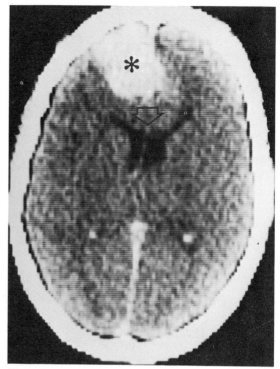

Figure 13.6.

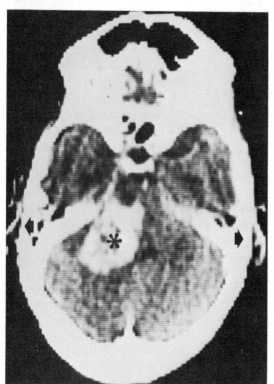

Figure 13.7.

Figure 13.5. Computerized axial tomogram showing large glioma in right parietal lobe (marked by black arrow). Note the gross displacement of the ventricles away from the glioma (open arrow)

Figure 13.6. Computerized axial tomogram showing large frontal meningioma (marked by asterisk). Note the displacement backwards of the ventricles (marked by arrow)

Figure 13.7. Computerized axial tomogram showing large acoustic neuroma (marked by asterisk). The black arrows point to the two ears

neoplasm and also surrounding blood vessels, particularly if he is dealing with vascular neoplasms such as meningiomas or haemangioblastomas. Very occasionally it is necessary to inject contrast material into the ventricles (ventriculography) or even occasionally into the subarachnoid space (cisternography) in order to detect such lesions as small acoustic neuroma or to outline the size of a pituitary tumour.

GENERAL PRINCIPLES OF TREATMENT OF INTRACRANIAL NEOPLASMS

Once a patient is suspected of suffering from an intracranial neoplasm he is referred to the regional neurosurgical/neurological unit for assessment and possible treatment. If raised intracranial pressure has been detected it is usual to give dexamethasone to counteract this dangerous condition. This often gives more time for investigation and allows treatment to be planned rather than rushed by a rapidly deteriorating situation. Once the neurosurgeon has amassed all the evidence he must decide whether the patient should undergo surgery or other forms of treatment. Where possible, attempts are made at removal of the tumour and in some cases (*see below*) complete cure may be effected. This however nearly always refers to extrinsic tumours, whereas with intrinsic tumours partial removal may be all that can be achieved. In general terms neurosurgeons in the United Kingdom aim at quality of survival rather than length of survival. That is to say that they may well prefer to leave some tumour behind if removal of that area meant producing a crippling neurological deficit in the patient. Where possible, surgery is planned on a routine operating list and the patient will be pretreated with dexamethasone and made as fit as possible for surgery. It is important to counter the harmful effects of dexamethasone on the stomach by giving regular 4-hourly antacids (magnesium trisilicate or aluminium hydroxide).

Upon return from surgery the patient will need very careful supervision. It is important that anaesthetists awake patients very quickly in the operating room in order to establish a baseline for subsequent clinical observation by the nurse and doctor. It must be remembered that a patient is not safe simply because he has had his neoplasm removed, because a postoperative haematoma may develop which will be every bit as dangerous as that occurring in a head injury and will need subsequent re-operation. Furthermore postoperative swelling of the brain due to oedema may occur and this will also need early recognition and energetic treatment, not only with dexamethasone but possibly with intravenous

20 per cent Mannitol. Some patients undergoing major surgery within the posterior fossa may have difficulty with respiration and will need to be maintained on intermittent positive pressure ventilation for variable postoperative periods. Usually there are no problems of feeding once the patient is conscious after operation on a supratentorial neoplasm. Operations in the posterior fossa may have led to some imbalance of the nervous supply to the pharynx and it is possible that nasogastric feeding may be necessary.

TYPES OF TUMOUR

Glioma

There are two types of supporting (i.e. glial) cell of the brain — astrocytes and oligodendrocytes. Each of these may give rise to intrinsic malignant tumours.

(1) Astrocytoma

With one notable exception (mentioned later) all astrocytomas must be regarded as intrinsic and malignant neoplasms. They may occur anywhere in the brain although the highest frequency is found in the cerebral hemispheres. They grow steadily and many of them produce damage to the brain as much by local destruction as by space-occupying effects. Those in the cerebral hemispheres can occur in any age group but tend to occur more frequently in the more elderly. Based upon their histological nature, they are graded I to IV with grade I the least malignant and grade IV (also called glioblastoma multiforme) being the most malignant. Irrespective of treatment the histological grading has direct significance in relation to the prognosis in that it is very rare for any patient with a grade IV astrocytoma to survive more than twelve months following detection, whereas patients with grade I astrocytoma may survive many years. The best treatment is removal of the neoplasm where possible although if the tumour is in a vital area of the brain the surgeon may content himself with confirming the diagnosis by drilling a burrhole and aspirating a needle biopsy. External irradiation is given to the tumour and the surrounding brain and **cytotoxic drugs** (such as CCNU) may also be used. It has to be admitted however that the results of treatment are extremely disappointing at the present time.

The notable exception to the above account is the juvenile cerebellar astrocytoma. This tumour occurs in children and young adolescents and may be solid, or cystic with a small nodule in the wall of the cyst. These tumours have a different histological pattern from the ones mentioned above and have a

Cytotoxic agent A substance acting as a cellular poison.

very much better prognosis. In fact even with partial excision it has been known for children to survive 20 years or more. Surgery is designed to completely remove the tumour where-ever possible and x-irradiation is not usually given in view of the benign nature of this tumour.

(2) Oligodendroglioma

Much of what has been said about the astrocytomas can apply to the oligodendroglioma, the major difference being that they tend to be more slowly growing than astrocytomas.

Meningioma

These tumours arise from the fibrous connective tissue of the dura and underlying arachnoid mater. The maximum incidence of these tumours is along the lines of the great venous sinuses, in particular the falx and sagittal sinus and the tentorium and the lateral sinus. They are rather variable in their consistency, some being extremely vascular and others rather hard and tough. The vast majority are histologically benign and tend to grow slowly. From these statements it might be concluded that patients with meningioma may be cured. This is indeed partially correct. However, many meningiomas when detected are already adherent to vital structures particularly at the base of the brain such as the optic nerves, carotid arteries and cranial nerves. Wherever possible, surgery is by total excision although it may not be possible to remove all the meningioma without producing a crippling neurological deficit. In these latter circumstances the surgeon may well elect to partially remove the neoplasm, knowing that the tumour may continue to grow and he may well have to perform further surgery at a later date. In general terms it is obviously better for a patient to have a meningioma rather than a glioma.

Ependymoma

These tumours arise from the lining cells of the ventricular system and therefore can occur anywhere within that system although the maximum incidence is in the 4th ventricle. They are malignant tumours and invade outside the ventricular system into the surrounding walls such that it is rarely possible to remove totally an ependymoma. They are partially radiosensitive and radiotherapy is usually given after surgery.

Medulloblastoma

The precise origin of this neoplasm is uncertain, though from its name one might surmise that it arose from the cells

N

within the medulla. These tumours almost always arise in and around the walls of the 4th ventricle and the majority will grow back into the cavity of the 4th ventricle. They tend to occur in children and young adolescents and it is unusual to encounter them over the age of 15 years. They are highly malignant tumours which grow rapidly. Wherever possible attempts at full removal are carried out and this is followed by radiotherapy since these tumours are radiosensitive. Medulloblastomas tend to metastasize within the cerebro-spinal fluid pathways and therefore irradiation is not only given to the site of the original tumour but also to the whole of the midline of the brain and vertebral column in an attempt to destroy any metastatic cells that may have become detached from the tumour.

Acoustic neuroma

This is a histologically benign neoplasm arising in the 8th (acoustic) nerve. These neoplasms grow and enlarge within the cerebellopontine angle (this is the potential space between the side of the pons, the superior surface of the cerebellum and the posterior part of the petrous bone into which the 7th (facial) and 8th nerves are running). When small they produce their effect by disturbance of the 8th nerve but as they enlarge they upset structures around the cerebello-pontine angle and ultimately when they are very large, displace the pons leading to hydrocephalus. Ideally these tumours should be detected when they are small and surgery is relatively simple. When they are very large the operation becomes much more hazardous but the results of surgery have been steadily improving even for large neoplasms even though it may be necessary to sacrifice the 7th nerve during surgery. Technically this is one of the most difficult operations in the whole of neurosurgery. However, the prognosis for the patient following successful removal is excellent, provided damage has not taken place during surgery to the blood supply of the pons.

Haemangioblastoma

These are benign neoplasms which are extremely vascular. They occur within the cerebellum and brainstem where they produce space-occupying problems. In addition 40 per cent of them secrete a hormone (erythropoietin) which stimulates the bone marrow of the body to overproduction of red cells. In 10 per cent of cases there is a strong family history and this is often associated with other tumours elsewhere in the body (when this happens it is called the von Hippel—Lindau complex).

Pituitary neoplasms

The pituitary gland is situated within a small bony cavity lying on top of the sphenoidal air sinus called the pituitary fossa. The normal pituitary gland is about the size of a small broad bean and is connected to the brain above it by the pituitary stalk. It is down this stalk that hormones are sent from the undersurface of the brain to the pituitary gland, giving it instructions to make and release the various hormones. Some of these hormones have a direct action throughout the body, but the majority act through target endocrine glands. Pituitary tumours are benign and they produce their effects in one of two ways.

(1) Compression of the optic nerves and chiasm

The optic nerves and chiasm are situated immediately above the pituitary gland and when the tumour enlarges out of the pituitary fossa, these structures are compressed and stretched. This leads to both a reduction of visual acuity and a bitemporal hemianopia such that the patient cannot see on the outer halves of the fields of vision.

(2) Endocrinological effects

Neoplasms may produce problems by either undersecretion or oversecretion.

(a) *Undersecretion* These neoplasms are usually called chromophobe adenomas and are endocrinologically inert. However, they compress the normal pituitary gland to one side leading to a generalized underfunction of the gland. This will result in all the target glands being affected and diverse effects such as **amenorrhoea**, impotence, anaemia, general loss of energy, some loss of secondary sexual hair and pale skin. When the visual pathways are upset, surgery is essential to restore vision and when large these tumours are usually removed through a frontal craniotomy. Following surgery in about 50 per cent of cases the pituitary gland resumes normal function but in the other 50 per cent it may be necessary to give the patient replacement pituitary hormones.

(b) *Oversecretion* (i) *Acromegaly:* This condition is due to a tumour producing excess quantities of growth hormone. This will lead to thickening of bones, in particular the hands, feet and face. In addition there may be enlargement of the thoracic and abdominal viscera, early **atheroma** of the blood vessels of the body and a pituitary stimulated diabetes mellitus. At the present time it is felt that surgical removal, either by frontal

Amenorrhoea Pathological absence of the menstrual discharge (i.e. due to a cause other than pregnancy, lactation or the menopause).

Atheroma Fatty degeneration of the walls of arteries.

craniotomy or transsphenoidal approach, is the treatment of choice although it may be necessary to give the drug bromocryptine as an adjuvant to surgery in order to suppress completely the excess growth hormone. (ii) *Prolactinoma:* These tumours produce excess prolactin, a hormone which in the female is necessary for lactation. In high levels this hormone will render the patient amenorrhoeic and infertile and also may stimulate the breasts to discharge fluid. Provided the tumour is small and there is no visual disturbance, the treatment of choice is by the drug bromocryptine which renders the prolactin level normal. Occasionally, with large prolactinomas, surgical removal may be necessary. (iii) *Cushing's tumours:* Cushing's syndrome is delineated by hypertension, increasing weight and **striae** over the trunk and is due to an increase of hormones from the adrenal cortex. Fifty per cent of patients with such a syndrome are due to primary dysfunction in the adrenal cortex but 50 per cent are due to increased production of the adrenocortical stimulating hormone from a tumour in the pituitary (**basophil** adenoma). In the latter case the surgical treatment is removal of the tumour though it may also be necessary to perform bilateral adrenalectomy later.

Craniopharyngioma

These are curious neoplasms which are thought to arise from Rathke's pouch. Early in the developing embryo the brain and upper alimentary tract are connected by this Rathke's pouch. In a very small number of patients it is thought that these remnants can give rise to craniopharyngiomas. Since Rathke's pouch is on a line between the undersurface of the brain, pituitary stalk and pituitary gland, it is along this line that craniopharyngiomas develop. They produce their effects both by compression of the chiasm and by compression of the pituitary gland leading to hyposecretion of the pituitary. They can become manifest at any age though tend to occur more in children and these children, since growth hormone is suppressed early, tend to remain very small. Treatment is by surgical removal if possible and where not wholly possible, it is followed by irradiation. Children who fail to grow will need replacement with pituitary hormones, in particular growth hormone.

Metastases

Striae Lines on the abdomen due to stretching.

Basophil A tissue which takes the stain of basic (alkaline) dyes.

As stated in the opening section, metastases may occur from any malignant primary tumour elsewhere in the body although the most common sites have already been described. In general terms surgery is not undertaken in patients who have metastases, particularly if they are multiple both within the body and the brain. However certain neoplasms have a relatively good prognosis in the body and if a solitary metastasis occurs within the brain, then surgical removal may be successful. Such neoplasms are renal carcinoma, thyroid carcinoma and breast carcinoma.

Subarachnoid haemorrhage

INTRODUCTION

By definition subarachnoid haemorrhage (SAH) means the presence of blood within the cerebrospinal fluid which is situated in the subarachnoid space lying between the pia and arachnoid mater. It is usual to separate subarachnoid haemorrhage into primary and secondary. Secondary subarachnoid haemorrhage can occur following a head injury or following a stroke, in which case the blood usually tracks into the ventricles and appears in the subarachnoid space once the CSF has left the 4th ventricle. Secondary SAH will not be discussed further.

Primary SAH is a relatively common condition with approximately 17 new cases per 100 000 population occurring annually. Following investigation by cerebral angiography it has become clear that the most common cause of SAH is a ruptured intracranial aneurysm, with another large group in whom no obvious cause has been found although such patients may have systemic hypertension. Ruptured arterio-venous malformations (angiomas) form the third biggest group, and finally there is a miscellaneous group due to rupture of blood vessels on the surface of intracranial tumours or in patients who have generalized bleeding disorders.

CAUSES AND SYMPTOMATOLOGY

Aneurysm

The blood supply to the brain is through the two internal carotid arteries and the two vertebral arteries. Shortly after entering the skull these vessels form an anastomotic circle of Willis situated at the base of the brain. The vast majority of aneurysms occur on the anterior part of the circle of Willis formed from the two internal carotid arteries. Aneurysms occur at sites of bifurcation of the various arteries involved in the circle of Willis (internal carotid artery, posterior communicating artery, anterior communicating artery and the middle cerebral artery). Only a small proportion occur on the posterior circle of Willis in relation to either the vertebral or vasilar arteries. It is rare for aneurysms to present as a space-occupying lesion; the majority of aneurysms rupture when they are about the size of anything between a small pea and a broad bean.

In about 10 per cent of patients there may be two aneurysms or more, although only one aneurysm will have actually bled. Aneurysms do occur in children and adolescents and it is thought that these juvenile aneurysms are due to an intrinsic weakness of the arterial wall at the site of its bifurcation. However the majority of ruptured aneurysms occur in the age group of 33 to 35 years at a time when atheroma is developing in the intracranial vessels. In these cases it is thought that the atheroma leads to weakening of the arterial wall which gradually gives way and an aneurysm develops which sooner or later ruptures causing a subarachnoid haemorrhage.

At the time of haemorrhage the patient usually complains of a blinding sudden headache following which he may either remain conscious (non-coma-producing haemorrhage) or lose consciousness rapidly (coma-producing haemorrhage). Of the latter group a small proportion may die very quickly and medical treatment is designed for all survivors. Following the haemorrhage patients will develop signs of meningitis, due to the presence of blood in the cerebrospinal fluid, with continuing headache, neck stiffness and pain down the vertebral column often associated with a mild degree of pyrexia. In addition blood vessels in the region of the ruptured aneurysm may develop spasm and in this event the blood flow through them may be diminished. If this falls below a critical level, ischaemia of that region of the brain may develop which will cause neurological signs such as contralateral weakness of the limbs, speech disorders and visual field deficit. In order to counteract the effects of spasm many patients may develop a reactive systemic hypertension in an attempt to push more blood through the narrowed arteries and capillaries.

Following a SAH the majority of patients slowly improve, gradually losing their meningism although they may be left with the problems of spasm and ischaemic deficit of the brain.

Pyrexia Fever.

Further rupture of intracranial aneurysm may occur most frequently between 7 and 14 days after the original haemorrhage. Blood in the subarachnoid space tends to prevent the circulation of CSF and many patients develop hydrocephalus, which usually settles after surgery.

Arteriovenous malformation

Arteriovenous malformations (AVM) are collections of blood vessels occurring in the brain at almost any site. There are many more blood vessels than is normally necessary for supplying that area and often blood is shunted straight from arteries into the veins causing an arteriovenous fistula. AVMs tend to enlarge and when they do they parasitize the supplying arteries which themselves get bigger and deliver more blood to the angioma. If the AVM is on the surface of the brain it may cause epilepsy for many years before a haemorrhage occurs. If the AVM is on the surface or just beneath when it ruptures it will lead to SAH, but those AVMs deep within the brain when they rupture will lead to an intracerebral haemorrhage. In either event they may well produce neurological deficit, either due to spasm or more particularly due to the destructive influence of an intracerebral haemorrhage. AVMs are less liable to early further rupture than intracranial aneurysms. The symptomatology of rupture is very similar to that of a ruptured aneurysm.

MANAGEMENT OF SUBARACHNOID HAEMORRHAGE

Initial management and investigation

Immediately following a SAH the patient should be admitted to hospital. In the unconscious patient it will be necessary to ensure that the airway is adequate. Following a neurological history and examination, a lumbar puncture is performed to confirm or refute the diagnosis of SAH. The diagnosis is confirmed by the finding of a blood-stained CSF which after centrifugation will show yellow staining in the supernatant fluid (xanthochromia). It is at this stage that a decision is taken as to whether to refer the patient to the Regional Neurosurgical Unit or not. It is accepted now that 75 per cent of patients, who survive their haemorrhage following neurosurgical operation upon their aneurysm, can resume their old occupation. However, it must be pointed out that such surgery is still fraught with difficulty and various factors work against success. In particular it should be mentioned that patients over the age of 65 years usually have rather hardened arteries that do not take kindly to surgery and it is usual to treat such patients by non-surgical methods. Further-more some neurosurgeons feel they should not operate on patients who have severe pre-existing systemic hypertension. Other serious medical conditions such as a previous myocardial infarction, diabetes mellitus or severe chest disease, may rule out surgery. If patients remain comatose for more than 7 days after the haemorrhage it is felt by the vast majority of neurosurgeons that it would be dangerous to operate and these patients are treated medically.

It is usual to transfer the patient to the Regional Neuro-surgical Unit two or three days after the haemorrhage. During this time in the district general hospital it is essential that the patient is kept quiet, flat in bed with one or two pillows only, and allowed only very restricted visiting. It is important however to make sure that the patient is adequately hydrated. It is often difficult to ensure this in a patient who is drowsy and complaining of headache but if this is not done, de-hydration can compound the problem of spasm of cerebral vessels and lead to a worsening neurological deficit. If the patient cannot take sufficient fluids by mouth, these must either be supplied by intravenous or nasogastric regimes, and a minimum of at least 1.5 litres a day should be supplied. Simple oral analgesics may be given to control headache, though it is wise to avoid the more powerful analgesics such as morphia or pethidine.

Upon arrival at the neurosurgical unit the patient is assessed. Provided he or she is reasonably fit, cerebral angiography is performed either by direct puncture of the arteries in the neck or by catheterization via the femoral artery (*Figure 13.8*). This is an unpleasant test for the patient and it is usual to perform it under general anaesthetic. Since the majority of aneurysms occur on the anterior part of the circle of Willis, bilateral carotid angiography is always performed and depending upon whether these are negative for aneurysm and on the age of the patient, a decision is taken as to whether to perform vertebral angiography as well. This decision varies from one neurosurgical unit to another and strict guidelines cannot be laid down within the compass of this book but in general terms it is unusual to undertake vertebral angiography in a patient over the age of 55 years.

Surgical treatment of aneurysms

The principle of surgery for ruptured aneurysms is to prevent further haemorrhage from the aneurysm by either removing it from the circulation by clipping the neck flush to the parent vessel (*Figure 13.9*) or by reinforcing the wall of the aneurysm with various synthetic materials. In addition

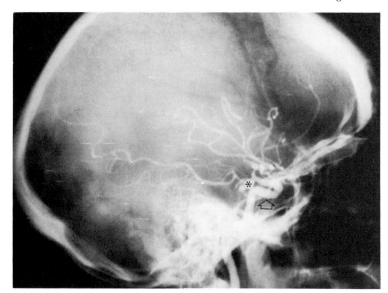

Figure 13.8. Preoperative angiogram. Aneurysm of posterior communicating artery (marked by asterisk). The internal carotid artery is marked by an arrow

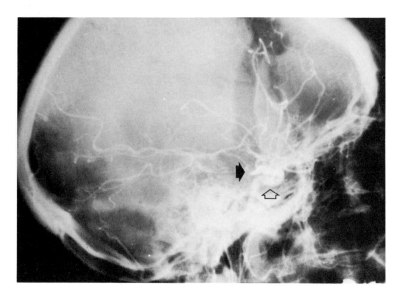

Figure 13.9. Postoperative angiogram of same patient as in *Figure 13.8*. The internal carotid artery is marked by an open arrow, and the black arrow points to aneurysm clip. The aneurysm is no longer visible

proximal ligation of the parent vessel may be performed provided there is adequate collateral circulation through the circle of Willis. This treatment can only be successful for aneurysms of the internal carotid artery by proximal common carotid ligation, or for aneurysms of the anterior communicating artery by proximal ligation of one of the anterior cerebral arteries. However, many neurosurgeons now feel that proximal ligation is no longer adequate and favour direct attack upon the aneurysm.

The timing of surgery is critical. If the surgeon operates too early he may well provoke further spasm with ischaemia and even infarction of the brain, and if he operates too late there may be a further fatal rupture of the aneurysm. It is usual therefore to judge each patient individually but in practice this means that the majority of operations for intracranial aneurysm are performed between the 6th and 12th day after the haemorrhage.

Operative access to the aneurysm is gained through a **craniotomy** and the neck of the aneurysm and parent vessel are carefully dissected using the advantages of the operating microscope. To minimize the dangers of rupture during dissection, many neurosurgeons favour dropping the systemic blood pressure during this critical phase and raising it once the aneurysm has been safely dealt with. If it is possible, a metal clip is closed around the neck of the aneurysm thereby making it totally safe (*Figure 13.9*). If this is not possible either cotton wool or lintine or acrylic cement is placed all the way around the aneurysm including the body of the aneurysm (fundus) as well as the neck to reinforce the wall. It is accepted that this treatment is second-best compared to clipping the neck.

The postoperative phase may be very difficult. Skilled nursing and medical care are essential. The cerebral vessels in a patient following a subarachnoid haemorrhage from a ruptured aneurysm are extremely sensitive and intolerant of surgical manipulation. Even more so than before surgery, they may react by going into spasm and leading to ischaemia and even possibly infarction of the brain. Upon return from surgery, a baseline level of observations must be established so that observation will indicate whether the patient is improving or deteriorating. There is no known method that is completely effective in abolishing spasm. If the surgeon suspects that this complication may arise, the patient will be started on dexamethasone 4 mg six-hourly. This is effective in reducing the swelling around ischaemic areas and preventing the vicious circle of spasm that may develop leading to ischaemia, which in turn leads to swelling which finally leads to further compression and spasm of the arteries. If the patient has a low level of consciousness and is suspected of suffering from brain swelling, then intravenous agents such as 20 per cent Mannitol may be used intermittently. The maintenance of normal blood gases is essential and it is particularly important for the nurses to make sure that the airway is adequate. If the patient is experiencing respiratory problems, then it may well be necessary to take over the ventilation by intermittent positive pressure respiration. The patient will need an adequate fluid in-put and if after the first few days he is unable to take fluid orally then it is usual to pass a nasogastric tube and feed the patient this way. Following

Craniotomy (1) Any operation on the skull; (2) the cutting away of a part of the skull.

aneurysmal surgery many patients are in an extremely volatile condition and their neurological and conscious level may change rapidly and therefore accurate observation is essential so that complications may be dealt with early.

The difficult postoperative phase may last up to five days by the end of which time if the patient is doing well he will continue to improve and there should not be any further major problems. If he has not done well then unfortunately infarction may well have taken place and it will be a question of rehabilitating a patient with a continuing neurological deficit. The only complication that may continue chronically after aneurysmal surgery is hydrocephalus. This is common in aneurysmal patients but usually settles either spontaneously or with sequential lumbar punctures over several days. In a small proportion of patients it does not and in these it is necessary to insert a ventriculoatrial shunt. Before finally mobilizing the patient, it is usual to perform a check angiogram on the side upon which the operation has been performed to ensure that the aneurysm is completely obliterated from the circulation (*Figure 13.9*). This is important for the surgeon both in checking his technique and in helping him give the patient an accurate prognosis. If the aneurysm is still filling it will be necessary to re-operate and adjust the clip. Needless to say, if an aneurysm has been wrapped, check angiography is unnecessary since it is obvious that the aneurysm will still be filling upon the angiogram though the surgeon will be relying on the wall being thickened by the synthetic material with which he wrapped the aneurysm. Depending on the degree of neurological deficit or otherwise, the patient can be mobilized and sent home or may need a further period of hospital rehabilitation. For a patient without neurological deficit and a successfully clipped aneurysm it will be possible to return to his old occupation two to three months after the initial haemorrhage, though patients with neurological deficit will obviously need a much longer period of rehabilitation.

Surgical treatment of AVM

Only the management of angiomas that rupture will be discussed here. The initial management and investigation are identical to that for aneurysms. Following angiography the neurosurgeon will discuss the prospects or otherwise of surgery (*Figure 13.10*). Although the early recurrent re-bleed rate is less than for aneurysms, it has become evident recently that AVMs will eventually re-bleed often with a fatal haemorrhage. It is this information that has persuaded neurosurgeons to completely excise AVMs wherever possible. However, AVMs may occur in very important areas of the brain and

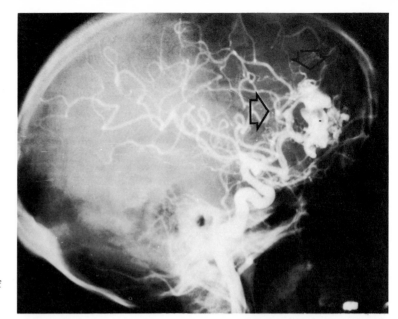

Figure 13.10. Preoperative angiogram of AVM situated in frontal lobe — marked by arrows

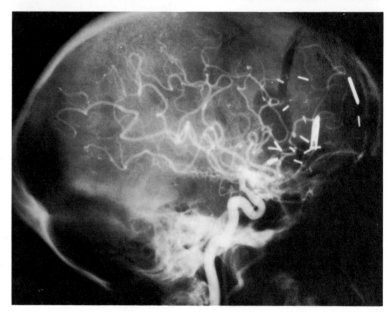

Figure 13.11. Postoperative angiogram of same patient as in *Figure 13.10*. The AVM has been excised and is no longer visible. Metal clips have been placed across the feeding arteries and can be seen

removal may result in crippling neurological deficit and the surgeon has to balance this against the danger to life of a further haemorrhage. If there is a large haematoma in relation to the rupture of the AVM and this is life-endangering in its own right, it is usual to remove the haematoma and AVM at the one operation. The decision to operate upon an AVM or not is a very personal and subjective one on the part of neurosurgeons.

The operation is performed through a craniotomy and an incision made around the AVM, usually just inside the normal brain, and gradually the large arteries and veins are ligated and the AVM excised. Since this results in a cortical scar, the neurosurgeon by operating does not really alter the likelihood or otherwise of epilepsy in AVM, and any such operated patient will need anticonvulsant therapy. Here again it is usual to perform a check angiogram to ensure that all the AVM has been excised (*Figure 13.11*). If it has not it is the practice of most neurosurgeons to return and remove that area left behind. Rehabilitation is as for aneurysms depending upon the state of the patient and in particular his neurological condition.

Medical management of aneurysms and AVMs

If for the reasons listed previously it is felt that surgery is not indicated in a patient, then it is usual to confine the patient to bed from between four to six weeks and at the same time once the initial acute phase of fourteen days has passed to ensure the patient is **normotensive** for his age by, if necessary, giving hypotensive treatment. Rehabilitation after that is gradual and hopefully one allows the patient to resume normal activities. However in the face of an untreated AVM and more particularly an aneurysm, it is difficult to allow the patient free physical activity due to the fear of recurrent haemorrhage.

Spinal cord compression

INTRODUCTION

The spinal cord is the continuation of the brain from the medulla starting at the level of the foramen magnum at the base of the skull and extending down to the conus medullaris at the 1st lumbar vertebra. The spinal cord is comprised of grey matter (containing **neurones**) which are situated centrally surrounded by an outer core of white matter (containing fibres). The spinal cord varies in its size, the main factor

Normotensive Having a normal blood pressure.

Neurones Nerve cells.

being the amount of grey matter. The grey matter is largest where there is a large anterior horn whose cells are involved in voluntary movement in the limbs; therefore the spinal cord is largest between C5 and T1 (where the arms are supplied) and between L1 and S1 (where the lower limbs are supplied).

Due to the fact that the spinal cord grows but little at a time when the vertebral column is growing rapidly during childhood and adolescence, the neurological level does not correspond with the vertebral level; for example, at the top of the spinal cord the neurological level of C1 does correspond with the vertebral level of C1. By the time the mid-thoracic region is reached the neurological level of T6 is approximately level with the vertebral level of T4 and by the lower end of the spinal cord the neurological level of S2 is level with the vertebral level of L1. This discrepancy must always be kept in mind and when referring to a level one must make it clear whether one is talking about a neurological level, or a skeletal level with reference to the vertebral bodies.

The spinal cord is surrounded by the same three membranes (pia, arachnoid and dura mater) that enclose the brain. There is a subarachnoid space between the pia and arachnoid mater which is in direct continuity with the subarachnoid space within the posterior fossa of the skull. Spinal cord compression can arise therefore in any of these three spaces and is referred to as: (1) extradural, i.e. the compression lies between the dura and the vertebra; (2) intradural extramedullary, i.e. the lesion lies inside the dura but outside the spinal cord; (3) intradural intramedullary, i.e. the lesion lies within the spinal cord.

These three types of compression may lead to slightly different neurological pictures but in general terms these distinctions are largely academic and it is more important in the clinical sphere to recognize three types of compression categorized by the speed of onset. These are IMMEDIATE, ACUTE and CHRONIC. These subdivisions are not to be thought of too rigidly and in particular it must be stated that a chronic compression may well become acute or immediate at any stage. However, the subdivisions do, by and large, allow some form of categorization so that a fairly complex subject may hopefully be made more easy to understand.

IMMEDIATE COMPRESSION

This type of compression is almost inevitably the result of trauma to the vertebral column. It can occur as a result of a fracture and/or dislocation in a previously normal vertebral column or may occur due to collapse of a bone diseased either by weakening (osteoporosis) or metastasis from a malignant tumour elsewhere in the body or infection (pyogenic or tuberculous). On the whole the thoracic vertebral column is better protected and certainly better splinted after trauma due to the action of the rib cage than the cervical or thoracolumbar junction. These latter areas are particularly vulnerable and it is at these areas that the major neurological problems occur.

Cervical spine

The cervical spine is particularly vulnerable in cases of trauma. The majority of accidents occur as a whiplash effect with alternating severe flexion and extension. Such injuries can occur in road traffic accidents, sports injuries and falls downstairs or upon slippery ice on the pavement. The spinal cord is either irreparably damaged at the moment of fracture/dislocation such that it will never ever recover (complete lesion), or it is partially damaged in which case it may recover (incomplete lesion). If there is instability after the injury to the cervical spine and the patient is moved without due precaution, an incomplete recoverable lesion may be converted to a complete irrecoverable lesion. This is a real tragedy. The first aid of such cases is very important and it behoves doctors, nurses and ambulance personnel to treat such cases adequately. If an injury to the cervical spine and/or spinal cord is suspected by weakness in the limbs and/or pain in the neck, the patient must be laid flat, though if he is unconscious attention must also be paid to his airway. If possible a firm collar must be fitted before moving the patient, or if this is unavailable, a temporary collar made of one of the larger daily newspapers may be fashioned. The patient must then be lifted flat into the ambulance and transported to the Accident and Emergency Department. Again, his transfer from ambulance into hospital must be performed with care and x-rays taken of the neck with the patient still immobile. If there is any question of instability on the x-rays, then skull traction must be immediately applied. Once this is done the patient is safe to be moved although it will need at least five people to do this adequately (one person looking after the neck and making sure the skull traction is applied properly and four people to lift the trunk and lower limbs).

Once the diagnosis has been made and a full neurological assessment carried out, the patient is admitted to the ward and continuing skull traction applied. Instability may be corrected surgically at a later date, usually by the anterior approach by anterior decompression and fusion but it is the nursing care of quadriparetic or quadriplegic patients that is so vital (this is discussed later). Unfortunately a lesion that is complete at the time of injury will never improve and attention is directed to rehabilitation in a spinal injury unit. If the lesion is incomplete neurologically then there are reasonable grounds for expecting improvement over the coming months. There is no way that surgery can improve the neurological deficit; it can only stop it getting worse.

Thoracic spine

Many of the statements listed above for cervical spine trauma apply to the thoracic spine. Fortunately the arms will not be involved but here again it is important to make sure that an incomplete lesion is not converted to a complete one. It is very important to keep the patient flat and lift him properly as he is transferred by ambulance to hospital and thence to the ward. In the mid-thoracic region, it is usual to get compression fractures, the majority of which by themselves are not very serious, causing mainly pain but not usually causing severe cord compression or transection. However it is much better to err on the safe side and regard any lesion as potentially dangerous until proven otherwise.

ACUTE COMPRESSION

By this term is meant spinal cord compression developing over a period from a few days to a few weeks. It is important to stress at this stage that it is often difficult to distinguish between spinal cord compression at one particular level from transverse myelitis due to a non-compressive agent. If there is doubt then it is much wiser to assume that there is compression and investigate it accordingly, since on the whole there are very few treatments available for the various forms of transverse myelitis, whereas surgery may be beneficial for compression. It is important not to miss a treatable condition.

By far the most common cause of acute spinal cord compression is tumour. Most primary tumours develop insidiously and come within the terms of chronic although there may be acute exacerbations, and on the whole it is secondary malignant neoplasms that cause acute spinal cord compression. They do so by a metastasis settling in one of the vertebral bodies and then gradually growing into the extradural space and leading to extradural compression. The most common primary sites for such metastases are carcinoma of the bronchus, carcinoma of the breast and carcinoma of the prostate.

Infection in bone may lead to the development of an abscess usually in the extradural space from either pyogenic infection, or less commonly in the United Kingdom today, tuberculous infection. More rarely, spontaneous haemorrhage may occur in either the subdural or extradural spaces and again this leads to compression.

In the majority of cases the patient will complain of pain in the back at the level of the tumour for some days followed by a pain around the body caused by radiating pain along the appropriate nerve root (girdle pain). This is followed over a period of only a few days by the rapid onset of a **paraparesis** involving both motor and sensory function, and ultimately the bladder is affected and the patient develops acute urinary retention.

If there is to be any neurological recovery then there is a real urgency for decompression of the spinal cord. Once the bladder function has been impaired, if there is to be any return to normality of bladder function in either sex and sexual potency in the man, then surgical decompression must be carried out within 12 hours from the onset of the cessation of bladder function. Following admission, such patients must be assessed neurologically and generally. Plain x-rays may often indicate destruction of one or more vertebral bodies due to the presence of a metastasis. A myelogram is performed by injecting iodine containing contrast material into the subarachnoid space in the lumbar region and this is screened on a tilting table to see precisely where the compression lies, although this can often be surmised from the neurological level. If the myelogram confirms the clinical findings, the patient will need urgent surgery by removal of the spines and laminae at the appropriate level (decompressive laminectomy). It may not be possible to remove all the tumour but at least the spinal cord must be given room to resume its more normal course so that neurological recovery may be allowed even though further treatment such as radiotherapy, cytotoxic therapy or antibiotics, depending on the primary cause, may be needed as well. Here again, skilled nursing care for the quadriplegic or paraplegic patient is needed (*see later*).

CHRONIC COMPRESSION

One of the major problems with chronic compression is that it may develop so insidiously that it is often missed until a very late stage by which time the patient has developed severe neurological deficit. The early symptoms which might suggest the development of chronic spinal cord compression

Paraparesis Imcomplete paralysis of the legs and the lower part of the body.

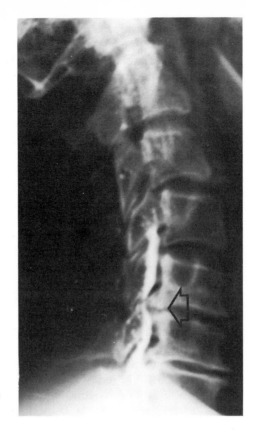

Figure 13.12. Myelogram of cervical region showing spinal cord compression due to osteophytes on either side of disc space — indicated by arrow

are a 'cotton-wool' feeling on the soles of the feet, some stiffness in the lower limbs and unsteadiness of gait, coupled with some reduction in fine movements of the hands.

The most common cause of chronic spinal cord compression is due to cervical spondylosis with other causes being spinal tumours, syringomyelia and chronic infections. Since these all have different problems of diagnosis and treatment, they are discussed briefly but separately.

Cervical spondylosis

Cervical spondylosis as characterized by radiological changes upon plain x-ray is common in the adult population over the age of 40 years. Only a small proportion develop severe secondary changes with protrusion of osteophytes (spurs of bone) into the spinal cord which will lead to spinal cord compression. These patients will develop a progressive compression at one or more levels in the cervical spine and eventually they may become so disabled that they are confined to a chair existence and are unable to feed and dress themselves. Once a neurological examination has been carried out it is essential to undertake myelography which is done by the injection of contrast material through the space laterally between C1 and C2. The dye is then screened throughout the cervical canal and the number and degree of protrusions into the spinal cord delineated (*Figure 13.12*). Although the spinal cord may be decompressed posteriorly (cervical decompressive laminectomy), much better results are obtained by operating anteriorly by an approach across the soft tissues of the neck and drilling out and curretting the osteophytes anteriorly (this is called anterior cervical decompression and fusion, and is often known by the name of the innovator, Cloward). Since this leaves a hole at the level of excision of the disc space, it is usual to fill this hole with a **dowel** of bone cut from the iliac crest.

Tumour

As in the skull and brain, the more chronic the tumour the more likely is it to be a histologically benign one, though not invariably so. The degree of deficit will depend upon whether it occurs in the cervical or thoracic regions. The two most common benign tumours presenting in this fashion are either a meningioma arising within the dura or a neurofibroma arising within a spinal nerve root. Their presence is confirmed by myelography done either by the high cervical or lumbar route and followed by surgery (*Figure 13.13*). Exposure is gained by a decompressive laminectomy over the site, the dura is opened and the tumour excised. The results of such surgery, particularly if done with the aid of the operating microscope are excellent even in a patient who may be very severely disabled before surgery.

Syringomyelia

This condition produces intramedullary expansion of clear, colourless fluid within the spinal cord. Syrinxes usually occur in the cervical spinal cord though may extend further down into the thoracic cord. The collection of fluid is situated centrally within the spinal cord and may or may not be in communication with the CSF as it leaves the 4th ventricle in the medulla. Such is the location of a syrinx that it usually interferes firstly with the fibres carrying pain and temperature sensation from the arms into the central spinal cord. These fibres cross from one side to the other within the spinal cord and it is at this point that they are damaged by a syrinx. The patient therefore loses awareness of these sensations and tends both to burn himself and injure himself without noticing it. Later, since the syrinx is central, grey

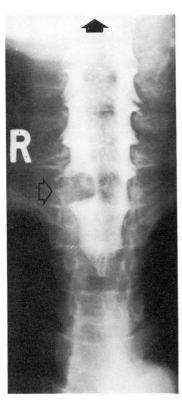

Figure 13.13. Myelogram of cervical region showing filling defect due to neurofibroma (open arrow). The black arrow points to the head

Dowel A pin fixed to the base of something (e.g. a tooth) to plug it in.

Syrinx A tube.

matter tends to be involved and wasting and weakness occur. Ultimately the syrinx may distend so much that it affects the long tracts and the lower limbs may be involved, particularly with regard to a weakness and spasticity.

The vast majority of syrinxes are congenital and may be associated with other abnormalities in either the brain, spinal cord or surrounding bones. The diagnosis is made by either water soluble myelography or by injecting air into the subarachnoid space. The treatment is by surgery. A decompressive laminectomy is made over the segment which contains the syrinx. The dura is opened and an incision is made in the spinal cord in the midline and the syrinx drained. This treatment will be effective for either a communicating or non-communicating syrinx, although some surgeons would favour putting a plug of material at the exit from the 4th ventricle for communicating syringomyelia. The results of such treatment are variable. Some patients are greatly benefitted, others are stopped from deteriorating and others deteriorate further in spite of all treatment.

MEDICAL AND NURSING CARE OF PATIENTS WITH SPINAL CORD DAMAGE

Good nursing plays a particularly important role in the care of patients with spinal cord damage. It is important to appreciate four facts:

(1) The patient who has lost the use of arms and legs or is unable to move adequately or not at all. He therefore cannot turn himself.

(2) Such a patient may well have lost skin sensation and will be unaware of the development or poor circulation in his skin, whereas the normal skin will protest by the development of pain. Furthermore the skin itself, by being deprived of its normal sensation, is rendered even more liable to damage. Such skin left short of blood for more than 2 hours will proceed to cell death and a pressure sore will develop.

(3) Following spinal cord damage, the bladder will cease to work properly. The majority of patients will initially be in urinary retention and since the sensory side of the bladder is diminished, they will not be aware of this, compared with the patient with acute urinary retention due to prostatic hypertrophy who although unable to open his bladder would be acutely aware of the discomfort. Adequate bladder drainage is vital.

(4) The psychological and morale aspects of a patient
disabled by spinal cord disease are severe, particularly
so in the acute traumatic lesion where at one moment
the patient was healthy and mobile and the next
paralyzed.

These four facts are fundamental to good nursing for such
patients. Patients must be moved frequently for prevention
of pressure sores and there is no more fitting monument to
good nursing than to see a patient nursed in a ward without
a pressure sore who has had severe neurological deficit for
many months. On the whole, turning a patient every two
hours is not a difficult procedure for the majority of patients,
using two nurses. However the patient with an unstable
cervical spine will be on continuous skull traction. It is usual in
these cases to place such a patient on a swivelling bed called
a Stryker frame such that he can be alternatively nursed at
two-hourly intervals either on his front or on his back. It is
important to ensure that the sheets are dry and not wet from
either sweat or urine. The skin must be kept clean, dry and
dusted with talcum powder at frequent intervals.

It is important to move the limbs though this is mainly
within the realm of good physiotherapy but nurses can play
their part here. It is particularly important to encourage
patients if they experience some neurological recovery, if
only for the sake of morale. It is a wonderful boost to a
patient if he can see a previously paralyzed limb begin to
move.

As soon as it is recognized that the patient is in acute
retention, a catheter must be passed and free bladder drainage
instituted. In a patient with a complete lesion this will be
continued for some months although an automatic function
may develop later in the bladder. For a patient who is experiencing recovery, it is usual to wait until the patient is
at least sitting in a chair and beginning to walk before removing
the catheter. It is to be hoped that he or she will start passing
urine normally. However it is important, after the patient has
passed water for a few days, to perform a check on residual
urine to ensure that the bladder is empty (in this test the
patient empties his bladder, a catheter is then passed and the
amount of urine left behind after micturition measured). If
the amount left is less than 100 ml the patient can be left to
his own devices. If it is more than 100 ml it is usual either to
give drugs to increase bladder tone or possibly to return the
catheter for a few more days.

The psychological morale aspects are very important and
the nurses are perhaps best placed to help such patients.

To the patient with a complete lesion after 48 hours there is no point in giving false hope. The doctors will need to explain the situation to the patient and then give him hope along the lines of adequate rehabilitation. However no patient, however well adjusted, can accept such information immediately and the doctor's words will need reinforcement by the nurses to help the patient through a very difficult time. It is important for the patient who is lying flat to be able to see what is going on around him. Prismatic spectacles, which can bend light through 90°, can be worn so that even though he looks up at the ceiling, the patient may see someone standing by his bed, read a book or watch television. Patients who are improving need constant encouragement since rehabilitation may well be prolonged and the nurse must regard herself as much a member of a rehabilitation team as someone who is initially concerned with the primary care.

Lumbar and sacral nerve root compression

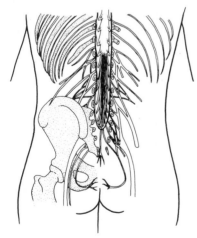

Figure 13.14. Conus medullaris (end of the spinal cord) and cauda equina (lumbar and sacral roots)

In an adult the spinal cord ends at the level of the body of the 1st lumbar vertebra. This is the fundamental fact which must be remembered in order to understand the difference of a presentation of lesions above and below that level.

What happens when spinal cord and cervical or dorsal roots are irritated or compressed has been already described.

Below the L1 vertebra there is no spinal cord. There are only lumbar and sacral nerve roots floating in the cerebro-spinal fluid, contained in the meningeal sac (*Figure 13.14*). When looking at these multiple roots one is reminded of a well groomed pony's tail. No wonder that the ancient anatomists described and named this structure 'cauda equina', which translated means 'horse's tail'.

The sac containing the cauda equina is made up of the arachnoidal and the dural matter and is called the lumbo-sacral theca. The roots are composed of nerve fibres. Some of these fibres originate in the spinal cord above, and run downwards. These are the motor fibres. Other fibres are sensory, transmitting the various modalities (various kinds) of sensations into the spinal cord.

Every root leaves the spinal canal by a gap between two adjoining vertebral bodies called the intervertebral foramina.

Each root is therefore 'mixed', i.e. it contains motor and sensory fibres and innervates a specific muscle, or group of muscles and a specific area of skin.

Similarly, such stretched reflexes, i.e. tendon reflexes, as knee jerk or ankle jerk depend on the integrity of one nerve root. The knee jerk for instance is mediated by the L4 root; the ankle jerk by the S1 root.

Loss of conductivity of the S2/S5 roots results in urinary and faecal incontinence.

LUMBAR DISC PROTRUSION

This is the only variety of so-called 'disc lesions' to be described.

Structure

The intervertebral disc is a fibrocartilaginous structure sandwiched between two vertebral bodies. Lumbar discs are larger, more massive than dorsal and cervical discs. The outer layer of the fibrocartilage is more condensed and eliptical in structure, containing the more loosely arranged central part. The outer part of the disc forms the so-called capsule which is further reinforced by the anterior and posterior longitudinal ligaments of the whole spinal column.

The capsule may become attenuated by stretch or even some of its fibres may be torn by a more violent strain of the lumbar spine.

The deeper part of the fibrocartilage degenerates in many people because it is poorly nourished and subjected to frequent mechanical strains and minor traumas over the years.

Any weakened area of the capsule may allow for the degenerated inner disc material to bulge into the spinal canal and irritate and compress one or more of the lumbar or sacral roots (*Figure 13.15*).

Sometimes a tear of the capsule may allow the disc material to protrude a long way, resulting in a bulky localized mass.

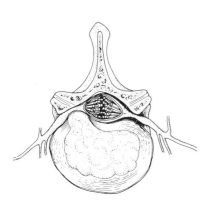

Figure 13.15. Protrusion of lumbar intervertebral disc, through a tear of the annulus fibrosus (capsule)

Single root lesions

Fortunately a protrusion is usually restricted to one inter-vertebral disc, and at least initially affects only one spinal root.

The largest number of protrusions occur at the last inter-vertebral disc, that is the one between the L5 and the sacral bone. The lumbosacral disc protrusion, being the commonest, results in compression of the S1 root, which traverses over it downwards to reach the foramen between the 1st and the 2nd bony segment of the sacrum.

'Sciatica'

The pain resulting from S1 root lesion is felt in the buttock, posterior aspect of the thigh and in the calf. It may even spread around the lateral ankle and along the lateral border of the foot into the little toe.

The S1 root is the main component of the sciatic nerve, hence this pain is called 'sciatica'.

This familiar name for any pain at the back of the leg was used for a long, long time before the existence of protrusion of the lumbar disc was recognized. It should also be remembered that not every 'sciatic' pain is due to a disc protrusion.

S1 root syndrome

A most simplified summary describing the S1 root lesion is listed as:

(1) Lumbosacral back ache.
(2) 'Sciatic' pain in the leg.
(3) Lost or diminished ankle jerk.
(4) Lost or diminished sensation to pin prick of the skin roughly corresponding to the distribution of pain.
(5) Some weakness of muscles, moving the foot downwards (plantar-flexion).

Lumbar roots

It is understood that each lumbar root is involved in its specific 'syndrome' of symptoms and signs.

The commonest of the lumbar roots involved in disc protrusion is the L5 root. This root traverses over the disc between the L4 and L5 vertebrae. It then leaves the spinal canal by the intervertebral foramen between the L5 and S1 bony components of the spinal column.

L5 root syndrome

The pain is still in the buttock, but in the thigh it is more lateral than the S1 root pain. Below the knee it radiates to the anteromedial aspect of the lower leg. Not infrequently it affects the dorsal aspect of the foot and radiates into the big toe.

This pain is also frequently called 'sciatic pain' despite the difference between it and the classic sciatic distribution.

There is a weakness or even a complete paralysis of the muscles moving the foot upwards. This type of paralyzed foot is named a 'flaccid drop foot'.

Sensation to pin prick is depressed or absent in the skin overlying the shin, dorsum of the foot and the big toe.

While treating the patient conservatively the appearance of motor weakness or even the slightest urinary difficulties call for emergency investigation by radiculography and radical treatment by surgery. (*Further reference later*).

L4 root

The loss of knee jerk related to the L4 root was already mentioned. The pain in the leg is anteromedial in the thigh and rarely extends beyond the knee. The L4 root takes part in the formation of the femoral nerve and should not therefore be called 'sciatica'.

For details of the L4 root syndrome and for symptoms and signs related to higher lumbar roots, a more advanced neurological textbook should be consulted.

TREATMENT

It must be categorically stated at the beginning that not every patient with lumbosacral backache and/or pain referred to the leg is necessarily suffering from a disc *protrusion*.

Secondly, not every patient with a disc protrusion should necessarily be treated by excision of the protrusion and evacuation of the disc material.

Probably no more than 10 per cent of all these patients will require surgical intervention in the neurosurgical centres (or orthopaedic centres) after failure of conservative measures.

Non-surgical treatment

This is not carried out by the neurological surgeons. Physicians, neurologists and the orthopaedic surgeons are mainly involved in the treatment by conservative measures.

O

Bed-rest on a hard mattress combined with analgesics, physiotherapy, traction by legs or pelvis with elevation of the foot of the bed or the wearing of a plaster of Paris jacket are all used and are frequently effective.

Nursing note

(1) The nurse will be familiar with the problems of skin protection of immobilized patients.

The foot up, head down position of the patients on traction brings up the difficulties of using bed pans and urine bottles. Some patients have insuperable difficulties of urination and defaecation even lying horizontally.

It is suggested here that less harm, if any, results from taking the patient to the toilet on a sanitary chair, than struggling, straining and spilling urine, under the 'strict' bed-rest orders.

Constipation is almost a rule, unless the diet and bowel function are constantly remembered.

While lying on a hard mattress for a number of days, the patient should be allowed to adopt his or her most comfortable position.

(2) The nurse must be aware of warnings of 'Danger!'

   (a) Acute exacerbation of pain despite the rest or rest and traction regime.

   (b) Suspicion of motor weakness, particulary of the up and down movements at the ankle.

   (c) The slightest suggestion of a developing urinary dysfunction.

These are advanced warning signs which the nursing staff must immediately report to the responsible surgeon.

The authors regard these signs to be a warning of the development of a major, possibly disastrous, compression of one or many roots of the cauda equina. It may be due to the rapidly progressing size of the protrusion or the presence of a spinal neoplasm mistakenly diagnosed as a disc protrusion.

It becomes the duty of a surgeon to institute *urgent* investigation leading to a likely emergency surgical treatment.

Radiological investigations

It may be argued that radiological investigations should have been referred to much earlier in this section. However, it is deliberate for reasons now to be described.

Routine lateral, axial and oblique x-rays of the lumbar spine are usually taken during the first examination of the patient in the out-patient department or at the time of the patient's direct admission to the hospital.

The purpose of these x-rays is to exclude evidence of bone destruction by neoplasms or inflammation; to show the degenerative and hypertrophic changes of bone, cartilage and ligaments; to show the presence or absence of any developmental bony **dysraphism**; finally, to assess the thickness of the disc structure which may be no more than suggestive of a disc protrusion.

There is no direct radiological evidence of an actual protrusion.

Radiculography

If after a period of conservative management (say 3 to 6 weeks) the condition of the patient is still unsatisfactory, radiculography should be performed. At present the water soluble iodine contrast medium named metrizamide is used almost universally. The medium is introduced by a lumbar puncture. The patient is screened and x-rays are taken in several projections. The protrusion of the disc is revealed and accurately localized (*Figure 13.16*). Neoplasms are shown up either by partial outline of the tumour or by more complete block to the passage of the medium.

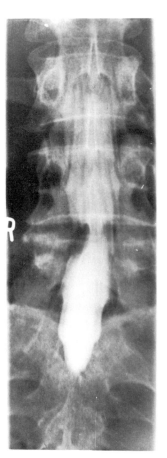

Figure 13.16. Radiculogram — protrusion of L4/L5 disc on the right

Nursing note

(1) Patients should be asked about any allergic reactions in the past and they have to be skin tested for allergy to iodine compounds.

(2) Nervous or emotionally disturbed patients may require premedication by diazepam or other sedative.

(3) The medium is absorbed from the CSF into the circulation and excreted in the urine in 4 to 6 hours.

(4) During the whole of that time, the patient's head must be kept well above horizontal. If possible the patient should sit up comfortably propped up. Even though the inflammatory reaction of the arachnoid to metrizamide is slight, some patients may develop headaches, lumbar muscle spasm, and they occasionally have spasms of the muscles of the legs.

This is controlled as a rule by an intravenous or intramuscular injection of diazepam, 5—10 mg.

Dysraphism Defective fusion.

SURGICAL TREATMENT

Indications

(1) Failure of conservative orthopaedic treatment in a proven case of disc protrusion.

(2) Recurrence of disabling symptoms for the second or the third time.

(3) Development of the warning signs already mentioned. This is an urgent situation.

The aims of surgical treatment are the removal of the protrusion and a thorough cleaning-up of all fibrocartilage from the depths of the disc space; and complete decompression of the affected root or roots.

Surgical methods

(1) *Fenestration* This operation consists of the excision of the ligamentum flavum attached to the lamina, above and below the level of protruding disc. Some overlapping bone of laminae is usually also trimmed.

(2) *Hemilaminectomy* Removal of the lamina on one side together with the ligament, if more room for surgical manoeuvres is required.

(3) *Laminectomy* This consists of bilateral removal of the laminae and ligaments with or without the removal of the spinous process. Rarely more than one lamina must be removed to expose the lesion adequately.

The real issue in all these operations is to remove enough of the bony lamina with the ligaments to give an easy access to the root or roots in question. Unnecessary removal of bone may result in formation of more massive epidural fibrosis (scarring), which may become harmful.

On the other hand more extensive laminectomy of two, three or four laminae may be essential for the removal of tumours or in the presence of gross narrowing of the lumbar spinal canal.

Nursing note

This is essentially the nursing of a patient with freshly sutured lumbosacral muscles and skin. The patient has a severe discomfort and a backache. He will require strong analgesics or even hypnotics for probably 24 or 48 hours.

Patients are usually nursed in lateral position with a pillow behind the dorsal spine. They are turned two-hourly and the skin over the recently dependent hip must be gently massaged.

Some patients prefer to lie on their abdomen and chest, which is allowed.

On average, patients turn themselves and adopt the most comfortable position from the second or third postoperative day.

During the first 24 hours there may well be difficulty in passing urine and very rarely, these days, a urinary retention.

Bowel motion becomes a real problem around the 5th day, but most patients of the authors are by then already mobilized and out of bed and physiotherapy is in progress.

Sutures are removed on the 10th day and many patients are then ready to be discharged home with instructions regarding physiotherapy.

Out-patient follow-up is timed at four to six weeks after discharge from the hospital. Most patients are then advised to return to work, unless it involves heavy lifting, prolonged stooping, crouching or standing or even walking for long distances. For some of these patients three to six months' rehabilitation period or retraining to another occupation may be necessary.

Lumbar spondylosis

Pathology

Multiple degenerative and hypertrophic lesions of the lumbar spine may develop in late middle-age or in more elderly patients.

The degeneration affects several discs and intervertebral joints, with the formation of multiple osteophytes. In addition the bone forming the (articular) pedicles and laminae, as well as the ligamenta flava and ligaments of the intervertebral joints, become hypertrophic. Together, these pathological structures encroach upon the intervertebral foraminae and the spinal canal. Canal stenosis is now radiologically evident. Some people are even born with smaller than average size of the spinal canal. In them symptoms may develop much earlier than in others.

Symptoms

'Claudication of the cauda equina'

The symptoms consist of what was named originally claudication of the cauda equina. That means that when the patient walks for any given distance he develops pain in the leg or legs. The pain is followed or preceded by numbness in various parts of the legs or buttocks or genital areas. Eventually weakness of the muscles also develops laterally or bilaterally. The pain and, to begin with, the other signs, subside when the patient rests, only to reappear on further exertion.

The exact mechanism of these claudication-like symptoms is not agreed. It is assumed that entrapment of various nerve roots of the cauda equina is responsible, but why symptoms fluctuate is debatable.

Treatment and nursing

The treatment of this condition is by extensive lumbar laminectomy decompressing the various roots. The last three to four lumbar laminae are usually removed, together with all the associated ligaments.

Nursing of these patients is similar to that with any patient after laminectomy with even greater vigilance regarding the skin, hips, buttocks and other pressure points of the lower limbs.

Some elderly patients require physiotherapy to prevent or treat chest complications.

Catheterization by an indwelling catheter may occasionally be required for a few days. In patients with advanced urinary disturbances already present preoperatively, a more prolonged bladder drainage may be necessary followed by intermittent two- to four-hourly release of the clamped catheter. Advice from a urologist with experience of neurogenic bladder is valuable.

Nowadays this condition is more frequently named by a long descriptive and more accurate title, namely 'Intermittent Lumbosacral Multiple Radiculopathy'.

NEOPLASMS OF THE CAUDA EQUINA

General classification by position and histological nature of neoplasms in the lumbar area of the spinal canal does not materially differ from what already has been described in connection with the spinal cord.

It should only be mentioned that spinal dysraphism which occurs in the lumbosacral region more frequently than elsewhere is sometimes associated with congenital tumours, such as epidermoids, dermoids and **lipomas**.

Apart from the skeletal tumours previously mentioned, one meets in the region of the cauda equina two neoplasms of infancy and early childhood, namely the highly malignant neuroblastoma and the benign ganglioneuroma. These tumours arise in the retroperitoneal region from the sympathetic nervous system and may grow through the intervertebral foramen or foramina into the lumbosacral spinal canal. The cauda equina is thus compressed by an extradural tumour and this may occasionally be the very first presentation of an unrecognized retroperitoneal mass.

Basically, there are two neoplasms to be considered in relation to the cauda equina.

(1) Ependymoma.
(2) Neurofibroma.

Clinical presentation

All neoplasms are expanding lesions. They may enlarge more rapidly or more slowly. Their presentation is characterized by a progressive disturbance of function of some/all roots of the cauda equina. Backache may be present, but pain in the leg or legs is more frequent than the 'lumbago'. Weakness usually affects more distal groups of muscles and gradually spreads up to the proximal muscles. Whether the weakness is unilateral or bilateral to begin with, the trend is to become progressively more severe and end in a complete bilateral paraplegia. The paralyzed muscles are flaccid.

The knee and ankle tendon reflexes are absent and the scrotal and anal reflexes also disappear.

The skin becomes insensitive to pin prick and temperature and possibly even to touch in the distribution of the various **dermatomes** of the various roots. Eventually, sensory deficit may be established in all the lumbar dermatomes. Analgesia in the S2 and S5 dermatomes, i.e. the perianal and genital skin, develops usually parallel to the development of urinary retention which is followed by a dribbling incontinence.

Cauda equina paraplegia described above should never be seen. The presence of the compressive tumour *must* be diagnosed sufficiently early for it to be removed before any advanced neurological deficit becomes established. Only lack of awareness of the existence of these expanding tumours, or the neglect to use the existing diagnostic facilities may explain, though not excuse, an established cauda equina paraplegia.

Lipoma A benign fatty tumour.

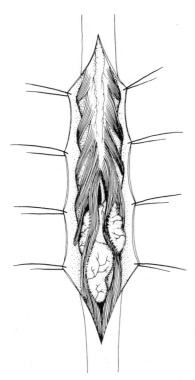

Figure 13.17. Ependymoma of the cauda equina

Ependymoma (*Figure 13.17*)

In the lumbosacral theca an ependymoma seems to be different, both with regard to the histological appearance and the long-term prognosis. While the ependymomas in the posterior fossa and in the third ventricle are of relatively high malignancy, those in the cauda equina are almost benign. Histologically they are of the mixopapillary variety and originate from the ependymal remnants in connection with the filum terminale (a vestigeal neural tissue).

Total excision of the mixopapillary ependymoma supplemented by local radiation is almost always curative.

Subtotal removal is usually followed by radiation to the whole of the spinal axis, right up to the posterior fossa. Frequently, a cure or a very prolonged remission is achieved.

The more malignant type of this tumour called ependymoblastoma behaves more unpredictably, but is rarely found in the region of the cauda equina.

Neurofibroma

As elsewhere in the spinal canal these tumours are single or multiple. The great majority of the neurofibromas in the lumbar theca are single and entirely benign. About 20 per cent of spinal neurofibromas are situated in this lower segment of the spinal canal.

Removal by a laminectomy, together with the root from which it originates, effects a permanent cure.

Nursing note

The nursing of patients with paraplegia due to a lesion of the cauda equina does not differ very materially from that already described with regard to compression or traumatic transection of the spinal cord.

Nevertheless it must be remembered that unfortunately the reflex-autonomic bladder function does not develop in lesions of the cauda equina. Frequent voiding of small amounts of urine or dribbling incontinence is the dreaded sequence of a caudal paraplegia. The help of a urologist must be sought from the very beginning and utmost care must be exercised to prevent urinary infection.

REFERENCE

Jamieson, K. G. (1971). *A First Notebook of Head Injury*. London: Butterworths

14 Thoracic surgery

B. J. Bickford

It is only possible in this chapter to give a very brief outline of the practice of thoracic surgery.

ANATOMY AND PHYSIOLOGY

The thorax is a mobile but rigid cage which is narrow above at the thoracic inlet, but wide below, where the diaphragm separates it from the abdominal cavity. The lungs, encased in the pleural membranes, fill most of the chest; the heart lies to the left of the midline and the mediastinum, which contains the trachea and oesophagus, the large arteries and veins connected with the heart, the thymus gland and numerous lymph nodes. The phrenic and vagus nerves traverse the whole length of the mediastinum and are subject to interference by disease or injury. The heart is enclosed in its own serous cavity, the pericardium (*Figure 14.1*).

We live under the weight of the air above us; this amounts to a weight of more than 14 lb on every square inch of body surface (760 mm Hg). The lungs, which are largely composed of the spongy alveolar tissue in which exchange of oxygen and carbon dioxide takes place between the blood and inbreathed air, remain inflated only because air can enter them through the air passages and because they are attracted by the suction effect of the empty pleural cavities to the inner aspect of the chest wall, to which they conform in shape. In inspiration the movement of the ribs and diaphragm increases the volume of the chest and so the lungs fill with air. They empty in expiration by a passive process. The whole mechanism of respiration depends on the stability of the chest wall, the maintenance of the vacuum in the pleural cavities, the patency of the airways and the pressure of the atmospheric air. In addition it is necessary that the lungs themselves are able to effect satisfactory gas exchange by being themselves healthy. In disease, or after injury, any of these components of respiration may be affected adversely and proper understanding of the pathology and treatment of chest disease means that we must take all these factors into account.

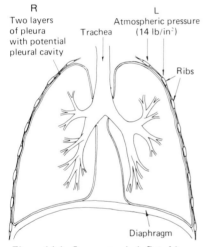

Figure 14.1. Lungs remain inflated in the body because of suction ('negative pressure') in the pleural cavity and the pressure of air entering through the trachea and bronchi.

R
Two layers of pleura with potential pleural cavity
Trachea
L
Atmospheric pressure (14 lb/in²)
Ribs
Diaphragm

SOME EFFECTS OF DISEASE AND INJURY ON THE LUNGS

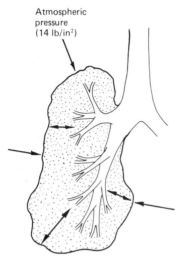

Atmospheric
pressure
(14 lb/in²)

Figure 14.2. Lung removed from the body collapses because of inherent elasticity and the pressure of the atmosphere

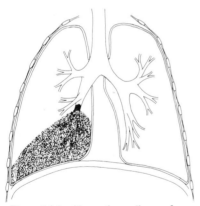

Figure 14.3. Absorption collapse of right lower lobe due to bronchial obstruction with normal blood flow to lung

Emphysema (1) A common chronic disease of the lungs characterized by breathlessness due mainly to difficulty in breathing out; it is associated with distension of the small air passages and air sacs in the lung; or (2) the presence of air in the body tissues (surgical emphysema).

It goes without saying that disease processes which affect the lungs widely necessarily lead to inefficient respiration. The most common is chronic bronchitis, which is associated with atmospheric pollution and with cigarette smoking. Excessive production of mucus in the bronchi is combined with swelling of the lining of these passages which obstructs the smaller ones; there is some degree of spasm of their muscular walls and often chronic infection as well. **Emphysema** is often associated with chronic bronchitis, but not always. By a combination of weakness of the alveolar walls and trapping of air in them when air cannot escape through narrowed **bronchioles** in expiration, the walls of the alveoli undergo progressive breakdown. This results in relatively large airspaces in the lung instead of innumerable small ones. Not only is gas exchange eventually deficient, but the reduction in capillary blood vessels obstructs the flow through them and leads to right heart failure. Diffuse fibrosis from inhalation of mineral dusts at work ('pneumoconiosis'), and other rarer conditions such as fibrosing alveolitis lead to much the same effect. Serious interference with pulmonary gas-exchange is reflected in a lowered tension of oxygen and a raised carbon dioxide tension in the arterial blood.

Collapse of the lung is a term which most unfortunately has two distinct meanings. It can imply that the lung merely becomes smaller when it is emptied of air through pressure on its surface. The pressure may be of the atmosphere if there is an open wound in the chest, or it may be due to accumulation of air or fluid in the normally empty pleural cavity. The lung also has a certain elasticity of its own which tends to make it collapse if not inflated (*Figure 14.2*). This *compression* or *relaxation* collapse does not greatly reduce lung function unless it is severe. *Absorption collapse* is due to obstruction of a bronchus without interference with the flow of pulmonary artery blood through the lung. The air in the affected area is absorbed by the blood and cannot be replaced because the bronchus is blocked (*Figure 14.3*). The lung therefore becomes solid and functionless. Function will, of course, be restored if the block is relieved. A whole lung, a lobe, a segment or smaller portions of lung may be involved. Examples of blocking agents are tumours, inhaled foreign bodies and retained secretions in the bronchi. With absorption collapse it is inevitable that some blood will be returned to the systemic circulation without having been reoxygenated in the lung. This can result in cyanosis if a whole lung is involved.

Paradoxical respiration is observed when the chest wall loses its stability, usually as a result of multiple fractures of the ribs. The term paradox implies a reversal of the normal movement in respiration. When an area of chest wall is freed from its attachments, it is unable to move outwards in inspiration because of the atmospheric pressure acting on it. It will thus seem actually to fall in when the other ribs move out; the reverse will happen during expiration. The result is a severe reduction in efficiency of respiration, and it can be very serious in a person who already has, for example, chronic bronchitis.

The epithelium lining the bronchi is ciliated columnar in type, with many mucus-secreting glands. These produce a film of mucus which moistens the lining and entraps small particles of dust, etc. The cilia move the mucous film up to the larynx, whence it is either swallowed or coughed up. If there is an excess of secretions the ciliary mechanism may be unable to cope; this is especially serious if the patient is unable to cough because of pain or instability of the chest wall. Bronchial secretions will then be retained in the lower parts of the bronchial tree, and obstruction of the lumen will result in absorption collapse, usually of the lower lobes. This may happen in a very short space of time.

It must be remembered that the control of coughing and respiration in general is located in the respiratory centre in the medulla oblongata. This is highly sensitive to the level of carbon dioxide in the blood. It loses its sensitivity if there is a chronically high level of CO_2 in the arterial blood (e.g. in advanced chronic bronchitis). Opiates and barbiturates are powerful depressants of the respiratory centre and must be used with much discretion when there is evidence of chronic lung disease; the same caution applies after operations on or injuries to the chest. A dose of morphine which can be easily tolerated by the normal patient may produce disastrous ill effects in the circumstances described.

SURGICAL DISEASES OF THE CHEST

(1) Diseases of the chest wall

Perhaps the most common are the congenital deformities of *pectus excavatum* ('funnel chest') and *pectus carinatum* ('pigeon chest'). These are unsightly and not surprisingly are a source of embarrassment and distress to adolescents in particular. Unfortunately surgical correction, which involves division of cartilages and the sternum, with elevation on some form of internal strut, is not very satisfactory. The immediate

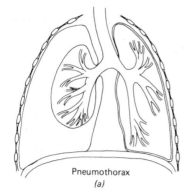

Pneumothorax
(a)

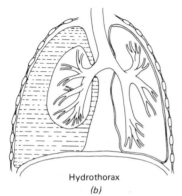

Hydrothorax
(b)

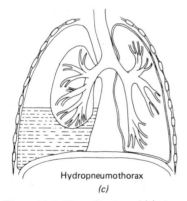

Hydropneumothorax
(c)

Figure 14.4. The collection of (*a*) air, (*b*) fluid, or (*c*) air and fluid in the pleural cavity collapses the lung by compression but does not necessarily expel all the air from it

Sequestrum A piece of dead bone detached from healthy bone, as in the centre of an area of necrosis.

Chyle Milky-white emulsified fat in the lymph vessels of the small intestine.

Bulla A blister.

correction may be good, but the deformity is all too apt to recur with time.

Neoplasms of the ribs are rare; they may be malignant (*chrondrosarcoma*), when wide excision is required. Any large defect in the chest wall will cause severe paradoxical movement unless it is beneath the scapula and reinforcement of the deficiency by an inert prosthesis will be required.

Infections of ribs and cartilages are rare, but may demand surgery if **sequestra** form. *Actinomycosis* rarely causes an abscess in an intercostal space, as does a neglected empyema ('empyema necessitans').

(2) Diseases of the pleura

These mainly originate in the lung, less often in the chest wall or beneath the diaphragm. Air collecting in the pleural cavity is termed a *pneumothorax*. A collection of blood is a *haemothorax*, of **chyle** a *chylothorax*, of air and fluid a *hydropneumothorax*, of air and blood a *haemopneumothorax*, and of air and pus a *pyopneumothorax* (*Figure 14.4*).

A pneumothorax means that air has entered the pleural cavity from the outside, through a wound, or from some lesion in the lung. *Spontaneous penumothorax* is due to rupture of an air-containing bleb (or **bulla**) on the surface of the lung. It occurs mainly in exceptionally tall, thin young people or in older chronic bronchitics. Treatment is first by intercostal drainage (p. 326), but if the condition recurs several times operation is necessary. The leaking bulla is ligated or stitched, and the parietal layer of the pleura stripped from the inner chest wall so that the lung will adhere to it and prevent any recurrence. In patients unfit for operation, adhesions produced by iodized talc powder put into the pleural cavity ('pleurodesis') may suffice.

Haemothorax is usually the result of trauma; it may accompany a 'spontaneous' pneumothorax if an adhesion tears as the lung collapses. Blood in the pleural cavity often does not clot and can be removed by aspiration. If it clots ('clotted haemothorax') removal by open operation is advisable to prevent later fibrosis with fixation of the ribs.

Pleural empyema is almost always secondary to infection in the lung. While this may be a simple pneumonia or a lung abscess, it is possible that it is associated with a lung cancer; this must therefore be excluded in adults. In babies, staphylococcal pneumonia often causes acute pyopneumothorax which needs prompt relief by intercostal drainage. In adults the best way to treat an empyema is aspiration and injection of an appropriate antibiotic until the cavity is sterile. It is seldom possible to clear the cavity completely of fibrin and the relatively simple operation of decortication of the lung is required to allow the lung to expand fully. This is preferable to treatment either by intercostal drainage or by rib resection, but water-seal drainage will be necessary if there is a leakage of air into the pleural cavity — 'bronchopleural fistula' (p. 329).

Neoplasms of the pleura are rather rare; fibromas occur and are prone to recurrence locally. **Mesothelioma** of the pleura is a malignant tumour for which no treatment is effective. It is associated with exposure to asbestos dust, especially at work.

(3) Diseases of the lung

Congenital abnormalities most often take the form of greatly distended lobes in children ('lobar emphysema'), or cysts which are prone to infection and which may have a blood supply direct from the aorta. Surgical removal is required.

Foreign bodies such as peanuts, beads and other small objects may be inhaled into the bronchi, especially by children. They can usually be removed by bronchoscopy (p. 321).

Lung abscesses seldom need surgery; *bronchiectasis* is an irregular dilatation of bronchi mainly secondary to ineffectively treated pneumonic infections. It tends to involve the lower lobes of the lungs and there is usually chronic infection with copious purulent sputum, often offensive smelling. If medical measures (postural drainage and antibiotics) fail and the disease is sufficiently localized, removal of the affected lobes or segments may be advisable.

Pulmonary tuberculosis rarely requires surgery, which is usually excision of an unhealed area of diseased lung.

Lung cancer, or *bronchial carcinoma,* is now the most common form of cancer in men and the second most common in women, in this country. It is about 3 times more common in men than women and is known to be strongly linked with heavy cigarette smoking. It is most commonly a **squamous cell carcinoma**, but **adenocarcinoma**, anaplastic carcinoma and the highly malignant 'oat-cell' carcinoma also occur. Symptoms occur relatively late in the disease; the most important is haemoptysis. The growth may obstruct a bronchus and an attack of 'pneumonia' which recurs or fails to clear up may be its first sign. It may invade the ribs and cause pain, and the rare **Pancoast tumour** causes severe pain by involving the brachial plexus at the apex of the chest; if so surgery is impossible. Lymph nodes in the mediastinum or the neck are frequently involved; they may enlarge so as to obstruct the superior vena cava or the oesophagus. As blood

Mesothelioma A tumour arising from the pleura, pericardium or peritoneum due to the presence of asbestos.

Squamous cell carcinoma A carcinoma of scaly, or flattened, cells.

Adenocarcinoma A carcinoma of gland-like structure.

Pancoast tumour A tumour at the apex of the lung which involves the brachial plexus and cervical sympathetic chain and so produces a characteristic syndrome of neurological changes affecting the arm and the eye on the involved side.

from the lung drains into the left atrium, blood-borne metastases from a cancer in the lung are easily carried over the whole body; secondary deposits are often found in the brain, the liver, in the bones, the adrenal glands and the skin. The left recurrent laryngeal nerve may be involved, causing a hoarse voice, and the phrenic nerve may be interrupted, leading to paralysis of one dome of the diaphragm. Surgical removal of the lung containing the growth (sometimes it is possible to remove only a lobe of the lung) gives the only real hope of cure. However, the age of the patient, the discovery of widespread disease, and poor pulmonary function mean that only about 15 per cent of the total number of sufferers of this disease can be offered an operation. Some of these will be inoperable when the chest is open, some will die after operation and about half the survivors will die in the year after apparently successful surgery on account of metastases which were not obvious earlier. In spite of these dismal facts, surgery is well worth while in the minority of patients who appear likely to benefit from it.

Non-malignant tumours of the lung are rare. The most frequent is bronchial adenoma, which is not beyond suspicion of malignancy on occasion. It should be treated as if it were a cancer, but the outlook for long-term survival is much better.

(4) Diseases of the mediastinum

These are uncommon. *Dermoid cysts*, which are really teratomas, are found beneath the sternum. They can be very large and tend to become infected. They may contain teeth, hair and other tissues. They should be removed.

Myasthenia gravis is a disease causing muscular weakness and is of uncertain cause. Removal of the thymus gland (thymectomy) may be helpful when medical measures with neostigmine etc. fail. The result is unpredictable and sometimes all the resources of the Intensive Care Ward are needed for postoperative weakness leading to respiratory insufficiency.

Neurofibromas and ganglioneuromas arise in connection with the nerves issuing from the spinal canal. They form beside the vertebral bodies in front of the necks of the ribs. They are usually benign, but may become very large and should be removed. *Hodgkin's disease* may cause very great enlargement of lymph nodes in the mediastinum. Surgery is only required in order to obtain a diagnosis by biopsy. The operation for this should be as small as possible. *Retrosternal goitre* is not a neoplasm, but a downward enlargement of the thyroid gland behind the upper part of the sternum. It tends to cause dangerous obstruction of the trachea and should

Teratoma A type of tumour (may be benign or malignant) derived from more than one of the embryonic germinal layers.

be removed. This can usually be done through the conventional thyroidectomy incision in the neck. Rarely, the sternum must be split or a formal thoracotomy performed in order to remove a huge goitre.

SYMPTOMS OF CHEST DISEASE

The leading symptoms of chest disease are cough, sputum, haemoptysis, pain, shortness of breath (including wheeziness) and loss of weight. Cough may be dry, spasmodic or 'bovine' (i.e. without any explosive character which suggests paralysis of a vocal cord). Sputum may be mucoid, i.e. a sticky jelly, clear or greyish; but it can be purulent, yellow or green and sometimes offensive in odour. Haemoptysis, or blood in the sputum, may be profuse or just a streak. In any event it must never be ignored and the patient must be investigated thoroughly. Lung cancer is the main disease that must be excluded. Pain in the chest may occur on deep breathing or coughing. It is then termed 'pleuritic' and reflects disease in the lung. If constant, progressively worsening, and interfering with sleep, it can be an ominous sign of advanced lung cancer. *Shortness of breath* ('dyspnoea') may be of any degree of severity up to the point of complete inability to do anything. It may be spasmodic and accompanied by a mainly expiratory wheeze ('asthma'); if there is a wheeze which can be heard in inspiration also, it indicates obstruction of a major air passage; it is then termed 'stridor'. *Weight loss* occurs especially in lung cancer, pulmonary tuberculosis and other chronic lung diseases.

THE INVESTIGATION OF CHEST DISEASE

To operate on a patient with chest symptoms in the hope of being able to find the cause is a futile exercise. Detailed investigation is therefore necessary before a patient can be advised that an operation is necessary. Some idea of the diagnosis can be obtained by careful history-taking supplemented by the traditional methods of inspection, palpation, percussion and auscultation with the stethoscope. The presence of bronchospasm, pleural fluid, consolidated lung or pneumothorax, can be inferred with reasonable accuracy. More elaborate methods are required, however, and the chief of these is radiography (*Figure 14.5*). This includes the standard 6 foot (184 cm) film, with the patient facing away from the tube. A directly lateral film helps to give precision in locating any abnormality. Tomography will provide

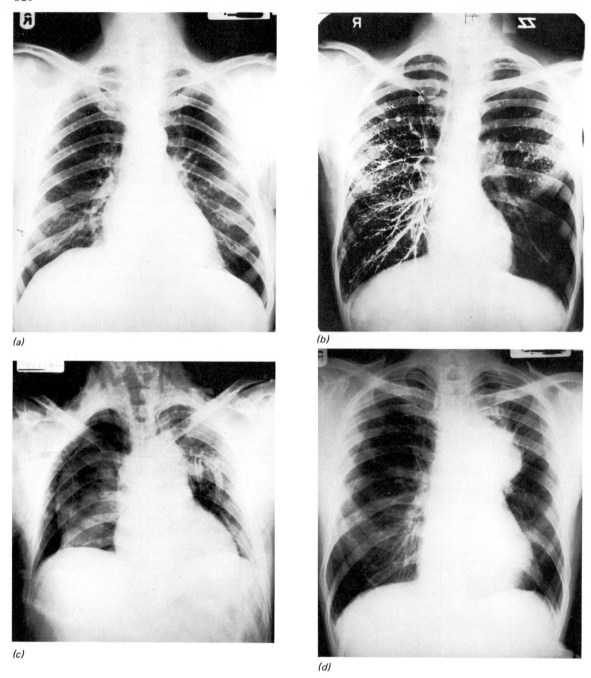

(a)

(b)

(c)

(d)

Figure 14.5. (*a*) Posteroanterior radiograph of normal chest. Note outline of heart with aortic 'knuckle' above due to arch of aorta. The lung fields are clear. The right dome of the diaphragm is slightly higher than the left because of the liver beneath it. (*b*) Right bronchogram. The bronchi of the right lung are outlined by opaque material introduced into the trachea. There is a little opaque 'dye' in alveoli on the left side. The appearances are normal. (*c*) Anteroposterior view of chest in patient with severe thoracic trauma. There is a pneumothorax and a partially de-aerated lung on the right side; intercostal drainage tubes have been inserted into both pleural cavities. There is much air in the soft tissues of the mediastinum, chest wall and neck. (*d*) Posteroanterior film of chest showing a large carcinoma in the hilar region of the left lung. In the film the hilum appears much enlarged. It was not possible to treat this patient surgically because of the extent of the tumour. (The x-ray films in this chapter and in Chapter 21 are reproduced by courtesy of Dr J. H. E. Carmichael)

information about x-ray densities at different depths in the chest, and with these pieces of evidence a very good idea of the disease process present (if any) can be obtained. Less good evidence can be obtained in ill patients by portable films in the ward, and less useful still are the films obtained with the patient lying down when he is unconscious or severely traumatized. *Bronchograms* outline the bronchial tree when a suitable oily medium is introduced into the trachea; *angiograms* outline the pulmonary arteries and the aorta when an opaque medium is injected into the heart through a cardiac catheter. This is more useful for cardiac than general thoracic diagnosis.

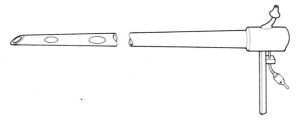

Figure 14.6. Rigid bronchoscope

Bronchoscopy is of great value when there is the possibility of bronchial obstruction by a neoplasm or a foreign body. The traditional bronchoscope (*Figure 14.6*) is a tapered hollow tube with side holes near its end and with a distal light. It can be passed through the larynx and the orifices of all the larger bronchi can be seen; a telescope with an angled

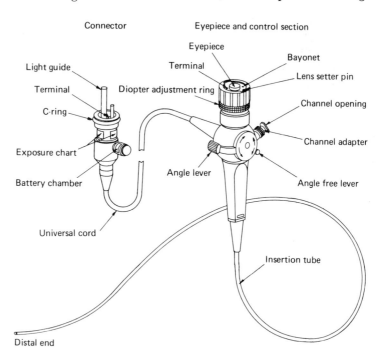

Figure 14.7. Flexible fibre-optic bronchoscope

lens will give a good view of bronchi not in the direct line of vision. A recent invention is the flexible fibre optic broncho-scope (*Figure 14.7*) which is much slimmer and which can be directed into branches of the bronchial tree which can never be seen with the metal instrument. Both instruments can be passed under local or general anaesthesia; local anaes-thesia is perfectly adequate for the flexible instrument, but general is preferable for the older one. For surgical diagnosis, both instruments may have to be used and a general anaes-thetic seems preferable. Biopsies may be obtained with either instrument and are an important part of the investigation.

Sputum cytology may be helpful in the diagnosis of lung cancer. A negative result does not prove the absence of a carcinoma and a positive one needs confirmation by other means.

Pulmonary function tests, which give information as to the amount of air that can be breathed in and out of the lungs, the rate at which it flows in the air passages and its distribution in the lungs, are always required before chest surgery is undertaken. *Blood gas analysis*, performed on arterial blood, is more useful after operation than beforehand. Suffice it to say that disturbed values are in general a warning that any chest operation will be poorly tolerated. The normal values for the partial pressure of oxygen (Po_2) are 10 to 13.3 kPa (75–100 mm Hg) and for Pco_2 4.7–6.0 kPa (35–45 mm Hg).

THORACIC SURGICAL OPERATIONS

Thoracotomy is the generic term for the operation of opening the chest; the commonly used incision is a long one, more to the back than the front of the chest and curving round the angle of the scapula. The 5th or 6th space is entered and the ribs are widely spread apart. This can be done in children and young adults without fracturing them, otherwise it is best to divide or excise a short length of either the 6th or 7th rib. When the incision is closed, the ribs are restabilized and the thick muscles which had been divided are sutured. Intercostal drainage is always established before the incision is closed; if 500 ml of fluid is put into the water-seal bottle as a matter of routine, it will be easy to see how much blood or fluid has drained from the chest after operation. (If the fluid level is 5 cm above the bottom of the bottle when it contains 500 ml of fluid, it is evident that for every rise in level of 1 cm 100 ml of fluid has collected. A paper or tape strip stuck on the outside of the bottle will make reading the level simple.

Lung resection. Removal of the whole lung is called *pneumonectomy*. Each lung is divided into lobes (upper, middle and lower on the right; upper and lower on the left). More or less well developed fissures separate the lobes and the lobes themselves are subdivided into segments, though usually there are no marks of separation between these. It is possible to remove one or more lobes of the lung (*lobectomy*), and many of the individual segments can be removed (*segmental resection – segmentectomy*). Smaller portions of lung can be removed by *local excision* or *wedge resection*. All major lung resections follow the principle of identifying the *hilar* artery, bronchus and vein, dividing them and closing the stumps securely. After pneumonectomy the empty pleural cavity fills up with air and fluid which gradually clots and becomes 'organized'. After lobectomy the remaining lobe expands to occupy the vacant space; after both types of operation the mediastinum tends to move over to the side of the operation to compensate for the loss of lung tissue.

Parietal pleurectomy. This procedure of stripping the parietal layer of the pleura from the chest wall has been described as the treatment for recurrent spontaneous pneumothorax (p. 316).

Decortication of the lung (from Latin *cortex* = bark) has been mentioned as useful in clotted haemothorax or sterilized empyema (p. 317). It consists in removal of fluid, clot and fibrin deposit. The lung will be found to be bound down and constricted by a fibrin layer on its surface. With care this can be removed from the pleural surface of the lung; during this process the lung gradually expands and resumes more or less completely its normal appearance. The parietal pleura is usually greatly thickened and has also to be removed.

Rib resection was formerly widely used in the drainage operation for the treatment of empyema but now this is employed usually only as a last resort. A length of about 5 cm of rib is removed — in many cases it is preferable to remove portions of 2 ribs. The lowest part of the empyema cavity is chosen for this. Drainage is likely to be prolonged, and healing rarely takes place in less than 3 months — this is the essential disadvantage of the method of treatment. In the final stages the opening tends to narrow down before the lung has expanded fully to obliterate the pleural space; therefore it is prudent to be radical at the outset and to fashion a 'stoma' by suturing the edges of the skin to the thickened pleura. This means that no drainage tube will be required, at least not until the final stages of healing. This, incidentally, is the only circumstance in which it is permissible to leave a chest wound open or with a drainage tube not connected to a water-seal. The reason is that the lung is covered with a thick layer of pleura so that it is unable to be collapsed by atmospheric pressure. When an 'open' tube has to be used for drainage, great care must be taken that it cannot get 'lost' by disappearing into the chest. This can happen all too easily, and any such tube must at least be prevented from doing this by having a safety-pin through its outer part; this in turn should be secured to the skin by adhesive tape.

Thoracolaparotomy implies opening of the thoracic and abdominal cavities; this is usually done by a long incision in either the 6th or 8th space crossing the costal margin into the abdomen.

Median sternotomy is used mainly for operations on the heart, but sometimes for access to the anterior mediastinum.

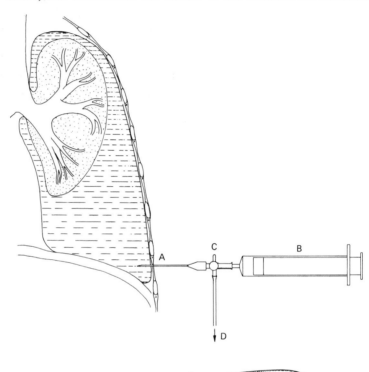

Figure 14.8. Diagram showing the technique of pleural aspiration. A, aspirating needle (may need to be of wide bore); B, aspirating syringe (20 ml); C, three-way tap; D, graduated collecting vessel

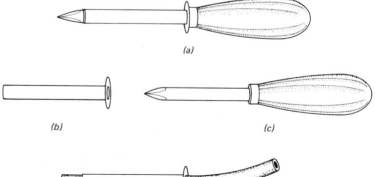

Figure 14.9. Equipment needed for intercostal drainage. (*a*) Trocar and cannula assembled; (*b*) cannula; (*c*) trocar; (*d*) tubing must be able to be passed through cannula

A vertical midline incision is made and the sternum divided, preferably with a pneumatically driven saw which is designed not to injure the soft tissues. The divided sternum must be securely refastened when the incision is closed.

Some important minor procedures must also be noted. The commonest is *pleural aspiration*, done preferably under local anaesthesia with the patient sitting up. The needle must be of wide bore, but care must be taken not to injure underlying viscera with it. It is best to connect the needle to the syringe with a 3-way tap; the syringe must be at least of 10 ml capacity and larger if there is a big collection of fluid (*Figure 14.8*). Air must not be allowed to enter the chest. If there is a large collection of fluid or air it is usually unwise to remove more than about 1000 ml at one session. A sample of any fluid removed must be collected in a sterile container and sent for laboratory examination (bacteriology or cytology).

Intercostal drainage is required when pleural collections reform rapidly after aspiration, or are too thick to remove

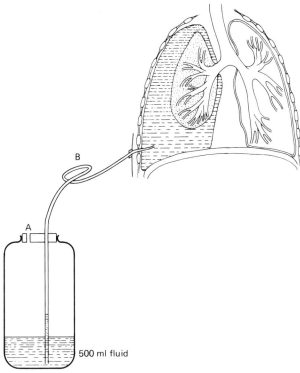

500 ml fluid

Figure 14.10. Diagram illustrating water-seal and intercostal drainage. Tube from patient is connected to tube ending just below water in bottle (about 2–3 cm). Bottle should be wide rather than narrow to prevent air entering vertical tube in inspiration. Mark level of known volume of fluid in bottle (for example 500 ml) when tube is connected. Drainage may be estimated by measuring increased depth of fluid. Many corks have a second tube which should be removed unless it is required for suction. A, Hole for second tube (only required for suction); B, loop of tubing to allow patient movement

through a needle. A rather larger area of chest wall is infiltrated with local anaesthetic and a needle confirms that the correct site has been chosen. An incision about 1 cm long is made and a wide-bored trocar and cannula is pushed cautiously into the pleural cavity (*Figure 14.9*). The trocar is removed and the cannula is blocked by the gloved finger. A tube which has already been matched for size with the trocar is then pushed into the pleural cavity through it. A Malécot catheter on an introducer will do, but the eyes become rather easily blocked. A simple transparent plastic tube is better, and should have a side hole near its end. It must not be pushed in too far. The tube is clamped and the trocar removed. It is then connected to a water-seal bottle (*Figures 14.10, 14.11*). A suture is placed in the edges of the small incision, to be used to close it when the tube is removed. Another suture is tied round the tube to stop it from slipping out accidentally. A combined catheter and trocar is available commercially, but its use is not advised because it is easy to push it in too far causing serious damage to vital structures in the chest.

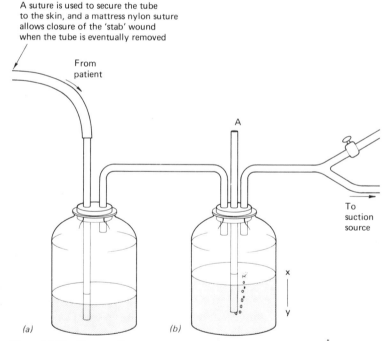

A suture is used to secure the tube to the skin, and a mattress nylon suture allows closure of the 'stab' wound when the tube is eventually removed

From patient

A

To suction source

X

Y

(a)   *(b)*

Figure 14.11. Diagram illustrating water-seal drainage with suction. The water-seal bottle is connected to a source of suction with an intermediate bottle as shown. This bottle ensures that suction is never more than the depth of the third tube and its cork is below the surface of the water (regulating bottle). Excessive bubbling can be regulated by a side tube partially closed with a screw clamp. Distance x–y is the maximum suction possible before air is drawn through tube (A); B, gate clip to be adjusted so that only a few bubbles of air are drawn through A

Pleural biopsies are obtained simply with a notched needle similar to that used for renal or liver biopsy. This can also be used to biopsy enlarged lymph nodes and other masses.

Lymph nodes in the root of the neck are quite often involved in disease processes originating in the chest. Most often they are the 'prescalene' nodes above the medial end of the clavicle. It is a simple small operation to expose these nodes through a small incision and to obtain a sample for histological examination.

Mediastinoscopy is an extension of the same idea. Through a short transverse incision in the front of the neck a mediastinoscope, which is much like an oesophagoscope but shorter, is pushed down into the mediastinum behind the sternum and in front of the trachea. The operation must be conducted with care, but it is usually possible to identify lymph nodes and to obtain biopsies from them.

The two last named procedures are diagnostic ones, chiefly useful in elucidation of obscure diseases in the chest; in the case of lung cancer, a biopsy containing cancer cells will weigh very heavily against a major operation.

POSTOPERATIVE CARE IN THORACIC SURGERY

Thoracic surgical operations threaten the patient's life by making breathing and coughing painful. Patients have to be nursed with the greatest care especially during the critical first 48 hours after operation. Especial care must be paid to pain relief, help with expectoration of sputum and to accurate fluid balance. Young, basically fit patients tolerate abnormal situations much better than the elderly and bronchitic. It is always wise to ensure that a patient's condition is as good as it can be before undertaking an operation.

Relief of pain after surgery is most important, but often difficult to achieve. Morphine and its derivatives are the most useful drugs in the early stages. As has been explained they have the great disadvantage of depressing the respiratory centre and the cough reflex. Rather than giving a large dose to begin with, it is better to start with a smaller dose of 10 mg of morphine or 50 mg of pethidine (for an adult) and to repeat these or smaller quantities as needed.

Assistance with coughing is of basic importance and must commence when there is even the smallest amount of sputum to be raised. Warning the patient before operation that this may be a difficulty helps to secure co-operation later. Relief of pain, and support of the wound area with the palm of the hand helps materially, as does firm but sympathetic encouragement to cough. When sputum remains in one part of the bronchial tree, it no longer initiates the cough reflex. If the patient is tipped on his side, sputum will often move a little so that it can be effectively coughed up. This is the principle of postural 'drainage' used in the treatment of bronchiectasis. Usually it is right to place the patient on his 'good' side, so that the lung on the operated side is uppermost. In the case of a pneumonectomy, however, there is only one lung, and the patient must ideally lie on his operated side to cough. Sputum becomes sticky in dry atmospheres or if the patient is short of fluid. *Humidification* of the inspired air therefore aids expectoration. This may be done by the patient inhaling steam from boiling water in an 'inhaler' before attempting to cough. It is useful to add compound tincture of benzoin ('Friar's Balsam') to the water. Children are conveniently nursed in an oxygen tent into which cold atomized water is blown. If all efforts to help a patient to cough up his sputum fail it will be necessary to suck it out by the use of a bronchoscope. Either type of instrument can be used, and this assistance must not be delayed until the patient becomes exhausted. It may have to be repeated, and if so a tracheostomy must be considered (*see* page 94). After this, sputum may be removed by suction catheter as often as required. Retained sputum tends quickly to become infected and antibiotics may be required.

Attention to *fluid balance* is important. As patients may come to the operating theatre already somewhat short of fluid it is important that all losses sustained during these long and sometimes traumatic operations should be accurately replaced. At one time there was a tendency to under-replace such fluid losses, but this is now generally recognized to be unwise. With large areas of the body open to the air for a long time, invisible losses of water are larger than was once appreciated. As some exudation of fluid takes place into the chest after operation and as the patient may not be able to drink adequately for some time it is always wise to maintain an intravenous regime after major surgery on the chest. Losses of blood, plasma or electrolyte-containing fluid can then be replaced with reasonable accuracy and the amount required can be equated with the urinary output, haematocrit and haemoglobin levels and blood chemistry figures. After very major operations it is wise to insert a central venous pressure cannula (p. 82) and a bladder catheter so that overloading the circulation is avoided and the exact urinary output is known.

After all thoracotomies, intercostal water-seal drainage must be established; after lung resection it is wise to have two tubes connected to individual bottles. One should have its end at the apex of the chest, the other in the lower part.

The object is to allow air to escape easily and fluid to drain. Unless there is a major air leak (shown by bubbling in the water seal on ordinary breathing) *no intercostal drainage tube should ever be disconnected without being clamped*, otherwise the immediate effect will be a pneumothorax with collapse of the lung. Nor must the water-seal bottle be raised above the level of the bed in case potentially infected fluid from it should enter the chest. If there is a large air leak the result of occlusion of the tube will be the rapid and alarming escape of air into the tissues of the chest wall, neck and face ('surgical emphysema').

COMPLICATIONS OF THORACIC SURGERY

In principle these are no different from those of other operations. Drainage tubes should not be removed until both air leak and drainage have ceased, otherwise they will merely have to be reinserted. Late, slowly accumulating collections of fluid and air may have to be aspirated by needle and syringe. Infection within the chest may not respond to antibiotics and an intercostal drain, perhaps with later rib resection, may be required. Superficial infection of the operation wound may occur, but total **dehiscence** of a thoracotomy wound is fortunately rare.

The most serious complication of lung resection is failure of the stump of the divided bronchus to heal, often as a result of disease in the wall. This produces a direct communication with the pleural cavity, a bronchopleural fistula. This is usually signalled by a small haemoptysis 7 to 10 days after operation. The danger of the fistula is that if the patient should lie with the diseased (operated) side uppermost, he will start to cough if the fistula is small, but if it is large he will be in danger of inhaling fluid into his other lung. The danger is particularly great after pneumonectomy, the mortality of a bronchopleural fistula then being high. At any suspicion of such a fistula the patient must lie continuously on the operated side until the pleural cavity has been drained.

INJURIES OF THE CHEST

These are of great importance and their rational management involves the application of the principles which have been outlined. The typical injury in which the chest is damaged is the road accident with sudden deceleration of the occupants of a car, but falls, severe blows, crushing injuries and wounds may all involve the chest.

Open wounds are rather rare in this country. They may result from stabs or bullet wounds. The lung is frequently damaged, but sometimes the heart, the great vessels, the

Dehiscence Gaping; usually applied to an operational wound that has come apart.

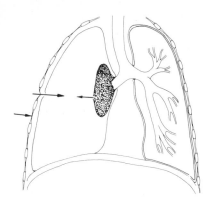

Figure 14.12. A stab wound of the chest sucks air in from the atmosphere. Air also escapes from puncture of the lung leading to tension pneumothorax

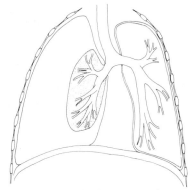

Figure 14.13. Tension pneumothorax displaces the mediastinum compressing one lung greatly and the other partially

spinal cord and the upper abdominal organs may be injured. It is almost certain that there will be a pneumothorax, air entering the pleural cavity from the chest wall wound and/or from the injured lung (*Figure 14.12*). It is likely that the wound will be valvular, allowing one-way passage of air; pressure will build up in the pleural cavity, the lung on this side will be compressed and the mediastinum shifted to the opposite side thus embarrassing the other lung as well (*Figure 14.13*). Such a 'tension' pneumothorax needs urgent relief if life is to be saved. A wide bore needle is effective in emergency, but an intercostal tube is an urgent requirement.

Open wounds of the chest make a communication between the atmosphere and the pleural cavity. This is obvious when one hears air being sucked into the chest in inspiration. The first necessity is to seal the wound, even if temporarily, by firm pressure. Normal surgical toilet is required for the wound, but it is not necessary as a rule to explore the chest widely unless there is evidence of considerable bleeding or a large air leak.

Blunt, or closed injuries of the chest present different problems. The simplest type of injury is fracture of one rib, without instability. This can cause severe pain on a deep breath or a cough. This may not matter too much in a young person, but can be serious in an elderly or bronchitic patient. Strapping the chest has been traditional, but is of doubtful help. In fact it may severely limit chest expansion if it is tight enough to relieve pain, and thus may easily do more harm than good. In practice probably the best treatment is adequate analgesia and instruction of the patient on how to support his painful chest with his hand when he coughs. If there are several fractures, and especially if they are double or if the sternum is fractured together with ribs or cartilages on both sides a special situation arises. As explained in *Figure 14.14* the loosened area of chest wall becomes unstable and exhibits paradoxical movement on respiration. This has a serious effect on respiration and treatment is not easy. One solution is to apply a compression bandage, but this limits chest expansion too much to be more than a first-aid measure. A method of treatment which fell out of use because of the extensive exposure of tissues required to be effective is surgical fixation of the 'flail segment' by pins, wires or pegs. This was superseded by endotracheal intubation and artificial ventilation of the lungs with a mechanical respirator. This, however, cannot be continued without a tracheostomy for more than a few days without causing serious damage to the larynx. It is found that the chest wall seldom becomes sufficiently stable for unaided respiration in less than 2 weeks, and the long period of mechanical ventilation is not well tolerated by

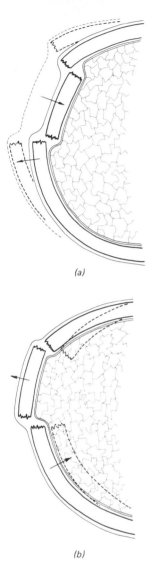

(a)

(b)

Figure 14.14. Paradoxical respiration with double rib fracture. (*a*) Inspiration: normal rib moves out, mobile rib moves in. (*b*) Expiration: normal rib moves in, mobile rib moves out

patients over the age of 60 years. It is also known that a certain number of troublesome strictures of the trachea occur after ventilator treatment. The question of early surgical fixation of the unstable chest wall is therefore being reconsidered at the present time, though it is generally agreed that the most important early treatment of these seriously injured patients is tracheal intubation and ventilation of the lungs by hand if no machine is available. Once this has been done the situation can be assessed calmly and a rational plan of action formulated.

Multiple rib fractures may occur in the posterior parts of the upper ribs as a result of a severe fall or blow on the shoulder. Although they may not be stable and deformity may be considerable, the scapula protects the injured chest wall from the weight of the atmosphere and disability is correspondingly slight.

Any rib fracture may cause puncture of the lung with either a pneumothorax or surgical emphysema of the chest wall.

Very severe blows on the front of the chest, especially in young persons may lead to rupture of the aorta or of a bronchus. Rupture of the aorta may be rapidly fatal, but sometimes the strong outer coat of the vessel may contain the blood, at least for a time. A wide mediastinal shadow on the x-ray should lead to suspicion of this injury; if confirmed by aortography early surgery must follow. A ruptured bronchus usually produces a huge air leak with tension pneumothorax or massive surgical emphysema. Again early surgical repair is necessary.

It must not be forgotten that any patient with severe chest damage may have other injuries as well, for example a rupture of the spleen or liver. Head injuries and upper limb fractures are more common accompaniments of chest injuries than fractures of the legs or pelvis.

Rupture of the diaphragm allows abdominal contents to enter the chest; it is more common on the left side, where the stomach, spleen and much of the small intestine may find their way into the pleural cavity. Surprisingly, this causes little immediate disturbance and the condition may not be diagnosed until weeks, months or years after the accident. The tear in the diaphragm must be repaired surgically.

A NOTE ON CARDIAC SURGERY

While sometimes thought exotic this is a very firmly established branch of surgery. Conditions amenable to surgery are grouped as congenital or acquired. A large variety of abnormalities may occur during the complex development of the heart, with its division into four chambers and the separate pulmonary and systemic circulations.

Incomplete separation of the left and right sided chambers results in the septal defects ('holes in the heart'), which can readily be repaired. The aortic, pulmonary, and less often the mitral valves, may be stenosed and if there is a ventricular septal defect with obstruction to the outflow from the right ventricle (Fallot's 'tetralogy') the venous blood is 'shunted' directly into the aorta. This is one form of the 'blue baby' syndrome. Operations to remedy this by direct repair mean that the heart must be opened, and arrangements made to receive the venous blood, oxygenate it and pump it back into the aorta or one of its branches. A number of types of 'heart-lung machine' are now available. These operations demand excellent exposure of the heart through a median sternotomy (p. 325) and it is necessary to make the blood unclottable by administering heparin, which is neutralized by protamine while the operation is being concluded. Some palliative operations, e.g. the Blalock operation, in which blood from the subclavian artery is diverted into a pulmonary artery in cases of Fallot's tetralogy — and this triumph was the development which gave the impetus to effective treatment of congenital heart disease — can be performed without interfering with the heart. They alleviate the condition without actually restoring normal anatomy.

Conditions not directly involving the heart are patent ductus arteriosus and coarctation of the aorta. The ductus arteriosus is a connection between the left pulmonary artery and the aorta which is normal in the unborn baby; if this persists after birth surgical ligation is carried out. Coarctation of the aorta is an abnormal constriction of the aorta usually just below the origin of the left subclavian artery; this may be excised or the lumen enlarged by a plastic operation.

Acquired heart disease is concerned mainly with the repair, or more often the replacement, of valves damaged by rheumatic heart disease, bacterial endocarditis and other conditions. The damaged valve is replaced by an artificial 'prosthetic' valve made of plastic material and metal, or by a valve wholly or partly of human or animal origin. More recently much attention has been paid to the by-passing of obstructed coronary arteries in symptomatic ischaemic heart disease (angina of effort). A length of saphenous vein from the thigh is commonly used; the mortality rate of the operation is low and the early results encouraging, but it is not possible to assess the long-term effectiveness of the procedure at the present time.

Cardiac transplantation, for the hopelessly diseased heart causing crippling disability, is undoubtedly feasible, but at the present stage of development it is unlikely to be practicable outside a few centres which can devote special study and facilities to the procedure.

15

Orthopaedic surgery and traumatology

C. J. E. Monk

INTRODUCTION

A hundred years ago Orthopaedic Surgeons were mainly concerned with the correction of deformities in children. This work in fact gave the name to Orthopaedics which literally means the rearing of straight children. In those days Orthopaedic Surgeons spent most of their time correcting the bow leg and knock knee deformities due to tuberculosis and rickets. There were also the late results of poliomyelitis which again caused severe deformities. During the early twentieth century the work of the Orthopaedic Surgeons spread to include the treatment of fractures and other injuries. This work was greatly increased during and after the First World War. Because of this extra load of trauma which has been added to the work of the Orthopaedic Surgeons we now, in the Health Service, refer to the speciality as Orthopaedics and Traumatology and in the vast majority of hospitals in Britain this work is carried out by the Orthopaedic Department. This chapter deals briefly with the main conditions seen, firstly in the Orthopaedic Department and secondly in the Accident and Emergency Department. Since the Orthopaedic Surgeons treat patients of all ages we will be discussing the orthopaedic conditions and injuries of children in addition to those of the elderly. Space does not permit us to give more than the outline of the principles of the treatment.

ANATOMY AND DEVELOPMENT OF THE SKELETON

Anatomy of bones

Most bones have a shaft and two ends which form joints with other bones. A joint is often referred to as an articulation, so the parts of the bone which come into contact with other bones are called the articular surfaces. These surfaces have to be smooth to ensure easy movement and for this reason they are covered by a smooth layer of cartilage referred to as articular cartilage.

Anatomy of joints

The ends of bone are held together by a fibrous envelope called the capsule of the joint. This capsule has thick strong bands of fibres in it called ligaments which prevent the joint from moving the wrong way — for example, the ligaments of the knee allow it to bend (flex) and straighten (extend) but not to angle inwards and outwards. Where these ligaments are very obvious or important they are given special names, e.g. the medial ligament of the knee or the lateral ligament of the ankle.

Lining the inner side of the capsule is a layer of special cells capable of secreting an oily fluid which lubricates the joints. The cells are called synovial cells and the fluid is called synovial fluid.

In some joints special pieces of cartilage separate from the articular cartilage are found. The reason for their presence is not known for certain, but it is thought that they help the bones to articulate more closely. Examples are the medial and lateral semilunar cartilages (menisci) of the knee joint and the cartilage of the temporomandibular joint.

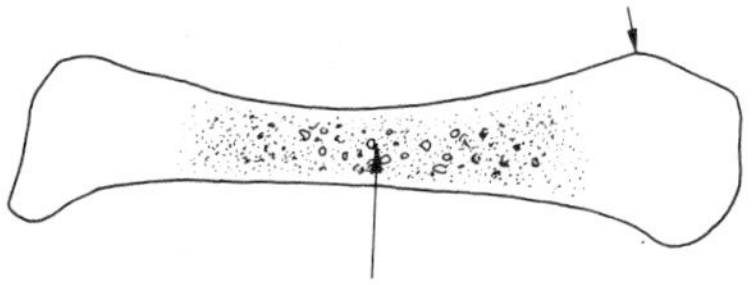

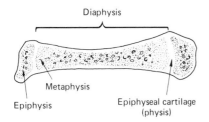

Cartilage outline of bone

Area of ossification

Figure 15.1. Process of ossification in the pre-bone cartilaginous templates

Diaphysis

Metaphysis

Epiphysis

Epiphyseal cartilage (physis)

Figure 15.2. Secondary centres of ossification at the ends of the bone

Template A mould or cast.

Development of bones and joints

During intrauterine life, the skeleton is developed from the mesodermal layer of the embryo. The outline of the bones is laid down first as a cartilage **template**; this is pre-bone cartilage, not to be confused with articular cartilage. During the later months of pregnancy these pre-bone cartilaginous templates begin to ossify or become bone. This process starts in the centre of the shafts and moves towards the ends (*Figure 15.1*).

At birth most bones are ossified in their shafts but not at their ends. During the first few years of life secondary centres of ossification appear in the pre-bone cartilage at the ends of bone (*Figure 15.2*). This leaves an area of unossified cartilage between the centres of ossification for shafts and ends of the bone. This area is referred to as the physis (or epiphyseal cartilage). That part of the bone (the shaft) developing between the physes is sometimes termed the diaphysis. These two areas outside the physes (the ends) are called the epiphyses and the part of the shaft next to the physis the metaphysis. This is the area of greatest ossification during growth and also the area of greatest blood flow.

ORTHOPAEDIC CONDITIONS IN CHILDREN

Congenital conditions

Congenital means present at birth and there are three main conditions which involve the Orthopaedic Surgeon.

(1) Club foot;
(2) Congenital dislocation of the hip;
(3) Spina bifida.

(1) Club foot

Some children are born with deformities of the feet. Any deformity of the foot is referred to as a talipes. There are two main deformities of the foot.

In the first the foot is turned downwards and inwards. A downward deformity at the ankle is referred to as an equinus deformity and an inward deformity of the foot is referred to as a varus deformity so this condition is referred to as congenital talipes equinovarus or CTEV for short.

All variations of severity are seen. Some of the milder types correct on their own and do not require any active treatment. Others are severe and require repeated manipulations and later operations to correct the contracture on the medial and posterior side of the ankle joint and foot. It is difficult to tell at birth how severe a case is but some indication of its severity can be gauged from the shape and position of the heel. If this is small and markedly turned in, the prognosis or outlook is poor. If soft tissue operation is required the foot is then immobilized in a plaster cast for six weeks before allowing manipulation to continue. It is important that all these children with CTEV, no matter how severe it is, are followed up and examined periodically at least until they are walking confidently and, in severe cases, until they are fully grown.

The other deformity seen is that in which the foot is turned outwards and upwards. This is referred to as congenital talipes calcaneovalgus. Calcaneo means 'heel down', valgus means turned away from the midline.

This deformity is less severe than CTEV and seldom if ever requires more than manipulative treatment.

All manipulative treatment and splintage of these congenital club feet is carried out in the Physiotherapy Department.

(2) Congenital dislocation of the hip

The hip of newborn infants in some individuals is lax and can be easily put in and out of joint. This condition is usually diagnosed at birth by the Paediatrician who then seeks the help of the Orthopaedic Surgeon. In the vast majority of cases these hips can be kept in joint merely by holding the thighs abducted and flexed, that is in the Lorenz or 'Frog' position. This is achieved by using double nappies which provide a large amount of cushioning between the thighs or by the use of a Craig splint which is a plastic splint put on over the nappy. All babies whose hips are thought to be in any way suspect are treated like this and followed-up for a minimum of six months. Unfortunately x-rays taken at birth are not of much use in deciding whether the acetabulum or socket of the hip joint will develop normally. However, in the vast majority of cases x-rays taken at six months do show enough bone development for us to decide whether the hip has developed normally. Some cases are not encountered until the child starts walking when he or she is noticed to have a limp. These cases require traction on the affected limb to overcome the shortening of the limb, followed by manipulation of the hip to reduce the dislocation. Plaster fixation in the Lorenz position is then used for several months until the x-rays show that the acetabulum is developing normally.

Very occasionally now we find patients whose hips are still dislocated after the age of three or four years. Each case has to be assessed on its merits but often, particularly if both hips are out of joint, it is decided that it is better to leave them out of joint than to attempt to put them back because in many cases reduction results in a stiff hip which causes more disability than a dislocated hip.

(3) Spina bifida

The lower spine of newborn infants is sometimes found to have failed to have developed properly. In normal development the bone of the spine grows around the spinal cord and forms a protective tube. In cases of spina bifida this growth of the bone around the cord is incomplete. The lack of closure of this tube varies in degree from child to child. In some the spinal contents, both cord (myelocele) and coverings of the cord (meningocele) are visible at birth. In others a small gap in the back of the neural arch (bony canal) can be seen on x-rays but this has no effect on the child. It is important to realize that a percentage of normal children have a very mild degree of spina bifida. If the neural tissue or its coverings are exposed there may be interference with sensation or motor power in the lower limbs. This ranges from a small area of anaesthesia (lack of sensation) or weakness of a few muscles to complete paralysis of the lower limbs (paraplegia). The treatment of these children consists of closure of the exposed spinal tissue and plastic operations to obtain skin cover and, later, orthopaedic treatment of the deformities and weakness of the legs. The object of treatment from the orthopaedic point of view is to get the child walking and able to stand and sit.

Infections of bones and joints

(1) Osteomyelitis

The ends of the long bones in children are especially liable to infections which reach the bone via the bloodstream. They usually follow the establishment of infection elsewhere in the body, e.g. sore throat, boils and sinusitis. The usual bacterium causing osteomyelitis is the *Staphylococcus aureus*. The infection settles in the metaphysis which is the growing part of the bone and rapidly sets up the formation of an abscess. This abscess may spread to the soft tissues around the bone or may spread to the joint nearby. It also spreads along the bone and may cause death or necrosis of the bone by cutting off its blood supply. If it does this an area of bone becomes devitalized and is referred to as a sequestrum. The periosteum or lining of the bone does not die and lays down new bone around the dead bone. This new bone is called involucrum. Before the use of antibiotics (during the Second World War) many children used to die of the septicaemia associated with osteomyelitis. Death from osteomyelitis is now a rare event mainly because these children are treated by antibiotics as soon as the infection has been diagnosed. It is important that a blood specimen be taken for bacteriology before antibiotics are given because at the outset of the disease the staphylococci are circulating in the blood and can be identified and their antibiotic sensitivity established. However, if the antibiotics have already been given the blood is usually clear of staphylococci and the decision as to which antibiotic to use is difficult to make. If the infection spreads to the tissues or to the nearby joint it is important that these be drained surgically. In some Orthopaedic Units immediate operation in osteomyelitis is advised but with the effective antibiotics now available many Orthopaedic Surgeons wait twenty four hours to see if the infection can be brought under control by antibiotics before advising operation.

(2) Septic arthritis

Septic arthritis in children may be caused by a blood-borne infection as seen in osteomyelitis or by a wound of the joint which allows infection to enter it. In either case the joint becomes swollen, hot and painful and aspiration or drainage reveals the presence of pus. The treatment is the same as for osteomyelitis — mainly the giving of antibiotics and if necessary the drainage or redrainage of the pus from the joint.

One exception to this rule is the hip joint. Since this joint is deeply situated it is often impossible to tell whether or not it is infected. In cases in which infection is suspected immediate operation is advised to visually inspect the joint and drain the pus if present.

Conditions of the hip during later childhood

(1) Perthes' disease

This is a condition which affects mainly boys and occurs between the ages of 4 and 12 years. Most of these patients are brought to the clinic because they have been limping and complaining of pain in the hip. Clinical examination shows that the hip is usually 'irritable' and by this is meant that the hip is painful to move and the muscles around it go into spasm on attempted movement. The child is noted to be reluctant to take weight on the affected hip. The diagnosis is made on the x-ray appearance and in this the epiphysis for the upper end of the femur becomes abnormal. The architecture becomes denser, it later becomes disorganized and finally it gradually returns to normal. The cause of the condition is believed to be necrosis of part or all of the capital epiphysis due to interference with its blood supply. The whole process of recovery of the hip may take up to eighteen months to two years to occur. The treatment of the condition has not been standardized throughout the country. Some centres do not treat Perthes' disease other than by resting the child during the time that the hip is irritable which may be anything up to six weeks. In these centres the child is then allowed to run free and use the hip normally. In other centres Perthes' disease is treated by altering the hip position so that more of the capital epiphysis becomes contained in the acetabulum. This is done, either by providing the child with a splint which holds the leg in abduction and internal rotation, or by operating on the upper femur and altering its shape to achieve the same containment of the head. The third method of treatment is to provide the child with a caliper which ensures that as he walks he does not take weight on the affected hip. This caliper is known as a weight-relieving caliper and is the method used in one of our hospitals. The object of treatment is to ensure that the upper end of the femur, when fully developed, is as close to normal as possible. This is because, if any deformity of the head of the femur results, there will more likely be the onset of osteoarthrosis in early adult life.

(2) Slipped upper femoral epiphysis

This condition occurs usually between the ages of 10 and 15 years. In it the epiphysis of the upper end of the femur loses its normal relationship to the diaphysis of the femur and comes to lie more posterior and lower than normal. The condition may occur gradually over the months or may occur suddenly with a fall. Again, the child presents with an irritable hip and a limp or is unable to walk because of a recent fall. The position of the epiphysis is gauged by x-rays, particularly a lateral x-ray. The treatment depends on the length of time for which the condition has been developing. If the condition is acute the alignment of the epiphysis to diaphysis is restored by manipulation and the epiphysis held in position by pins passed up the neck of the femur. If it is chronic the hip is protected until the position has become stabilized and then a corrective operation is done at a level between the trochanters, in order to realign the leg up with the hip in its normal position.

Scoliosis

If you look at a normal spine from the side you will see that there are a series of gentle curves in it. There are curves convex forwards in the cervical and the lumbar regions; these curves are referred to as lordoses. There are curves convex backwards in the thoracic and the sacral region; these curves are called a kyphoses. In addition to these two normal types of curve we sometimes find an abnormal curve to one or other side which is referred to as a scoliosis. This condition of scoliosis may develop for no obvious reason (idiopathic) or may be secondary to nerve and muscle disease (paralysis or spasticity) or may be due to congenital abnormality in the vertebrae themselves.

visible curvature of the spine and to distortion of the ribs with the formation of the so-called rib hump and (b) physiological — affecting the breathing because the distortion of the chest cage may be so marked that lung expansion is interfered with. For these reasons Orthopaedic Surgeons consider that it is unwise to allow a curve to develop to more than 30° or 40° and these children are kept under observation in the clinic and their spines x-rayed periodically. The less severe curves are treated by means of a Milwaukee brace which is a brace supporting the head and resting on the iliac crests. It also has corrective side-pulling straps to press on the rib cage. If a curve progresses in spite of treatment with a Milwaukee brace, operation is advised and the spine is straightened by means of Harrington rods and a spinal fusion is carried out in order to prevent relapse.

Cerebral palsy

This term is used to describe those conditions seen in childhood in which muscle tone is increased or co-ordination or voluntary movement is interfered with due to changes in the brain. The majority of these children present with delay in the normal development during the early years of life and later with increased tone in either one limb (monoplegia), or the upper and lower limb on the same side (hemiplegia), or both lower limbs (paraplegia or diplegia), or all four limbs (quadriplegia). From the orthopaedic point of view the treatment is usually concentrated on the lower limbs and is concerned with the correction of the deformities which these children develop: (a) they develop adductor spasms of the hips which tend to force the thighs together and give rise to the so-called scissor gait; (b) the flexors of the knee become relatively over-powered and cause flexion contractures of the knee; and (c) the plantarflexors of the ankle become more powerful than the dorsiflexors so the child tends to walk on his toes with his knees bent and his hips adducted. Treatment is by physiotherapy, which helps the child to develop a walking pattern, and orthopaedic operations usually in the form of tendon lengthenings to overcome the contractures of the joints. Occasionally the loss of function of the hand can be improved by lengthening the over-acting flexor muscles of the thumb and fingers.

ORTHOPAEDIC CONDITIONS IN ADULTS

A lot of the work of Orthopaedic Surgeons in adult clinics is associated with the late results of trauma, i.e. correction of deformities due to malunion of fractures and the treatment of tendons, ligaments which were damaged by trauma often in association with fractures. These are covered elsewhere in this book. There are however many pure orthopaedic conditions seen in adult clinics and a representative selection will be discussed here.

Degenerative joint disease

With the gradually rising age of the population as a whole, the incidence of degenerative joint disease is increasing. The joints undergo a progressive wearing-out (of the articular cartilage) and roughening of the bone underlying the cartilage, giving rise to the changes of osteoarthrosis. In the past this used to be referred to as osteoarthritis but the newer term is preferable if only to avoid the anxiety that the term arthritis causes in the minds of some patients. Degenerative arthrosis may appear for no obvious reason and be thought to be idiopathic or it may follow some other condition of the joint which has rendered the articular surfaces uneven. Common conditions doing this are congenital dislocation, Perthes' disease, slipped upper femoral epiphysis, fractures and rheumatoid disease. In these cases the osteoarthrosis is referred to as secondary. Clinically, the patient presents with a joint which may be deformed slightly but which is painful on movement and has a restricted range of movement. X-rays show the classic four signs of degenerative arthrosis: (1) narrowing of the radiological joint space which is in fact due to erosion of articular cartilage, (2) sclerosis or increased density of bone in the region of the degenerative arthrosis, (3) osteophytes or excess bone formation at the edges of the joints, and (4) cysts which appear in the bone adjacent to the worn joint. The joints commonly affected are the knee, the hip, the big toe metatarsophalangeal joint and the thumb carpometacarpal joint. In secondary arthrosis the joints affected with rheumatoid, i.e. the elbow and the ankle, are also included.

Treatment

In the early stages pain can be relieved and the movement improved by physiotherapy in the form of short-wave diathermy, which warms the joints, and mobilization exercises. If the joint is a weight-bearing one, e.g. hip, knee or ankle, pain can be relieved by taking some of the body-weight off the joint by means of using a walking stick. Pain-killing tablets are also useful. If the condition progresses and it often does, it may be necessary to advise operation on a degenerative joint and then three types of operation are available.

(1) *Arthrodesis* This means the complete stiffening of a joint and is done by removing the joint surfaces and allowing the two bones which form the joint to unite just as though it had been a single bone with a fracture.

(2) *Osteotomy* The bone is cut in two and the joint surfaces realigned to alter the lines of stress going across the joints.

(3) *Arthroplasty* This means remaking of a joint and this can be done either by removing the joint surfaces and allowing movement to take place as in the Keller arthroplasty of the big toe or by replacing one or both of the bone surfaces forming the joint in the form of a hemiarthroplasty, for example Moore's arthroplasty of the hip or as a total joint replacement as seen in the hip in the Charnley type of hip replacement. In this the plastic socket and metal ball are inserted into the pelvis and femur respectively and a new joint created.

Recent advances in the techniques of replacement of joints have led to a great increase in the number of operations done for degenerative joint disease.

Rheumatoid disease

Rheumatoid disease is basically an inflammation of synovial tissue. This tissue lines the inner side of the capsules of joints and also the inner sides of tendon sheaths so that rheumatoid disease is characterized by swelling of joints and tendon sheaths. The disease process in a joint eventually affects the articular surface and leads on to roughening and degenerative arthrosis as mentioned in the previous section. In the tendon sheaths the disease causes stiffness, may cause triggering of the tendons and eventually causes rupture of the tendons. These ruptures are commonly seen in finger extensor tendons, the rupture occurring as they glide over the wrist. In addition to the joint and tendon effects of rheumatoid disease there are also effects on the patient as a whole. There is often a severe degree of anaemia, there is general debility and marked muscle wasting. The number of patients with rheumatoid disease is increasing as the average age of the population increases and they will provide a large part of the work of the Orthopaedic Surgeons in the closing quarter of the twentieth century.

Cervical and lumbar spondylosis

These conditions, which probably form the largest single group of conditions seen in Orthopaedic clinics, may be considered as degenerative disease of the spine. Patients with disc degeneration may present with pain in the spine or with pain in the spine associated with pain or with pins and needles radiating down from the neck to the upper limbs or from the lumbar spine to the lower limbs. Often this condition is brought to light by unusual activity such as moving furniture or a heavy bout of gardening after a period of rest. On examination the patient is found to have a restricted range of movement in the neck or the lumbar spine but on neurological examination there is no deficit or motor or sensory loss in the relevant limbs. This distinguishes these groups of conditions from those due to disc prolapse which is an acute phenomenon usually in younger people and is described in Chapter 13. However the secondary changes to disc degeneration may include the laying down of new bone at the edges of the vertebral bodies in such a position that as a late development the patient is found to have a neurological problem. The treatment of cervical and lumbar spondylosis depends on the severity of the symptoms. If severe the patient is confined to bed and the area rested by traction. Traction implies a pulling force, applied either to the legs in lumbar spondylosis or to the head in cervical spondylosis, in order to diminish the movement of the spine in the relevant site. Less severe types of cervical or lumbar spondylosis may be treated in a collar or back support or, if there is no obvious aggravation of the pain on movement, by a course of short-wave diathermy and gentle exercises. Operative treatment is seldom indicated.

Deformities

(1) Hallux valgus

One of the commonest deformities seen in adults is a valgus or outward angulation of the big toe. This is often associated with the development of soft tissue thickening and inflammation on the inner side of the big toe metatarsophalangeal joint. This soft tissue thickening is referred to as a bunion. Minor degrees of hallux valgus can be treated by altering the footwear so that the prominent head of the metatarsal is not rubbed, but more severe degrees require correction and this is done by the Keller's arthroplasty in which the proximal third to a half of the proximal phalanx of the big toe is excised and the prominent head of the metatarsal shaved down. In this way the deformity is corrected and the bony prominence causing the bunion is removed.

(2) Dupuytren's contracture

This is a common condition causing the contracture of the joints of the fingers particularly the ring and little fingers. It is due to a contracture of the fibrous tissue of the palm. The tendon is not affected. As the contracture increases the finger, usually the ring or little finger or both, becomes progressively flexed and if untreated will become permanently flexed into the palm. Treatment is by excision of the thickened, contractured palmar fascia and then by mobilization of the fingers. It is important to operate on these cases early before the contracture of the joints has proceeded to a point at which it cannot be corrected. The proximal interphalangeal joint is the joint most commonly, irreversibly affected.

Bone and joint infections

In the past, chronic osteomyelitis due to staphylococcal infections and tuberculous osteomyelitis were common. These two conditions are now rare in Great Britain but are seen commonly in other countries. The problem of tuberculous infection was that it was remarkably difficult to eradicate and the treatment was very time-consuming. However we now have antibiotics which do attack the tubercle bacillus and the treatment follows similar lines to those of acute osteomyelitis in children, only the whole picture is less dramatic and acute. Most cases respond to antibiotics and operative interference is limited to those cases in which abscess formation is seen. In tuberculous infections it is the spine and hip joints which are commonly affected. Acute septic arthritis still does occur in adults but the picture is much less acute than that seen in children and for this reason the diagnosis is often delayed. The treatment follows the same lines, namely aspiration of drainage followed by antibiotic therapy. Resolution is usually complete but occasionally the infection persists and leads on to fibrous or bony stiffening of the joint (ankylosis).

TRAUMATOLOGY

Introduction

In this section we will discuss the diagnosis and treatment of injuries of: (a) bones — fractures; (b) joints — dislocations, subluxations, sprains, penetrating wounds, effusions and haemarthroses; (c) tendons; and (d) nerves.

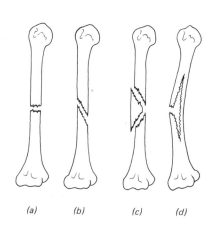

(a)   (b)   (c)   (d)

Figure 15.3. Examples of bone fractures: (*a*) transverse, (*b*) oblique, (*c*) comminuted, and (*d*) greenstick fractures

FRACTURES OF BONES

Any break in any part of a bone is called a fracture. This includes breaks in the fine network of bone threads (trabeculae) within the bone as well as those in the hard shell (cortex).

Classification

There are many descriptive terms applied to fractures (*Figure 15.3*) but for practical purposes there are two main types of fractures.

(1) Simple or closed fractures — in this type the bone has broken but there is no contact between the broken ends and the exterior, i.e. the skin or mucosa over the fracture is still intact. This means that there is no danger of infection entering the fracture from the outside.

(2) Compound or open fractures — in this type the fracture is open to the exterior either because the skin has been injured at the same time or because the bone ends have penetrated the overlying skin or mucous membrane. In this type infection of the fracture is likely.

This classification into simple and compound types is the most important distinction in fractures. Several other descriptive terms are used. A fracture is said to be 'complicated' when some important structure other than the bone is involved, for example, a blood vessel or a nerve. The term 'comminuted' fracture implies that there were more than two fragments or pieces resulting from the fracture. In pathological fracture the bone in which it has occurred was diseased or abnormal. The amount of force necessary to produce the fracture in these cases is usually less than with normal bone.

Diagnosis

Signs of a fracture
The most common signs of fracture of a bone are:

(1) deformity — the limb may be of abnormal shape if the fracture has marked angulation or displacement;
(2) loss of function — there is usually weakness of muscle action distal to a severe fracture;
(3) tenderness — this is the most dependable sign of a fracture as the bone is tender to pressure no matter how small the fracture is; and
(4) abnormal mobility — when the patient attempts to move the limb, movement is seen where there is normally none (compare with dislocation).

In the past some authors have mentioned crepitus as a sign of a fracture. Today, with the advantage of good radiological facilities, it is not justified to attempt to elicit **crepitus** as it is usually painful to the patient.

Radiology
Anyone suspected of having a fracture should have the injured part x-rayed. In most cases — with the exception of fractures of the scaphoid bone and an occasional undisplaced or stress fracture — the fracture will show up on a radiograph.

Treatment

There are three main phases in the treatment of any fracture: realignment, immobilization and protection.

Realignment
Some fractures are not displaced or angulated and therefore do not need realignment. Some, however, have been displaced or angulated to such a degree that the position is not acceptable. In these the angulation or displacement (or both) has

Crepitus A grating noise produced when two rough surfaces are rubbed together.

to be reduced, the procedure being termed 'reduction of the fracture'.

There are two main methods of fracture reduction – closed and open. By closed reduction is meant manipulation (usually under general anaesthesia) or traction which may be gentle and continued for several hours or days. In an open reduction the fracture is approached surgically and the bones realigned under direct vision.

Because open reduction inevitably converts a simple to a compound fracture, most surgeons reserve open reduction only for those fractures which cannot be treated by closed reduction.

Immobilization

Having realigned the fragments of bone, it is then necessary to hold them in place until the processes of repair have led to union of the fracture. Union is said to have occurred when the fracture is no longer mobile and gentle stressing of the fracture does not cause pain. The time taken for this to occur varies according to which bone is fractured and with the age of the patient.

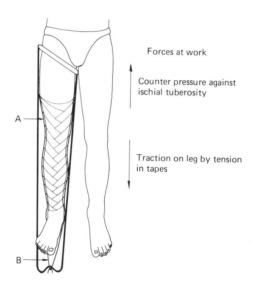

Forces at work

Counter pressure against ischial tuberosity

Traction on leg by tension in tapes

Figure 15.4. Diagram showing the use of traction for immobilization of a fracture of the femur. A, Strips of Elastoplast held in place by bandages; B, tapes attached to Elastoplast and tied over end of splint

Various methods of immobilization are used. They are divided into external and internal methods. The external methods are splintage, plaster of Paris casts and traction. Traction means exerting a pull in the line of a limb and, as mentioned above, it can be used as a method of reduction as well as a method of immobilization of fractures (*Figure 15.4*).

Internal methods require a surgical operation for insertion and consist of plating, screwing and the use of rods placed within the medullary canal of the bone. Again, the same objection applies to internal fixation as to open reduction — its use converts a simple to a compound fracture. Most surgeons prefer to use external fixation if at all possible. Some fractures are unsuitable for external fixation, however, either because the cast or splints cannot hold them (for example, fractures of both forearm bones) or because the size of the cast necessary to hold the fracture would be deleterious to the general condition of the patient (for example, fractures of the neck of the femur in the elderly).

Protection

Once a fracture has united, the patient may start to move the limb but full use (for example, taking full weight on a recently fractured leg) must be avoided until the bone has regained its pre-fracture strength. When this has occurred the fracture is said to be consolidated. While waiting for consolidation the fracture is protected by means of splints, calipers and crutches. The splints and calipers can be removed for exercises aimed at mobilizing the joints usually done in the physiotherapy department.

Treatment of compound fractures

Because of the danger of infection, compound fractures are surgical emergencies. The patient is taken to the operating theatre as quickly as possible and the wound is cleaned and either sutured or closed in such a way that any communication between the fracture and the exterior is cut off. The fracture is later treated on its own merits.

To illustrate the principles mentioned above, an example of the diagnosis and treatment of a fracture will be given.

Colles' fracture

Colles' fracture is probably the commonest fracture seen in fracture clinics. It occurs usually in the middle-aged and elderly and consists of a fracture of the lower end of the radius and of the ulna styloid process. It is sustained by falling on the outstretched hand and the displacement of the lower radial fragment is backwards and towards the radial side.

The patient is anaesthetized and the fracture reduced by gentle traction in the line of the limb for about 1 minute to loosen up the tightened tendons and then by manipulation of the fragment towards the palm and towards the ulna side of the forearm. This is usually easily achieved because there is some degree of comminution of the dorsal part of the fragment. Once the fracture has been reduced the forearm is immobilized with the wrist flexed and turned to the ulnar side. The immobilization can be achieved either with splints of aluminium, which are held on with Elastoplast, or by means of plaster of Paris.

The author prefers the use of splints because these can be easily tightened as the swelling subsides over the first 2 weeks following the injury. Plaster of Paris cast is satisfactory but should be changed after 10 to 14 days in order to take up the slack which has resulted from the reduction of the swelling. Most Colles' fractures unite within 4 to 5 weeks, so the plaster or splint is removed at 5 weeks, and if the fracture area is not tender to moderate pressure and there is no sign of movement on straining, immobilization is discontinued and the patient treated with a supporting bandage. After another 2 to 3 weeks movement has usually returned and the patient can be discharged from the clinic.

Complications of fractures

Complications of fractures may occur either at the time of injury or during the healing process.

Complications at the time of injury include haemorrhage and shock (discussed in Chapter 12), damage to nerves causing paralysis distal to the fracture, and infection which is seen usually with compound fractures and may threaten the health of the patient or may interfere with healing.

Complications of fractures during the healing process include (1) malunion when the fracture may unite in a displaced or angulated position; (2) delayed union if a fracture has not united within the period of time that union normally takes; and (3) non-union where there is no sign of union occurring after a specific period of time (in lower limb bones in 1 year). In practice both delayed union and non-union are usually treated by bone grafting.

INJURIES TO JOINTS

DISLOCATIONS AND SUBLUXATIONS

If the bone ends forming a joint are displaced so that no contact remains between their articular surfaces, the joint is said to be dislocated. If they are displaced but there is still some contact between their articular surfaces the joint is said to be subluxated. The old name for a dislocation was 'luxation' so a subluxation is 'almost a luxation'.

Quite often a dislocation or a subluxation is associated with a fracture; the whole is then referred to as a fracture dislocation or a fracture subluxation.

As in the case of fractures, dislocations may be either simple or compound.

Diagnosis

Signs

The most common signs of joint dislocation are: (1) deformity — this is common but, in the case of dislocation of the shoulder joint, may only be obvious if the joint is examined from behind; (2) loss of function — the patient has difficulty moving the limb distal to the dislocation; (3) pain on attempted movement of the joint; and (4) loss of normal mobility — the normal movement of the joint is lost.

Radiology

Radiography usually shows the dislocation or subluxation but must be taken in two planes (usually anteroposterior and lateral) because the displacement may not be obvious if inspection is carried out from only one angle.

Treatment

The principles of treatment of a dislocation are the same as those for treatment of a fracture. The only difference is in the time taken for the repair processes.

Most dislocations can be reduced by manipulation under a general anaesthetic. Occasionally some structures (for example, a tendon) obstruct reduction and open reduction is then necessary. Tearing of ligaments may require operative repair (*see later*).

The capsule and ligaments have usually been stretched, torn or separated from their bone attachments. After reduction the joint must be immobilized until they have undergone repair. The length of time necessary for this repair is of the order of 3 to 4 weeks as against 3 to 4 months for some fractures.

The joint should be protected from strain for 3 to 4 months after a dislocation — again a shorter period than for a comparable fracture.

Recurrent dislocation

If a dislocation is not immobilized for a sufficient time, the capsule and ligaments may not regain their full strength and attachment to bone. This will lead to a weak joint which will redislocate more easily if subjected to strain. This is seen commonly in the shoulder joint and may constitute a grave disability especially in a patient whose occupation depends on strong shoulder and arms (for example, a steel erector).

Example of treatment of a dislocation

One of the commonest dislocations seen in clinics today is dislocation of the shoulder. This usually occurs in young men as either a sports injury in rugby football or as the result of falling onto the shoulder.

On examination, the patient is found to have lost the normal outline of his shoulder (*Figure 15.5*) and the head of the humerus is usually palpable below the coracoid process in the front of the shoulder.

Radiographs should always be taken before reduction of the dislocation in order to ascertain whether a fracture of the head of the greater tuberosity of the humerus has occurred at the same time.

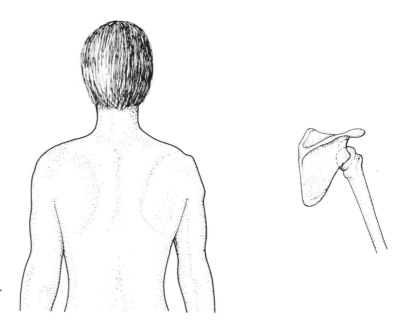

Figure 15.5. Dislocation of the shoulder. Diagram showing the characteristic loss of normal contour of the shoulder

Reduction of the dislocation is done usually under general anaesthesia. Gentle traction in the line of the limb is kept up for about one minute and then, with traction applied, the head of the humerus can usually be manipulated around the inferior edge of the glenoid fossa. Reduction is usually sudden and visible and once the dislocation has been reduced, movement of the upper limb is again full to passive testing. The arm is then immobilized by means of a collar and cuff sling which holds the forearm across the chest and a body bandage or Elastoplast strapping which keeps the upper arm against the side of the chest. A cotton wool bandage is placed in the axilla for comfort. This immobilization should be kept up for at least 3 weeks in a young person. Thereafter, gentle mobilization is allowed, but the shoulder should not be strained for 2 to 3 months following a dislocation.

OTHER INJURIES TO JOINTS

Penetrating wounds

It is common in road traffic accidents for sharp objects, such as broken glass, to penetrate joints. It is important to realize that the synovial cavity has been opened because of the danger of infection entering the joint and causing septic arthritis.

The presence of synovial fluid in the wound and air in the joint cavity (as seen on a radiograph) are helpful signs.

Treatment is by surgical exploration, cleansing and repair of the capsule and synovium.

Sprains and tears of ligaments

Ligaments may be strained when abnormal forces act on the joint: if the force is great enough, the ligaments tear and the joint subluxates or dislocates. It is important to realize that this displacement of the joint may only last 1 to 2 seconds so that when the patient is seen in the casualty department, the joint is back in position but the ligaments are damaged.

There is pain over the affected ligament and it is tender. Stretching the ligament causes pain. If the patient is given a general anaesthetic and the joint is examined, it is possible to subluxate or dislocate the joint in cases of ligament tears. This can be demonstrated by taking a radiograph while the joint is under strain (strain-view radiography).

Sprains are treated by supporting the joint with strapping. Tears of ligaments are usually treated by immobilizing the joint in a plaster of Paris cast until the ligament has undergone fibrous repair or as in the case of some special ligaments (for example, the lateral ligaments of the knee and ankle) operative repairs have been carried out.

Synovial effusions

The natural response of the synovium to injury (strain, contusion or laceration) is to increase the production of synovial fluid. This gives rise to a fluctuant swelling which takes up the shape of the synovial cavity.

Most effusions reabsorb with the passage of time. If they persist or become tense, they should be aspirated.

Haemarthrosis

Severe injuries may lead to bleeding into a joint. This is seen particularly in fractures in which the articular surfaces of the joints are involved and in severe tears of capsules and ligaments.

It is customary to aspirate effusions of blood into joints as reabsorption is not as dependable as in the case of synovial effusions.

Complications of dislocations

Damage to neighbouring nerves is seen particularly in the shoulder joint where the circumflex nerve is injured leading to paralysis of the deltoid muscle. Damage to sciatic nerves leads to paralysis of the leg in dislocations of the hip.

There is often a fracture of one of the bones forming the joint in addition to the dislocation (*Figure 15.6*). This is seen in dislocations of the shoulder (fracture of the greater tuberosity of the humerus) and in dislocations of the hip (fractures of the acetabulum).

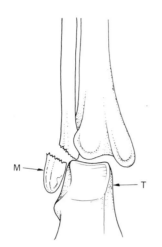

Figure 15.6. Diagram of a radiograph of fracture subluxation of ankle joint. M, Lateral malleolus fractured; T, talus displaced

INJURIES TO TENDONS

Tendons may be damaged by incised wounds or by spontaneous ruptures which are seen particularly in degenerate tendons. Incised wounds of tendons are seen particularly in lacerations of wrist and the back of the ankle region in which the tendo Achillis is damaged. Lacerations of the palm and fingers also are associated with damage to the flexor tendons of the fingers.

Treatment

Most tendon injuries can be sutured at the time of treatment of the overlying skin laceration. However, the flexor tendons of the fingers are a special case because these tendons run in fibrous flexor sheaths and there are two tendons to each finger. If these are repaired at the time of the injury subsequent fibrosis leads to adhesion between the two tendons and between the tendons and the sheaths. This leads to stiffness of the fingers. In order to prevent this most surgeons suggest that the tendons are not repaired at the time of injury but that the skin is sutured and allowed to heal. Approximately six weeks later the tendon injury is treated by replacement of the whole tendon with a graft tendon taken from some other part of the body where a tendon is found that is not of important use, for example the palmaris longus tendon in the forearm or one of the extensor tendons to the toes. In this way adhesion between tendon and sheath is avoided.

MENISCUS INJURIES

There are two menisci in each knee, a medial and a lateral. These are structures shaped like the segment of an orange and composed of fibrocartilage. Their function is not fully understood but they may act as 'washers' to enhance the fit of the lower end of the femur onto the upper end of the tibia. They tend to be damaged in twisting injuries of the knee and this may result in a tear of the meniscus which is referred to as a 'torn cartilage'. This injury is particularly common in football players and miners. Since the cartilage has no blood supply its capacity for repair is very poor and most patients are advised to have a torn cartilage removed so that the fragments of the cartilage do not interfere with joint movement. The medial cartilage is more often torn than the lateral. After the operation the patient's knee is usually rested on a back splint for two weeks before allowing gentle movements to restart. In young people the results of menisectomy are very good but in persons over thirty-five years occasional swelling and instability are seen in later years.

NERVE INJURIES

The peripheral nerves in the limbs are often damaged and usually in combination with other injuries such as tendon lacerations. The injury results in immediate loss of muscle power in the muscles supplied by the injured nerve and in sensory loss in the skin supplied by that nerve. If the wound is clean the nerve can be sutured at the time of closure of the skin. If it is dirty then the nerve ends are marked by a black silk suture and the skin is closed and the patient is treated with antibiotics. When the inflammation has all settled (six to eight weeks later) the wound is re-explored and the nerve ends approximated after excision of all scar tissue. The results of nerve suture are good in motor nerves, e.g. the radial nerve or the lateral popliteal nerve, but less satisfactory in sensory nerves. Occasionally a large area of nerve is damaged and in these cases some form of bridging of the gap is done by means of a nerve graft taken from elsewhere in the body. In addition to laceration of the nerves the nerve may be damaged by contusion which may merely cause loss of function for a few weeks or if the axon, the actual impulse-carrying structure at the centre of the nerve sheaths, is damaged recovery will take longer. Three terms are used to describe the degree of injury: (1) neuropraxia is concussion of the nerve without loss of continuity of its structure, (2) axonotmesis is breaking of the axon cylinder so that regrowth has to occur and (3) neurotmesis, which is cutting of the whole nerve so that repair is necessary.

After nerve repair the site of repair must be protected from distraction and this is usually done by immobilizing the relevant limb in a plaster of Paris cast. As repair continues the position of the limb is gradually returned to the normal by means of serial plaster casts.

16

Burns

D. O. Maisels

INTRODUCTION

The old saying that beauty is only skin deep is almost as far from the truth as the equally common fallacy that burn injuries are an affliction of the skin only. A serious burn will not only affect such underlying structures as the tendons, joints, muscles, nerves, blood vessels and even bones by direct thermal damage, but also the systemic effects of burns can have serious and lethal consequences in every body system. In this chapter, however, attention will be confined in the main to the important features of the structure and function of the skin only, followed by a consideration of the causes, pathology and treatment of burns.

Anatomy of skin

The skin which covers the whole body surface, consists of two main layers, the epidermis and the dermis (*Figure 16.1*). Although the epidermis, which is stratified epithelium, is in itself a complex structure, it can for practical purposes be regarded as a sheet of cells, several layers thick, which is constantly being replaced from below upwards. Thus as new cells are formed in the deepest layer, the oldest ones are

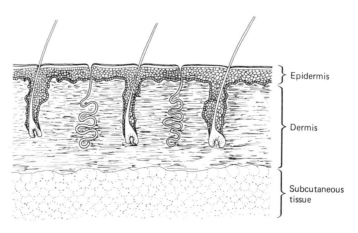

Figure 16.1. The structure of skin

Epidermis

Dermis

Subcutaneous tissue

shed from the surface. Below the epidermis lies the dermis which again is a complex structure consisting mainly of specialized connective tissue cells. An important difference between epidermis and dermis is that while the former can replace itself by multiplication of the cells, if the dermis is damaged or destroyed it is replaced by granulation tissue which in turn becomes scar tissue. In addition to these two main layers, the skin contains important appendages, that is, sweat glands and hair follicles with their sebaceous glands. These appendages develop as downgrowths from the epidermis into the dermis and not only are the layers of cells which form them continuous with the epidermis, but they also retain the proliferative abilities of the epidermal cells. The dermis is supplied by a rich capillary bed of blood vessels and lymphatics as well as a network of sensory nerves and their specialized endings. Finally, a passing reference should be made to the special cells concerned with the manufacture and transport of pigment.

Function of skin

The skin is the largest organ in the body with functions as important to survival of the whole organism as any of the other organs or systems.

By virtue of its waterproof qualities the epidermis prevents the body from becoming waterlogged if immersed and also prevents it from drying out in dry atmosphere. Thus it is concerned with the important function of water regulation. Similarly, because of the rich blood supply and the presence of sweat glands, temperature regulation of the body is effected through the agency of the skin. The sweat glands are concerned with excretion, while vitamin D is produced in response to ultraviolet light; pigment protects against too much sun and the epidermis forms a barrier against infection, while the sensory nerves constitute one of the main sensory organs for the transmission of information about the environment to the rest of the body.

INCIDENCE AND AETIOLOGY OF BURNS

In the field of traumatic surgery there can be few more challenging situations than that presented by the patient with an extensive burn. Certainly there is none where the share of the burden of treatment falls more heavily upon the nursing staff. But considering the problem of burns from the point of view of the community at large, it offers no less a challenge. An idea of the magnitude of the problem is given by the realization that about 12 000 people in England and Wales require hospital treatment for burns each year and of these approximately 700 die from their injuries. Many of these patients are small children who are scalded by pulling teapots, cooking pans, and so on, onto themselves or whose clothes are ignited at unguarded fires and electric radiators. While various Acts of Parliament have gone some way towards the prevention of these tragedies by laying down rules about fire-guards, flame-proof clothing and the like, there remain a great number of children who are burned in a moment of carelessness or thoughtlessness on the part of the parents. And who can legislate for the natural curiosity of children who investigate the mysteries of electrical appliances?

In adults, burns are commonly divided into industrial and domestic. Not surprisingly, the bulk of the former occur in men and the responsibility for their prevention rests heavily upon the firms concerned.

Domestic burns, on the other hand, are the predominant variety in women, though there are many men who are burned at home as well.

In common with many other diseases it is possible to identify predisposing causes of burns as the first stage in their prevention and elimination. Studies, carried out in the Liverpool Regional Burns Centre, established the presence of a predisposing factor in no less than 25 per cent of all the adult admissions. Of these patients the largest single group were the epileptics who composed 11 per cent, but cerebro-vascular disease, physical disabilities and other degenerative processes in the elderly all played their part. What emerged is that it is not only children who are in need of special care and protection against burning. There are many adults equally at risk, not least among them being the epileptics, the old and the infirm.

PATHOLOGY

Causes

Burns are subdivided into different groups according to their cause.

Thermal burns

Thermal burns are the commonest and therefore the most important type of burn injuries. They are of two varieties: scalds and burns. The former are the result of contact with hot fluids, such as water, tea, soup, fat, tar and so on, as well as injuries caused by steam which are usually classified as scalds. Burns, on the other hand, are caused by flames and contact with hot objects such as electric irons, stoves, fire-grates, and molten metals. Generally burns tend to be deeper than scalds though this is not always the case.

Chemical burns

Chemical burns are most frequently caused by strong acids or alkalis although here again there are many exceptions to the rule, and in addition to the local effects of the burn one must bear in mind the possibilities of systemic effects of absorbed chemicals on the kidneys, liver and other vital organs.

Electrical burns

Electrical burns are the result of damage following the passage of a current through the tissues. There is always an entrance and an exit burn and the damage may be far more extensive than the area of skin destruction. Electric burns can be difficult to treat because of vascular changes which may result in late extension of the area of destruction either from bacterial invasion of devitalized tissues or from thrombosis of vessels and consequent ischaemic necrosis of tissue.

Radiation burns

Radiation burns are of various types. Those following irradiation treatment are very superficial and in the acute phase do not present any special problems in management. However, the irradiated skin becomes atrophic and many years later may undergo simple necrosis or malignant degeneration. Similar changes may follow accidental or careless overexposure of the skin to diagnostic radiographs and present difficult and special problems in treatment. Severe acute irradiation burns are unlikely to follow the explosion of a nuclear weapon because anybody close enough to sustain them would almost certainly be killed by the heat, the explosion or the acute effects of severe irradiation. Circumscribed acute irradiation burns have occurred in accidents with nuclear reactors and linear accelerators and the resulting destruction of, for example, a hand, has been very severe indeed.

Measurement of severity of burns

The severity of a burn is measured in two ways, that is by depth and by extent.

Depth

In the past there have been numerous complicated systems for the description of the depth of a burn. In clinical practice, however, there are only two types and these form the basis of the current description of burns as being superficial (partial thickness — first degree) or deep (full thickness — second degree). In superficial burns the deeper layers of the dermis are spared and since this area contains the bases of the sweat glands, hair follicles and sebaceous glands there are numerous epithelial 'islands' from which healing can take place. The epithelium grows out from these islands and soon covers the whole surface to reconstitute the intact epithelial covering over the dermis. In deep burns, on the other hand, the full thickness of the skin is destroyed and no epithelial islands remain. Healing can only take place from the edges and is usually so prolonged that skin grafting is necessary to repair the defect.

Extent

The other important factor in burns is their extent. Obviously, the severity of the burn injury will be proportional to the surface area involved and it is of the utmost importance in planning treatment to be able to measure the extent of the burn. Perhaps the simplest and most popular method for measuring extent is the 'rule of nine' in which areas of the body are divided into sections measuring 9 per cent or multiples of 9 per cent of the total body surface (*Figure 16.2*). Furthermore, the patient's outstretched hand represents roughly 1 per cent of his body surface. The rule of nine is not applicable to children for, as is well known, the head of a baby is relatively enormous compared with that of an adult. As the child grows his trunk and limbs gradually enlarge relative to the size of the head so that special charts and tables varying with age are required for measuring surface areas in children.

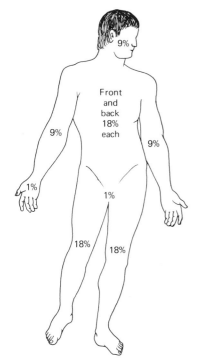

Figure 16.2. 'The rule of nine'

PATHOLOGICAL CHANGES RESULTING FROM BURNS

Local effects

The fact that the depth of a burn will vary with the intensity and duration of the causative agent is so self-evident as to require no enlargement.

It must also be obvious that the age of the patient and the thickness of the skin in the burned area is of equal importance.

It has already been noted that in superficial burns the surface epithelium and upper layers of the dermis are destroyed. The epithelium growing out from the surviving bases of hair follicles, sweat and sebaceous glands will re-establish an intact surface in approximately 2 to 3 weeks. If the burn has been treated by exposure, the dead tissues and coagulated exudate which form the crust will flake off and leave a healed and virtually unscarred area of skin. If, however, a superficial burn becomes infected, the surviving epithelial islands in the dermis may be destroyed and the burn consequently converted to one of full thickness. Since the skin appendages penetrate into the dermis for varying distances, the deeper the destruction in a superfical burn the fewer will be the surviving epithelial elements and consequently the greater the danger of the burn becoming converted to a deep one by bacterial invasion.

The situation in deep or full-thickness burns is quite different. Here the whole thickness of the skin is destroyed and converted to a layer of tough, leathery slough. In the viable tissue immediately below the slough the normal processes of repair produce a layer of granulation tissue, and eventually the slough separates leaving a characteristic pink, granulating surface. Epithelialization here can only take place by the ingrowth of epithelium from the wound edges and if the area is large it may take months. This ingrowth of epithelium gradually slows down and ceases and in certain cases the wound may not heal at all. It is in such cases that after 10 or more years malignant changes may supervene to produce a squamous cell carcinoma.

But even in a short period of weeks or months, the deeper layers of granulation tissue mature into a scar which in turn gives rise to contractures.

General effects

Shock

The first and most pressing general effect of a serious burn is that of burn shock, for it is this phenomenon which, if unrecognized or untreated, will kill the patient in a matter of hours or days after burning.

A simple concept of the mechanism of burn shock comes from an understanding of the pathological processes at work. Immediately beneath the tissues destroyed by the burn lies a layer, usually of subcutaneous tissue, in which the capillaries have been damaged but not destroyed. As a result of this damage the permeability of these capillaries increases which permits the escape or leakage from them of large quantities of protein-rich fluid containing the same amounts of electrolytes as the plasma. Some of the fluid will appear at the burn surface as exudate or blister fluid, the rest escapes into the intercellular spaces and produces oedema in the affected area.

The amount of fluid which may escape in this way is proportional to the extent of the burn and in large or moderate sized burns may be very large indeed. The first effect of this fluid loss is to produce a relative haemoconcentration and the body attempts to compensate for this by mobilizing fluid from the rest of the body and by absorption of fluid from the gut. Because the blood volume is reduced, the vascular spaces in the splanchnic bed and in the skin contract and by these methods the body attempts to compensate for the fluid loss.

In all but minor burns, however, these compensatory methods are inadequate and unless supplemented by treatment the patient passes into a state of peripheral circulatory failure because of the reduction in blood volume.

The increased capillary permeability is maximal in the early hours after burning and then there is a gradual recovery in the course of the first 36 to 48 hours. Consequently, the amount of fluid which is escaping from the circulation will follow a similar pattern and after 48 hours oedema fluid will begin to be reabsorbed into the vessels.

Red cell destruction

Obviously a number of red blood corpuscles will be destroyed in the burned tissues, but others in the deeper, surviving capillaries will be damaged. As a result of this the circulation will contain cells of increased fragility which will undergo lysis and release haemoglobin into the plasma and urine. In certain cases, for reasons which are still not understood, the red cell destruction may amount to as much as 25 per cent of the red cell mass.

This red cell destruction has two effects. First it may give rise to an anaemia which is of no importance in the average case since the cause of the shock is reduced circulating blood volume rather than a reduction in number of cells. Second and more important, however, is the effect the free haemoglobin may have upon the kidneys giving rise to **oliguria** and eventually, if unchecked, to renal failure.

Renal failure

Lysis The breakdown of cellular material into a fluid state.

Oliguria Urine output below the normal level.

Perfusion The passage of fluid through an organ or tissue.

Inadequately treated peripheral circulatory failure results in renal failure in burns in the same way as it does in shock from other causes. Adequate **perfusion** of the kidneys is vital to their normal function. As has been stated above, free haemoglobin in the plasma can further impair renal function. Reference should also be made to the unusual case of renal failure with a high urinary output. Here the kidneys secrete large volumes of dilute urine with a fixed specific gravity while the blood urea rises and the patient's condition deteriorates.

Infection

While renal failure is a feature of the shock or early phase of burn pathology, infection appears later. With greater understanding of the shock phase and its treatment, few patients fail to survive this period.

Infection remains the greatest problem in the management of burns and is responsible for most deaths.

An extensive burn is the largest wound known and offers the greatest portal for entry of bacteria. In superficial burns this is obviously an immediate problem but in full-thickness burns the leathery slough presents an effective barrier against bacteria for a limited period. Very soon, however, as it softens and moistens, it provides an ideal site for bacterial growth and becomes an enormous reservoir of bacteria which can pass across the interface between slough and underlying viable tissue.

The bacteria concerned in burn infections include all the common ones but those which require special mention are the β-haemolytic streptococci, the staphylococci, Gram-negative organisms such as *Pseudomonas aeruginosa* and, of course, *Clostridium tetani*. Apart from their local effects in the wound, where they may cause further tissue destruction and delay healing, the organisms or their toxins may be absorbed into the body and give rise to septicaemia, 'toxaemia', bacterial shock and eventually death. Infection is today the most common cause of death from burning and despite the advent of antibiotics and other potent therapeutic measures, remains a problem of the first magnitude.

Respiratory burns

Especially in patients who are burned in confined spaces such as home, caravan fires, and so on, the inhalation of smoke and fumes may cause respiratory damage. Plastic materials, which are now widely used in furnishing, are the source of extremely toxic fumes when burned in house fires. Very occasionally one sees laryngeal obstruction from oedema of the cords, but pulmonary oedema, passing on to infection, is common. Quite recently too it has been realized that the lungs may suffer damage from any large burn irrespective of the inhalation of toxic fumes, and indeed this effect has been described also after severe injuries of other types. It appears that the lungs in these cases behave as 'target organs' for as yet unrecognized toxins.

Water loss

It has been seen above that one of the functions of the skin is control of the water balance. Burned skin is incapable of performing this function and in large burns enormous quantities of water may escape through the burn and lead to dehydration. This process occurs even through the apparently dry leathery slough of a full-thickness burn and must be borne in mind when planning treatment. It continues until the wound is healed by epidermis.

Gastrointestinal effects

Acute ulcers of the stomach, duodenum and, less commonly of other parts of the intestinal tract, may occur occasionally in burns and catastrophic haemorrhage calling for urgent surgical control of the bleeding.

Other general effects

In many respects the metabolic response of the patient with an extensive burn is similar to that of the postoperative patient with the important difference that it continues for a longer period. Because of the catabolic response his nitrogen balance will become severely disturbed in addition to which he will be suffering a constant drain from the protein-rich exudates from his wounds.

Infection leads to suppression of the bone marrow and anaemia and the 'pseudodiabetes' of burns serves as a further drain on the patient's reserves.

Finally, there is the psychological trauma of the accident, the treatment, prolonged illness and the disfigurement, accentuated perhaps by magnesium deficiency, so that the patient with an extensive burn can provide the very greatest challenge for the attendants, and has rightly been described as constituting a continuing emergency.

TREATMENT

The treatment of burns may most readily be considered in three phases, each with its own objectives and problems, although there is overlapping between phases in many respects.

The shock phase

The objective here is the immediate saving of the patient's life, for it has been seen above how an untreated patient may die of burns shock in a matter of hours or days. It has also been seen that the basis of burns shock is oligaemia so that the anchor of treatment resides in the maintenance or restoration of the circulating blood volume.

The first stage in treatment of any condition is diagnosis and burns are no exception to this general rule. On admission to hospital, the diagnosis of the extent of the burn as described above and an estimate of the patient's age and weight, are the first steps, for with this knowledge one can plan his resuscitation. Burns of 10 per cent or less in children and of under 15 per cent in adults can generally be managed with oral fluids only. A careful watch must nevertheless be kept to ensure that the patient is getting – and retaining – adequate volumes of replacement fluid.

In burns of greater extent an intravenous infusion and usually also an indwelling catheter are essential, in order to monitor the urinary output which provides a valuable guide to the success of the resuscitation programme. There are numerous formulas for the amount of fluid replacement in the shock phase but the most satisfactory is the one based on the extent of the burn and the weight of the patient. It has already been seen that the fluid loss is maximal soon after burning and gradually declines over the next 36 to 48 hours. To keep pace with this loss, the largest amounts are infused in the early hours after burning, the rate being tailed off towards the end of the shock phase. The choice of fluid for replacement varies a great deal from centre to centre, but since it seems most logical to replace that which is being lost one may conclude that the best fluid is plasma. In addition, however, to the extra fluid required as replacement therapy, the patient will also need his normal daily fluid requirements. These may be given by mouth, but in patients with large burns, excessive oral fluids in the early stage may lead to vomiting so that this amount of fluid may have to be given intravenously in the form of dextrose.

However, no formula is perfect. At best it can only serve as a rough guide to treatment. Regular and frequent checking on the patient's progress is essential in order to modify treatment as and when required. The best guides are an assessment of the patient's general condition, his pulse rate and blood pressure (if the site of the burning does not preclude this latter measure) and his urinary output. Needless to say, intake and output charts are essential and careful watch is kept on the urine not only for its volume but also its specific gravity, the presence of albumin or haemoglobinuria which suggest renal damage, and also the presence of sugar.

Special tests include the measurement of the central venous pressure and of the packed cell volume which serves as a guide to the degree of haemoconcentration. In certain situations measurements of the blood gases are made to assist in the diagnosis and treatment of impaired pulmonary function and of metabolic acidosis.

Pain is not usually a major problem in deep burns during the shock phase for the nerve endings will have been destroyed in the skin. Partial-thickness burns may be extremely painful and require morphine. This is best given intravenously, in frequent, small doses.

Healing phase

Having brought the patient safely through the shock phase, one is faced with the task of healing his wounds. This treatment, of course, commences during the shock phase but resuscitative measures must take precedence at that time.

Once again the first problem is diagnosis, for treatment will differ for superficial and deep burns. Diagnosis of depth is helped by the knowledge of the history of the burns — for example flash burns and scalds are usually superficial while electrical burns and those sustained when clothing catches fire are deep. The appearance of a superficial scald and of the leathery slough of a deep burn are so different as to pose no difficulty. There are many cases, however, in which even an experienced observer cannot be certain of the depth of the burn. The 'pin-prick' test, in which sensation is tested for, is only reliable if positive, that is, if the area retains sensation, indicating that the burn is superficial.

In superficial burns all that is required is to prevent infection in order to allow spontaneous healing to proceed normally. There are two main methods of achieving this.

Exposure method

The exposure method entails exposing the burned area to the atmosphere to encourage the formation of a dry crust or eschar. Bacteria flourish in conditions of warmth, moisture and darkness and, therefore, by providing the opposite conditions, the exposure method discourages bacterial growth.

This method is most suitable for burns of the head and neck and of single surfaces of trunk or limbs. In circumferential burns the lower surfaces tend to become moist and macerated, but recent experiments with special equipment, in which the patient is kept suspended on a cushion of air, promise to overcome these difficulties.

In superficial burns the dry eschar will separate after 2 to 3 weeks leaving a healed surface.

With deep burns, on the other hand, the eschar begins to separate at 2 to 3 weeks leaving pockets of exudate and granulating wounds. At this stage the exposure method is no longer applicable and dressings are required.

Eschar The dry scab that forms on an area of skin that has been burned or the superficial layer otherwise destroyed.

Great nursing care and ingenuity are demanded with the exposure method if it is to be used properly and the patient maintained in reasonable comfort.

Closed treatment

Closed treatment implies the application of dressings from the earliest possible time. It is mandatory in certain burns as suggested above and is becoming increasingly widely used with the advent of potent antibacterial dressings such as mafenide hydrochloride or acetate (Sulfamylon). The latter is a sulphonamide which is not only effective against the common Gram-positive bacteria but also against Gram-negative organisms such as *Pseudomonas aeruginosa* which in recent years have emerged as the most difficult and lethal of the organisms occurring in burns. Another popular and excellent agent is silver sulphadiazine cream (Flamazine) which contains both sulphonamide and silver nitrate.

The principles of burn dressing are gentle cleaning of the loose slough and debris with a bland solution such as hydrogen peroxide. A non-adherent dressing is then applied with copious amounts of dressing to soak up exudate and firm, but not tight, application of crêpe bandages.

These agents must be applied every second day but it is not necessary in every case. In many cases of superficial and moderate sized burns all that is required is **tulle gras** or Carbonet, plain or impregnated with an antibiotic.

In deep burns when the slough begins to separate at 2 to 3 weeks, efforts are made to hasten the process and to achieve a clean granulating surface which will accept skin grafts. To this end the wounds are dressed with eusol and paraffin or chlorhexidine cream and, if the granulations are pale and oedematous, hypertonic saline or sodium sulphate will improve their condition. In recent years the use of heterografts, that is grafts from another species, has gained wide acceptance. The material most widely used is split-thickness pig skin which is used as a dressing material which is changed every four or five days. It both protects the wound and prepares it for acceptance of autografts.

At each change of dressing any loose slough is snipped away using scissors and dissecting forceps. Frequent swabs are taken to keep a check on the bacterial flora present in the wound so that appropriate antibiotics may be prescribed where indicated. In the absence of systemic signs and of β-haemolytic streptococci, antibiotics are not used.

The β-haemolytic streptococcus is capable of great tissue destruction and should be eliminated, and skin grafts will certainly fail if applied to a wound infected with this organism.

Skin grafting

Deep burns will require skin grafting once the granulations are satisfactory and the wound free of β-haemolytic streptococci. *Pseudomonas aeruginosa* has also an adverse effect on

Tulle gras A coarse-meshed gauze soaked with a soft paraffin preparation.

grafts but is only of importance in very gross infections with copious discharge. Medium-thickness split skin grafts are cut from any available unburned donor site using a skin graft knife or electric dermatome (*Figure 16.3*). The grafts are applied to the granulating wounds and held in place with dressings or simply exposed, depending largely upon the site to be grafted.

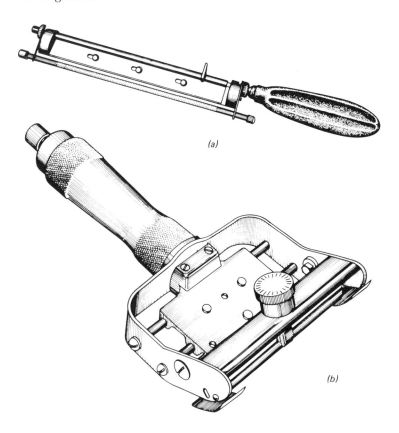

(a)

(b)

Figure 16.3. (*a*) A hand knife for skin grafting; (*b*) an electric dermatome

Extensive burns may require more than one grafting session because of lack of adequate donor sites and here repeated 'crops' of graft will have to be taken from the same sites once they have healed.

Homografts
Autografts are grafts taken from the patient. Homografts are those taken from another person and these have a limited part to play in the treatment of burns. They will, of course, only survive for 3 or 4 weeks at most before being rejected, but may be used to gain time in the extensively burned or very ill patient and to supplement autografts as a temporary measure.

Prevention of infection

The most important single factor in the general care of a patient with burns is the prevention of infection. This means not only that the most scrupulous attention should be paid to aseptic dressing techniques but that all the techniques of barrier nursing should also be applied to prevent cross infection from other patients and from attendants. This ideal can only be achieved in the most modern and sophisticated units but it should be aimed at everywhere.

Because of the rapid development of resistance and the huge reservoir of bacteria in the slough, antibiotics have not on the whole fulfilled their promise in the treatment of burns. Nevertheless, they have their place in the treatment of septicaemia and of established infections of the respiratory and urinary tracts.

Nutrition

The metabolic effects of burns have been considered above. The patients will require a diet providing in the region of 16.8 to 21.0 kJ (4000–5000 calories) per day together with adequate protein, iron, vitamins and trace elements. In the early stages the patient may be unable to take adequate amounts by mouth and will require supplements by naso-gastric tube or intravenously.

Anaemia must be avoided and where necessary blood transfusions should be carried out. It is customary to transfuse large burns in the later stages of the shock period to compensate for red cell destruction and to start the patient on the healing phase with an adequate level of haemoglobin.

Morale

Surviving a burn is a prolonged, painful and demanding process for the patient and it behoves his nurses and medical attendants to pay the greatest attention to making him as comfortable as possible, ensuring a good night's rest and offering him continuous and cheerful encouragement in boosting his morale and assuring him not only of his eventual recovery but also of his return to society as a useful and presentable member.

Treatment of special sites and types

Circumferential burns Deep circumferential burns of the limbs with underlying oedema may act like a plaster of Paris cast in impeding the circulation and should be managed in the same way, that is by splitting. This is easily achieved with a scalpel and requires no anaesthetic for the burned skin is already devoid of sensation. In the same way, circumferential burns of the chest can interfere with respiration and should be dealt with similarly.

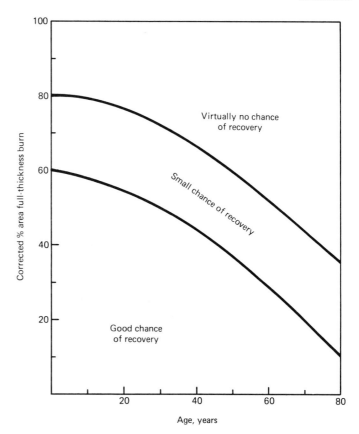

Figure 16.4. An indication of the mortality rate in relation to age of the patient and the size of burns

Eyes Burns of the eyes are uncommon but burns of the lids may result in contractures which lead to exposure, drying and ulceration of the cornea and eventual blindness. A careful watch must be kept to see that the eyes are closed during sleep and at the first sign of exposure the lid contractures are released and grafted.

Hands Burns of the hands are of special importance, for incorrect treatment can easily lead to permanent, crippling deformities. They are generally treated in plastic bags to encourage movement and maintain function. If dressed every effort is made to keep the metacarpophalangeal joints flexed to 90 degrees and the interphalangeal joints extended. Where tendons and joints are involved early surgery involving grafts or flaps is indicated.

Primary excision Primary excision means excision of the burned tissue within the first few days after burning. It is the treatment of choice for circumscribed deep burns and for isolated burns of the hands, the resultant defects being repaired by skin grafts. Primary excision and grafting of large burns have been tried in order to shorten the healing phase and to prevent infection but the magnitude of the surgery has resulted in a mortality rate which is as yet unjustifiable. On the other hand, tangential excision, that is carefully shaving off the dead tissue with a skin graft knife until viable tissue is reached and then applying either autografts or pig skin, is being increasingly used to hasten healing and reduce scarring.

Mortality

The mortality rate of burns is proportional to the age of the patient and the extent of the burn. As will be seen in *Figure 16.4* it rises very steeply with increasing age so that an old person is unlikely to survive even a 10 per cent full-thickness burn.

Reconstruction and rehabilitation phase

As indicated above, the process of rehabilitation commences during the healing phase. It is then that the physiotherapist and occupational therapist first come in contact with the patient to encourage movement, to prevent the onset of contractures by active and passive measures and to boost his morale.

Once he is healed the grafts and underlying scar continue to contract for months and the rehabilitation programme can be prolonged and taxing for all concerned.

Surgery is required for two main reasons in this period.

Release of contractures
Established mature scar contractures lead to deformities and limitation of joint movements. Their correction entails releasing the contractures, which inevitably opens up defects in skin cover which are replaced by thick free skin grafts or by flaps depending upon the particular circumstances. In the hand there may be need for release of contracted ligaments, resurfacing with flaps and/or grafting of tendons destroyed in the burn.

Cosmetic improvement
Burn scars and grafts tend to become hypertrophic, contracted and extremely disfiguring. Once they have matured, a process which may take anything up to 18 months, there

may be a place for cosmetic improvement by replacement with thicker grafts or flaps. On the whole, the results are less than satisfactory and patients should not be led to believe that they can be returned to their original appearance.

REFERENCES

Jackson, I. T. and Macallan, E. S. (1971). *Plastic Surgery and Burns Treatment.* London: William Heinemann

Laing, J. E. and Harvey, J. (1967). *The Management and Nursing of Burns.* London: English Universities Press Ltd

McGregor, I. A. and Reid, W. H. (1966). *Plastic Surgery for Nurses.* Edinburgh and London: Livingstone

Muir, I. F. K. and Barclay, T. L. (1974). *Burns and their Treatment.* London: Lloyd-Luke

17

Surgery of the skin

D. O. Maisels

Having acquired some knowledge of the structure and function of the skin in Chapter 16, one is in a position to consider a number of the more common lesions which may affect it. Bearing in mind its complexity, it is not surprising to find that there is a very great variety of conditions which may arise in the skin and these may be most conveniently discussed under several broad headings.

CONGENITAL CONDITIONS

Congenital defects of skin

Congenital defect of skin, sometimes referred to as congenital absence of skin, is probably commoner than might be supposed from the number of recorded cases. It is usually seen in the scalp where the underlying bone is occasionally also deficient or absent. The lesion presents as an ulcer observed at birth and usually heals in a few weeks leaving a bald patch. The treatment consists of simple excision of the patch for cosmetic reasons.

Haemangioma

Haemangioma is perhaps the commonest of all congenital lesions and presents in three forms, differing from each other in appearance, natural history and treatment.

Strawberry naevus

As the name implies, strawberry naevus is reddish in colour, raised and nodular. It is first noticed within a few days of birth sometimes being preceded by a pale area in the skin. The lesion may grow very quickly during the early months but by about 6 months of age usually ceases to grow out of proportion with the baby. During the next year or so, pale areas develop in the naevus as the vessels which comprise it thrombose and by 3 to 4 years of age, over 90 per cent have disappeared spontaneously leaving no mark or only very fine scarring. Not surprisingly the parents of these children are alarmed by the appearance of the lesion and press for its removal. In most cases surgery is not indicated and should only be considered if the lesion continues to grow, fails to resolve by the age of 4 or 5 years or is interfering with function, as for example in the case of a large naevus on an eyelid which is obscuring the patient's vision.

These lesions occasionally ulcerate and this usually serves to hasten their resolution. Very exceptionally an extensive, ulcerating or bleeding naevus will demand surgical excision.

Cavernous haemangioma

Cavernous haemangioma differs from the strawberry naevus in being more deeply situated and therefore having a darker, bluish colour. It consists of large vascular spaces often with palpable feeding vessels and frequently fails to resolve spontaneously. Most of these lesions are only of moderate size and are well defined and may be treated by repeated diathermy coagulation or by excision. Occasionally, however, they are large, extensive and infiltrating and may involve the underlying muscles and bone. These can present very serious difficulties in treatment and should be investigated by angiography prior to surgery.

Port-wine stains

Port-wine stains are the common and familiar 'birth-marks'. They consist of fine capillary vessels in the dermis and do not resolve spontaneously. If small, they can be excised for cosmetic reasons but to exchange a port-wine stain for a skin graft is simply to exchange one blemish for another. Some surgeons have treated these lesions by tattooing them with pale pigments but this is not a very satisfactory method of treatment and has no real advantages over skilful cosmetic camouflage.

A port-wine stain in the distribution of the trigeminal nerve is sometimes associated with intracranial vascular abnormalities leading to mental deficiency, fits and other features. This constitutes the Sturge—Weber syndrome.

Lymphangioma

Lymphangioma is very similar to the cavernous haemangioma, consisting of large pools of lymph and dilated vessels. The affected area is swollen and oedematous but of normal colour. The lesion may infiltrate the muscles and interfere with function so that if, for example, the face is affected, in addition to the swelling, the patient will show the features of a facial palsy. This is a difficult condition to treat and all that can be hoped for is to reduce the magnitude of the deformity by extensive excisions of skin and subcutaneous tissues and the application of the principles of treatment of facial palsy.

Not infrequently one finds a mixed picture, both haemangioma and lymphangioma occurring together, perhaps compounded by a degree of neurofibromatosis. It is in these cases that one may see gigantism, that is, overgrowth of a whole limb or half a face together with the underlying bone, and satisfactory treatment becomes virtually impossible.

Neurofibromatosis (Von Recklinghausen's disease)

Neurofibromatosis is characterized by café-au-lait areas in the skin and subcutaneous tissues together with a number of other features. The neurofibromata present as discrete nodules and occasionally as large pedunculated masses which hang down from the skin of the face, scalp and so on. Lesions which are unsightly and the occasionally tender nodule may be excised. Sarcomatous degeneration can take place in the fibromata but, contrary to previously held views, there is no evidence that partial excision of these lesions will precipitate malignant degeneration.

Pigmented naevus

Pigmented naevi are the common pigmented birth-marks which may vary in size from that of a freckle to the giant pigmented naevus which may involve one-half or more of the body surface. There are three main types of pigmented naevi which are often only distinguishable from each other on histological examination, but since their natural history differs, some brief remarks are apposite.

Junctional naevus
Junctional naevus varies in size from a few millimetres to several centimetres, can be light or dark brown to black and is usually smooth, flat and hairless. Histologically the naevus cells are situated in the basal layer of the epidermis at the junction between epidermis and dermis. It may evolve into a compound naevus, an intradermal naevus or a malignant melanoma.

Although this lesion usually develops in the first few years of life it may appear at any age.

Compound naevus
Compound naevus is usually larger than the junctional naevus and may be very large. It tends to be dark brown or black, raised and nodular and is often hairy.

Histologically the naevus cells are both in the junctional zone and in the dermis. The compound naevus develops from a junctional naevus and commonly goes on to become an intradermal naevus, though it may develop into a malignant melanoma. Although this is the common naevus of children, it can occur at any age.

Intradermal naevus

Intradermal naevus is the common mole on adults but may be of varying size. It is often raised, dark and hairy. Histologically the naevus cells are in the dermis with very little or no junctional element. The intradermal naevus develops from the compound and only very rarely becomes malignant.

Treatment

It will be obvious from what has been said above that it is the junctional component of pigmented naevi which is potentially malignant. The junctional element is in a sense the immature form and is common in children before puberty when it is entirely benign. As the child matures the naevus seems to do the same so that in adults most naevi are of the mature intradermal type. If, however, they retain their junctional form, they are potentially malignant especially if traumatized.

Knowing this, one can formulate guidelines for treatment. Any pigmented naevus which undergoes rapid change in size, configuration or colour or which bleeds or ulcerates should be removed completely and examined histologically. There is no place for incisional biopsy, that is, the removal of part of the lesion, nor should it be cauterized, curetted or subjected to any other form of trauma which might stimulate malignant change in a junctional element. By the same token, any pigmented lesion subject to repeated trauma such as on the sole of the foot or where it can be rubbed by a belt or brassière strap should be removed.

Some naevi will require removal for cosmetic reasons. In adults these should be completely excised and the defect repaired by direct suture, a skin graft or flap, depending upon the size and local situation. In children before puberty there is a place for serial excision. This means removal of part of the lesion and suture of the wound. After about 9 months or a year the adjacent skin will be stretched or relaxed so that all or a further portion of the lesion can be excised and the wound sutured. It is quite safe to cut into a naevus in this way before puberty without fear of precipitating malignant change, but it should never be done in an older patient and, therefore, serial excision should be completed before puberty.

Adenoma sebaceum

Fibroadenoma(ta) Tumour of mixed fibrous and glandular structures.

Adenoma sebaceum is composed of **fibroadenomata** of the sebaceous glands in a typical 'butterfly' distribution over the nose and cheeks. This condition associated with lesions of the viscera, eye, bone and brain may give rise to fits and mental deficiency and the whole picture is known as tuberous sclerosis which is inherited as a dominant trait.

The skin lesions may be reduced by shaving them down with a knife or rotating abrasive cylinder for cosmetic reasons only.

Cutis hyperelastica

Cutis hyperelastica (Ehlers—Danlos syndrome), an inherited anomaly, is characterized by overproduction of elastic tissue and in the skin presents as the 'rubber-man'. Wounds heal very poorly leaving tissue paper scars.

Dermoid cysts

Dermoid cysts are small cystic lesions commonly occurring around the orbit and are closely applied to the bone. They are removed by simple excision.

Those occurring in the midline of the nose may have deep connections through the nasal bones and septum with the dura of the anterior fossa and should be excised with caution and care to ensure total removal or they will recur. Very occasionally the deep connection will demand an intracranial approach for its removal.

TUMOURS OF SKIN

Benign tumours

Squamous papilloma
Squamous papilloma is a simple tumour growing from the epidermis and projecting above the surface. It consists of a connective tissue core and is covered by fairly normal epidermis with a thickening of the stratum corneum which gives it a rough surface. A keratin horn is a simple squamous papilloma with an unusual amount of keratin on its surface which gives it the appearance of a horn. Occasionally there are early malignant changes present in the base of a keratin horn.

Treatment of these lesions is by excision and since they are usually small the wound can be closed by direct suture.

Seborrhoeic keratosis (senile wart)
In seborrhoeic keratosis pigmented slightly raised greasy lesions arise from the basal cells of the epidermis. They are common on the trunk, face and neck of older people, pieces

tending to flake off with minor trauma and cause slight bleeding. They are benign lesions but if troublesome can be readily shaved flat or curetted.

Keratoacanthoma (Molluscum sebaceum)

Keratoacanthoma, a lesion which may be multiple, has the features of a very rapidly growing carcinoma reaching a size of 1 to 2 cm in a few weeks. The typical lesion has a keratin plug in its centre which drops out and the lesion undergoes spontaneous regression over a period of several months, leaving a white pitted scar. It is a benign condition but because of the uncertainty of the diagnosis most authorities agree that it should be excised and submitted to histological examination to establish the diagnosis.

Sebaceous cyst (wen)

A sebaceous cyst is not really a tumour but may be considered in this section. It is a retention cyst due to the obstruction to the outflow from a sebaceous gland. Thus it always has an attachment to the skin surface at the punctum or opening. The cyst wall is smooth and contains sebum and not infrequently these cysts become infected and may discharge pus. Very occasionally this results in fibrosis and spontaneous resolution but usually repeated episodes of inflammation will follow.

Simple sebaceous cysts can be shelled out through a small incision. If they have been inflamed, the fibrosis may make them more adherent to surrounding tissues so that they have to be excised rather than simply shelled out.

Rhinophyma

Rhinophyma is a curious condition due to hypertrophy of the skin and sebaceous glands of the nose and adjacent cheeks. The nose becomes red with large, irregular lumps especially on the tip. It is commonly, and erroneously, associated with alcoholism with consequent distress to the unfortunate owner who seeks cosmetic surgical relief. This is obtained by shaving down the nose to more normal contours, the surface becoming re-epithelialized in about 10 days from the cut stumps of the numerous sebaceous glands.

Inclusion dermoids

Inclusion dermoids too are not true tumours. They result from a fragment of epidermis being driven below the surface, for example, by a prick from a sewing needle. The fragment survives, continues to grow and eventually forms a cyst which can be easily excised.

R

Hypertrophic and keloid scars

In a sense hypertrophic and keloid scars are benign tumours of the connective tissue of the skin. The hypertrophic scar is red, raised and itchy. Usually it gradually settles over the course of 12 to 18 months, becoming pale and flat. Surgical interference such as attempts at excision will usually result in recurrence of the hypertrophic scarring, often worse than the original. Certain individuals such as those with a very fair complexion have a tendency to produce this type of scar as do people of the pigmented races. Resolution may be hastened and recurrence following surgical revision prevented by small doses of x-rays. In recent years the use of intralesional steroids has been preferred to x-rays and gives equally satisfactory results. Continuous pressure for many months by specially made garments of elastic material contribute to the resolution of hypertrophic scars and are increasingly being used.

The true keloid merges with hypertrophic scarring and is probably best defined as hypertrophic scarring which fails to resolve after a couple of years and which may even go on enlarging. It is most common in pigmented people and can result from the most trivial scratch. Treatment of true keloid on the lines outlined above is still somewhat unsatisfactory.

Lipoma

Lipoma is a benign neoplasm of the subcutaneous tissues consisting of encapsulated mature fat. It is quite simply shelled out of the surrounding fat.

Premalignant lesions

Senile keratoses

Senile keratoses which occur most often on the face, neck and backs of the hands are sometimes referred to as solar keratoses. They are not uncommon in elderly patients and fair complexioned individuals who have spent years in sunny climates or exposed to the weather. They are scaly, red or pigmented and slowly progressive. Their importance lies in their potential for malignant change to a squamous cell carcinoma. Histologically they are characterized by changes in the epithelium with some dermal inflammatory infiltration. Isolated lesions can be excised but if they are multiple and extensive, being superficial, they are readily treated by shaving or planing off the epithelium and superficial layers of dermis.

In recent years they have been very successfully treated by the application of 5-Fluorouracil cream (5-FU) which is a chemotherapeutic agent which has a specific effect on abnormal cells.

Radionecrosis

Irradiation, either therapeutic or accidental, can give rise to skin changes which result in squamous carcinoma many years after exposure. The early changes of pigmentation and **telangiectasis** may after a number of years give way to scaling and ulceration which in time progresses to frank malignancy. Areas of radionecrosis are difficult to treat for the tissues tend to heal very poorly and skin grafts do not take well on a heavily irradiated bed. Consequently, following excision of a radionecrotic ulcer it is usually necessary to repair the defect with a flap which carries its own blood supply thus ensuring its viability.

Chronic ulceration

Reference has already been made above to the possible development of a squamous cell carcinoma in a burn which is allowed to remain unhealed for many years. Other chronic ulcers such as those associated with a discharging sinus from a chronic osteomyelitis are also potential sites of malignant change.

Bowen's disease and erythroplasia of Queyrat

The typical lesion of Bowen's disease is a pink, scaly patch which slowly increases in size. This condition is a carcinoma *in situ*, there being malignant changes in the cells of the epidermis superficial to the basement layer. It is premalignant in that if not excised, the malignant cells will break through the basement layer and the lesion then becomes an invasive squamous cell carcinoma.

Erythroplasia of Queyrat is an entirely similar lesion which occurs on the glans penis.

Lentigo maligna

Lentigo maligna, also known as Hutchinson's melanotic freckle, is a pigmented macule or a flat patch usually occurring on the face of middle-aged people, and usually slow growing. It consists of a proliferation of abnormal melanocytes or pigment cells at the junctional zone. A significant number of these lesions develop into frank malignant melanoma and they should therefore be excised.

Malignant non-metastasizing lesions

Non-metastasizing lesions are lesions which are malignant in the sense that they are locally invasive and destructive but they do not, except in the very rarest circumstances, metastasize to distant parts either by blood or lymphatic vessels.

Telangiectasis Small collections of dilated capillary blood vessels in the skin.

Basal cell carcinoma (Rodent ulcer)

Basal cell carcinoma is a common tumour which occurs most usually in middle age or later on the face. There are, however, many exceptions in that they are seen in other sites and younger patients. Broadly speaking there are three types of basal cell carcinoma. The cystic type is a rounded, pearly lesion with tiny blood vessels coursing over its surface. The ulcerating type characteristically has a central ulcer covered with a scab or crust which tends to come off and slight bleeding occurs. The edge of the ulcer is slightly raised or rolled. The third type is the least common. It is the 'grass-fire' type in which, as the advancing edge progresses, a thin covering of epithelium heals in behind it leaving a smooth, shining surface.

This tumour arises from the basal cells of the epidermis and, in addition to being capable of great skin destruction, it can invade the deeper structure and involve muscle, cartilage and bone.

These tumours respond to irradiation but surgery offers many advantages. Thus the excised specimen can be examined histologically in several planes to determine the adequacy of excision both in extent and in depth. Radiotherapy of the ears and eyelids may damage the underlying cartilage and radionecrosis developing many years after therapy can even progress to a squamous carcinoma. Finally, the cosmetic results of excision by a surgeon trained in plastic and reconstructive surgery are superior to those following radiotherapy.

5-Fluorouracil cream has recently found a place in the treatment of certain basal cell carcinomata in selected patients.

Dermatofibrosarcoma protruberans

Dermatofibrosarcoma protruberans is a rather unusual tumour which is mentioned only as being an example of a locally malignant connective tissue tumour. It arises in the dermis and enlarges by local invasion. Like the basal cell carcinoma it does not recur if completely excised.

Malignant metastasizing lesions

Squamous cell carcinoma

Squamous cell carcinoma is a malignant tumour which develops from the cells of the epidermis. It can arise in normal skin and frequently occurs in skin which has been damaged or altered in some way. Thus it can develop from a senile keratosis or an area of Bowen's disease, radionecrosis or chronic ulceration as seen above. Chemical irritation by arsenic, tars and soot can also be a predisposing cause.

These tumours can be exophytic, i.e. heaped up and nodular or ulcerating with a raised edge. They tend to metastasize to the regional lymph nodes and usually only later in their course to distant sites via the bloodstream.

Most, though not all, squamous cell carcinomata, respond to radiotherapy though, as for basal cell carcinomata, surgery offers many advantages. Excision of a squamous cell carcinoma needs to be somewhat more radical than that of a basal cell carcinoma, the line of excision being at least 2 cm beyond the margins of the tumour and well clear in depth. When the regional lymph nodes are involved they are removed by radical block dissection.

Malignant melanoma

Malignant melanoma is the malignant tumour arising from the pigment cells of the skin. It has already been seen how it can develop from a pre-existing junctional or compound naevus or from Hutchinson's melanotic freckle. It can also arise *de novo* and is extremely rare before puberty.

A history of any recent change in the size, colour or other feature of a pigmented lesion should be accepted as being significant and indicating at the very least early excisional biopsy.

The lesion is very variable in size and may be any colour from pink (the **amelanotic** type) to black. It may have a marginal slightly pigmented halo and be surrounded by a ring of small, dark satellites. The surface is usually raised and may be roughened, scaly or ulcerated.

Malignant melanoma is a strange and interesting tumour with many paradoxes. Thus, while it seems to be commoner in sunny climates such as Australia, the increased incidence of the tumour there is not confined to those parts of the body which are normally exposed to the sun. It behaves in an unpredictable fashion, and some of this behaviour may be due to the accumulating evidence of an immunological component of the disease.

Malignant melanoma metastasizes via the lymphatics and via the bloodstream. The sheet anchor of treatment is surgery for it is a very radioresistant tumour. Excision must be very wide, the margin on limbs and trunk being at least 5 to 7 cm clear of the tumour so that the resultant defect will require a skin graft for its repair. Most authorities are now agreed that radical lymph node dissection should be reserved for those cases in whom there is evidence of node involvement. Unless the node dissection can be carried out in continuity with the excision of the primary, it is best deferred for 3 weeks in order to allow any malignant cells which are in the lymphatics between the primary and the nodes to reach the

Amelanotic Without black pigment.

latter before excising them. Failure to allow this interval to elapse can result in secondary seedlings appearing in the intervening tissues.

Surgery has no place in the treatment of multiple, distant metastases which may be palliated by chemotherapy. Vaccination of superficial metastases with smallpox vaccine causes them to regress and can alleviate the patient's distress.

INFLAMMATORY LESIONS

Erysipelas

Erysipelas is an acute streptococcal infection of the skin which gains entry via a surgical incision, a trivial wound or the lesions of eczema and so on. On the face it has a typical 'butterfly' distribution across nose and cheeks. The affected area is red, hot and tender with a slightly raised edge which advances in an irregular manner. The regional lymph nodes are enlarged and the patient may become febrile and ill. Because of the nature of the causative organism the patient should be isolated and the local lesion treated with penicillin or other antibiotics to which it responds very well.

Cellulitis

Cellulitis is an acute spreading inflammation of the subcutaneous tissues which is generally caused by a haemolytic streptococcus or a staphylococcus. The affected part becomes red, swollen and tense and there may be **lymphangitis** and **lymphadenitis**. Pus is scanty but if untreated the condition can proceed to extensive sloughing of skin and subcutaneous tissues. Once again the patient is toxic and febrile and if untreated can develop **pyaemic** abscesses and septicaemia.

Furuncles

Furuncles (boils) are familiar lesions due to acute infection in a hair follicle. They will respond to antibiotics but once pus has formed they are in essence an abscess and drainage should be established by incision.

Progressive synergistic gangrene (Meleney's gangrene)

Progressive synergistic gangrene is an unusual condition usually following an operation for a deep infection such as drainage of an appendix abscess though it can develop from an apparently trivial skin lesion. It starts about a week after operation and is characterized by very extensive progressive

Lymphangitis Red streaks running up a limb and representing inflammation in lymphatic vessels.

Lymphadenitis Inflammation of the lymph nodes.

Pyaemia The presence of pus-producing bacteria in the blood leading to multiple abscesses.

necrosis of skin and subcutaneous tissues. The lesion is extremely painful and the patient becomes debilitated and emaciated. The bacteriological basis of this condition lies in the synergistic action of an anaerobic or **micro-aerophilic** non-haemolytic staphylococcus and an aerobic haemolytic staphylococcus. Antibiotics alone are ineffective in treatment as is packing with zinc peroxide paste. Wide surgical excision is the only effective treatment and healing can be accelerated by split skin grafting of the granulating wound.

Pilonidal sinus

The usual pilonidal sinus is found in the natal cleft between the buttocks and consists of ramifying epithelial-lined tracts. These tracts are found to contain hairs and frequent recurrent abscesses are the presenting feature of this condition. There are several theories about the origin of pilonidal sinuses, many believing they are due to hairs being driven into the natal cleft by the constant rubbing together of the buttocks aided by the fact that the microscopic scales on hairs point towards the free end of the hair. This configuration is similar to that on an ear of barley corn which can work its way up the inside of a jacket sleeve and lends support to the theory. Further evidence lies in the fact that barbers can develop pilonidal sinuses in the webs between their fingers caused by the hairs from their customer's heads. Treatment is a much vexed problem. Some authorities recommend simple drainage of the abscesses and keeping the natal cleft shaved to prevent recurrence but once there are fully developed ramifying tracts and chronic inflammatory tissue in the region this simple approach is unlikely to succeed. The best therapy then is wide excision of the area and, once the wound is clean and granulating, healing can be hastened by skin grafting.

Mention should be made of the congenital pilonidal dimple which is seen in this region. Some claim this is the origin of pilonidal sinuses and it may well be that this is true for certain cases.

Suppurative hidradenitis

There are two types of sweat glands, the first being the exocrine glands which are widely distributed over the body and secrete a thin, clear fluid. The second type, the apocrine glands, have a sexual connotation and are found in the axillae, breasts, groins and perineal regions. These secrete a thick fluid with characteristic odour. Suppurative hidradenitis is an acute or chronic infection of the apocrine glands and presents as multiple recurrent abscesses in the regions where

Micro-aerophilic Organisms which grow in an atmosphere of reduced oxygen.

the apocrine glands are situated, the axillae being the most commonly affected.

The only satisfactory treatment for this condition is wide surgical excision and repair by direct suture, skin grafts or flaps, depending upon the local circumstances.

SKIN REPLACEMENT

Any skin defect too large to close by direct suture will require repair by transplantation of skin from another area by one of two techniques. The first is free grafting in which the transplanted tissue is completely severed from its blood supply during transfer and the second is the use of flaps which retain their blood supply during transfer.

Free grafts

Free grafts consist of two types, the split skin or Thiersch graft and the whole skin or Wolfe graft which consists of the full thickness of skin but no underlying fat.

The thinner the graft the greater is the likelihood of it picking up a blood supply and 'taking' in its new situation. Thus this is the method of choice in burns and granulating wounds where conditions are not ideal. On the other hand, the thicker the graft, the better its wearing qualities and match for colour and texture so that in freshly excised wounds this would be the graft of choice for the palms of the hands, face and so on. Other factors to be considered in the choice of a free graft are that they tend to contract in inverse proportion to their thickness and that while split skin donor areas heal themselves, the size of a full-thickness graft may be limited because the donor area will itself have to be repaired.

The final decision on whether or not to use a free graft may also depend on the recipient bed. Bare cortical bone, tendons devoid of paratenon and heavily irradiated tissues will not support a free graft and in these situations a flap will be required.

The taking and application of split skin grafts have been mentioned in the chapter on burns. A full-thickness graft is usually cut to a pattern of the defect, care being taken to remove all the fat from its deep surface lest this interferes with its 'take'. In freshly excised wounds haemostasis is of the utmost importance in free grafting, for the interposition of any blood clot between the graft and its bed will prevent the development of vascular links between them which are vital to the survival and 'take' of the graft. Thus, in these

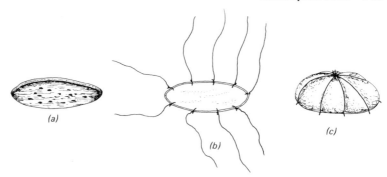

Figure 17.1. Free skin grafting. (*a*) The defect; (*b*) graft sutured in place with sutures left long; (*c*) sutures tied over a bolus of wool

situations, it is customary to suture the graft to the wound edges leaving the sutures long so that they may be tied over a bolus of wool or sponge to ensure haemostasis and prevent any shearing strains which could rupture the delicate new vascular connections (*see Figure 17.1*).

Flaps

Not only do flaps retain a blood supply during transfer, thus being essential for repairing avascular defects, but also they are thicker than free grafts since they include a layer of subcutaneous tissue. This added substance is useful in the repair of contour defects, for example, on the face and for extra durability such as the sole of the foot or heel in certain cases. Moreover, if tendons and joints are to function properly beneath a skin repair, a layer of fat is essential. There are two main types of flaps which require consideration.

Local flaps

Local flaps are those where skin is moved to an adjacent area and these have the advantage of being quicker and providing tissue of good match for colour and texture. The best examples are the rotation flaps (*see Figure 17.2*) which normally leave no secondary defect and the transposition flap in which the secondary defect may be sutured (*Figure 17.3*) or repaired with a split skin graft (*Figure 17.4*).

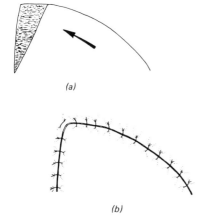

Figure 17.2. A rotation flap. (*a*) The triangulated defect and flap outlined; (*b*) flap rotated and sutured in place

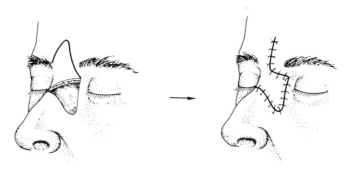

Figure 17.3. The glabellar flap. A transposed flap with direct suture of secondary defect

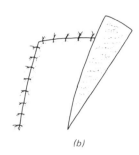

Figure 17.4. Transposed flap with secondary defect. (*a*) Defect and flap outlined; (*b*) flap transposed, skin graft on secondary defect

(a)   (b)

Distant flaps

Distant flaps are also of two main varieties, the direct and migrated flap, but they require a minimum of two stages for their transfer and therefore are more time-consuming. The cross-leg flap (*Figure 17.5*) is a good example of a direct flap. At the first stage the flap is raised and sewn into the defect. After about 3 weeks the flap will have developed adequate vascular connections in its new position to allow of severence of its base at the second stage.

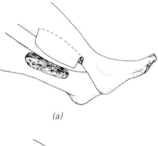

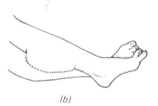

(a)   (b)

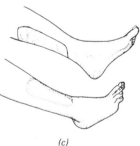

Figure 17.5. Cross-leg flap — an example of a direct flap. (*a*) Defect on right leg, flap on left one; (*b*) flap sutured into defect; (*c*) base divided and flap inset. Graft on flap donor area

(c)

The best example of a migrated flap is an abdominal tube pedicle. In this a strap flap is raised on the abdomen at the first stage and sutured to form a tube. At the second stage about 3 weeks later one end of the tube is divided and sutured to the wrist. After a further 3 weeks there will be an adequate circulation entering the tube from the wrist end to allow the other end to be detached from the abdomen. The flap can then be sewn into its intended destination, for example the face or leg, and after a further 3 weeks the wrist attachment can be separated at the fourth stage (*Figure 17.6*). It is clear that this is a protracted and complex programme calling for patience, fortitude and a modicum of acrobatic versatility on the part of the patient, and careful

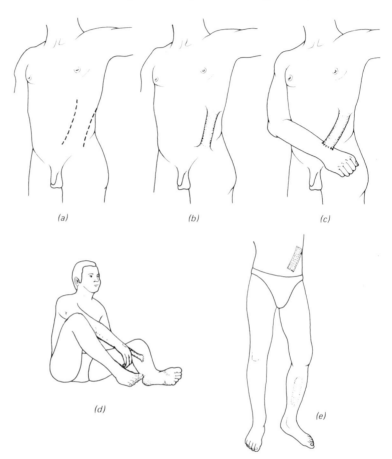

Figure 17.6. Abdominal tube pedicle to leg. A flap migrated via the wrist. (*a*) and (*b*) Strap flap outlined on abdomen, raised and tubed; (*c*) one end inset on wrist; (*d*) other end divided and inset on leg; (*e*) flap on leg, graft on donor area on abdomen. Sometimes this can be closed by direct suture

planning and sympathy from his surgeon. Where the base of the flap contains no large vessels it is known as a random flap and its length to breadth ratio will be limited. An axial flap is one which contains large feeding vessels such as the superficial temporals which supply a forehead flap. Axial flaps can consequently be designed much longer and narrower than random flaps and the base can be reduced to contain only the feeding vessels, i.e. an island flap. In recent years, with the advent of microsurgical techniques it has become possible to divide the feeding vessels of such an island flap and transfer it to another part of the body as a free flap. The possible advantages of this manoeuvre are of course obvious and enormous.

18

Diseases of the breast

Roger Brearley

The breast (*mamma* in Latin) develops as a group of glandular downgrowths of the dermis similar to sweat glands. The ducts radiate from a central cluster into the surrounding subcutaneous fat in which they are supported by a network of fibrous partitions. Breast formation may occur anywhere along a line running from groin to axilla (mammary line or milk line) and different species show different arrangements of number and position, two pectoral breasts being normal in man. Rudimentary breasts are present at birth in both sexes, but further development at puberty normally occurs only in the female.

BENIGN LESIONS

Congenital and developmental abnormalities

The following are congenital and developmental abnormalities of one or both breasts.

(1) Aplasia or absence.
(2) Hypoplasia or underdevelopment.
Both may be associated with a wider defect including lack of pectoral muscles and malformed ribs.
(3) Supernumerary (extra) breasts or nipples situated anywhere along the milk line – in the female they may develop at puberty and later lactate.
(4) In hyperplasia or hypertrophy (both terms are used) pubertal enlargement is accompanied by great deposition of fat causing the breasts to grow to gigantic dimensions.
(5) Primary retracted (or inverted) nipple, which becomes evident at puberty is due to shortness of the main ducts and their associated connective tissue in the nipple. Mild cases may be corrected by repeatedly pulling the nipple out. It is often bilateral, is a bar to breast-feeding and predisposes to abscess formation, but it has no serious significance. Retraction of a previously normal nipple, on the other hand, is commonly a sign of breast cancer.

Injuries of the breast

Because of its mobility and soft texture the breast commonly escapes injury, though bruising and haematoma sometimes occur. A severe localized blow may disrupt an area of fat, leading to death of cells and **extravasation** of fat globules outside the cells. This excites a foreign body reaction which is manifested as a tender, tense area followed later by fibrosis and sometimes calcification, giving rise to a small, hard and rather fixed lump resembling an early cancer. Injection of mineral oils (paraffin) or silicone oil to produce cosmetic enlargement of the breasts is reported from time to time. It is a highly dangerous practice and leads to the formation of lumpy granulomatous masses, sometimes complicated by chronic sinuses.

Infections of the breast

Acute infection with staphylococci is quite common. All other forms of infection are extremely rare, though tuberculosis, actinomycosis and syphilis can occur.

Acute staphylococcal infection can affect both sexes and all ages, but it is commonest during the early stages of lactation. At first a sector of the breast becomes swollen, hot and tender with throbbing pain. The patient is pyrexial and may experience a **rigor**. There is evidence that at this stage, in many cases, bacterial infection has not occurred and the lesion is simply engorgement of the affected area with milk, due to duct blockage or inefficient sucking by the baby. This leads to rupture of ducts and extravasation of milk which excites an intense, sterile, inflammatory reaction. Bacteria entering through the obstructed milk ducts or through cracks in the nipple gain access to the inflamed area and convert it to a septic inflammation. Ultimately tissue breakdown and pus formation occur, constituting an abscess which may burrow extensively in the fibrofatty compartments of the breast before pointing on the surface.

Management

Factors which help to prevent the condition include prenatal care of the nipples to ensure a satisfactory shape and freedom from cracks or retraction, a healthy baby able to suck effectively, and the avoidance of any practice likely to introduce staphylococci into the baby's mouth such as wiping it out with gauze swabs. Carriers of staphylococci should also be eliminated from the lying-in ward. In the early stage of

Extravasation Fluid escaping from its containing vessel (e.g. blood) or cavity (e.g. urine).

Rigor An extreme shivering fit.

congestion, reduction of the milk flow by diuretics, combined with efforts to drain the congested area by expression of the milk either manually or with an electric breast pump may avert the condition. If early bacterial invasion is present, an antibiotic effective against all strains of staphylococci should be prescribed. The presence of pus is indicated by exquisite local tenderness, brawny **induration** and loss of sleep through throbbing pain. Antibiotics are no longer sufficient, and given alone are positively harmful. The requirements now are to evacuate the pus and afford free drainage to all pus-containing cavities by breaking down fibrous **septa** between the loculi and to remove any sloughs which have formed. Antibiotics do not do any of these things, but convert sloughs and abscesses into sterile on nearly sterile foreign bodies. A chronic inflammatory granuloma results (antibiotic granuloma), forming an indurated fixed mass with oedematous, thickened overlying skin and enlarged axillary lymph nodes. Such a condition is extremely difficult to distinguish from an advanced infiltrative type of inflammatory cancer. It takes months to resolve, and may at any time break down, pointing and discharging pus for a while through one or more sinuses. Adequate drainage once pus has formed averts these troubles and antibiotics given after drainage hasten recovery. At the same time it is necessary to abandon breast-feeding and suppress lactation by administration of a powerful oestrogen in sufficient dose. Quinestrol (Estrovis) 4 mg (1 tablet) followed by a second tablet 48 hours later is probably the simplest if not the cheapest of many possible routines. If lactation has been truly suppressed, an effective antibiotic prescribed and pus properly evacuated, frequent dressings are not required and the breast should be left undisturbed for several days.

Mammillary fistula

Mammillary fistula is a condition in which small abscesses recur quite apart from lactation at one spot on the edge of the areola. It is due to blockage of a main duct in the nipple by epithelial debris, resulting from the presence of an abnormal duct lining composed of squamous epithelium. Often the nipple is also inverted. It may be treated by laying the affected duct open (as an anal fistula is treated), by excising the affected duct, or by excising all the main ducts entering the nipple.

Plasma cell mastitis is a great rarity. It is really a foreign body reaction due to extravasation of duct contents in a non-lactating breast. It leads to a fibrous lump and like traumatic fat necrosis, mimics carcinoma.

Induration The hardening of a tissue or organ due to disease.

Septa Thin partitions within or between anatomical structures.

Dysplasias of the breast (Mammary dysplasia)

The great increase in size and complexity of the female breast which occurs at puberty is followed at monthly intervals throughout reproductive life by alternate phases of proliferation and regression of the glandular tissue which accompany the menstrual cycles. In addition, pregnancy and lactation may lead to further growth of ducts and secretory **acini**, followed ultimately by return to the resting state. Proliferation of the gland is called hyperplasia, the opposite is involution and both are under hormonal control. When these changes proceed in an abnormal or disordered fashion the condition is spoken of as dysplasia. Common microscopic features of dysplasia include fibrosis, proliferation of ducts or duct linings and cyst formation. Changes may be widespread throughout the breasts or patchy, giving rise to lumps, and various aspects of dysplasia may predominate. The resulting conditions used to be grouped under the name 'chronic mastitis', but the term is thoroughly misleading and has now been largely abandoned. The following clinical forms are commonly encountered.

Fibroadenosis

In fibroadenosis the three microscopic features mentioned above are all in evidence and the breasts are nodular and painful, especially premenstrually. Rubbery enlargement of the axillary glands may also be found. It is a disease of young **nulliparous** women and seldom persists beyond two pregnancies and lactations.

Pill nodularity

Young women taking an oral contraceptive may develop diffuse nodularity which disappears when the pill is stopped. The incidence of true fibroadenosis may be reduced, however. The long-term effects of oral contraceptives on established benign breast disease are not known but histologically the epithelium shows great cellular activity.

Painful breasts (Mastalgia)

Mild premenstrual discomfort in the breasts is very common. At times, both duration and intensity may be much greater than this and occasionally pain and tenderness are of crippling severity.

Examination usually reveals some nodularity but it is not invariable. If the pain is cyclical fibroadenosis is often present; more continuous pain may accompany duct ectasia (*see below*). However, both conditions may be painless and the cause of mastalgia is unknown though its disappearance after the menopause suggests a hormonal mechanism.

Acinus The basic unit of any glandular structure. It consists of secreting cells gathered round a small central tubule, which ultimately drains into a large collecting duct.

Nulliparous Never having given birth.

There is no certain remedy and initial success may be followed by relapse. Measures recommended include a well-fitting brassière; a diuretic in the premenstrual phase; androgens (also cause hirsutes and voice changes); progesterone; contraceptive pills; bromocriptine (may cause nausea and increased fertility); danazol (causes amenorrhoea and infertility).

Drugs which cause profound disturbances of the endocrine system need to be used with caution in the management of a benign condition.

Cystic disease

Multiple symptomless small cysts are commonly seen throughout the breast in specimens removed for a variety of conditions, benign or malignant, or examined at post-mortem, and must therefore be regarded as normal. Larger cysts are usually found in the second half of reproductive life (ages 30 to 50 years) and may be single or multiple. They give rise to a rounded, smooth, tense and fairly mobile swelling which can usually be felt to fluctuate. They are regarded as a form of dysplasia though on rare occasions a carcinoma may be associated. They contain turbid fluid of various colours ranging from yellow through brown to green.

Opinions vary as to the correct treatment; some authorities favour excision but aspiration is gaining in popularity. However, all would agree that every breast lump should be positively identified and eliminated, but aspiration achieves these ends, provided three conditions are observed: (1) the lump must disappear completely; (2) the aspirated fluid must not contain old or fresh blood in appreciable amounts; (3) there must be a careful follow-up and the lump must not recur. Failing these conditions, immediate excision must be performed.

Sclerosing adenosis

Sclerosing adenosis is a microscopist's diagnosis. It is an area of involuting breast embedded in fibrous tissue and gives rise to a lump which is likely to be removed for histological examination.

Duct stasis (Duct ectasia)

The accumulation in the ducts of shed epithelial cells and their breakdown products together with small amounts of milk and secretions of the resting gland leads them to become distended with thick material of pasty consistency, varying in colour between black, brown, green and cream. Such distended ducts may give the breast a knotty consistency and they may also discharge their contents intermittently from the nipple. Evidence of duct stasis is often encountered when removing a cyst. In itself the condition does not require any treatment and may be regarded as within the range of normality in women over 30 years of age. More severe degrees of the condition may cause blood-stained nipple discharge, nipple retraction and peripheral abscesses.

Nipple discharge

The commonest cause of discharge from the nipple is lactation and the fluid discharged is milk. Coming after the birth of an infant, it poses no diagnostic problem. Small quantities of milky fluid may appear at other times, and such fluid is also milk. It is seldom sufficiently persistent or copious to call for treatment. Black, brown, green or creamy discharge is due to duct stasis. Treatment is required only if the quantity and duration of the discharge are sufficient to constitute a serious nuisance. It may then be possible to identify and remove the duct or segment of the breast responsible. The black discharge of duct stasis does not owe its colour to old blood, which is not normally found in this condition, and black discharges should be submitted to an occult blood test.

Benign tumours

Discharges which are either serous and golden or blood-stained (bright red or tawny) constitute a third group. They arise either from a duct papilloma or a carcinoma. Papillomata are either single tumours 5 to 15 mm in diameter, occupying a dilated cystic portion of a main duct under the areola, where a soft swelling may be palpable, or multiple, microscopic papillomata of wider extent. Usually the discharge comes from a single duct orifice which can be located at operation provided the discharge has not been recently expressed. When discharge is due to carcinoma, it is almost invariable to find a lump which in its own right, quite apart from any discharge, would be recognized and treated as a carcinoma. Failing such a finding the cause of the discharge is likely to be a benign condition and is treated by identification and excision of the appropriate duct or segment, followed by microscopic examination of the specimen.

A benign tumour presenting as a solid lump may be a fibroadenoma, giant fibroadenoma **lipoma** or sebaceous cyst. The last two conditions, sometimes dubbed the universal tumours, will not be considered further.

Lipoma A benign fatty tumour.

A fibroadenoma is a mobile, rounded, firm and rubbery tumour, usually single and of extreme mobility so that it can be made to shoot about under the finger like a piece of ice in a tumbler. For this reason it has also been called 'a breast mouse'. It consists of clusters of proliferating ducts wrapped in dense whorls of connective tissue (two microscopic types – hard or pericanalicular and soft or intracanalicular – used to be recognized, but both appearances may be seen in the same tumour), and is absolutely benign. It is common in the late teens and early twenties but may occur at any time during reproductive life, the average age being 33 years. The treatment is by surgical removal through a small incision and usually it shells out easily, having a well-formed capsule of loose areolar tissue.

A giant fibroadenoma is a very rare tumour usually found in older women (average age: 45 years). It has a large number of other names, including serocystic tumour of Brodie and cystosarcoma phyllodes. Structurally it resembles a soft fibroadenoma. It may attain huge size so that the overlying skin and breast tissue are stretched to the point of giving way, exposing the tumour, when it may be mistaken for a fungating cancer. Usually it is completely benign and may be cured either by enucleation or by simple mastectomy. On occasions malignant change takes place, resulting not in carcinoma but in sarcoma.

Diseases of the male breast

All the diseases of the female breast so far described, as well as carcinoma described below, may occur on rare occasions in the male.

The breast tissue may become swollen, tender and inflamed during the first 2 weeks after birth in both sexes (neonatal mastitis) and although this is due to hormonal causes it may become secondarily infected and proceed to suppuration. Similar changes may occur at puberty (pubertal mastitis) followed in girls by the onset of normal development. In males it may also occur in late middle age (involutional mastitis).

Enlargement of the male breast to resemble the female form is known as gynaecomastia. It may result from many causes including hormone administration (for example, stilboestrol), secreting tumours of testis, adrenal, pituitary or even certain bronchial carcinomas, liver disease, starvation and obscure diseases of the central nervous system, and it may be a feature of Cushing's syndrome and Klinefelter's syndrome. In many cases no cause can be found and often the enlargement is unilateral.

Enucleation The separation of an organ from its capsule, or a tumour cleanly from the surrounding tissue.

CARCINOMA OF THE BREAST

Any of the tissues constituting the breast may be the source of a malignant tumour and the possibility of sarcoma arising in a giant fibroadenoma has already been mentioned. The vast majority of malignant breast tumours, however, are carcinomas arising from the epithelium of the ducts and alveoli.

General facts

Carcinoma of the breast has been known to all races throughout history and is not confined only to the human species. It is rare before 35 years of age and first appears after the age of 50 years in more than one-half of those affected. As men and women throughout the world live longer, the number of cases of carcinoma has increased. It is more common in those who have lactated little and late, and comparatively rare in communities where early marriage and prolonged lactation are usual. There are therefore considerable variations between different countries, incidence being high in Europe, especially in Great Britain, and low in Japan and Chile. These variations mainly reflect differences in the proportion of women over 40 years of age in the population and in social patterns of marriage, pregnancy and lactation. The risk is also greater among women with affected relatives and very slightly so among those previously suffering from fibro-adenosis. Studies of the urinary excretion of hormone metabolites show that not all women follow the same pattern and certain patterns are associated with increased risk of cancer. Trauma is not thought to increase the risk at all.

Untreated breast cancer always kills. About one-half of those affected are dead in 3 years, but a few may survive well beyond 5 years.

Clinical features

Breast cancer is first detected as a lump and almost always this is painless. As yet there is no way suitable for population screening, which will detect growths too small to feel, though there are special radiological techniques (mammography) and skin temperature measuring methods (thermography) which will do so at great trouble and expense. For the moment, therefore, the best way of increasing the frequency of early diagnosis is by educating women to carry out regular and effective self-examination.

The following types of lump may be encountered.

Scirrhous type

The lump is small, often only 1 to 2 cm in diameter, hard, and peripherally situated (most frequently in the upper outer quadrant). From an early stage it shows signs of fibrous attachment to its surroundings, especially skin, nipple and the fascia of the pectoralis major muscle. As a result, the skin over the lump may be dimpled or the nipple retracted either all the time, or in certain positions of the breast, or on moving the lump either with the examining finger, or by contracting the pectoralis major. An extreme version of this is found in very elderly women. The lump remains small though it may ultimately ulcerate, but the spread of the growth and its attendant fibrosis is accompanied by contraction of the fibrous tissue so that the breast is drawn up into a little hard puckered knot, sometimes even seeming to disappear. This is known as the atrophic scirrhous type.

Soft bulky type

The lumps of the soft bulky type are usually less peripheral, larger (often 4 to 5 cm in diameter) and of a rubbery softness which may make them difficult to distinguish from a cyst. The fibrous tissue reaction which they excite is much less marked than in the case of the scirrhous type and therefore the tell-tale signs of attachment are far less easily detected. Microscopically some show recognizable papillary patterns, some are merely very cellular and soft (so-called medullary or encephaloid type) while some produce mucus (colloid type).

Diffuse type

A growth of the diffuse type is a widely infiltrating lump which spreads throughout the breast causing it to become generally hard and immobile. It is usually in an advanced stage when first recognized. Sometimes the cancer cells excite an inflammatory reaction and the breast becomes red, hot and painful, resembling acute mastitis. This is called inflammatory cancer and is probably the most rapidly and uniformly lethal of all forms of the disease.

Paget's disease

Paget's disease is a destructive malignant eczema which eats away the nipple. A carcinoma also occurs separate from the nipple — often it is a peripherally placed scirrhous growth and it may precede, accompany or follow the nipple change. There are also cancerous changes in the linings of the main ducts within the nipple. It is a disease of older women and usually arises after 60 years of age.

Eczema A non-contagious inflammatory skin condition.

Spread

From its site of origin breast cancer spreads by local infiltration, by lymphatic pathways, by the bloodstream, and (later) across body cavities.

Local infiltration

Local infiltration and the fibrous reaction it causes, are the cause of the signs of attachment to surroundings already listed. As local spread proceeds, the lump may become fixed to chest wall, skin or nipple while infiltration of the dermal lymphatics causes the skin to become first thickened and pitted like orange peel (peau d'orange), then fixed and leathery over a wide area (cancer en cuirasse — cuirasse, a leather armour breast-plate). Cancerous nodules appear in the skin and later ulceration follows, either over a wide area, or over the area of the tumour (fungation).

Lymphatic spread

Tumour cells entering the lymphatics of the breast pass mainly to the lymph nodes in the axilla which are accessible to palpation, or through the medial ends of the intercostal spaces to those lying along the internal mammary vessels which are not accessible. From both sites they drain into the supraclavicular glands which are palpable and ultimately with the lymph stream into the subclavian veins. Uninvaded glands draining a cancer-containing breast are often rubbery and enlarged. Early invasion causes little alteration but later the glands become stony hard, and later still, matted together and fixed to adjacent structures. At this stage, signs of lymphatic blockage appear, particularly brawny oedema of the arm.

Blood-borne spread

Blood-borne spread results from invasion of veins in the breast, axilla or neck and carries the disease to the lungs and beyond them to all parts of the body. Such distant deposits are called metastases. No organ is exempt, but the bones and lungs are especially liable and after these, the liver and the serous linings of the chest and abdomen. Lung deposits lead to loss of pulmonary function with progressive dyspnoea; bony deposits produce destruction of bone which causes long bones to break (pathological fracture) and vertebrae to collapse. Vertebral collapse causes persistent pain, kyphosis and sometimes paraplegia. Serous deposits cause malignant effusions (pleural effusion or ascites) and liver deposits cause irregular hard enlargement of the liver and, later, jaundice with liver failure. Sometimes metastasis reaches the brain, the picture being that of a cerebral tumour. Deposits in the lungs and bones may be detected radiologically. Radioisotope scanning may also be used to detect deposits in bones and the liver and ultrasound scanning may also show them in the liver.

Diagnosis and treatment

The experienced clinician can frequently make a nearly certain diagnosis on clinical grounds alone, but with small early growths (and some others) this may not be possible. The problem may be solved by needle biopsy (possible at the outpatient visit), operative excision biopsy, with immediate frozen section or with macroscopic naked eye diagnosis of the excised piece, or with wound closure and later paraffin section. Preoperative staging is an aspect of diagnosis which also critically affects the choice of treatment (as well as its probable outcome). Two systems are widely used. One evaluates numerically the tumour extent (T), lymph node involvement (N), and distant metastasis (M). The other recognizes four stages.

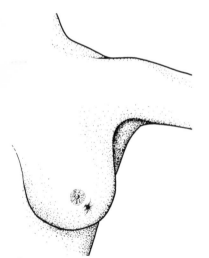

Figure 18.1. Stage 1 of breast cancer

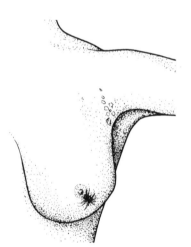

Figure 18.2. Stage 2 of breast cancer

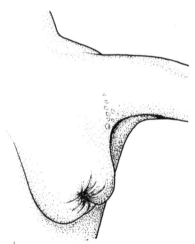

Figure 18.3. Stage 3 of breast cancer

Stage 1 small growth (up to 2 cm) confined to the breast; skin attachment absent, or present only immediately over the tumour.

Stage 2 growth larger or attached to fascia, or to skin over a larger area or skin infiltration or mobile involved axillary glands.

Stage 3 local growth and lymphatic spread more advanced; skin attachment over 6 cm across with or without oedema or ulceration, fixity to chest wall, fixed axillary glands or oedema of the arm.

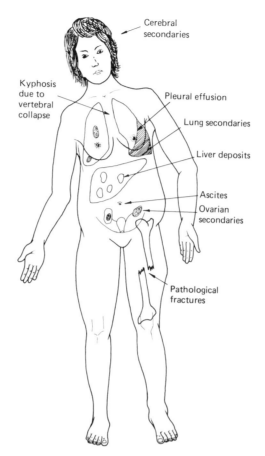

Figure 18.4. Stage 4 of breast cancer

Stage 4 any local conditions early or late but distant metastases present.

All growths in stages 3 and 4 and most in stage 2 will ultimately kill, but in many cases, judicious treatment will lead to considerable prolongation of life and avoidance of discomfort. Effective treatment of stage 1 growths leads to prolonged survival in a high proportion of cases.

The methods of treatment available fall into four main groups: (1) surgical removal of the tumour; (2) irradiation by x-rays or other ionizing radiations; (3) alteration of the hormonal environment; and (4) administration of cytotoxic drugs.

Surgical removal

Most women fear the disfigurement of losing a breast or even a portion of one. Comfort, reassurance and the company of another patient who is making a good recovery from a similar operation will help. The nature and extent of the proposed operation should be made clear as far as this can be known in advance.

During the last 30 years operable breast cancer has been variously treated in different centres by radical mastectomy (removal of breast, pectoral muscles and axillary contents) alone, or with pre- or postoperative radiotherapy, super-radical mastectomy (with removal of internal mammary and supraclavicular lymph nodes), simple mastectomy with irradiation of the axilla, simple mastectomy with axillary dissection, simple mastectomy alone, and simple removal of the lump, with or without irradiation. In growths of equal stage, all these methods give broadly similar results (65 per cent 5-year survival and 45 per cent 10-year survival in Stage 1 — not all the deaths being due to cancer). In some series, the results of the simpler operations have even proved to be better and it may be that when the axillary glands are not involved it is better not to damage them by excision or x-rays. In such growths, there is little danger of local recurrence and mortality results from the appearance of distant metastases. It is thought that small deposits of tumour cells may lie dormant for many years, or even for ever, held in check by some immunological mechanism in which the axillary glands play a part. At the present time comparative trials of different surgical policies are going on in many centres, but radical mastectomy is no longer the most frequently performed operation for early breast cancer in Great Britain, its place having been taken by extended simple mastectomy (Patey's operation), simple mastectomy with irradiation, and, for stage 1 growths, simple mastectomy alone, or simple removal of the lump.

Postoperative care

Patients are soon ambulant and serious complications are rare. Collection of serum within the wound is sometimes troublesome if drainage has not been effective. Oedema of the arm and stiffness of the shoulder are rare unless pre-operative radiotherapy has been given, and it is not necessary in the first week to demand vigorous shoulder movements.

Irradiation

Irradiation with x-rays is no substitute for surgery in operable growths, but it may be combined with operation either pre- or postoperatively with the aim of destroying outlying tumour cells, or as the sole treatment of the axilla in McWhirter's method. In advanced growths it will cause marked and often prolonged regression and is useful when fungation threatens. It is the best initial treatment of inflammatory cancer. It is also very useful in the form of a single concentrated dose applied to a painful bony metastasis or pathological fracture.

Hormonal methods

Almost any measures which upset the hormonal balance of the body may induce regression and such measures include oöphorectomy, adrenalectomy, destruction of the pituitary by implanting a seed of radioactive yttrium, the administration of oestrogens (stilboestrol, ethinyloestradiol), oestrogen antagonists (drostanolone — Masteril; tamoxifen — Nolvadex), progestogens (norethisterone — SH 420), adrenal steroids (cortisone, prednisolone), or possibly androgen analogues (nandrolone phenylpropionate — Durabolin). The choice of agent is not entirely governed by science, but good regression of disseminated disease occurs in about 40 per cent of cases. When relapse occurs, a further regression may be obtained with a new agent. Oestrogens, in particular, frequently give marked regression in women over 60 years of age.

Cytotoxic drugs

Cytotoxic drugs, like hormonal measures are only employed for the treatment of disseminated disease. Their action in the body resembles that of x-rays in that they are injurious to multiplying and dividing cells, including tumour cells, bone marrow, intestinal mucosa, skin and hair follicles. Doses sufficient to induce tumour regression can cause loss of hair and **leucopenia**. The patient may need a wig and dosage of the drug must be controlled by regular white cell counts.

Leucopenia (Leukopenia) A diminished number of white cells in the peripheral blood which may arise from bone marrow depression following the administration of cytotoxic drugs, associated with decreased resistance to infection.

19

Endocrine surgery

Paul Atkins

The endocrine system is composed of a number of glands. In this account, the prominence given to an individual gland reflects its importance in clinical practice rather than its physiological importance. The gastrointestinal tract for example is a source of many hormones but as yet their relevance to the clinician in most instances has not been determined. The endocrine disturbances described are those affecting the thyroid, parathyroid, adrenal, pituitary, testis, ovary and pancreas (*Figure 19.1*).

An endocrine gland is sometimes called a ductless gland, or a gland of internal secretion. This is because its secretion, a chemical substance called a hormone, is not conveyed along a duct but passes directly into the bloodstream. The bloodstream carries hormones widely throughout the body. Organs and tissues respond to specific hormones commonly by alterations in their functional state, but structural changes may also

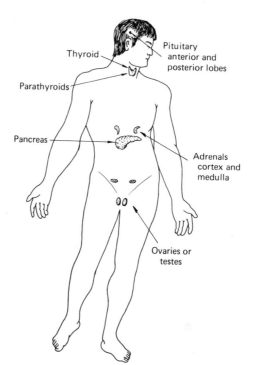

Figure 19.1. The position of endocrine glands

occur. Physiologically the anterior lobe of the pituitary is the most important endocrine gland, since it secretes hormones which stimulate many other glands in the system. To prevent overstimulation of the other 'target glands' there is a 'feedback' mechanism, so that when the hormone level in the blood

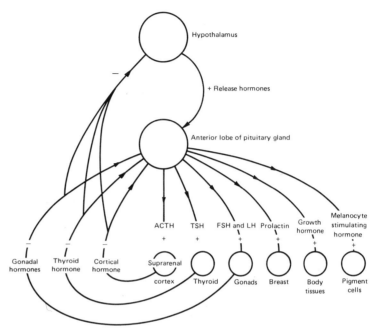

Figure 19.2. The pituitary drive and the feedback mechanism shown by the full circles. ACTH, adrenocorticotrophic hormone; TSH, thyroid-stimulating hormone; FSH, follicle-stimulating hormone; LH, luteinizing hormone

exceeds an optimum for a particular gland, the pituitary drive to that gland is reduced (*Figure 19.2*). Additional control of the anterior pituitary gland is brought about by release hormones secreted by the hypothalamus.

THE THYROID GLAND

Anatomy and physiology

The thyroid gland, which weighs 25 g in the adult, lies at the root of the neck. It consists of two lobes joined by an isthmus, the latter overlying the upper rings of the trachea or windpipe. The thyroid gland has a good blood supply and lymphatic drainage. The recurrent laryngeal nerves which supply the vocal cords and the parathyroid glands lie close to the thyroid gland.

The thyroid gland is made up of a very large number of small, spherical sacs called acini or vesicles (*Figure 19.3*). These acini are lined by a single layer of cells and contain a substance called colloid, which is a storage form of thyroid hormone. When the gland is active, two things occur: the cells lining the acini increase in size and number, and colloid drains away as it is converted to the active form of hormone and secreted. The greatest periods of activity occur in childhood, at puberty and during pregnancy.

The thyroid gland's functions are to make and supply the body tissues with thyroid hormone. These functions are regulated by the pituitary. An essential component of thyroid hormone is iodine; this is absorbed from the diet, concentrated

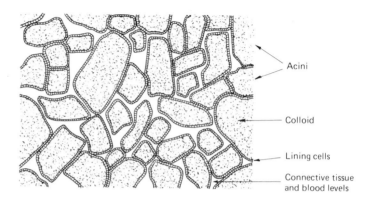

Figure 19.3. Microscopic appearance of the thyroid gland

within the gland, and utilized in the synthesis of thyroid hormone. In accordance with the body's needs, thyroid hormone is released into the bloodstream to reach the tissues and stimulate normal growth and development.

'C' cells also occur in the thyroid gland. Their function appears to be quite separate from the rest of the thyroid gland. They secrete a hormone called calcitonin which lowers the serum calcium level.

Pathology

Thyroid disease is much more commonly seen in women than in men. It is also more common in some areas of the world than others: this is almost entirely a reflection of the low iodine content of the water in these areas.

Developmental abnormalities

Failure of thyroid development

In a child of normal parents the thyroid gland may not develop or its development may be incomplete (hypoplasia). In areas where there is iodine deficiency infants may be born with goitres to parents who themselves have goitres. In both instances insufficient thyroid hormone is formed and this infantile form of hypothyroidism is called cretinism.

Ectopic thyroid, thyroglossal cyst and fistula

During fetal life the thyroid gland develops as a downgrowth from the midline of the anterior wall of the pharynx. Remnants of this are left as the thyroglossal tract. Normally in the adult this is fibromuscular tissue only. Rarely, thyroid tissue may develop anywhere along the thyroglossal tract from the base of the tongue to the isthmus of the thyroid gland. More commonly, a cyst may form in the line of the thyroglossal tract, usually below the level of the hyoid bone. A thyroglossal fistula results from infection of such a cyst or from an attempt to treat it by drainage.

Goitre

An enlargement of the thyroid gland is called a goitre. Simple goitre is not uncommon in the female in the late teens and should probably be regarded as little more than a physiological response to the increased activity that occurs in the endocrine system at this time. Goitre, however, is also closely related to iodine deficiency in the diet and in those areas of the world where the iodine content of the water is low, there is a particularly high incidence. This explains why goitre is common in Switzerland, the Himalayas and in Derbyshire in Great Britain (endemic goitre). A shortage of iodine leads to a shortage of thyroid hormone. Consequently, the pituitary secretes more thyroid-stimulating hormone which results in the thyroid gland enlarging in an effort to produce more thyroid hormone. Although a lack of iodine in the diet provides the most obvious way in which a goitre occurs, it is easy to appreciate that anything which interferes with the production of thyroid hormone will lead to an increase in the pituitary drive and to the formation of a goitre (sporadic goitre). Hence, a failure on the thyroid's part to utilize iodine correctly, either because of congenital malfunction or because of interfering substances (called goitrogens), will lead to enlargement of the gland.

The thyroid gland responds by a uniform enlargement in the younger person, but beyond the age of 30 years the gland responds in a patchy fashion. The areas of the thyroid which show this overgrowth, or hypertrophy, form nodules.

Complications A large goitre may compress and displace the trachea, particularly when it has enlarged downwards into the chest — a so-called retrosternal goitre. Occasionally compression is brought about suddenly by haemorrhage into an area of the gland which has become cystic and the patient may become acutely breathless. A multinodular goitre may produce too much thyroid hormone and the patient suffers from thyrotoxicosis. Rarely, a multinodular goitre may undergo malignant change; a solitary nodule is rather more likely to show this change.

Prevention The importance of iodine deficiency in the aetiology of goitre has been widely recognized. In some countries, where there is a particularly high incidence, successful attempts have been made to prevent goitre occurring by adding iodide to table salt and to flour.

Thyrotoxicosis

Thyrotoxicosis occurs when the thyroid gland secretes an excessive amount of thyroid hormone into the blood. Thyrotoxicosis occurring in patients under the age of 30 years is often called Graves' disease. When it occurs in patients over the age of 40 years who have a nodular goitre, it is sometimes termed 'secondary thyrotoxicosis'. Although there is considerable similarity in these two groups, there are minor differences in symptomatology and the cause is different.

Graves' disease The cause is often not apparent but sometimes an emotional shock appears to precipitate the disease. The normal pituitary control of the thyroid gland mediated by TSH is overridden by a pathological stimulator. This thyroid-stimulating antibody unlike TSH continues to be produced despite high circulating thyroid hormone levels. The antibody (LATS) is produced by lymphocytes. In Graves' disease the thyroid is smoothly enlarged, soft and vascular. The acini contain little colloid because, as soon as the thyroid hormone is formed, it is secreted. The overactivity of the gland is reflected by the cells which line the acini being taller than normal and showing considerable papillary enfolding.

Secondary thyrotoxicosis A similar pattern of hyperplasia is seen, but instead of being general throughout the gland, it occurs in patches; usually these overactive areas of the gland are not the nodules but the tissue between. The nodules are more often degenerative, cystic areas. Rarely, a single nodule occurring in the thyroid may be the only overactive area and the rest of the gland may be underactive.

Thyroiditis

Thyroiditis suggests an inflammation of the thyroid gland. In fact, simple inflammation of the gland as a response to infection is very uncommon, but three diseases called thyroiditis are recognized. Hashimoto, De Quervain and Riedel have all given their names to separate diseases.

Hashimoto's disease It is believed that the patient forms antibodies to thyroglobulin (the storage form of hormone) and to the epithelial cells lining the acini. Possibly because of these antibodies, the thyroid gland is destroyed and replaced by lymphoid and fibrous tissue. The disease is commonest in females between the ages of 30 and 50 years.

Riedel's disease Riedel's disease is an extremely rare form of thyroiditis in which not only the gland, but the surrounding structures are involved by fibrous tissue.

De Quervain's disease De Quervain's thyroiditis is more common. It is probably caused by the mumps virus.

Hypothyroidism

Hypothyroidism occurs when the thyroid gland secretes too little thyroid hormone into the blood. Minor degrees of hypothyroidism are not uncommon and frequently go unrecognized. Hypothyroidism is more common in women than in men. Hypothyroidism occurs in infants when there is a failure of thyroid development or when there is a failure of the gland to synthesize thyroid hormone, usually due to iodine deficiency. In adults, Hashimoto's thyroiditis, removal of too large a part of the gland, complete destruction by radiotherapy or excessive use of drugs given for thyrotoxicosis may all lead to hypothyroidism. The most severe form of hypothyroidism is termed myxoedema.

Thyroid carcinoma

Thyroid carcinoma is rare, but is more common in areas where goitre is endemic. It is more common in women than in men. Carcinoma occurring in young patients is usually well differentiated, which means that under the microscope the growth looks very similar to normal thyroid tissue. In the older patient, the growth is usually quite unlike normal thyroid tissue and grows rapidly. Carcinoma in the older patient tends to invade the surrounding structures and in the younger patient it spreads by the lymphatics and bloodstream. The metastases of some of the well-differentiated growths function as normal thyroid tissue.

Clinical presentation and diagnosis

Developmental abnormalities

Ectopic thyroid Thyroid at the base of the tongue may lead to difficulty in swallowing and breathing while thyroid tissue in the line of the thyroglossal tract is likely to be mistaken for a thyroglossal cyst. It is important for the surgeon to remember that this may be the only thyroid tissue. Consequently if it is found necessary to remove it replacement therapy with thyroxine will have to be commenced.

Thyroglossal cyst and fistula Despite being of developmental origin a cyst does not usually present until the teens or early adult life. It is a midline cystic swelling which may move on protruding the tongue. Often the patient comes to the doctor because the swelling has become infected. This is apt to be diagnosed as an 'infected sebaceous cyst' and drained resulting in the development of a thyroglossal fistula.

Goitre

The patient usually attends the doctor because she has noticed a swelling in the neck. Difficulty in breathing and a tightness in the neck may also be complaints. Less commonly, the patient may have noticed difficulty in swallowing. Occasionally the gland may have grown from its normal position in the neck into the chest. This is especially likely to lead to congestion of the veins of the neck. A very occasional presentation is a patient who complains of acute breathlessness with a history of rapid enlargement of one side of the thyroid. This presentation is brought about when a haemorrhage occurs into a cystic part of the gland. Apart from the obvious enlargement of the gland, patients who have goitres may sometimes show evidence of either overactivity or underactivity of the gland.

Thyrotoxicosis

Thyroid hormone stimulates metabolism and thus many of the clinical features of thyrotoxicosis can be explained on the basis of an increase in metabolism. Others may be due to an overactive sympathetic nervous system. The symptoms in Graves' disease and secondary thyrotoxicosis are similar. In Graves' disease, however, the brunt of the disease is borne by the nervous system and the eyes are commonly affected, whereas in secondary thyrotoxicosis, the cardiovascular system is particularly affected. In Graves' disease the patient, invariably a woman, complains of a feeling of anxiety and general irritability. She may have noticed an increase in her appetite, but despite this, a loss in weight. An inability to tolerate hot weather and profuse sweating is common. The patient may complain of palpitations. She will probably have noticed a swelling in the neck. The patient may have noted that her periods have become scanty and on questioning, it may be apparent that there has been an increase in frequency of daily bowel actions and of micturition. Examination reveals a patient who is invariably anxious and jumpy, with hot moist palms, a rapid pulse rate and a tremor of the outstretched hands. A goitre is usually present; it is soft and diffuse in Graves' disease unlike secondary thyrotoxicosis where the goitre is nodular. The eyes may be prominent and there are various tests which may be done to demonstrate this. In severe cases, the eye muscles become paralyzed. In secondary thyrotoxicosis, the symptoms already described may be present but atrial fibrillation, detected as an irregularity of the pulse and heart failure are often the leading features, and the eye signs are much less obvious.

Thyroiditis

In Hashimoto's disease an enlargement of the thyroid, which is often rubbery, and symptoms of hypothyroidism are usually the prominent features. In Riedel's thyroiditis symptoms such as difficulty in breathing and swallowing arise when the trachea and oesophagus become involved with fibrous tissue. In De Quervain's disease the patient experiences an acute episode. The thyroid is painful and tender and the temperature is raised.

Hypothyroidism

In infants and children hypothyroidism or cretinism gives rise to obvious mental and physical retardation. The infant is lethargic, slow to feed and constipated — there is great delay in reaching all the developmental milestones. The appearance is characteristic — the face is coarse and sallow and the tongue lolls from the mouth. The fontanelles are more widely open and the hair is thin and dry. The abdomen is distended and there is often an umbilical hernia. The hands and feet are squat and there may be deposits of myxoedematous tissue particularly in the supraclavicular areas. The pulse is slow and the temperature subnormal.

In adults, severe hypothyroidism is termed myxoedema. Symptoms of hypothyroidism are not always very obvious, but a general slowing down occurs throughout the body. Lethargy and aches and pains in the limbs and joints are common. The patient always feels cold and, despite a poor appetite, her weight increases. Great difficulty in thinking and a poor memory may be noticed. The skin becomes dry and the hair falls out. Constipation is invariable and this can be so severe that intestinal obstruction is mimicked. Disturbances in menstruation are common and libido may be lost. Examination shows an overweight patient with dry skin and coarse, falling hair. The face is sallow and there is a general coarsening of the features by myxoedematous tissue. This at first sight appears to be oedema, but it does not pit on pressure. The patient is found to have a slow pulse and may even be found to have a lowered temperature. In the most severe cases coma can occur.

Carcinoma

Usually the patient notices a slowly growing nodule in one lobe of the thyroid; or the patient, who has had a long-standing goitre, notices that one nodule has begun to increase more rapidly in size. Sometimes metastases, spreading by the bloodstream lead to pain in the bones and to shortness of breath. Undifferentiated carcinomas can grow very rapidly and the trachea and the oesophagus can be compressed, resulting in breathlessness and difficulty in swallowing. The recurrent nerve can be similarly invaded by growth and hoarseness results.

Special diagnostic measures

Investigations performed on a patient with thyroid disease have two main aims: the first is to delineate the anatomical extent of the gland, and the second is to show whether the gland is functioning normally. When abnormal, it is determined whether the gland is overactive or underactive.

Radiology Straight radiographs of the neck and the upper part of the chest may show that the trachea has been pushed over to one side or compressed and narrowed by a thyroid enlargement. If the gland extends into the chest, this is seen as a shadow in the upper part.

Radioactive iodine scan Radioactive iodine or technetium is concentrated in the thyroid in exactly the same way as ordinary iodine. It is consequently possible to give a patient a drink containing a minute amount of radioactive iodine and to map out the thyroid gland by using a special instrument which detects the concentrated radioactive iodine. Normally, iodine is evenly concentrated throughout the gland. If the uptake is uneven, it is an indication of some abnormality such as the presence of a cyst or carcinoma. A small proportion of carcinomas have functioning metastases and these will be apparent if the whole body is scanned after radioactive iodine has been given.

Thyroid and thyroid-stimulating hormones The most obvious way to determine whether a patient's thyroid is acting normally is to measure the end result, that is, the amount of thyroid hormone in the blood. Both thyroxine and tri-iodothyronine which make up circulating thyroid hormone can be estimated. Normal values are: thyroxine 60—160 nmol per litre; tri-iodothyronine 1.4–3.5 nmol per litre. Thyroid-stimulating hormone may also be measured (normal level 0–7 mU per litre). The pituitary gland increases its output of TSH if the thyroid gland is failing to produce sufficient hormone — for a while normal thyroid hormone levels may be achieved with TSH set at a higher level. Measurement of TSH therefore finds its greatest use in the patient suspected of having early hypothyroidism. TSH levels may also be measured after an injection of thyrotrophin release hormone — extremely high levels are seen in hypothyroidism.

Uptake of iodine and secretion of thyroid hormone The ability of the thyroid to remove iodine from the blood and concentrate it within the gland is increased when the gland is overactive and when it has been starved of iodine. The rate at which hormone is secreted is increased in the overactive gland, but decreased in the patient with an iodine-deficient goitre. Radioactive iodine can be used to follow these departures from normal. A small dose of radioactive iodine is given by mouth and, at varying times after this, the uptake in the thyroid gland is measured. By taking a blood sample at 48 hours and measuring the protein-bound radioactive iodine, a measure of the thyroid hormone released is obtained; this is a particularly useful test in the underactive gland.

Indirect tests Indirect tests are based on the effects that a departure from the normal thyroid state can have on the body. The serum cholesterol, the basal metabolic rate, the electrocardiogram and a sophisticated measurement of the ankle jerk can all, at times, be useful. The most consistently used of these tests at present is the serum cholesterol, which is raised in the presence of hypothyroidism (normal 3.6–7.8 mmol per litre).

Thyroid antibodies In patients suspected of having Hashimoto's disease, the blood may be examined for thyroid antibodies. Their presence is good evidence that the patient is suffering from the disease.

Treatment

A combination of medical and surgical treatment is commonly used in thyroid disease. The lines of treatment available and their indications are briefly described, before certain aspects of treatment are considered in more detail. It will be apparent that often the same object can be achieved in a number of different ways. As might be expected, the emphasis placed on alternative lines of therapy varies from centre to centre.

Antithyroid drugs

A number of drugs interfere with the synthesis of thyroid hormone. The most commonly used drug in this group is carbimazole. All patients with thyrotoxicosis are given antithyroid drugs either as definitive therapy or as part of a preoperative preparation. They are extremely effective in bringing the disease under control, but relapse of thyrotoxicosis after discontinuing the drugs is common. Continuing enlargement of the gland, rashes, sore throats and, very rarely, depression of the bone marrow, are complications which may occur.

In thyrotoxicosis iodine has a beneficial effect by temporarily reducing the rate at which thyroid hormone is secreted; it also makes the gland less vascular and surgeons make use of this action by using iodine for the final 2 weeks before thyroidectomy. Iodine on its own, however, is not adequate therapy for thyrotoxicosis. In children iodine may be used to bring about regression of a simple goitre.

Removal or destruction of the gland

Surgery Operative removal of the thyroid gland may be partial or total; if it is total, hypothyroidism will occur. Total thyroidectomy is consequently performed only when the thyroid is the site of malignant disease. The usual operation performed for goitre and thyrotoxicosis is a partial thyroidectomy. This operation achieves two objects, namely removal of a lump in the neck and reduction of circulating thyroid hormone.

When surgery is undertaken for a thyroglossal cyst or fistula, the thyroid gland is left undisturbed; however an important part of the operation is to ensure that the whole of the thyroglossal tract is removed. The tract is therefore traced up to the base of the tongue and the middle third of the hyoid bone is removed.

Radioactive iodine Radioactive iodine is concentrated within the thyroid gland. Although no damage occurs to the gland when tracer doses are used for diagnostic purposes, destruction of the gland can be induced by larger doses. This destructive action can be utilized for the treatment of thyrotoxicosis, for the treatment of functioning secondary thyroid carcinomas and as an alternative to surgery for the treatment of some primary carcinomas. Radioactive iodine is only used in benign disease in the older patient since there is a potential risk of inducing malignant disease and causing genetic damage. After radioactive iodine, hypothyroidism is a common complication and must be treated with thyroxine.

Radiotherapy External irradiation is another way in which the gland may be destroyed. Its use is confined to the treatment of carcinoma.

Thyroid hormone replacement and pituitary suppression

In hypothyroidism, the thyroid's decreased hormone output can be replaced by thyroxine tablets. This is extremely effective, and provided the dosage is correct there are no complications (0.15 mg to 0.2 mg is adequate replacement therapy for most adults). Since pituitary drive tends to cause growth of the thyroid, it is probably advantageous to suppress this with thyroxine in adolescent goitres and it is certainly of benefit in Hashimoto's disease and in carcinoma.

Indications for the various types of treatment are summarized in Table 19.1.

Table 19.1   Indications for medical and surgical treatment

Type of treatment	Indication
Antithyroid drugs	
Carbimazole	As definitive treatment in young patients with mild thyrotoxicosis
	As preoperative preparation in majority of thyrotoxic patients
Iodine	Final phase of preoperative preparation of thyrotoxic patients
	Goitres in children
Gland removal and destruction	
Surgery	Large nodular goitres especially when they lie in the chest or press on the trachea
	Majority of patients with moderate and severe thyrotoxicosis
	Differentiated carcinomas
	Limited operations to obtain thyroid tissue for microscopic examination in Hashimoto's disease and anaplastic carcinoma
Radioactive iodine	Thyrotoxicosis recurring after surgery and occurring in patients too ill for surgery
	According to some, in all patients over the age of 45 years with a small toxic gland
	In functioning metastases
	As an alternative to surgery for a functioning primary carcinoma
Radiotherapy	Anaplastic carcinoma in the elderly
Thyroxine replacement and pituitary suppression	Hypothyroidism
	Adolescent goitres
	Hashimoto's disease
	Carcinoma

Thyroidectomy

Preoperative preparation It is essential that, at the time of operation, the patient be euthyroid, that is, that thyroid hormone in the blood is at an optimum level. To achieve this in thyrotoxicosis, carbimazole in a dosage of 30 mg per day is given for about 6 weeks. If at the end of this time the patient's disease appears to be controlled, potassium iodide in a dosage of 60 mg three times daily is substituted during the final 2 weeks before operation. Before the operation, the vocal cords are always inspected to ensure that both recurrent nerves are intact.

Operation The gland is approached by making a transverse incision in the neck. In a partial thyroidectomy the isthmus of the gland and all but 4 g of either lobe are resected, while

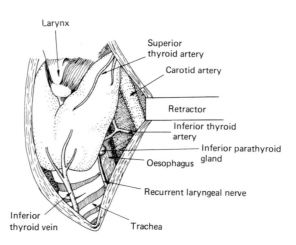

Figure 19.4. The thyroid gland at operation

in a total thyroidectomy, all the gland is removed. Particular care is taken to preserve the recurrent nerves and the parathyroid glands (*Figure 19.4*). The skin is usually closed with clips and the wound is always drained.

Postoperative management On return to the ward, the patient is sat up as quickly as her general condition allows. Routine observations of pulse, blood pressure, respiration and temperature are made. Drains and dressings are inspected for evidence of excessive bleeding. Half the skin clips or sutures are removed on the second postoperative day and the remainder on the following day. Drains may usually be removed on the second postoperative day. If the postoperative course is uncomplicated, the patient is discharged on the fourth postoperative day.

Complications In the early postoperative period breathlessness, hoarseness, tetany and a thyroid crisis can occur. Breathlessness may not be directly related to the operation, but it is important to exclude the presence of a haematoma in the closed spaces of the neck. Such a collection may lead to compression of the trachea, especially if the latter is soft, as may be the case when the patient has had a large goitre. The haematoma must be evacuated as rapidly as possible. A particularly harsh form of breathing (stridor) or a hoarse voice occurs when the surgeon has inadvertently damaged the recurrent nerve. If both nerves have been injured, urgent tracheotomy is required since the vocal cords adopt an almost closed position. It is routine practice to examine the vocal cords before and after the operation. Tetany occurs if the parathyroid glands are damaged. It is due to a fall in the calcium level of the blood; treatment is by calcium administration, intravenously at the beginning and then orally along with vitamin D which increases absorption from the gut and mobilizes calcium from the bones.

A thyroid crisis is an ultra-acute form of thyrotoxicosis occurring after surgery. It is very rarely seen now and only occurs when a thyrotoxic patient has had insufficient antithyroid medication before operation. The patient is sedated, cooled and given propranolol, iodine and steroids.

Follow-up Late complications of thyroidectomy are recurrent thyrotoxicosis and hypothyroidism. The former is relatively uncommon. It is usually treated with radioactive iodine, though further surgery or antithyroid drugs may be preferred. Hypothyroidism is not uncommon; it occurs even more commonly as a complication of radioactive iodine therapy. Hypothyroidism is somewhat insidious in onset and may not be recognized by the patient; because of this, patients should be checked periodically for 2 years after thyroidectomy for benign conditions. Thyroxine 0.15 mg to 0.2 mg per day orally is effective treatment. After malignant conditions have been treated, the follow-up should be lifelong so that recurrent disease may be promptly treated.

THE PARATHYROID GLANDS

Anatomy and physiology

There are normally two pairs of parathyroid glands and they usually lie in the neck, close to the posterior surface of the thyroid gland. The parathyroid glands are small oval bodies commonly covered in fat. When examined under a microscope, the gland is seen to consist of many small cells with large nuclei. Larger cells containing granules are also present. Like the thyroid, the parathyroid has an excellent blood supply.

The hormone secreted by the parathyroid gland is called parathormone; its effect is to increase the amount of calcium circulating in the blood. The parathyroid responds directly to the blood calcium level — parathormone is secreted when the calcium level falls below the optimum and secretion is suppressed when the level is above it. The pituitary does not influence parathyroid activity.

Pathology

Disease of the parathyroids is recognized, either because insufficient parathormone is secreted, or because too much hormone is secreted. Insufficient parathormone is almost invariably the result of a surgeon removing parathyroid glands, or damaging their blood supply when removing part of the thyroid gland. The resulting fall in blood calcium makes the nerves hyperexcitable. Hyperparathyroidism results when a tumour, usually benign, arises in a parathyroid gland, or when an overgrowth (hyperplasia) of all the glands occurs. Usually tumour formation or hyperplasia occurs without an obvious precipitating factor. Hyperplasia may occur however as a response to a persistently low serum calcium brought about by renal failure. Even more rarely, a tumour may develop in one of these hyperplastic glands. The high level of parathormone can lead to decalcification of bone and cysts may form, having the appearance of a growth. Sometimes fractures occur, particularly collapse of the vertebrae in the spine, although by no means all patients have evidence of bone disease. More commonly there is evidence of increased deposition of calcium within the body. This may be in the form of deposits within the substance of the kidney, as kidney stones, and as deposits occurring in the conjunctivae and around joints.

Clinical presentation and diagnosis

Hypoparathyroidism

Following a thyroidectomy, the patient may notice tingling and numbness of her lips and fingers. If the blood calcium is particularly low, severe cramps are felt in the hands and feet. The hand may adopt a position in which the fingers remain extended but the wrists flexed. In the most severe cases, difficulty in breathing and spasm of the eye muscles leading to double vision occur.

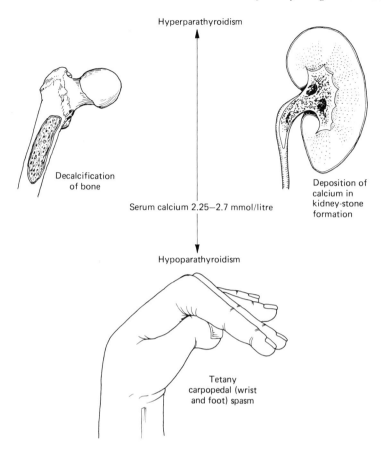

Figure 19.5. Major features of parathyroid disease

Hyperparathyroidism

The commonest presentation of this rare disease is a patient with recurrent renal stones. Less commonly the patient may present because of bone pain, fractures, weakness of muscles and generalized lethargy. Chronic peptic ulceration and pancreatitis are sometimes associated with hyperparathyroidism.

The commonest symptoms of parathyroid disease are seen in *Figure 19.5.*

Special diagnostic measures

The parathyroids are intimately concerned with calcium metabolism and the most useful investigation in parathyroid disease is measurement of the blood calcium level (normal: 2.25–2.7 mmol/litre). A low level is found in hypoparathyroidism and a high level in hyperparathyroidism. The serum calcium measurement should, however, be repeated on a number of occasions. In hyperparathyroidism more calcium than normal is excreted in the urine and therefore urinary calcium should also be measured (normal: less than 7.5 mmol in 24 hours).

In hyperparathyroidism radiographs may show de-calcification of the bones and fractures. Radiographs of the urinary tract may show calcium deposited in the kidneys, or stones in the kidneys.

It is now possible to measure parathormone levels. By introducing a catheter in the leg and running it up into the main veins of the neck it is possible to obtain venous samples from different sites. The sample taken from nearest a tumour is likely to have the highest parathormone level. This technique is helpful in localizing a tumour and is particularly useful if the neck has been previously explored and the anatomy distorted.

Treatment

Hypoparathyroidism
Tetany may be abolished by an intravenous injection of 10 ml of 10 per cent calcium gluconate, given slowly. After this, oral calcium up to 5 g per day and vitamin D as calciferol up to 5 mg per day are given as this mobilizes calcium from the bones.

Hyperparathyroidism
The treatment of hyperparathyroidism is surgical. A para-thyroid tumour is removed, or most of the parathyroids if hyperplasia is the cause. Occasionally the parathyroid tumour is not found in the neck but in the chest.

The postoperative management of a patient who has had a parathyroidectomy is very similar to management after thyroidectomy. However, after parathyroid glands have been removed, it is usually necessary to give calcium and vitamin D by mouth. Initially it may be necessary to give intravenous calcium.

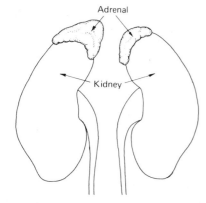

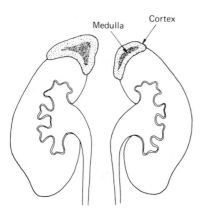

Figure 19.6. The adrenal glands

THE ADRENAL GLANDS

Anatomy and physiology

There are two adrenal glands. Each lies in close proximity to the upper pole of a kidney (*Figure 19.6*). The glands are triangular in shape and yellow in colour. The gland consists of an outer part called the cortex and an inner part called the medulla. The cortex and medulla, though structurally composing one gland, are functionally separate. The glands are extremely vascular.

The cortex, secretes three types of hormone which are concerned with carbohydrate metabolism, salt and water retention and the development of secondary sexual characteristics. Glucocorticoids, of which cortisol is the most important, are the ones concerned with carbohydrate metabolism. They increase blood glucose at the expense of protein synthesis and increase the deposition of glycogen (a storage form of glucose) in the liver. Glucocorticoids are important in the body's resistance to stress. Their secretion is regulated by ACTH. Mineralocorticoids, of which aldosterone is the most important, lead to more efficient conservation of sodium by the kidney but with a proportionate loss of potassium. Aldosterone is secreted in response to an intermediate stimulant renin which is produced by the kidney when the sodium concentration of urine within it is low. Adrenal sex hormones — the ketosteroids — are normally produced in very small amounts compared to the gonads.

The adrenal medulla secretes adrenaline and some noradrenaline. Hormone secretion is stimulated by stress. Adrenaline and noradrenaline have many actions but the most important is on the cardiovascular system. The heart rate and output are increased and the majority of small vessels constrict, leading to a rise of blood pressure. In stress there is some interaction between the medulla and cortex. Adrenaline adds to those stimuli on the anterior pituitary gland which cause it to produce ACTH. This in turn leads to secretion of cortisol. The medulla also appears to work more efficiently in a high cortisol environment.

Pathology

The adrenal cortex

Overgrowth (hyperplasia) and tumours of the cortex lead to an excessive output of cortical hormones. Depending upon which hormones are secreted, various disease syndromes will result.

Cushing's syndrome (*Figure 19.7*) is due to an excessive output of glucocorticoids. This may be due to the presence of tumour in the adrenal gland but more commonly it is due to hyperplasia of the glands brought about by excessively high levels of ACTH. Rarely, a patient may present with a clinically recognizable pituitary tumour. An ACTH-like substance is occasionally produced by non-endocrine tumours such as carcinoma of the lung and this causes hyperplasia of the adrenals in the same way. Women are affected by Cushing's syndrome more commonly than men and, though it may occur at any age, the highest incidence is between the age of 20 and 40 years.

Conn's syndrome and the adrenogenital syndrome are both extremely rare. The former is usually due to a benign growth.

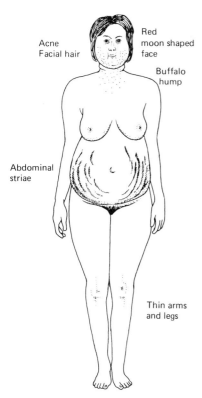

Acne
Facial hair

Red moon shaped face

Buffalo hump

Abdominal striae

Thin arms and legs

Figure 19.7. The main features of Cushing's syndrome

Oversecretion of aldosterone leads to retention of sodium and water and decrease in body potassium. In the adrenogenital syndrome, excessive secretions of androgens or masculinizing hormones will cause different symptoms at different ages. Sometimes the excess androgens are produced not from a tumour, but because of a failure in the normal process of hormone synthesis.

The adrenal medulla

Tumours of nerve cells (ganglioneuroma or neuroblastoma) occur. Ganglioneuromas occur at any age, neuroblastomas only in infancy and childhood. The former tumour is benign, the latter highly malignant. Neither tumour secretes hormones.

A tumour of the cells which produce adrenaline and noradrenaline, called a phaeochromocytoma, may rarely occur. It is commonest between the age of 30 and 40 years and may occur in either sex.

Adrenal insufficiency

Adrenal insufficiency can occur from haemorrhage into both glands as part of an overwhelming infection or other stressful situation, from tuberculosis, and from secondary deposits of growth. Sometimes atrophy of the gland occurs because the patient has developed antibodies to his own adrenal cortex. Perhaps the most important cause of adrenal insufficiency, however, is the therapeutic use of steroid hormones for diseases, such as rheumatoid arthritis or asthma. Their use leads to a depression of the pituitary drive to the adrenal glands, allowing them to atrophy. Normally in stressful situations of illness or operation, the adrenal cortex increases its secretion of hormones, but this response may not occur in patients who have been treated with steroids.

Clinical presentation and diagnosis

Cushing's syndrome

In Cushing's syndrome, the patient gradually puts on weight and the body configuration changes. The face becomes moon-shaped and fat is deposited on the back of the neck and shoulders in a way that has led to a description of it as a 'buffalo hump'. The arms and legs remain thin. The face is often red due to polycythaemia (an increase in the number of red cells) and striae or lines due to stretching appear on the abdomen. Fractures, particularly of vertebrae, are frequent. Acne and growth of facial hair are common. The effects of high blood pressure or muscle weakness usually bring the patient to the doctor.

Conn's syndrome

In Conn's syndrome patients suffer from high blood pressure, general weakness and lassitude.

Adrenogenital syndrome

If excessive androgens are secreted during intrauterine life, a female child will be born with male characteristics. If excessive secretion of androgens takes place in early childhood, the masculinization of a female child and precocious puberty in a male child will occur. When the secretion of androgens takes place after puberty, a deepening of the voice, a growth of hair on the face, acne and reduction of female secondary sexual characteristics occur.

Ganglioneuromas, neuroblastomas and phaeochromocytoma

The presence of a lump in the abdomen or widespread secondary disease in the case of neuroblastomas, leads to medical advice being sought. Phaeochromocytoma is characterized by sudden attacks of high blood pressure, rapid pulse rate and sweating. Patients struck by a sudden attack show signs of acute anxiety and complain of a severe headache.

Adrenal insufficiency

Adrenal insufficiency may be of sudden or gradual onset. Collapse and a low blood pressure are the prominent features of suddenly occurring adrenal failure. When there has been long-standing insufficiency, other symptoms of what is known as Addison's disease are present: namely, lassitude, weight loss, pigmentation of skin and mucous membranes and, commonly, abdominal colic.

Special diagnostic measures

Investigations are designed to show the anatomical extent of the adrenal gland, secretion abnormalities and their effects on the body.

A tumour of the adrenal gland may be seen on soft tissue radiographs. Displacement of the kidney by the tumour may be better shown by an intravenous pyelogram and an abnormal vascular pattern in the tumour may be seen in an arteriogram. A venous sampling technique similar to that used in the localization of a parathyroid tumour may be utilized to locate an adrenal tumour — it is particularly appropriate in the investigation of a phaeochromocytoma.

Direct measurements of adrenal secretions in the blood and their breakdown products in the urine, are used to elucidate the various syndromes. For example, in Cushing's disease the plasma cortisol level and its excretion products in the urine are high and remain high even at night when, normally, plasma cortisol shows a fall. Similarly in phaeochromocytoma, the urinary excretion products of adrenaline and noradrenaline are raised.

Varied effects on the body occur as a result of secretion abnormalities. In Cushing's syndrome sugar may be found in the urine and decalcification of bone and fractures may be seen on radiographs. In adrenal insufficiency and in Conn's syndrome, electrolyte abnormalities occur.

Treatment

Removal of one adrenal gland is practised when it is the site of a tumour and of both when there is bilateral hyperplasia. When, rarely, a pituitary tumour is the apparent cause of Cushing's syndrome the pituitary is removed or ablated by radiotherapy. Cortisone is used in the treatment of the adrenogenital syndrome, when it is due to a failure of hormone synthesis.

Surgical excision

Preoperative management In the normal patient subjected to the stress of a major operation, cortisol secretion increases tenfold from 30 to 300 mg per day. Patients undergoing adrenalectomy are therefore given intramuscular injections of hydrocortisone sodium succinate 100 mg 8-hourly. The first injection is given with the premedication. Provided there is no complication, steroid dosage may be progressively reduced and changed to the oral route until a normal maintenance dose is reached — 20 to 40 mg hydrocortisone or its equivalent as cortisone acetate. Fludrocortisone 0.1 to 0.2 mg per day, a synthetic steroid with actions akin to aldosterone, is also required to conserve sodium.

Specific preoperative therapy Metyrapone may be given to patients with Cushing's syndrome. It reduces cortisol levels by interfering with its synthesis. Patients undergoing operation for phaeochromocytoma are treated with phenoxybenzamine as this helps to control hypertension by relaxing arteriolar constriction thereby increasing the circulatory capacity. Propanalol is also given as this reduces the heart rate and the risk of arrhythmias.

Operation Although the adrenal gland may be removed through an incision similar to that used for the removal of the kidney, it is more usual to approach the gland through the abdomen.

Postoperative management After removal of the adrenal gland it is essential to record the pulse and blood pressure with great care, since hypotension is not uncommon. Replacement therapy with hydrocortisone given intravenously may be required and when a phaeochromocytoma has been removed, noradrenaline is sometimes required though adequate transfusion usually avoids this.

Follow-up If both adrenals have been removed, replacement therapy with cortisone must be life-long. Cortisone dosage must be increased during periods of stress occasioned by intercurrent illness or operation.

THE PITUITARY GLAND

Anatomy and physiology

The pituitary gland lies in the skull. It is a small, oval structure attached to the base of the brain. It is rather a complex structure of which the anterior lobe is the most important. Three types of cell are present in the anterior lobe.

The anterior lobe of the pituitary secretes stimulating hormones. These promote growth and stimulate the thyroid, the adrenal cortex, the ovary or testes, the lactating breast and melanocytes responsible for pigmentation of the skin. The posterior lobe of the pituitary secretes hormones which raise the blood pressure and reduce the output of urine, a so-called anti-diuretic effect. They also cause contractions of the uterus at the end of pregnancy.

Pathology

The bodily changes which occur in disease of the anterior lobe of the pituitary gland occur because of the secondary effects abnormal levels of stimulating hormones have on target organs and glands.

Overactivity
Oversecretion may result from overt tumours, microscopic tumours and from increased cellular activity of hormone-secreting cells.

Underactivity
A tumour of non-secreting cells by its expansion depresses the function of secreting cells — and an underactive state called hypopituitarism occurs. Hypopituitarism may rarely occur in women if a difficult delivery is accompanied by massive blood loss. Even more rarely, hypopituitarism may

be due not to a pituitary tumour but to a tumour arising in anatomical proximity to it.

The posterior lobe of the pituitary gland is less commonly involved by disease. It may however be damaged in a patient who sustains a head injury and lack of antidiuretic hormone leads to the patient producing large volumes of unconcentrated urine — a condition known as diabetes insipidus.

Clinical presentation

Tumours of the pituitary gland may encroach on the optic nerves and cause a particular type of blindness while a rise of intracranial pressure may cause headache and vomiting.

Overactivity
Increased growth hormone secretion results in gigantism in childhood and acromegaly in adults — the latter is characterized by enlargement of the hands, feet, nose and lower jaw. The skin is thickened and the lips and tongue may be noticeably enlarged. Enlargement of internal organs, e.g. the heart, also occurs. Hypertension is common and diabetes may develop.

Increased ACTH levels appear to be responsible for Cushing's syndrome of the type associated with bilateral adrenal hyperplasia.

Non-pregnant women sometimes present with a syndrome that mimicks the situation that appertains in the woman who is breast-feeding — namely the breasts secrete milk and there is amenorrhea. Increased levels of prolactin but normal FSH and LH levels are found.

Underactivity of the pituitary gland
Failure of lactation, reduction of secondary sexual characteristics with amenorrhea, loss of libido, and infertility result from depression of prolactin FSH and LH. Hypothyroidism results from depression of TSH. General weakness and hypotension occur from ACTH depression. Failure to grow occurs in childhood as a result of growth hormone depression. Some patients are particularly pale due to lack of MSH.

Isolated stimulating hormone deficiencies
Suppression of FSH may occur and be responsible for infertility.

Growth hormone may also sometimes appear to be the only stimulating hormone which is absent.

Special diagnostic measures
Measurement of the secretions of the many endocrine glands influenced by the abnormal pituitary drive are used to

elucidate the complex syndromes of pituitary disease. Straight radiographs of the skull show pressure changes. More sophisticated radiological techniques are available for showing the position and size of tumours.

Treatment

Pituitary tumours are removed by surgical excision, destroyed by radiotherapy, or a combination of treatments is used. Hypopituitarism results in most instances. To keep the patient with hypopituitarism in good health the hormones secreted by target glands are prescribed, e.g. cortisone acetate 37.5 to 50 mg per day, thyroxine 0.2 mg per day and appropriate androgens or oestrogens. After surgery, posterior lobe extract (pitressin) may be necessary for a few months to provide antidiuretic hormone.

Specific therapy for apparent single hormone abnormalities is available. Extracts of growth hormone may be given. Bromocriptine may be prescribed to inhibit the release of prolactin and clomiphene may be used to stimulate FSH release.

THE GONADS

THE TESTES

Anatomy and physiology

The testes are paired oval bodies which lie in the scrotum. The testis is largely composed of tubules which pass from the anterior to the posterior aspect of the gland. Here they join a number of wider ducts which enter the epididymis, which is a single convoluted channel, this subsequently becoming the vas deferens. Lying between the tubules in the testis are groups of cells called interstitial cells.

The duct system is concerned with the production and transport of developing spermatozoa. The interstitial cells have an endocrine function and secrete testosterone. This hormone is responsible for the male secondary sex characteristics and it also stimulates the build-up of protein in the body. The anterior pituitary secretes two gonadotrophic hormones: the former in the male follicle-stimulating hormone (FSH) and luteinizing hormone (LH) stimulates spermatogenesis and the latter testosterone secretion.

Pathology and clinical presentation

Ablation

Removal of the testes before puberty leads to a failure in the development of the secondary sexual characteristics. If the

T

testes are removed after puberty, the patient will be sterile, but will retain normal secondary sexual characteristics.

Hormone-secreting tumours

Only a very few tumours of the testis secrete hormones. One tumour, known as a chorionepithelioma, produces chorionic gonadotrophin. This hormone is normally produced by the placenta and, indeed, the Aschheim–Zondek test for pregnancy may be positive. The tumour is highly malignant and spreads to the lungs via the bloodstream. As a result of hormone secretion, there may be enlargement of the breasts. Another tumour which secretes hormone is the interstitial cell tumour; it is an exceptionally rare tumour, but if it occurs in childhood, testosterone is likely to be secreted and cause precocious puberty. When it occurs in adult life, oestrogens are more usually secreted. This has a feminizing effect.

Treatment

When the testis contains a tumour, **orchidectomy** is performed. Radiotherapy has little effect on these endocrine-secreting tumours, but cytotoxic drugs are of help in the treatment of chorionepithelioma.

Carcinoma of the prostate gland and the endocrine system

Carcinoma of the prostate is a common disease in the elderly male. Unfortunately, by the time symptoms are sufficiently disturbing to bring the patient to the doctor, the disease is usually advanced and beyond the scope of a radical surgical excision. Obstruction to urinary outflow may be relieved by resecting part of the gland by the transurethral route, but this is in no sense a curative operation for cancer. Fortunately, carcinoma of the prostate responds well to alterations in the hormone environment. The growth of a prostatic carcinoma is stimulated by androgens which are secreted by the testes and adrenal glands. Alteration in the hormone state is brought about by removal of the testes, by adrenalectomy or by destruction of the anterior pituitary. More commonly, instead of removing the source of androgens, oestrogens are given. The drug most frequently used is stilboestrol 15 mg per day. This is a synthetic oestrogen which has a feminizing effect and suppresses the anterior pituitary production of hormones stimulating the testis. Occasionally, in advanced disease, cortisone is used to reduce the anterior pituitary drive on the adrenal glands.

Orchidectomy Surgical removal of a testis.

THE OVARIES

Anatomy and physiology

There are two ovaries. Each ovary is oval in shape and in the adult female measures just over 4 cm in its longest diameter. The ovary lies within the pelvis, in close proximity to the uterus and Fallopian tubes, being attached to the back of the broad ligament. The outer surface is white and scarred from previous ovulations. The centre of the ovary is composed of vascular connective tissue, but the outer cortex contains numerous Graafian follicles.

The ovary's most obvious function is to discharge an ovum from a Graafian follicle every month from puberty to the menopause. During this process an endocrine function is also fulfilled, for, as the Graafian follicles mature, they secrete oestrogen. One follicle discharges a mature ovum, but the majority degenerate. After the ovum has been discharged from the follicle, the latter is converted to a yellow structure called a corpus luteum. This then secretes progesterone. Usually, the corpus luteum persists until a few days before the next menstrual period and then degenerates. During pregnancy, however, it continues to develop up to the third month. Pituitary FSH is responsible for the maturation of the Graafian follicle while LH is responsible for the persistence of the corpus luteum.

Oestrogen is responsible for the development of the generative organs and the secondary sexual characteristics. It causes the endometrium of the uterus to proliferate during the first half of the menstrual cycle. Progesterone is responsible for the secretory changes in the endometrium during the second half of the cycle; the withdrawal of progesterone leads to menstrual bleeding. During the first few months of pregnancy, progesterone is necessary for the maintenance of the fetus.

Pathology and clinical presentation

Endocrine-secreting tumours

There are two hormone-secreting tumours; the granulosa cell tumour and the arrhenoblastoma. They are uncommon. Both tumours are solid, though they may contain cystic cavities. They are yellowish grey in colour. The tumours are usually benign, but may be malignant. The granulosa cell tumour secretes oestrogen. If the tumour occurs in childhood, precocious puberty occurs, secondary sexual characteristics are developed and menstruation takes place. In adult patients **menorrhagia** is usually the only symptom, though carcinoma

Menorrhagia Excessive menstrual bleeding.

of the uterus is sometimes associated with a granulosa cell tumour of the ovary. In patients after the menopause menstruation may recur.

The arrhenoblastoma is an even rarer tumour which secretes masculinizing hormone. Very occasionally the tumour shows the appearance of seminiferous tubules, but usually the differentiation is not so great. Interstitial cells may be present. At first the patient develops amenorrhoea and the secondary sexual characteristics regress. Subsequently **hirsutism**, a deep voice and enlargement of the clitoris occur.

The treatment of endocrine-secreting tumours is to remove the affected ovary.

Carcinoma of the breast and the endocrine system

In a small proportion of patients with advanced carcinoma of the breast, regression may occur if the hormone environment is altered. This may be achieved either surgically, or medically. In the premenopausal patient, removal of the ovaries is sometimes beneficial. Removal of the adrenal glands and the pituitary may have the same effect. The adrenals are removed surgically, but the pituitary may be destroyed by irradiation. Less good, but worthwhile results may occur if androgens such as durabolin 25 to 50 mg i.m. once a week are given. An anti-oestrogen, tamoxifen 20 to 40 mg per day, may also be prescribed. In older patients oestrogens, e.g. stilboestrol 15 mg per day, may be beneficial.

Some help in predicting the value of hormone therapy may be obtained by assaying the tumour for oestrogen and progesterone receptors. Tumours with high ER + Values tend to fare best from endocrine ablation and anti-oestrogen medication.

THE PANCREAS

Anatomy and physiology

The pancreas is a large vascular gland which lies deeply in the middle of the abdomen.

Most of the secretions of the pancreas enter the duodenum and are concerned with the digestion of food. The gland is also an endocrine gland, however, and the hormones secreted are insulin, glucagon and gastrin. Insulin causes the blood sugar to fall, while glucagon causes it to rise. Gastrin stimulates gastric secretion.

Hirsutism Excessive bodily growth of hair.

Pathology and clinical presentation

Overactivity of the endocrine cells of the pancreas is rare but, as might be expected, tumours of the cells producing insulin give rise to attacks which simulate those due to an overdose of insulin, while tumours which form from the cells producing gastrin may give rise to recurrent peptic ulceration. Under-activity of the cells producing insulin causes diabetes mellitus. The role of glucagon in this condition is not clear.

Treatment

In insulin-secreting tumours, the tumour is removed, while in gastrin-secreting tumours, it is probably more important to remove the whole of the stomach, so that no hydrochloric acid is present to cause peptic ulceration. The treatment of diabetes mellitus is entirely medical.

20 Surgery of the head and neck

P. M. Stell

For purposes of anatomy and surgery the term 'head and neck' does not include the contents of the skull, which are usually assigned to neurosurgery; furthermore the ears, nose, sinuses and larynx and pharynx are almost exclusively the province of the ear, nose and throat specialist and will not be described in this book. Apart from the neck, the parts to be discussed here therefore are the skin of the head and face, the mouth and the salivary glands.

ANATOMY

Skin

The skin of the face and neck resembles the skin elsewhere, except for the lips, which are of surgical importance, and do differ from skin elsewhere in being covered by thin, relatively transparent, squamous epithelium so that they appear pink.

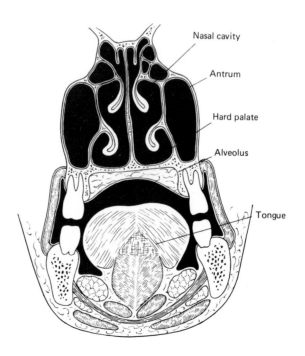

Figure 20.1. Antrum, nasal cavity and mouth

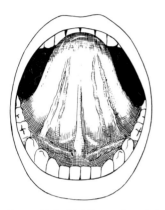

Figure 20.2. Mobile portion of the tongue

Mouth

The mouth (*Figure 20.1*) has a roof consisting of the alveolus, which forms the floor of the maxillary antrum, and the hard palate, which forms the floor of the nose. The floor of the mouth extends on each side medial to the mandible, and is limited in the midline by the massive bulk of the tongue; its side walls are composed of the buccal mucosa, or cheeks. The whole cavity is lined by squamous epithelium, with many small salivary glands within the epithelium.

The tongue has an anterior mobile portion (*Figure 20.2*), and a posterior part (or base) which lies within the pharynx; it consists of numerous muscle bundles, covered by squamous epithelium containing taste buds.

Posteriorly the mouth leads into the pharynx, and at the junction of the two lie the tonsils.

Salivary glands

The salivary glands (*Figure 20.3*) have several components: the major glands called the parotid and submandibular glands, and the minor glands, which are collections of very small glands, already referred to, in the mucosa of the mouth. The parotid gland lies immediately anterior to the ear in the substance of the cheek (*Figure 20.4*). The facial nerve, which supplies the muscles of the face, runs through its substance dividing it into a superficial and a deep lobe which makes surgery of the gland difficult. The saliva produced by its acini drains via a duct which opens into the mouth opposite the upper second molar tooth. The submandibular glands lie inferior and medial to the body of the mandible. Their salivary secretions drain upwards to enter the mouth immediately beneath the tip of the tongue.

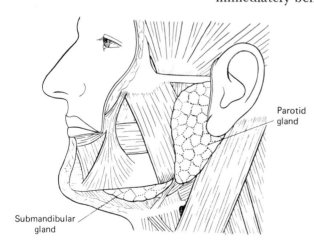

Figure 20.3. Major salivary glands

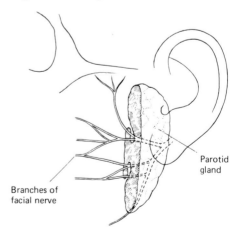

Figure 20.4. Parotid gland and facial nerve

Neck

The neck supports the heavy and highly mobile head; its central vertebral column is therefore surrounded on all sides by a thick layer of muscles. Anterior to this thick layer of muscles lie the other important structures of the neck — the midline viscera, that is, the tongue, larynx, pharynx, trachea and thyroid gland and on each side the carotid sheath covered by the sternomastoid muscle. The spaces of the rest of the neck are filled in by fatty tissue, with salivary tissue in the upper parts of the neck, interspersed richly with lymphoid tissue, and the whole encased in layers of fascia.

The vertebral column and its surrounding layer of muscles are of little surgical interest but the other tissues will now be described in more detail.

Midline viscera

In the centre of the neck lie the pharynx, larynx, trachea, tongue and thyroid gland. The pharynx consists of three parts: the nasopharynx lying posterior to the nose and closed inferiorly by the soft palate; the oropharynx, continuous above with the nasopharynx, anteriorly with the oral cavity and inferiorly with the hypopharynx; and the hypopharynx which lies lateral and posterior to the larynx and leads into the oesophagus. The nasopharynx contains the adenoids in

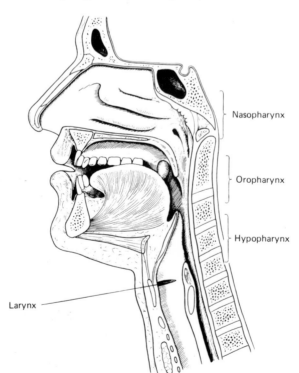

Nasopharynx

Oropharynx

Hypopharynx

Larynx

Figure 20.5. Larynx and pharynx

the middle of its posterior wall, and the oropharynx has the tonsils on its lateral wall; the adenoids and tonsils are collections of lymphoid tissue of surgical importance in childhood.

The larynx produces sound (phonation); it also has other functions, notably preventing the inhalation of food. The larynx leads downwards into the trachea, part of which lies in the root of the neck (*Figure 20.5*).

On each side of the trachea lie the lobes of the thyroid gland, which are described in Chapter 19.

Carotid sheath

Immediately lateral to the midline viscera lie the carotid arteries, the internal jugular vein and the vagus nerve encased in the carotid sheath. The common carotid arteries enter the neck at the thoracic inlet, just behind the medial end of each clavicle. They run vertically upwards, giving off no branches until they reach the level of the hyoid bone, where they divide into the internal and external carotid arteries. The internal carotid artery continues upwards, without giving off any branches, and enters the skull, through its base, to supply the brain. The external carotid artery, however, divides up into a large number of branches which supply blood to all the structures of the neck and to the head except the contents of the skull.

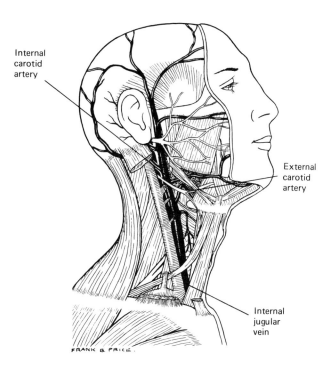

Internal carotid artery

External carotid artery

Internal jugular vein

FRANK G. PRICE.

Figure 20.6. Carotid arterial system and internal jugular vein

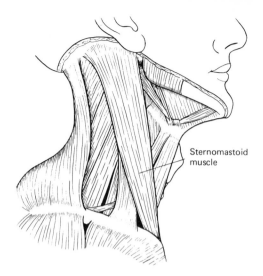
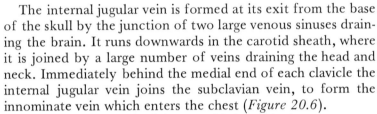

Figure 20.7. Muscles of the neck

The internal jugular vein is formed at its exit from the base of the skull by the junction of two large venous sinuses draining the brain. It runs downwards in the carotid sheath, where it is joined by a large number of veins draining the head and neck. Immediately behind the medial end of each clavicle the internal jugular vein joins the subclavian vein, to form the innominate vein which enters the chest (*Figure 20.6*).

The third structure of the carotid sheath is the vagus nerve which arises in the medulla, leaves the base of the skull and runs through the neck towards its destination in the thoracic and abdominal viscera. In the neck it gives off branches to the pharynx and at the root of the neck on the right side the recurrent laryngeal nerve, the main motor and sensory nerve of the larynx. On the left side, the recurrent laryngeal nerve arises at the level of the aortic arch and runs upwards in the tracheo-oesophageal groove to reach the neck.

The sternomastoid muscle The carotid sheath is covered by the sternomastoid muscle, whose function is to flex and rotate the head, and which forms a prominent mass in the lateral part of the neck, dividing it into the anterior triangle above, and the posterior triangle below (*Figure 20.7*). The posterior triangle consists of little but fat and blood vessels, but the anterior triangle contains the submandibular salivary gland.

Lymphoid tissue

Three hundred of the body's 800 lymph nodes are contained in the neck and arranged in groups (*Figure 20.8*), the highest of which is a circle round the upper part of the neck draining the skin of the scalp and face, the tonsils, the nose, sinuses

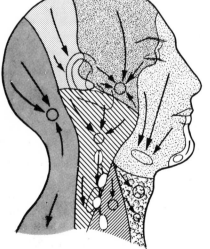

Figure 20.8. Lymphatic system of the head and neck

and floor of the mouth and the lips. Efferent lymph channels run downwards from these nodes to a large chain in the carotid sheath known as the jugular chain. The jugular lymph trunk finally drains into the internal jugular vein low in the neck.

Fascia

The contents of the neck are bound together by layers of fascia. The muscles surrounding the vertebral column are covered by the prevertebral fascia, while the front of the neck is covered by an investing layer of fascia which splits to include the sternomastoid muscle. The pharynx is covered laterally and posteriorly by a layer of fascia, which continues downwards into the mediastinum behind the pharynx and oesophagus, forming the retro- and parapharyngeal space. Attached to the larynx is the pretracheal fascia, which splits to enclose the thyroid gland, and also continues downwards into the mediastinum, anterior to the trachea. Structures within this fascial layer, including the thyroid gland, move up and down when the patient swallows.

PHYSIOLOGY

The principal functions of the mouth are eating and speaking. In eating, food introduced into the mouth is chewed by the teeth to convert it into a semi-solid mass called a bolus. This bolus is then propelled backwards into the pharynx by the mobile part of the tongue, where it is pushed downwards by the base of the tongue, and is then carried down the oesophagus by peristalsis. Speech consists of two phases: phonation in which a sound is produced by the larynx, and articulation in which the sound so produced is modified by the lips, tongue and teeth to produce recognizable speech.

The function of the salivary glands is to produce saliva. Unlike all other glands connected with the digestive tract they are not motivated by hormones, and are stimulated solely by nervous reflex action. Their resting secretion is nil, so that we wake up in the morning with a dry mouth. Food placed in the mouth stimulates the afferent side of the salivary reflex, and the glands are stimulated to produce saliva; it is also said that the sight, thought and smell of food have the same effect, as shown in experiments on dogs, but this is uncertain. Saliva is a watery matter with a few substances dissolved in it — an enzyme ptyalin, which helps in the early stages of food breakdown, mucus and several inorganic compounds, including calcium and sodium. About 1500 ml of saliva are produced every day, although this figure may vary.

PATHOLOGY

It will be obvious from the above anatomical description that there is a rich variety of tissue present in the head and neck; and in each of these tissues a variety of diseases can occur. The pathology of these diseases is as follows, subdivided into the tissue of origin.

(1) Skin:
>   branchial cyst;
>   dermoid cyst;
>   tumours.

(2) Subcutaneous tissue:
>   lipoma.

(3) Nerves:
>   **neurofibroma**;
>   **neurilemmoma**.

(4) Blood vessels:
>   arteries — carotid body tumour (chemodectoma);
>   veins — haemangioma.

(5) Lymph glands and lymphatics:
>   congenital — cystic **hygroma**;
>   lymphadenitis — secondary to acute or chronic non-specific inflammation of the ear, nose or throat; primary acute infections (infectious mononucleosis, toxoplasmosis); specific chronic inflammatory diseases (tuberculosis, syphilis);
>   tumours — primary (**reticulosis**, Hodgkin's disease, lymphosarcoma, reticulum cell sarcoma, follicular lymphoma, leukaemia); secondary — any malignancy anywhere may metastasize to the nodes in the neck but the common sites are nasopharynx, hypopharynx, lung, stomach;
>   miscellaneous — sarcoid.

(6) Salivary tissue: the submandibular gland, and the tail of the parotid gland, included in the neck. Common diseases of the salivary glands include:
>   inflammation — specific (mumps); non-specific (usually secondary to calculi);
>   calculi (much commoner in the duct of the submandibular gland); and
>   tumours — benign (90 per cent) ('mixed tumour' sometimes called pleomorphic adenoma); malignant (10 per cent) (adenoid cystic carcinoma, cylindroma).

(7) Thyroid gland:
>   multinodular goitre;
>   solitary adenoma;
>   carcinoma;
>   thyroglossal cyst.

These are all considered elsewhere.

Neurofibroma A benign tumour composed of nervous and fibrous tissue.

Neurilemmoma A benign tumour arising from a nerve sheath.

Hygroma A benign cystic tumour of lymphatic tissue.

Reticulosis Disease of the reticuloendothelial system (i.e. the lymph nodes, spleen and bone marrow). It is part of the body defence mechanism against infection.

(8) Larynx and pharynx:
   laryngocoele;
   pharyngeal pouch.
   Both conditions may present as swellings in the neck and therefore are considered here.
   Other diseases of the pharynx and larynx are dealt with in ear, nose and throat textbooks.
(9) Mouth:
   ulceration — **aphthous ulcers**; dental trauma; syphilis and tuberculosis; carcinoma;
   infection — **Vincent's angina**;
   tumours — papilloma, carcinoma.

DIAGNOSIS

A large number of diseases can arise from the different structures within the neck; they virtually all present with a lump in the neck, and this is a common clinical problem for the surgeon. This section will deal with the investigations which are done to establish a diagnosis in such a patient. The usual steps of history, clinical examination, laboratory investigations, radiology, endoscopy, and possibly biopsy must be adhered to.

History

The age of the patient is important — below the age of 20 years a neck mass is probably inflammatory or congenital in origin, between 20 and 40 years of age it could be an inflammatory process or a reticulosis, and above the age of 40 much the most likely cause is malignancy.

The lump may have appeared suddenly and be continuously painful, when it is likely to be inflammatory; it may be painless and have been present for a few weeks, when it is probably malignant; it may have been present for months, when it is probably tuberculous; or it may have been present for years when it is likely to be something unusual such as a carotid body tumour.

Certain swellings in the neck communicate with the mouth, pharynx or larynx; they therefore contain fluid, air or food, and fluctuate in size. Lumps which fluctuate in size include a laryngocoele, which is continuous with the larynx, a pharyngeal pouch, low on the left side of the neck which fills on eating, a branchial cyst, and a submandibular calculus

Laryngocoele An air-containing pouch connected with the cavity of the larynx.

Aphthous ulcers Shallow painful erosions, usually of the mouth.

Vincent's angina An acute ulcerated and membranous infection of the tonsil.

which causes pain and swelling of the submandibular gland with eating.

Since the swelling of the neck may well be secondary to disease elsewhere, the patient should be asked about symptoms of local disease in the head and neck, and elsewhere. He thus may have a history of unilateral **epistaxis** or deafness if an enlarged lymph gland is secondary to carcinoma of the nasopharynx.

Common diseases which metastasize via the thoracic duct to the lymph nodes of the neck are carcinoma of the stomach and bronchus, and the appropriate symptoms will then be present.

Finally there may be generalized symptoms such as fever in inflammatory lesions, and loss of weight in malignancy.

Examination

The mass itself is examined first to find out its site, shape, size, fluctuation and fixation to surrounding tissue. A few lesions can be diagnosed definitely from their site — for instance, a midline swelling above the larynx which moves when the tongue is protruded is almost certainly a thyroglossal cyst. Lumps arising from the thyroid gland are usually obvious by their position, and move on swallowing — as do all masses within the pretracheal fascia including laryngocoeles and tumours of the laryngeal cartilages.

Shape, size and consistency of a mass give little help in its diagnosis. It is said that Hodgkin's lymph nodes feel rubbery, and that malignant nodes feel hard, but this is a very variable impression. Masses which fluctuate have already been mentioned above.

A mass which invades surrounding structures is almost certainly malignant. The rare carotid body tumour, which lies in the upper part of the neck, can be moved from side to side, but not up and down.

The areas which drain lymph to the nodes of the neck are then examined carefully — the scalp, ears, nose, nasopharynx, mouth (particularly the alveolingual sulcus because tumours here may be missed); the pharynx and larynx must usually be examined with mirrors by an ear, nose and throat specialist.

The rest of the body is now examined, particular attention being paid to the axillae, groins, liver and spleen if reticulosis is suspected, and the upper abdomen and testes if a visceral malignancy is thought to be the basic cause of an enlarged node in the neck.

Epistaxis A nose-bleed.

Laboratory investigations

The following laboratory investigations may be needed.

Haematology

It is usual to estimate the haemoglobin content, on general grounds, the erythrocyte sedimentation rate (ESR) which may be raised in malignancy and tuberculosis, and the white cell count and differential, which is abnormal in leukaemias and in infectious mononucleosis. Diagnosis of the latter is confirmed by the Paul—Bunnell test.

Bacteriology

In acute infections such as tonsillitis, a throat swab will show the responsible organism, usually the haemolytic streptococcus, if the infection is bacterial.

In syphilis, the usual serological investigations should be done.

Two skin tests may be needed—Mantoux test in tuberculosis and Kveim test in sarcoid disease.

Radiology

Two radiographs are done as a routine: a plain radiograph of the neck and a chest radiograph. Others may be needed in special circumstances.

A plain radiograph of the neck may demonstrate many different conditions: calcification in tubercular nodes, cervical ribs, stones in the submandibular gland, compression or deviation of the trachea by a thyroid mass, a laryngocoele, and the presence of air in a pharyngeal pouch.

A chest radiograph may show tuberculosis, enlargement of the mediastinal glands in reticulosis, or a primary carcinoma of the lung. Any of these diseases may be the primary cause of a mass in the neck. In addition, a chest radiograph is needed as part of the assessment of the patient's general health.

Special radiographs which may be needed include a barium swallow and meal to show up a tumour of the pharynx, oesophagus or stomach; an intravenous pyelogram if a renal tumour is suspected; a carotid angiogram if the mass is thought to be a carotid body tumour, or if it involves the common or internal carotid artery.

If the mass is in the thyroid gland, or is a secondary from a primary carcinoma of this gland a thyroid scan will be needed.

Endoscopy

The primary cause of an enlarged node in the neck often lies in the nasopharynx or hypopharynx so that these areas require examination under anaesthetic.

Biopsy

Biopsy is seldom indicated or justifiable in arriving at the diagnosis of the cause of a lump in the neck. The purpose of a biopsy is to confirm and not to establish a diagnosis, which will virtually always be made by clinical examination detailed above. Furthermore, there is the danger of dissemination of a malignant tumour. Most carcinomas of the upper respiratory tract have a reasonably high cure rate when treated by radiotherapy or surgery, but if a secondary lymph node is operated upon and the tumour spreads within the tissues of the neck, the possibility of cure is drastically reduced.

MANAGEMENT

Before considering the management of individual conditions the pre- and postoperative management common to all operations on the neck will be considered; any special points will be discussed as they arise.

GENERAL OPERATIVE MANAGEMENT

Preoperative preparation

Skin

It is important, particularly in men, to shave the neck before operation. If an extensive operation, such as a radical neck dissection, is to be done, the skin over the mastoid process and over the chest down to the nipple must also be shaved.

Feeding tube

After many operations on the head and neck, the patient may be unable to swallow for a few days and a nasogastric tube must often therefore be passed before the operation.

Position of the patient

For virtually all operations in the neck, optimum access must be gained by extending the neck. If the operation is on the centre of the neck, this is done by placing a sandbag between the shoulders, but if the operation is on the side of the neck, e.g. a radical neck dissection, the sandbag is placed under the shoulder on the same side to extend the neck and to turn it to the opposite side.

Postoperative care

General care

The usual care of all major operations is needed. Many patients have temporary interference with their swallowing after neck surgery, and need feeding via a nasogastric tube; it is also usual to leave an intravenous infusion running after the operation and continue this until the next morning to ensure sufficient intake of fluid. Feeding by mouth or by tube can usually begin the first day after the operation, however major, because the occurrence of paralytic ileus is very unusual after a neck operation. Similarly, electrolyte disturbances are less common after this form of surgery than after abdominal operations, but the electrolytes should be estimated every day or two for the first week; a postoperative check on the haemoglobin is also needed about the third day.

The neck is a difficult area to dress and dressings have very little useful contribution to make if the skin edges are closed properly. Therefore many neck surgeons no longer use them, but if dressing is used, it should be dispensed with as soon as possible after seepage of blood and serum has stopped.

It is very important in a neck operation to produce an invisible scar. It is usual therefore to sew up the skin with fine sutures of non-absorbable material, such as nylon, or to coapt the skin edges in a small collar incision with clips. In either case the strength of the wound depends on a sub-cutaneous layer of catgut sutures; the skin sutures or clips are therefore removed after 72 hours to ensure minimal scarring of the skin. When removing stitches, the cut stitch must be extracted from the skin by pulling towards the wound — pulling away from the wound disrupts its edges.

Most neck operations are carried out in a clean field, and unless the pharynx is opened into, for example, in a laryngectomy, postoperative antibiotics are not used, unless there is established infection of the wound, or the chest.

Drainage

It is vitally important after many neck operations that the skin flaps which were raised at the start of the operation heal by adhering to their underlying bed; they cannot do so if they are lifted away from this bed by blood or serum. It is common practice therefore to use suction drainage. A vacuum must be maintained on this system at all times, otherwise infection can easily be introduced. In smaller wounds, a simple wick type of drain is often used, and this must usually be removed on the first or second day after operation. One ligature is often left untied at the position of the drain; this is tied by the nurse, after removing the drain, so as to oppose the wound edges.

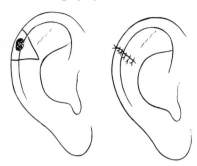

Figure 20.9. Wedge excision of a tumour of the auricle

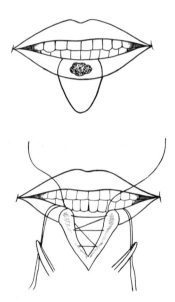

Figure 20.10. Wedge excision of a carcinoma of the lip

Furuncle A localized infection of the skin and subcutaneous tissue by *Staphylococcus aureus*.

Carbuncle An infection of the skin and subcutaneous tissue by *Staphylococcus aureus* in which there is diffuse necrosis of the subcutaneous tissue.

INDIVIDUAL CONDITIONS

The skin

The lesions of surgical importance on the skin can be classified as sebaceous cysts, dermoids, infections (**furuncles and carbuncles**) and tumours (basal or squamous cell carcinoma).

Sebaceous cysts

Sebaceous cysts are dealt with elsewhere (*see* page 377). They are removed surgically in the usual fashion. Inclusion dermoids occur round the bridge of the nose; they must be differentiated from encephalocoeles which are sacs of herniated meninges and brain. They are usually removed.

Infections

Infections of the skin of the face are potentially dangerous if the area around the nose and eyes is involved, because the venous drainage of this area has communications with the venous sinuses of the brain, particularly the cavernous sinus, so that thrombosis of this sinus can result. Fortunately such infection is now usually controlled by antibiotics.

Tumours

Tumours of the skin of the face are malignant, with the exception of the occasional papilloma. Tumours of the lip are always squamous cell carcinoma, and 9 out of 10 involve the lower lip, about its middle. This tumour occurs in elderly men, exposed to sunlight at work. The commonest tumour on the skin of the face is the basal cell carcinoma or rodent ulcer; squamous cell carcinoma occurs less often. Rodent ulcers usually occur within a triangle bounded by the ear, the outer canthus of the eye and the corner of the mouth. These tumours may be managed with radiotherapy, or may be excised, the resulting defect being closed by undercutting the surrounding tissue to allow closure of the defect by a full-thickness skin graft, or by a local flap of skin.

Tumours of the auricle by contrast are usually squamous cell carcinomas, and involve the rim of the auricle. At this site they are removed by a wedge excision (*Figure 20.9*). If the whole of the auricle is involved, it is excised and replaced by a plastic prosthesis.

Tumours of the lip are dealt with by radiotherapy or by a wedge excision (*Figure 20.10*), the defect then being closed primarily. Large tumours may require resection of a large part of the lower lip, which is then replaced by a flap taken from the upper lip. Because the skin of the rest of the lip is usually also affected by premalignant change, it is usually shaved off and replaced by a flap of mucosa from within the mouth.

The salivary glands

The following diseases commonly occur in the salivary glands.

Inflammation

Inflammation of the salivary glands (sialoadenitis) may be acute or chronic. Acute parotitis occurs in seriously ill dehydrated patients. Because of their dehydration the salivary flow is reduced, allowing organisms to track up the salivary duct. Acute infection of the submandibular gland is usually caused by blockage of its duct by a stone. Chronic inflammation of the parotid gland is also seen, associated with diminution of its secretions.

Virus infection of the parotid gland (mumps) is common.

Stones

The saliva contains several minerals, notably calcium, and since the submandibular duct drains upwards it is not surprising that stones fairly often form in it, leading to obstruction of the duct.

Tumours

Nine out of 10 salivary tumours affect the parotid gland, and 9 out of 10 salivary tumours are benign. The common benign tumour is the so-called 'mixed' tumour, which classically affects the tail of the parotid gland. It grows slowly over many years, and occasionally becomes malignant. The only malignant tumour of importance is the adenoid cystic carcinoma, or cylindroma, which affects usually the minor salivary glands within the mouth, particularly those of the hard palate.

Radiological investigation

Stones in the submandibular duct may be demonstrated by plain radiograph. Any mass in the parotid or submandibular gland is usually investigated by sialography, in which radio-opaque dye is introduced in the duct of the gland; subsequent radiographs then show up a filling defect in tumours, or dilatation of the ducts (sialectasis) in chronic infection. Occasionally the ability of the gland to secrete is measured by cannulating the duct and measuring the response to stimulation with pilocarpine; the response is reduced in chronic infection.

Acute sialoadenitis

In parotitis there is pain, swelling and redness over the parotid gland; pus is usually to be seen emerging from the parotid duct, and in addition to the dehydration and illness of the

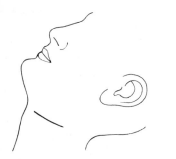

Figure 20.11. Incision for removal of the submandibular gland

intercurrent disease, the patient has a fever. Treatment is carried out by antibiotics, and drainage if the infection fails to respond rapidly.

Acute infection of the submandibular gland may spread within the tissues of the neck — the so-called Ludwig's angina. Apart from local pain, tenderness and swelling, there is then extensive cellulitis and oedema of the neck, and because of pressure on the larynx, also stridor. In that case a tracheostomy may be necessary, at the same time the infection being treated by antibiotics, and incision and drainage. After the acute phase, the diseased gland, with the stone in its duct, is removed.

Calculi

Stones usually affect the submandibular duct, and cause pain and swelling of the appropriate gland with eating. The stone can often be felt in the duct, within the mouth, and is usually demonstrated by a plain radiograph. If the stone is in the duct, it can be removed by an incision over it, within the mouth. If the stone is within the gland, however, the gland must be removed. This is done via an incision in a skin crease over the

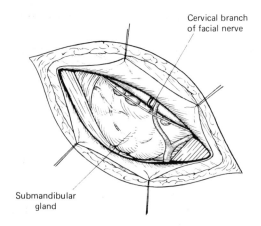

Figure 20.12. Exposure of the submandibular gland after elevation of the skin flaps

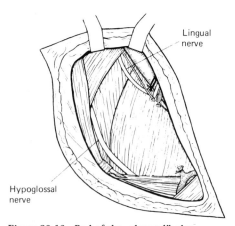

Figure 20.13. Bed of the submandibular gland after its removal

hyoid bone, so placed that the cervical branch of the facial nerve is not damaged (*Figures 20.11* and *20.12*). The gland is dissected, preserving the underlying hypoglossal and lingual nerves, and its duct is tied off (*Figure 20.13*). It is then removed and the skin closed.

Tumours

Mixed tumours of the parotid gland present as a slowly growing lump in the tail of the gland. There are usually no other symptoms, and the facial nerve is never paralysed by this tumour. The appearance of pain usually indicates malignant changes, as does a facial paralysis, but this is uncommon.

These tumours are treated by superficial parotidectomy, in which all the superficial lobe of the gland (from which these tumours virtually always arise) is dissected off the facial nerve, which is thus preserved with almost no risk of permanent paralysis. The alternative method of enucleating the tumour by blind dissection quite often causes facial paralysis and recurrence of the tumour, because small seedlings are left behind. Tumours of the minor salivary glands, usually adenoid cystic carcinomas, are treated by wide excision of the lesion within the mouth.

The mouth

The lesions of surgical interest in the mouth are ranulas, ulceration, infection and tumours.

Ranula

A ranula is a cystic swelling lying at the front of the mouth beneath the tip of the tongue. It is thought by some to be a retention cyst of one of the mucosal glands and by others to be a lymphangioma.

There are no symptoms of this swelling apart from its size. Ranula is difficult to remove with a guarantee that it will not recur, and it is usually therefore easier to marsupialize the cyst — that is, to remove the roof of the cyst, leaving its floor as part of the floor of the mouth.

Ulceration

There are several different causes of ulceration with the mouth.

Aphthous ulcers are small, about 5 mm in diameter, with a grey base; they are painful, and tend to occur in crops, usually on the inner surface of the lower lip. Their cause is unknown, and there is no specific treatment for them; they usually heal spontaneously in 1 to 2 weeks.

Dental ulcers usually occur on the lateral border of the tongue, due to trauma from jagged teeth or ill-fitting dentures. The treatment is that of the cause.

Agranulocytosis, that is relative or complete absence of white cells from the blood due commonly to leukaemia or chloramphenicol intoxication, may present with numerous small shallow ulcers within the mouth. The treatment is also that of the cause.

Syphilis and tuberculosis are both causes of ulceration in the mouth which are now rarely seen in this country.

Inflammation

Infections within the mouth include Vincent's angina and thrush. Vincent's angina is due to two bacterial organisms, a spirochaete and a bacillus. There are multiple small painful ulcers, usually affecting the gums. The condition is usually only seen in people who are in poor general health, in whom it can be highly contagious. The condition responds well to local painting of the ulcers with methylene blue, supported by systemic administration of penicillin. Thrush is due to infection by *candida* and is usually seen in patients treated with broad spectrum antibiotics. It is treated by withdrawal of antibiotics and the administration of nystatin.

Tumours

Small papillomas are occasionally seen in the mouth, but the most common and most important tumour is the carcinoma, which is always squamous in type. The common sites are the lateral border of the tongue, the inner surface of the cheek, and the lateral part of the floor of the mouth. About 40 per cent of these patients have an enlarged lymph node in the neck, classically the jugulo-omohyoid node, which lies just below the middle of the jugular chain.

Patients with this tumour are usually aware of its presence, and present because of this. There may also be difficulty in swallowing and referred pain to the ear on the same side. Because of the difficulty in swallowing there is often loss of weight. The diagnosis is confirmed by a biopsy. If the tumour lies close to the mandible, radiographs should be taken to show bone destruction.

These tumours may be treated either by surgery or by radiotherapy. If the tumour is fairly small and there is no bone erosion on radiographs of the mandible, there is a high chance of curing it by an implant of radium needles. A radical neck dissection is done if there are enlarged lymph nodes in the neck (*see below*). If the tumour is large, if it recurs after radiotherapy or if there is bone erosion, then it is treated surgically by a wide excision, including part of the tongue (hemiglossectomy) and usually part of the mandible also (hemimandibulectomy).

The neck

Some of the more important lesions within the neck will now be described.

Branchial cyst

This cyst which is probably not of congenital origin but due to an inclusion in a lymph node lies at the level of the upper part of the sternomastoid muscle, between the internal and external carotid arteries. It should be removed via a horizontal incision. The cyst is dissected out, taking care not to damage adjacent structures, particularly the internal and external carotid arteries, and the hypoglossal nerve.

Dermoid cyst

These cysts, due to the congenital inclusion of epithelium, occur uncommonly in the upper midline of the neck. They present in young adults, with an otherwise asymptomatic swelling, and are removed via a collar incision high in the neck.

Lipoma

A lipoma may present as a soft smooth subcutaneous swelling at any site in the neck. It is usual to remove it via a small horizontal incision.

Nerve tumour

Tumours arising from nerves include neurofibromas and Schwannomas. Neurofibromata are usually multiple, and associated with staining of the skin (café-au-lait spots), the syndrome of Recklinghausen. Schwannomas are solitary tumours arising from the nerve sheath of any of the nerves in the neck but more particularly the vagus.

Solitary Schwannomas may present because of a lump in the neck or, if the tumour arises from the vagus, with a swelling protruding into the pharynx. There are usually symptoms of involvement of the appropriate nerve: paraesthesia and numbness in its area of distribution if it is a sensory nerve, or paralysis if it is a motor nerve.

It is usual to remove such tumours through a horizontal incision.

Blood vessels

Carotid body tumour

A carotid body tumour arises from the carotid body, which is a small collection of nervous tissue, sensitive to changes in pH of the blood, lying in the bifurcation of the internal and external carotid artery. It grows very slowly, and rarely metastasizes, that is, it is a benign tumour. It is rare.

There are few symptoms of this tumour other than a slowly growing mass in the neck. The diagnosis is usually confirmed by a carotid angiogram.

It is sometimes justifiable to remove this tumour, but because it involves the internal carotid artery, there is a danger of death or hemiplegia after the operation. To protect the cerebral circulation, hypothermia and carotid by-pass may be needed.

Haemangioma

Haemangiomas may occur in the head and neck, particularly in the parotid region, where they form the commonest tumour of childhood. These tumours are described in more detail in Chapter 17.

Lymph glands and lymphatics

Lymphangioma (cystic hygroma) is described in Chapter 17.

Acute infection

Any group of lymph nodes may become enlarged as a result of infection of an area from which the node collects lymph. The commonest in practice is probably the jugulodigastric node, which enlarges in tonsillitis. The treatment of this is that of the underlying conditions, usually with antibiotics.

Acute enlargement of the lymph nodes also occurs in glandular fever and certain similar conditions. Glandular fever (mononucleosis) is thought to be associated with the Epstein–Barr virus; it is a disease of young adults, commonest in summer, and said to be spread by kissing.

The patient usually feels unwell, has a fever, and painful swelling of the lymph nodes of the neck, usually those at the middle or the upper end of the jugular chain, can be observed. Other lymph nodes in the axillae may be enlarged, as may also the liver and spleen. Pharyngitis is often found in these patients, with quite severe and persistent sore throat, and there is occasionally a rash, jaundice or polyneuritis.

The Paul–Bunnell test, a blood test showing antibodies to sheep's red cells, is positive in this disease. The lymphocyte count of the blood is also raised, with many abnormal cells and monocytes.

There is no medical or surgical treatment of this disease, which is allowed to burn itself out. This may take many weeks or months, during which time the patient feels generally unwell and lethargic.

Chronic infection – tuberculosis and syphilis

The lymph nodes may be secondarily infected from any chronic infection in the head and neck, particularly the tonsil. They may also be specifically involved by tuberculosis and syphilis.

Tubercular glands of the neck were once very common; recently this disease has become less common and has changed in character. Previously the infection in children was often observed to be of the bovine type spreading from cow to man via infected milk; the organism gained entry to the lymphatic system via the tonsil. In more technologically advanced countries, however, the most common infection is that of the human type, spreading from man to man by infected saliva. Furthermore, it is now found mainly in older people, in whom presumably the infection has lain dormant for many years, to become active again for some unknown reason.

A cervical lymphadenopathy also occurs in children due to a related organism, the so-called anonymous mycobacteria.

Tuberculous lymphadenitis usually presents with a mass in the neck, commonly affecting the upper end of the jugular chain. Initially there are no other symptoms, unless there is tuberculous disease present elsewhere, particularly in the lungs. After a lapse of weeks or months an abscess is formed, which may be either 'cold' or 'hot' — the former is due to tuberculous pus, the latter to secondary infection by pyogenic organisms. If cold, the abscess is usually of the 'collar stud' type, because it tracks between fascial layers, forming two abscess cavities joined by a narrow isthmus. Eventually, in either case, the overlying skin becomes involved, and the abscess bursts forming a discharging sinus which does not heal unless the infection is treated. In Great Britain today progress beyond the stage of a hard neck mass is unusual.

Tuberculous glands of the neck are now usually treated medically, by a combination of one or more of the following drugs: streptomycin, isoniazid or para-aminosalicylic acid (PAS). Surgery is seldom needed, but it may be necessary to excise locally any remaining enlarged nodes after medical treatment and abscesses may occasionally need to be drained.

Enlarged neck nodes are said to occur at any stage of syphilis — from a primary **chancre** within the mouth, to a snail track ulcer during the secondary stage and in the tertiary phase of the disease. This disease is now rarely seen in Great Britain, however.

Malignancy

The lymphatic system of the neck drains the entire head and neck; also because the thoracic duct ends in the internal jugular vein or the subclavian vein, lymph from the rest of the body may find its way into the cervical system. The lymph nodes of the neck may thus become involved by malignancy of virtually any part of the body; if this involvement is secondary to tumours of the head and neck, the disease is still treatable; if, however, it is secondary to visceral malignancy, it indicates widespread metastases.

Tumours at almost any site in the head and neck metastasize to the lymph nodes in the neck, but this happens at some sites more than at others, particularly the nasopharynx, and

Chancre The primary ulcer of syphilis.

the piriform fossa. At both these sites an enlarged node in the neck may be the first and only symptom of a carcinoma; the dangers of carrying out an open biopsy of such a mass before looking for the primary tumour have already been mentioned.

The lymphatic system of the neck can be described as being 'closed'. That is, lymph cannot spread from it in all directions, as in the abdomen, but can only spread in an orderly manner from one node to the next, ultimately leaving the system by one channel only, where it joins the internal jugular vein. For this reason carcinomas of the head and neck remain for a long time localized to the neck, and only in a late stage of the disease do they metastasize to a distance, usually the lungs. They can thus be treated, usually with a reasonable chance of success, by dealing with the primary tumour, and the nodes of the neck, if these are involved.

As regards treatment of the primary tumour, for example, in the larynx, pharynx or tongue, there are two possible forms of treatment — radiation or surgery. Either of these may be used in certain circumstances, but the relative merits of each will not be considered here. As regards lymph node involvement, however, there is little doubt that the treatment should be surgical, since radiotherapy seldom sterilizes carcinoma in a lymph node. The operation is called a radical neck dissection, and it may be carried out either in continuity with the removal of the primary tumour, for example, a laryngectomy, or may be done on its own after the primary tumour has been controlled by radiotherapy — for example, by the insertion of radium needles into a carcinoma of the tongue.

Operative treatment

It will be presumed here that the operation is being carried out on its own for a primary tumour which has been controlled by radiotherapy; in other words no other adjacent structure, such as the larynx, is being removed in continuity with the radical neck dissection. The operation is therefore carried out under a general endotracheal anaesthetic with the patient in the supine position, with his neck extended and turned to the opposite side, by a pillow under the ipsilateral shoulder; this position is very important to allow the surgeon easy access to the site to be operated on.

Various incisions have been described for this operation, but the most common one is a 'Y'-type of incision (*Figure 20.14*). After making the incision, skin flaps are raised up to the mandible, down to the clavicle, back to the trapezius muscle and forward to the midline (*Figure 20.15*).

The entire lymph-bearing area of the neck between these limits is then removed in one block; this involves removal not

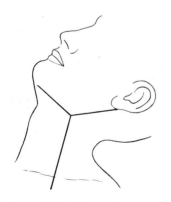

Figure 20.14. Skin incision for radical neck dissection

only of the lymph nodes and their surrounding fat, but also of the sternomastoid muscle, the internal jugular vein, and also the submandibular gland; the accessory nerve is inevitably divided. However, the carotid sheath, the vagus and the hypoglossal nerves are preserved.

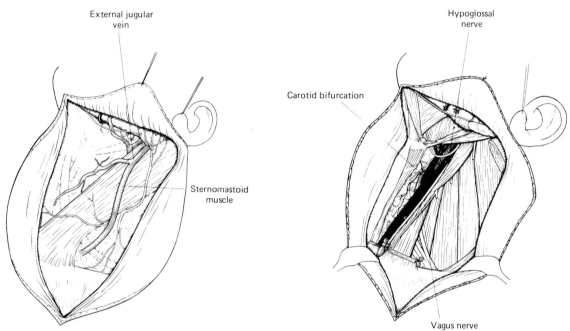

Figure 20.15. Radical neck dissection: view of the neck after elevation of skin flaps

Figure 20.16. Radical neck dissection: tissues of the neck after completion of the operation

At the end of the operation (*Figure 20.16*) a closed suction drain is stitched beneath the flaps, which are then closed.

Postoperative care

The general postoperative care of patients after neck operations has already been detailed above; all parts of it apply to radical neck dissection.

It is important to follow up patients after this operation, because of the possibility of recurrence of the tumour at the primary site, and because an enlarged lymph node may appear on the other side of the neck; both of these conditions require further treatment and the patient should be seen at monthly intervals for the first year and thereafter every 3 months or so.

Primary tumours

Primary tumours of the lymph nodes occur fairly often in the neck. The commonest of these is Hodgkin's disease, but reticulum cell sarcoma and lymphosarcoma also occur; the latter two may manifest themselves as primary involvement of the lymph nodes or may be associated with a similar tumour of the tonsil; furthermore, sarcomatous enlargement of the lymph nodes often occurs during the course of the leukaemias, particularly acute lymphatic leukaemia in children, and chronic lymphatic leukaemia in the elderly.

The disease is commonest in young adults, particularly men. A smooth rubbery enlargement of one or more glands of the neck can be observed. There is also often enlargement of nodes in the axillae and groins, and of the liver and spleen.

Generalized symptoms occur later in the disease — **pruritus** and fever — which may be intermittent of the wellknown but rare variety known as Pel—Ebstein fever. The patient also becomes weak due to anaemia. Laboratory investigations are otherwise usually normal; a chest radiograph sometimes shows widening of the mediastinum due to enlarged nodes there. The diagnosis is confirmed by biopsy.

The further investigation and treatment of this disease are discussed in Chapter 10.

Thyroid and parathyroid glands are discussed elsewhere (*see* Chapter 19).

Larynx and pharynx

Laryngocoele

Laryngocoele is an air-containing diverticulum arising from within the larynx just above the vocal cords, passing behind the thyrohyoid membrane to cause a swelling in the lateral part of the neck.

A swelling just above and lateral to the larynx can be found, which is fluctuant and painless, and sometimes disappears when it empties. It shows up on a plain radiograph of the neck as an air-containing space.

The cyst enlarges slowly and eventually either becomes infected or compresses the airway and should therefore be removed: after exposure via a collar incision the cyst is dissected free and divided at its neck where it emerges from the larynx.

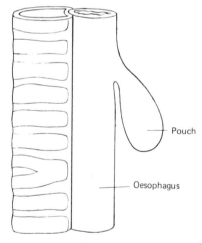

Figure 20.17. Pharyngeal pouch

Pharyngeal pouch

A pharyngeal pouch is a diverticulum, occurring in the elderly, which arises from the junction of the pharynx and oesophagus (*Figure 20.17*). The junction of the pharynx and oesophagus is guarded by a sphincter consisting of two sets of muscle fibres, one placed horizontally and the other obliquely; there is thus a gap, posteriorly, of unsupported mucous membrane.

Pruritus Itching.

It is thought that the diverticulum is caused by inefficient or ill-timed relaxation of the lower horizontal sphincter, allowing pressure to build up in this part of the pharynx, and herniating the mucous membrane outwards. The pouch so formed passes downwards next to the oesophagus, and compresses it.

This is a disease of the elderly, with long-standing and progressive difficulty in swallowing food, causing loss of weight. Food is regurgitated in an undigested form and tends to spill over into the trachea causing recurrent respiratory infections.

The pouch is clearly demonstrated by a barium swallow and the patient should also have an oesophagoscopy carried out to exclude the presence of a carcinoma within the pouch.

If the patient is fit, he should be treated for this condition by one of two operations.

The party wall between the pouch and the oesophagus can be divided by cutting **diathermy** via an endoscope. This is a satisfactory palliative operation for elderly frail patients.

Alternatively, the pouch can be removed by an external approach. It is usual to carry out an oesophagoscopy immediately before the operation, to wash out the pouch, and pack it with sterile gauze, so that it can be identified.

A collar incision is then made over the pouch, which is exposed by dissecting medial to the carotid sheath. The pouch is dissected out and removed and the defect in the pharynx repaired. It is also usual to divide the muscle fibres of the sphincter below it to prevent recurrence.

After the operation the patient is usually given antibiotics because the pharynx has been opened and he must be fed through a nasogastric tube for a week until the pharynx heals. He can then begin swallowing and needs no further treatment or follow-up.

Diathermy Intense local heat, generated in a blade or needle by a high frequency electric current, which may be used to seal bleeding vessels or cut tissues.

21

Surgery of the oesophagus

B. J. Bickford

ANATOMY AND PHYSIOLOGY

The oesophagus is a muscular tube which runs from the pharynx above to the stomach below. In the neck it lies behind the trachea, and in the chest it is in the posterior mediastinum behind the heart. It lies in front of the bodies of the vertebrae, somewhat to the right in the upper part of the chest, distinctly to the left lower down. The thoracic surgeon divides the oesophagus in the chest into thirds; the upper third is above the aortic arch, the middle above the inferior pulmonary vein and the lower below this again (*Figure 21.1*). The oesophagus enters the abdominal cavity through the oesophageal hiatus, which is a gap in the muscle tissue of the diaphragm. A very short length of the oesophagus is actually within the abdominal cavity. The junction with the stomach is referred to, rather imprecisely, as the 'cardia'.

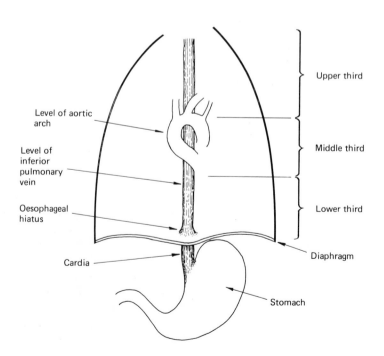

Figure 21.1. Diagram of anatomy of thoracic portion of the oesophagus. A very short length of oesophagus is in the abdominal cavity. This is attached to the oesophageal hiatus by the phreno-oesophageal ligament and ensures that there is an angle between the lower segment of the oesophagus and the fundus of the stomach

454

The wall of the oesophagus is mainly smooth muscle arranged in both longitudinal and circular fibres. The mucosa is stratified squamous in type, without glands. The transition to gastric mucosa is somewhat indefinite, and a certain amount of 'gastric' mucosa is often to be found above the cardia.

The cricopharyngeus acts as a sphincter at the upper end and the circular muscle coat acts as a rather weak one at the lower end. The oesophagus transmits food, drink and saliva by peristaltic action. The abdominal pressure is higher than the intrathoracic pressure at most times and to prevent reflux of gastric contents into the oesophagus during straining Nature provides a special mechanism at the cardia. The main component of this is the angle between the stomach and the oesophagus, which is maintained by the firm fixation of the lowest part of the oesophagus to the edges of the hiatus it passes through. The lower sphincter plays some part but it seems that the main thing which prevents reflux is compression of the cardia by the fundus of the stomach when the intra-abdominal pressure is raised (*Figure 21.2*). This mechanism is overcome in the act of vomiting, and also in 'burping' swallowed air.

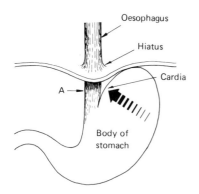

Figure 21.2. Diagram showing points in the anatomy of the cardia. The angle (A) between stomach and the lower part of oesophagus ensures that the cardia will tend to close when pressure rises inside the stomach. This is the main factor preventing reflux of gastric contents into the oesophagus

DISEASES OF THE OESOPHAGUS

Congenital disorders

Such disorders, apart from *oesophageal atresia* (p. 143), are rare. A *double lumen* or a *mediastinal cyst* lined with a gastric type of mucosa may occur. *Hiatus hernia* with reflux of gastric contents occurs in babies, presumably as a result of a weak attachment of the lower oesophagus to the hiatus.

Functional disorders

The most important is *cardiospasm* or *achalasia of the cardia*. Neither term defines the nature of the condition well; the gross abnormality of the oesophagus is variable but it does become dilated and shows no effective peristaltic contraction. The muscle coat in general is much thicker than normal, and the cardiac sphincter remains tightly contracted. Undigested food, particularly vegetable matter, accumulates in the oesophagus, and may cause attacks of 'pneumonia' through spill-over into the trachea at night. There is a distinct tendency to the development of a carcinoma after some years, probably as the result of stagnation of foodstuffs in the lumen. The cause of the condition is degeneration of the nerve cells in the oesophageal wall, but why this should happen is not known. In mild cases no treatment is required, but the disease tends to be progressive and relief is required sooner or later. Most surgeons believe that *myotomy* of the tight lower sphincter (Heller's operation) is the best treatment. There is some evidence that dilatation of the sphincter with an inflatable balloon filled with opaque solution and observed in the x-ray room is almost as good. However, neither method deals with the lack of motility in the oesophagus; in certain cases it seems better to excise the functionless organ and replace it by stomach or colon.

Diffuse spasm of the oesophagus may respond to oral diazepam, but sometimes myotomy is required.

Corrosive burns

Burns of the oesophagus follow drinking of fluids such as caustic soda, strong acids, bleach etc. This may be by accidental or by suicidal intent. Early treatment by prednisolone in high dosage with progressive reduction will prevent much stricture formation, but it must be used early. If a stricture forms it has to be treated by dilatation; if there is a severe burn the oesophagus shortens leading to a hiatus hernia and a 'peptic' stricture as well. Excision of the oesophagus may well have to be carried out if the stricture causes long-term difficulties.

Swallowed foreign bodies

Coins, bones, large lumps of unchewed meat and dentures etc. may stick above the aortic arch or in the lower third of the oesophagus. They can usually be removed at oesophagoscopy; on occasion it is safer to push them on into the stomach.

Perforation of the oesophagus

This is most often the result of a difficult oesophagoscopy or attempt at dilatation of a stricture. Except for minute tears in the cervical oesophagus surgery is always required as an urgency. The accident is almost always followed by severe pain in the chest or the back. X-ray investigation with a Gastrografin swallow is indicated to confirm the diagnosis and indicate the site of the leak.

Spontaneous rupture of the oesophagus

This may follow vomiting, especially after overindulgence in food or drink. It may be mistaken for a perforated peptic ulcer or a coronary thrombosis. The important physical sign

Gastrografin Water soluble radiographic contrast medium containing iodine, and especially formulated for gastrointestinal use.

in any oesophageal tear is the appearance of air in the tissues of the neck. This has a characteristic feel. Urgent surgery is required to repair the tear; if there is a long delay before operating the chances of recovery fade progressively, since there will always be a degree of infection in the mediastinum (*Figure 21.3*).

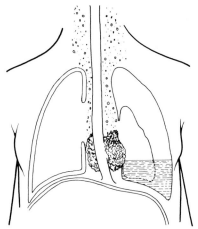

Figure 21.3. Perforation of the oesophagus leading to a mediastinal abscess, pyopneumothorax and air in the neck tissues

Hiatus hernia

This is not strictly an oesophageal condition, but is conveniently discussed here since the only organ importantly affected is the oesophagus. The condition is essentially due to widening of the oesophageal hiatus and weakening of the connective tissue which normally attaches the oesophagus to the edges of the hiatus. The precise cause is not known; hiatus hernia is seen in infancy, and again in middle-aged and elderly people. In babies, a period of strict avoidance of lying flat seems usually to effect a cure. This area is evidently a 'weak' point of body design, and the fact that it is seen most commonly in plump middle-aged women suggests that some 'degenerative' factor is partly responsible.

There are two types of hiatus hernia – 'sliding' or 'rolling' ('para-oesophageal'). The sliding type is much the commoner. The hiatus is unduly wide and the stomach finds its way up into the chest under the influence of the normally higher pressure in the abdomen compared with that in the chest. The gastro-oesophageal angle is straightened out and the most important mechanism for preventing reflux into the oesophagus is lost (*Figure 21.4*). Only the weak lower oesophageal sphincter remains. Some people with a hiatus

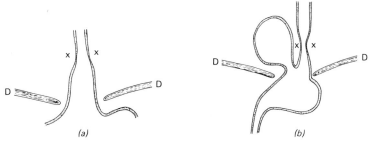

Figure 21.4. (a) 'Sliding' hiatus hernia; (b) 'rolling' or para-oesophageal hiatus hernia. Note that in (a) the gastro-oesophageal junction (XX) is above the hiatus in the diaphragm (DD) up into the chest through the enlarged oesophageal hiatus. Thus the normal oesophagogastric angle is no longer present and a rise in abdominal or intragastric pressure will allow free reflux into the oesophagus, while in (b) it stays in the normal position

hernia on x-ray have no real symptoms, but typically the complaint is almost entirely attributable to the effect of reflux of digestive gastric juice into the oesophagus, the lining of which is not designed to withstand it. The most characteristic symptom is a burning sensation behind the lower part of the sternum frequently accompanied by a bitter taste in the throat; both occur mainly when lying flat or stooping forward and are aggravated by spicy or fatty food. This is popularly referred to as 'heartburn'. Continued reflux results in chronic irritation of the lining mucosa of the oesophagus, perhaps with actual ulceration. The wall of the oesophagus becomes thickened and vascular. Fibrosis later results in shortening of the oesophagus and stricture formation. The patient will then complain of difficulty in swallowing.

'Rolling' or para-oesophageal hiatus hernia

This is relatively rare; some hiatal muscle fibres are intact, so that the cardia remains in place while the stomach turns over so that a large part of it, with the greater curvature and omental tissue, passes up into the chest, usually more to the right than to the left side (*Figure 21.4b*). Surprisingly, symptoms tend to be few, apart from shortness of breath after meals. There is a danger of strangulation, with vomiting and rapid dehydration needing early surgical relief.

Carcinoma of the oesophagus

This is a most serious complaint. It can affect any part of the oesophagus, but is most common in the lower third. Neoplasms here tend to be constrictive in nature and cause symptoms relatively early, whereas in the middle third of the organ they are soft and bulky, often invading the mediastinum before causing serious swallowing problems. Carcinoma of the cardiac end of the stomach surrounds the entry of the oesophagus into the stomach in a typical 'mushroom' shape. Most cancers of the oesophagus are of the squamous celled type; all those at the cardia are adenocarcinomas, as are a small proportion of those in the lower third of the oesophagus proper. Distant metastases are rather rare, probably because life is threatened by dysphagia at an early stage of the disease. Local lymphatics in the mediastinum and the pre-scalene nodes in the neck are involved, and metastases in the liver are common. Carcinoma of the cardia may spread widely in the peritoneal cavity.

SYMPTOMS OF OESOPHAGEAL DISEASE

Difficulty in swallowing ('dysphagia') is by far the most important symptom of oesophageal disease. Sometimes thought to be of 'nervous' origin, it is usually due to organic disease and must be regarded as such until proved otherwise. Dysphagia usually begins with difficulty in eating solids; liquids are then involved and in the final stages the situation is miserable in that even saliva cannot be kept down. If symptoms progress slowly, patients tend to minimize them by adjusting to softer diet. This may mislead the doctor also. Symptoms are little different whatever the cause of the obstruction. The patient may or may not have a good idea of the level of obstruction. A benign stricture causing dysphagia may have been preceded by a long history of heartburn, not necessarily severe. In achalasia (cardiospasm) dysphagia is often intermittent at first; the history tends to be long and the patient may bring-up food he has eaten several days earlier.

'Heartburn'

This is an important symptom which has already been described. It is also referred to as 'acidity' by patients, and clarification of what the patient actually means by these terms must be sought by careful questioning (p. 458).

Pain

Pain is an uncommon symptom in oesophageal disease. It may be felt during swallowing in some cases of localized spasm, and occasionally in patients with a malignant tumour.

INVESTIGATION OF OESOPHAGEAL DISEASE

Clinical examination is usually rather unhelpful in making a diagnosis. Weight loss may be obvious, and there may be other signs of malnutrition and in some instances actual dehydration. There may be enlargement of the liver, ascites and enlarged lymph nodes in the neck in advanced disease.

The opaque swallow

The most important radiological investigation is the opaque swallow, usually with barium paste; the plain chest x-ray must not be omitted. The barium swallow will show alterations in diameter and contour of the oesophagus as well as demonstrating any obstruction. The radiologist will detect abnormal peristaltic activity, and by tipping the head end of the table steeply down will be able to demonstrate whether there is any gastro-oesophageal reflux. Without this manoeuvre, many cases of reducible sliding hiatus hernia will escape detection. A watery opaque solution will be used when there is any suspicion of a perforation of the oesophagus.

Oesophagoscopy

This has in the past been performed with a simple rigid tubular instrument (*Figure 21.5*). Marks on the outside indicate how far (in cm) the end of the instrument is from the upper teeth. The cardia is usually reached at 40 cm. The instrument must be passed with great care as it is not difficult

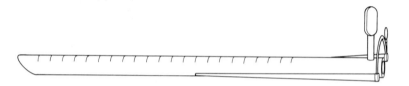

Figure 21.5. Oesophagoscope (Rigid Negus instrument)

to injure the delicate wall of the oesophagus if it is handled roughly. The flexible fibre-optic oesophagoscope is being used more frequently for diagnostic purposes. It has the advantage that it can be passed without a general anaesthetic; also the stomach can be inspected as well as the oesophagus. The rigid instrument may have advantages when a foreign body is being removed, a stricture dilated, or an inoperable neoplasm intubated although recent developments have allowed fibre-optic instruments to be used for these procedures also.

By passing a double or triple lumen tube attached to a recording manometer, it is possible to measure the pressure in the oesophagus at different levels. This is helpful in determining the cause of symptoms and in the diagnosis of specific diseases such as achalasia or oesophageal reflux. The degree of acidity of the oesophageal contents at various levels can also be recorded.

SURGICAL TREATMENT OF OESOPHAGEAL DISORDERS

Surgery is not indicated unless simpler means of treatment fail; organic obstruction of the oesophagus does, however, mean that active treatment is necessary.

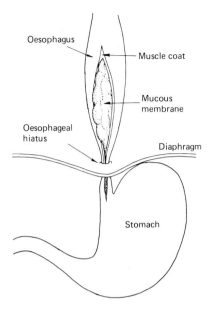

Figure 21.6. Heller's operation for cardiospasm (cardiomyotomy). A longitudinal incision is made in the muscular coats of the oesophagus reaching down to the cardia. The mucous membrane bulges through but is not damaged. Note the considerably dilated oesophagus

Heller's operation

This operation for achalasia has been briefly described (*Figure 21.6*). Through a thoracotomy the oesophagus is mobilized and the thickened muscle coat is divided carefully down to, but not through, the mucous membrane. It is important to extend this 'myotomy' onto the stomach and to make sure that the attachment of the oesophagus to the edges of the hiatus has been restored by suture, or reflux will result.

Repair of a hiatus hernia

This continues to be a matter of controversy. Chest surgeons regard a thoracic approach as preferable to an abdominal one as it is possible to visualize the anatomy so much better. If the stomach can be replaced beneath the diaphragm and the wide hiatus narrowed so as to stop it from slipping up again reflux will be stopped. The difficulty is that sutures may eventually cut out from the muscle into which they must be inserted; also, if the oesophagus is fibrosed as a result of severe reflux there will be shortening of the organ and tension on the repair. The repair is often supplemented by folding the stomach round the oesophagus in some way (Belsey Mark IV and Nissen operations). But the very nature of the condition makes it certain that a number of recurrences will take place after a time. In most series at least 85 per cent of patients are satisfied, and only 5 per cent unrelieved.

Resection of the oesophagus

This is indicated for neoplasms of the oesophagus and cardia. The usual operation for either site is virtually the same (oesophagogastrectomy *Figure 21.7*). The chief difference is in the length of oesophagus removed. Totally radical operations are poorly tolerated, but it is wise to remove as much of the oesophagus as possible in cases of carcinoma of this organ. The area is exposed by a thoracolaparotomy through the 6th or 8th space; some surgeons prefer a laparotomy followed by a right thoracotomy for growths in the middle third. The retained portion of stomach is brought up into the chest, or even into the neck, and anastomosed to the oesophagus. Great care is taken with this suture line, as damage to the tissues or to their blood supply may lead to a disastrous leak afterwards. After division of the oesophagus the vagi are interrupted and there is a tendency to dilatation of the stomach and to spasm of the pyloric sphincter. If the latter seems feeble at operation, it may be

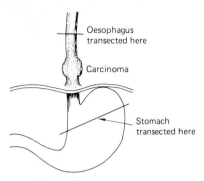

Oesophagus
transected here

Carcinoma

Stomach
transected here

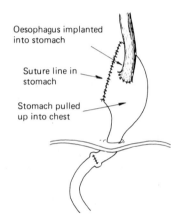

Oesophagus implanted
into stomach

Suture line in
stomach

Stomach pulled
up into chest

sufficient to stretch it digitally; if it is thick it will be wise to divide either the muscle coat (pyloromyotomy) or to perform a pyloroplasty. As there will be no efficient anti-reflux mechanism after oesophagogastrectomy, the patient should take a regular antacid in the hope of being able to prevent late stricture formation; this is always a risk with long survival, unfortunately.

Replacement of the oesophagus

This is indicated when there is disease in a length of the oesophagus which cannot be restored to normal functioning. Long caustic strictures, peptic strictures with hiatus hernia intractable to other methods and, rarely, cases of gross achalasia may be best treated in this way. The stomach is kept in its normal place beneath the diaphragm. The organ most suited to replace the oesophagus is the left part of the colon, i.e. the region of the splenic flexure with a variable length of descending and transverse colon (*Figure 21.8*). The colon segment depends for its nutrition on its own arteries and veins, so the greatest care must be taken not to injure them or obstruct them in any way. The colon can easily

Figure 21.7. Oesophagogastrectomy for carcinoma of lower oesophagus or cardia. After transection of the stomach and oesophagus the remainder of the stomach is pulled up into the chest through the oesophageal hiatus and the oesophagus is anastomosed to it

Figure 21.8. Diagrams to show method of colonic replacement of oesophagus. (1) Hiatus hernia with long stricture of oesophagus. (2) Colonic replacement of stenosed oesophagus.

A, Stenosed oesophagus;
B, Transverse colon with (C) hepatic and (D) splenic flexures;
X–X   lines of transection of colon (and
Y–Y   corresponding anastomoses with oesophagus and back of stomach);
E, Re-anastomosis of colon;
F, Colonic blood vessels

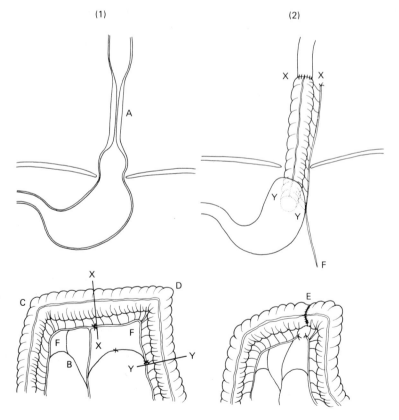

(1)   (2)

reach the neck if the lower end is anastomosed to the stomach below the diaphragm. The results of surgery are good; swallowing, which had been unsatisfactory beforehand, with the need for frequent dilatations, is much improved though often food goes down rather more slowly than normal. The operation of *colonic interposition*, as it is called, should not be performed in fat patients (in whom it is difficult to see the precise details of the blood supply to the colon) or in elderly patients (who may have atheromatous changes in the arteries). Before operation it is wise to 'prepare' the colon as for operation on the colon itself with wash-outs and antibacterial agents (kanamycin and metronidazole is a good combination).

Palliative surgery of the oesophagus

This is mainly concerned with the relief of dysphagia in patients who are not suitable for major surgery, or who are not sufficiently bothered by their complaint to need operation.

For benign ('peptic') stricture, which in the majority of instances is associated with a sliding hiatus hernia, dilatation of the oesophagus with soft graduated **bougies** at oesophagoscopy may suffice. This, however, tends to lead to more pronounced reflux, with gradual recurrence of dysphagia. If the procedure is only required once or twice a year the patient may well prefer this to a major operation. It is also true that many of these patients are in their 8th or 9th decade and on this count alone are not good subjects for surgery. Some patients can maintain an adequate 'swallow' by self-bougienage, swallowing a mercury-filled Hurst bougie daily or every few days at home.

Palliation for inoperable carcinoma is a difficult problem. If the patient is fit, it may be best to resect the neoplasm in the standard way even if there are secondaries in the liver. Survival may not be for long, but the quality of swallowing should be good. The same considerations apply to by-passing a malignant stricture with stomach, colon or jejunum. These are, however, very major procedures and may not be well tolerated. Palliative intubation with a gold-plated coiled wire tube (Souttar's tube) (*Figure 21.9*) can give good results if a wide enough tube can be pushed through the strictured area. There is a real danger of perforating the oesophagus in doing this, and this accident will almost certainly prove fatal. Various other forms of intubation exist, among them the Mousseau–Barbin plastic tube (*Figure 21.10*) or its modification by Celestin. This can be pulled down from the mouth after a small incision has been made in the stomach and a bougie pushed through the growth area from below. The redundant portion of tube is then cut off and the lower

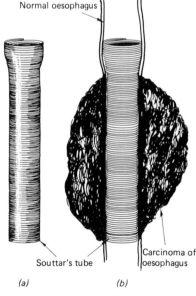

Normal oesophagus

Souttar's tube

Carcinoma of oesophagus

(a)   (b)

Figure 21.9. (*a*) Souttar's tube. (*b*) Souttar's tube relieves dysphagia after being passed through carcinomatous stricture of the oesophagus

Bougie Tapered, often flexible, surgical instrument for passing into and dilating body passages, especially if narrowed by stricture.

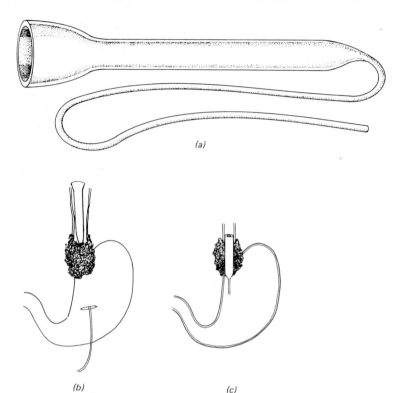

Figure 21.10. (*a*) Mousseau—Barbin tube. (*b*) The tube has been pulled down into the stomach by a small incision in the anterior wall. The cardiac end of the stomach is occupied by a carcinoma which blocks the lumen. (*c*) The tube has been cut off below the growth in the stomach and the incision in the stomach sutured

end of the tube is sutured to the wall of the stomach. This procedure may work very well provided the patient can be persuaded to keep to a really soft diet. It has the disadvantage of often producing severe gastro-oesophageal reflux, which cannot be controlled and is unpleasant for the patient.

RESULTS OF SURGERY FOR CARCINOMA OF OESOPHAGUS AND CARDIA

It is agreed that surgery for carcinoma of the oesophagus and cardia is palliative rather than radical in nature. Attempts at too radical extirpation result in physiological difficulties which make the quality of life unduly poor for the patient as well as leading to a higher mortality. Overall, perhaps 75 per cent of patients with cancer of the oesophagus can have the obstructing growth removed; with a cancer in the lower third the operative mortality is not more than 5 per cent. At higher levels removal tends to be less often possible and the mortality is considerably higher. In general a mortality of 12 to 15 per cent is likely. About 20 to 25 per cent of survivors will be alive 5 years later. For cancer of the cardia the results are much less good; only about 50 per cent will be resectable,

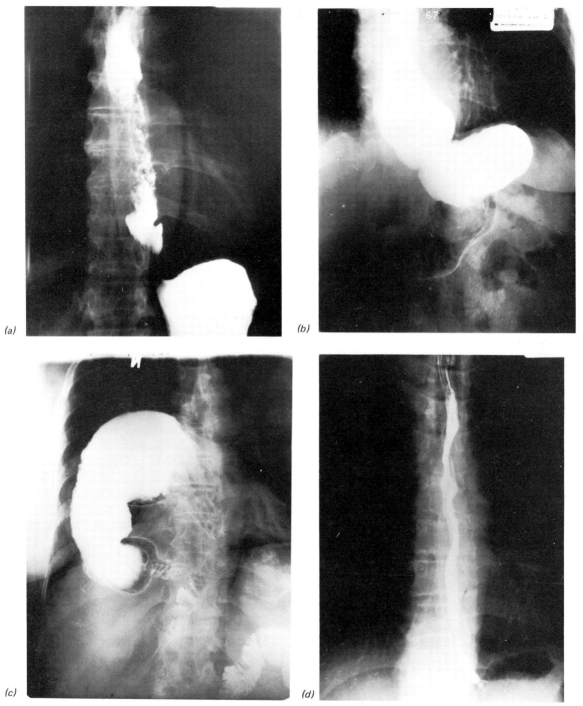

(a)

(b)

(c)

(d)

Figure 21.11 (a) Barium swallow film showing large filling defect in the mid-oesophagus due to extensive carcinoma. (b) Barium swallow with patient tilted head down (Trendelenburg position). There is a large sliding hiatus hernia with reflux into the oesophagus from the stomach. (c) Barium meal showing enormous para-oesophageal hiatus hernia with volvulus of stomach. The stomach occupies a good deal of the right hemithorax and is completely inverted. (d) Barium swallow: the oesophagus is outlined by radio-opaque barium paste. Curved impressions on the left side of the oesophagus are due to the aorta above and the left main bronchus lower down. Barium can be seen just entering the stomach beneath the diaphragm; there is air in the upper part of the stomach

and the 5-year survival will be about 10 to 15 per cent of survivors of resection. The results of elective intubation or by-pass are worse still, with a hospital mortality of the order of 20 per cent and an average postoperative survival of 5 months. Some of these patients will, however, have been able to swallow almost normally.

A NOTE ON FEEDING AFTER OESOPHAGEAL SURGERY

After an uncomplicated and well performed oesophageal resection there is no need to anticipate that a leak may occur from the anastomosis. It will certainly be wise not to give anything by mouth for at least 24 hours and one should not commence oral feeding in any event until peristaltic sounds can be heard in the abdomen with the stethoscope. The patient will have to have his main supply of fluid and electrolytes intravenously for at least the first 3 or 4 days after operation, and he should be warned about this beforehand. If he is well hydrated, he will be swallowing saliva and in the writer's opinion there is every reason to give small amounts of water every hour by mouth. To begin with, 30 ml is a convenient amount and this can be stepped up to 60 ml hourly the next day, then 90 ml and so on. Pain after swallowing may indicate a leak, and a Gastrografin swallow should be done if this is suspected. At 120 ml hourly, the feeds can be made more nutritious with milk, and genuine 'slops' can soon be given. It is most important that any food which does turn to a pulp in the mouth is not given for the first 14 days after operation. Total fluid intake in the first few days must be kept up to 2.5 to 3 litres each 24 hours; whether **hyperalimentation** should be used in all cases is a matter for debate. No doubt in theory this is proper, but it does introduce difficulties by requiring a long intravenous line and careful monitoring. In poor risk cases this will in any event be wise. It is true that unexpected complications may need prolonged intravenous feeding, and that there will be better control of the situation if this had provided calories and adequate nitrogen from the beginning. It is essential that no patient who is dehydrated, anaemic or hypoproteinaemic should be submitted to major surgery until this has been corrected.

It is not necessary to pass a nasogastric tube after oesophageal surgery; it makes the patient uncomfortable and serves no useful purpose. The one reason for a tube is if there should be slow emptying of the stomach. If the stomach is getting full it will readily be seen on the postoperative chest x-ray. This must be obtained daily at first, less often after

Hyperalimentation Excessive feeding; either by mouth in excess of the demands of the appetite, in which case it may be forced, or intravenously.

3 or 4 days. Delay in emptying of the stomach is liable to occur after oesophageal resection, as the vagus nerves have been divided and spasm of the pyloric sphincter may occur.

These remarks about feeding apply to cases in which an incision has been made in the oesophagus and sutured. More care should be taken after repair of a perforated or ruptured oesophagus, especially if there has been a delay of more than 6 to 8 hours before repair. Reliance will prudently have to be placed on intragastric feeding by a nasogastric tube, but in many instances greater security will be given by gastrostomy feeding until it is quite certain that the injured oesophagus has healed as shown by a normal Gastrografin swallow.

22 Surgery of the stomach and duodenum

John McFarland

ANATOMY AND PHYSIOLOGY

Anatomy

The stomach is the expanded upper part of the alimentary canal and lies in the upper abdomen. The oesophagus enters it at its upper end, just below the diaphragm, and this point is suspended by fascia and other tissues underlying and, partly covered by, peritoneum, the surface of which is a thin membrane of flat cells. Below this point the front and back of the stomach are almost wholly covered by peritoneum. Two coats of smooth (involuntary) muscle lie deep to this and the inside of the stomach is lined by mucous membrane. Its size and shape, when empty, is quite variable and depends mainly on the physique of the subject. In an adult food or fluid may stretch the stomach to a capacity of 1 litre or so, but distension to this degree would be uncomfortable for some people.

Towards the lower end of the stomach the muscle layer begins to thicken to where, at the pylorus, it forms a sphincter. Contraction of the muscle at this point can separate the stomach from the duodenum. This is a tube of constant diameter about 25 cm long. Unlike the stomach it lies behind the peritoneum for most of its length. The gross structure of the alimentary canal at the duodenum is continued through the small intestine. However, the duodenum terminates at its junction with the jejunum (the duodenojejunal flexure) and from this point the alimentary canal is again almost surrounded by peritoneum.

The stomach may be considered as having a fundus, body and antrum (*Figure 22.1*). The cardiac area is a small part of the fundus adjacent to the oesophagus; the pyloric canal is the distal part of the antrum. Although these divisions are not clear-cut on superficial inspection, they are important because of the different microscopic appearances of each part. The mucosa throughout consists of a surface epithelium of columnar cells. From this extend pits into which the gastric glands open. Two important cell types in the glands are

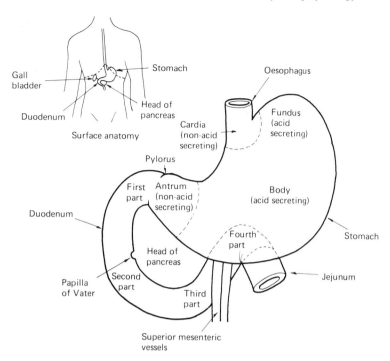

Figure 22.1. Diagram of anatomy and
divisions of the stomach and duodenum

zymogen (chief) cells (producing pepsinogen, converted by
acid to pepsin) and parietal (oxyntic) cells (producing hydrochloric acid). Zymogen and parietal cells are present in greatest
concentration in the body and are virtually absent in the
pyloric canal and cardiac areas. Secretion here is mainly of
alkaline mucus.

The muscle wall of the duodenum is similar to, but thinner
than, that of the stomach. The mucous membrane is covered
by mucus-secreting columnar cells as in the stomach. Pits
lined by similar cells extend towards the deeper layers. Deep
to the pits and connecting with them lie more mucus-secreting
cells (Brunner's glands) and into the lumen project numerous
villi (relatively long processes also covered with columnar
epithelium). These are characteristic of the whole small
intestine whereas towards the duodenojejunal flexure the
Brunner's glands disappear.

For the stomach and duodenum arterial blood supply
(from the coeliac axis of the aorta), venous drainage (to the
portal vein), and lymphatic drainage (to the para-aortic
nodes), are profuse. The autonomic nerve supply is from the

vagus nerve (parasympathetic) and the sympathetic nerve plexuses derived from the sixth to ninth thoracic spinal cord segments.

It is usual, but not invariable, for the bile and pancreatic ducts to have a common opening near the middle of the medial wall of the duodenum.

The stomach lies to the left and the duodenum to the right of the midline because of rotation of the foregut at an early stage in embryological development.

Physiology

The prime role of the alimentary canal is the absorption of food after reducing it to a suitably basic form.

Very little absorption occurs across the wall of the stomach but this muscular pouch has the important function of continuing the mechanical breakdown of food (which has already been chewed in the mouth) and of mixing it with gastric secretions. The two most important of these are hydrochloric acid and pepsin (an enzyme acting on proteins). These arise from the cells described above and the mechanism for this is two-fold. The nervous phase of gastric secretion is initiated by the sight, smell, taste or even thought of food. Nerve impulses pass from the brain centre to the stomach by way of the vagus nerve. There is a small continuous discharge of nerve impulses and even without these stimuli this results in the resting (or basal) secretion. The presence of food in the antrum of the stomach causes the liberation of a chemical, the hormone gastrin, from the mucosa which is carried through the body by the bloodstream. This has the particular effect of stimulating the parietal cells and the result is the hormonal phase of gastric secretion.

Simultaneously with this secretion, gastric muscular activity increases and, particularly in the antrum, circumferential waves of contraction pass down towards the pylorus. Periodically this opens to expel the fluid food homogenate (chyme) into the duodenum. This depresses gastric secretion, an effect mediated by the postulated hormone, enterogastrone.

Chyme is not held in the duodenum but the considerable activity of the muscular wall mixes it with secretions from Brunner's glands and bile and pancreatic enzymes. Absorption starts here but the much greater length of the jejunum and ileum makes them the most important site for this function.

PATHOLOGY

It is usual to consider diseases of the stomach and duodenum together. This has tended to emphasize the similarity of their pathology when, in fact, there are important differences. For example, carcinoma of the stomach is not uncommon but carcinoma of the duodenum is extremely rare. Nonetheless the stomach and duodenum usually act together and appreciation of their physiological concord is essential for a full understanding of the mechanisms and sequelae of their disease. Two examples of disordered pathology (pathophysiology) may be cited.

(1) Excessive vagal stimulation of the stomach (perhaps due to continuing mental stress) may lead to a high level of gastric secretion and may make the subject more vulnerable to duodenal ulceration.

(2) Gross pyloric stenosis will result not only in starvation but also in excessive fluid depletion as fluid, both that taken by mouth and that secreted from the mucosa, cannot pass on and will be vomited. Very large volumes of secreted fluids containing electrolytes may be involved with the result that the patient becomes dehydrated, sodium-deficient, potassium-deficient and **alkalotic**.

The gastric lesions most commonly encountered by the surgeon are gastritis, gastric ulceration and cancer. In the duodenum ulceration and its complications are the major problems. Other tumours of the stomach or duodenum are uncommon and primary cancer of the duodenum is virtually unknown (unless originating at the papilla of Vater). Congenital hypertrophic pyloric stenosis and duodenal obstruction due to atresia or to an annular pancreas are conditions presenting in infancy. The swallowed foreign body is usually a problem of childhood but may, rarely, cause trouble at any time. The surgical rearrangement of the upper alimentary tract may expose the area of operation in particular to possible ulceration or the patient generally to undesirable metabolic change.

Diseases of the stomach

Gastritis

Gastritis could be expected to mean inflammation of the stomach and in some circumstances this is the case. The cause is not usually an infective organism. Gastric acidity is bactericidal and, except as a terminal event, the stomach is very resistant to bacterial invasion. Irritable agents such as alcohol or excessive salicylates (aspirin) or, more acutely, a strong acid or alkali may cause an erosive gastritis. This condition may be associated with systemic disease such as uraemia. The superficial cell layer is lost and the raw surface bleeds readily. The process may extend in places to ulceration into the deeper layers of the stomach wall.

Alkalotic A state in which the body fluids and tissues are more alkaline than normally.

Two particular forms of so-called gastritis do not have such clear aetiology.

Atrophic gastritis is a condition in which the mucosa is extremely thin. Although it is characteristic of this situation that the submucosal vessels may readily be seen through this layer at gastroscopy, the diagnosis can only be confirmed by histological examination of a biopsy specimen. In some instances this type of atrophic gastritis may be associated with a deficiency of intrinsic factor, necessary for the intestinal absorption of vitamin B_{12}. This defect will interfere with red blood cell formation and cause pernicious anaemia (a type of **megaloblastic anaemia**).

Hypertrophic gastritis is the reverse. Mucosal thickness is excessive and this layer is thrown into large folds. An extreme form of this is giant hypertrophic gastritis (Ménétrièr's disease).

Gastric ulcer

Acute ulceration involving only the gastric mucosa is likely to heal unless an associated condition (for example, uraemia or a toxic/debilitating illness) is overwhelming. It may be manifest by the complication of bleeding if the ulcer should breech the wall of an artery.

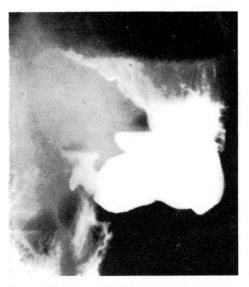 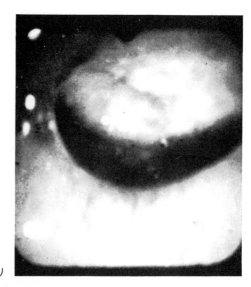

(a)   (b)

Figure 22.2. Gastric ulcer. (*a*) A barium meal radiograph showing a large ulcer crater on the lesser curve of the stomach. There is a fluid level in the crater with a gas shadow above. The duodenum is also deformed due to ulceration. (*b*) A photograph taken at gastroscopy showing the same ulcer. The edge of the crater is smooth and regular. The benign nature of the ulcer was later confirmed at operation

Megaloblastic anaemia Anaemia characterized by the presence of megaloblasts (large primitive red cells) in the blood.

Once the muscle layer has been eroded healing will be associated with some fibrosis and there is a tendency for the ulcer to become chronic. Chronic ulceration is more common in the duodenum than in the stomach (as much as 8:1) with

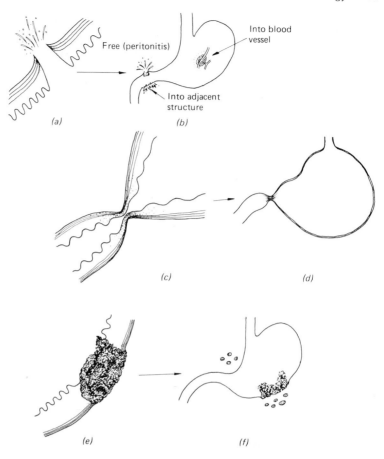

Figure 22.3. Possible complications of ulcer of the stomach and duodenum. (a) Penetration leads to (b) perforation which may be classified as free (peritonitis), into an adjacent structure (e.g. pancreas), or into blood vessel (haematemesis or meleana). (c) Stricture caused by excessive fibrosis leads to (d) stenosis (for example pyloric). (e) Carcinoma (rare in the stomach and almost unknown in the duodenum) which leads to (f) local extension and distant spread of carcinoma

a greater incidence in men (2:1) and a peak in the fifth decade of life. However, these figures have shown a change over the years and there is also considerable geographical variation. This may point to a dietetic or genetic basis of causation (**pathogenesis**) — a subject still open to a great deal of investigation and discussion.

Chronic gastric ulcers are usually situated along the lesser curve of the stomach (*Figure 22.2*). They may be multiple or they may coexist with a duodenal ulcer. When the mucosa is destroyed acid pepsin erodes the muscle wall and perforation may occur either into the peritoneal cavity (causing acute severe peritonitis), into an artery (causing bleeding into the stomach) or into the pancreas which lies against the posterior wall of the stomach (*Figure 22.3*). Microscopic examination

Pathogenesis The origin and development of disease.

W

of the ulcer shows inflammatory change with cellular infiltration and epithelial distortion evident at the edge and fibrosis most marked in the base.

Gastric carcinoma

Gastric carcinoma arises mainly in the fourth to sixth decades of life and the incidence is higher (3:2) in men. The aetiology is unknown but consideration must be given to the importance of genetic factors (geographical differences of incidence are quite striking) and environment, particularly with regard to diet.

There are certain situations with which an increased association of gastric carcinoma has been noted. Thus gastric polyps and gastritis with achlorhydria may be considered to be premalignant. However these are probably important in only a small proportion of instances and the dangers should not be overemphasized.

Carcinoma may arise at any point in the gastric mucosa but 70 per cent occur in the pyloric region. The preference for the lesser curve is not as marked as in benign ulceration. The histological appearance is of an adenocarcinoma but the cellular pattern may range from being well organized (similar to normal mucosa) to complete anaplasia (immature cells with no structural arrangement). The gross presentation may be in several forms.

(1) Ulcerating form may have started as a solid tumour which has undergone central necrosis. Raised irregular edges usually give this an appearance quite different from that of a benign ulcer.

(2) Polypoid form ranges from a small malignant polyp to a massive fungating growth.

(3) Spreading form is a lateral infiltration of the stomach wall without a local mass or evident ulceration. This may be local, most usually at the pylorus, where it spreads circumferentially causing stenosis. Alternatively it may spread diffusely throughout the body of the stomach causing this to be hard and rigid as a 'leather bottle'. This is known as linitis plastica.

(4) Early gastric carcinoma (EGC) is a term used to describe a tiny focus of cancer which involves only the gastric mucosa or submucosa. Diagnosis of lesions as early as this requires expert radiological, gastroscopic and histopathological teamwork. So far the highest yield of the intense and sophisticated mass screening necessary for this has been reported mainly from Japan where gastric carcinoma is particularly prevalent. The results of treatment are excellent particularly when compared

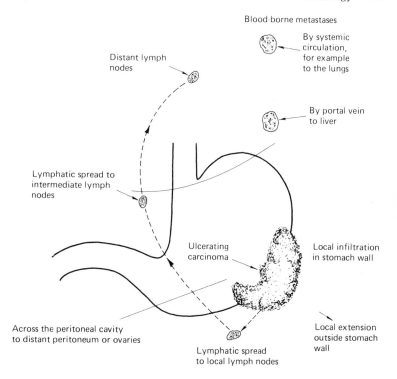

Blood-borne metastases

By systemic circulation, for example to the lungs

By portal vein to liver

Distant lymph nodes

Lymphatic spread to intermediate lymph nodes

Ulcerating carcinoma

Local infiltration in stomach wall

Across the peritoneal cavity to distant peritoneum or ovaries

Lymphatic spread to local lymph nodes

Local extension outside stomach wall

Figure 22.4. Diagram of possible spread of carcinoma of the stomach

with the dismal outlook for most forms of gastric carcinoma.

Spread of gastric carcinoma occurs commonly in four ways (*Figure 22.4*).

(1) Direct extension first within and then through the stomach wall leads to fixation and erosion of adjacent organs such as the pancreas or colon.

(2) Lymphatic spread, initially within the local lymph channels, may spread to the local lymph nodes at an early stage and then along the lymphatics accompanying the vessels to the para-aortic chain. A late stage is the involvement by way of para-aortic spread of a supra-clavicular lymph node, usually in the left side.

(3) In some cases spread may be by free passage of cells across the peritoneal cavity. Seedling deposits grow in the peritoneum of the abdominal viscera, notably the ovaries (Krukenberg tumour).

(4) Blood spread is initially by the portal vein to the liver. Hepatic metastases can grow rapidly to form a total tissue mass larger than the primary growth. Blood-borne metastases elsewhere (lungs, brain, bones) are usually a late event.

Other tumours

Other tumours of the stomach and duodenum are all uncommon. Mucosal polyps may occur in the stomach. Tumours of fat (lipoma), smooth muscle (leiomyoma), nervous tissue (neuroma) or blood vessels (haemangioma) may occur in the stomach or duodenum. These arise from connective tissue and if malignant are sarcomata.

Foreign bodies

A very wide range of objects may be swallowed, most commonly by children (e.g. toys or bits of blankets) or the mentally defective. If they do not lodge in or perforate the pharynx or oesophagus, they pass into the stomach. If this is normal it is unusual for the swallowed object to be retained there or cause trouble. An exception is a hair ball (trichobezoar) which consists of a mass of the subject's ingested hair. This striking problem is, however, very uncommon and usually occurs in women with the neurotic habit of hair-chewing.

Diseases of the duodenum

Duodenal ulcer

The incidence of acute duodenal ulceration is not known. This is because it cannot usually be demonstrated by radiology and, until recently, endoscopic inspection of the duodenum has not been possible. Acute ulceration may give rise to bleeding or perforation or progress to chronic ulceration.

Chronic duodenal ulceration may be a problem at any time of life but is mainly so from the third to sixth decade of life. Men are four times more commonly affected than women. The causative factors of acute ulceration are unknown, nor is it understood why there is progression to chronicity in some instances. Various factors have been extensively studied, most notably gastric acid secretion. This is commonly high in subjects with chronic duodenal ulceration. However, although duodenal ulcers do not occur in the absence of acid, individuals with acid production within the normal range may have every degree of duodenal ulceration and its complications. Clearly other factors must be concerned and poor blood supply, intrinsic defect of the mucosa or the inadequacy of its protective layer of mucus have been suggested.

Chronic duodenal ulcers occur most commonly in the first part of the duodenum. They vary in size but 1 cm is an average diameter. Microscopically non-specific inflammatory changes are evident, the sides are smooth and the base consists of granulation tissue on the muscle wall. Erosion deeper than this may broach a vessel, with resultant haemorrhage, or perforate the wall itself (*Figure 22.3*). In the latter case there will either be free perforation with spillage of duodenal contents into the peritoneal cavity or ulceration into an adjacent viscus (usually the pancreas). Which of these occurs will depend on the location of the ulcer. If the mucosa has been broached, healing will involve fibrosis ('scar tissue'). If the damage has been small, effects will be minimal, but if it has been severe or recurring, considerable deformity may result and will persist. If this is circumferential, stenosis will result. This is called pyloric stenosis and, although it is true that if the ulcer is exactly at the pyloric sphincter stenosis may be more likely and occur earlier, the actual point of hold-up is often in the duodenum.

Postoperative situations

Operative procedures are considered later but reconstruction, whether following gastric resection or 'drainage' is either in continuity (Billroth I; pyloroplasty) or as a by-pass (Billroth II; gastroenterostomy). In either event the mucosa in the area of the anastomosis may be involved with further ulceration (stomal ulcer). This may occur particularly if an operation intended to reduce acidity has been unsuccessful. Such ulceration follows the pattern and may lead to the complications of the benign ulceration already described.

Inadequate tissue removal in cancer cases may later be followed by local recurrence and, of course, the development of metastases in other sites is always possible. Later complications will certainly result when the whole stomach has been removed as the body has been deprived of its source of intrinsic factor and, unless the patient is treated by regular vitamin B_{12} injections, megaloblastic anaemia will develop.

Other problems may result from the inadequacy of the residual stomach in playing its part in the initial digestion of food. This will usually be manifest by the patient's failure to reach a normal weight or by late evidence of dietetic deficiency (**hypochromic anaemia**, low body calcium).

Too rapid a passage of gastric contents from the stomach, particularly when this is into the jejunum as in the Billroth II gastrectomy or gastroenterostomy, may give rise to uncomfortable symptoms following meals (abdominal distension, sweating, faintness and so on). The term 'dumping syndrome' is based on the mechanical explanation of these symptoms.

The incidence of serious diarrhoea after gastric operations is low but in some instances it may be very troublesome. It is most commonly seen after vagotomy with a drainage procedure and its mechanism is not clear.

Hypochromic anaemia Anaemia with decreased haemoglobin due to iron deficiency.

CLINICAL PRESENTATION AND DIAGNOSIS

Clinical presentation may be sudden and severe or insidious. Clearly distinction must be made both in history taking and clinical examination of the acutely ill patient (who may be in severe pain and 'shock') and the one who has a chronic condition.

In the upper gut catastrophies occur when ulceration is complicated by perforation or haemorrhage.

The acute abdomen

The 'acute abdomen' is the descriptive title for a symptom/sign complex caused by severe visceral disease usually with peritoneal involvement arising from one of many acute conditions (*see also* Chapter 26). As the name implies the diagnosis may only be resolved by operation. In perforation of a gastric or duodenal ulcer, the key point in the history is the sudden abdominal pain originating in the epigastrium and, later, spreading all over, sometimes with early emphasis on the right side. Two features are particularly notable when the abdomen is examined. These are the 'board-like' rigidity of abdominal wall (due to extreme spasm of the abdominal muscles following irritation of the parietal peritoneum by gastric contents) and the presence of gas (air) in the peritoneal cavity. Clinical suspicion of this may be reinforced by plain radiology and confirmed by needle aspiration of air and turbid fluid from the peritoneum.

Upper gastrointestinal bleeding

Upper gastrointestinal bleeding is manifested by external evidence, specifically the vomiting of blood either fresh or changed ('coffee-grounds') by gastric activity or the passage of changed blood mixed with the faeces (melaena) which are characteristically black and 'tarry'. Either of these indicates that haemorrhage is arising from a point in the oesophagus, stomach or duodenum. This may occur because acute, or chronic ulceration, or (less commonly) carcinoma, has eroded a blood vessel. Another important although uncommon origin is from oesophageal varices. Chronic blood loss from any of these may appear as 'occult' blood in the faeces (that is, only detectable by chemical testing). It is also important to appreciate that there may be a lag of several hours between a sharp bleed of considerable severity and evidence of this appearing as vomit or in the faeces.

The systemic response of the patient will depend essentially on the amount and rate of the blood loss. Chronic low grade loss may be suspected by the pallor of anaemia. The patient with an acute severe loss may have a low blood pressure and will have a rapid pulse and pallor as a result of the compensatory mechanisms of increased heart rate and peripheral vasoconstriction.

Non-acute presentation is based on consideration of the symptoms of 'indigestion', that is, pain, anorexia, acid regurgitation, flatulence, nausea and vomiting; and of the systemic signs, such as malnutrition, anaemia and weight loss.

Symptoms

Pain

In theory, it should be possible to diagnose gastric and duodenal ulcers by characteristic pain patterns. However, overlap of 'specific' features (for example, pain with the stomach empty for duodenal ulcer, with the stomach full for gastric ulcer) is the rule and pain without any demonstrable ulcer may also be quite severe. The very subjective nature of this symptom makes interpretation difficult but a common pattern is as follows. The patient experiences pain, rather poorly localized in the upper abdomen, which occurs between meals. It may be relieved by food, alkali medicines or following vomiting. Characteristically attacks persist for a matter of days or weeks and are followed by remission lasting months, or even years, but recurrence, at some time, is usual. Persistence of pain suggests severe disease, possibly with localized perforation. If there is reference to the back, pancreatic involvement may be signified.

Pain in gastric carcinoma usually has a late onset.

Anorexia

A poor appetite may be a reflection of the fact that food ingestion results in pain (for example, in gastric ulcer). Or it may be a major feature as in gastric carcinoma when it is usual for patients to have virtually no appetite.

Reflux into the oesophagus

The symptoms of reflux into the oesophagus range from nil to severe dysphagia due to stricture secondary to lower oesophageal ulceration. Retrosternal pain ('heartburn') due to irritation of the already inflamed oesophagus by gastric contents and regurgitation of this into the mouth ('waterbrash') may also occur. These usually imply too large an opening at the oesophageal hiatus in the diaphragm (hiatus hernia). However, reflux (demonstrable by barium meal radiography with the patient in a head-lowered position), may occur without an evident hiatus hernia. Hyperacidity or increased abdominal fullness may aggravate this situation.

Flatulence

A small amount of swallowed air in the stomach is normal. Troublesome symptoms of belching or gastric distension may arise when swallowing is excessive (often a reflex of which the dyspeptic subject is unaware) or gastric emptying is inadequate when there is pyloric spasm or frank stenosis.

Nausea and vomiting

Nausea may occur on its own, but will commonly be a precursor of vomiting or retching. Vomiting may be initiated by gastric stimulation or centrally in the hypothalamus, situated in the brainstem. Pyloric stenosis, whether due to benign or malignant obstruction, will inevitably cause persistent vomiting of all ingested food and fluid.

Signs

Malnutrition, anaemia and weight loss are non-specific. They may be indirect manifestations of benign disease of the stomach and duodenum and, unless, for example, there has been excessive blood loss, will usually be unremarkable in the early stages. They may assume greater significance in malignant disease when local symptoms may be minimal and weight loss, in particular, is a relatively early presenting symptom. However, clinical examination may be uninformative even when severe disease is present. With regard to the alimentary tract the clinician will be examining particularly:

(1) the mouth — a 'dirty' tongue, poor teeth or unpleasant breath may be significant;

(2) the abdomen — distension, excessive peristalsis or even a mass may be evident on inspection. Palpation may reveal, or confirm, a mass or elicit tenderness in the area of an ulcer, although this is not usually marked. The detection of splashing (succussion splash) on brisk palpation of the left upper abdomen indicates fluid and air contents and may indicate pyloric hold-up if a significant time has passed since the patient's last meal or drink; and

(3) the rectum — digital examination *per rectum* (p.r.) is important not only to exclude local disease but because information may be obtained relative to disease elsewhere, e.g. tenderness in pelvic peritonitis following an ulcer perforation or pelvic metastases from a gastric carcinoma.

Significant clinical findings in the abdomen may usefully be indicated in a simple sketch.

Special investigations

Special investigation of the stomach and duodenum may be carried out by: (1) radiology, (2) direct study of function, (3) indirect study, (4) endoscopy, and (5) biopsy.

Radiology

A plain film of the abdomen may give the expert a good deal of information, such as, the characteristics of the gastric air bubble or the presence of gas outside the alimentary canal and so on. However, maximum information is obtained only when the patient swallows a barium mixture (barium meal) which is opaque to the x-rays (*see Figure 22.2*). This is rather thick and if there is an obstruction which may not be easily cleared from the gut, a more fluid agent (Gastrografin) may be preferred although the radiological definition obtained is not so good. The walls of the stomach and duodenum are outlined and the radiologist who is watching these shadows concentrated on a television screen (image-intensified) is able to see the movement as well as the shape of these walls. This may be particularly important as disease in its earliest stage may be manifested by depression of motility or by muscle spasm. The radiographs subsequently available for inspection are 'stills' taken at important points in the screening.

Direct study of function

It has already been described how the ingested food is mixed by the muscle action of the stomach with the hydrochloric acid and pepsin secreted by the gastric mucosa. It would seem to be important for the doctor to know the output of these two substances when he is investigating possible disease and therefore the acid output level has been very extensively studied (pepsin output largely runs parallel to this). There are, however, two problems in the interpretation of the information; firstly, the difficulty of obtaining all the gastric juice secreted over a period and, secondly, the very wide variation in output by people known to be normal. Nonetheless, this information can be useful; perhaps most of all in investigating a patient who has had a previous operation. There are several variations in the technique of study, but a widely accepted method is as follows.

Gastric secretion study

Following an overnight fast the subject swallows a plastic tube with multiple perforations near its tip, which should be radio-opaque. The attachment of an additional very fine tube allows small quantities of air to be injected to clear the tube from the mucosa. Radiological screening ensures that the perforated length of the tube lies in the dependent part of the body of the stomach. The resting juice is then aspirated. Following this the juice is aspirated in 15-minute samples by either hand or mechanical suction. With the latter a negative pressure of 40 mmHg is suitable and constant checks are important. Three basal samples are collected. A subcutaneous injection of pentagastrin (6 µg/kg body weight) is given and six further samples are collected. If the test is done post-operatively and if it is important to test for the completeness of a vagotomy, insulin is injected intravenously (0.15 units/kg body weight) and six samples collected before proceeding to the pentagastrin injection (if these tests are done consecutively it is reasonable to collect, respectively, three, six and four 15-minute samples). Blood is taken for blood sugar levels which must fall below 2.2 mmol per litre (40 mg/100 ml) following the insulin injection. The patient may sweat profusely and even faint should the hypoglycaemia become too great. Oral or intravenous (50 per cent) dextrose solution should be readily available.

Table 22.1   The mean (and range) of basal and peak acid output (mEq/h) in normal subjects and patients with peptic ulcer*

	Normal		Duodenal ulcer		Gastric ulcer	
	Basal	Peak	Basal	Peak	Basal	Peak
Men	1(0–5+)	22(<1–45)	4(0–15+)	42(15–100+)	1(0–5+)	23(3–40)
Women	1(1–5+)	12(<1–30)	2(0– 5+)	32(15–100+)	1(0–2+)	10(1–30)

*From Baron and Lennard-Jones (1971)

Sample volumes, pH and titratable acidity to pH 7 or 7.4, are measured and from these the hydrochloric acid in milli-equivalents (mEq) per sample may be calculated. The basal acid output (BAO) is that for the hour before any stimulation.

The peak acid output following pentagastrin (PAO pg) may be obtained by doubling the sum of the two greatest consecutive 15-minute samples. Results from these tests are shown in Table 22.1.

Interpretation of the insulin test depends on assessment of the figures, increased volume with fall of pH (that is, increased acid) suggesting an incomplete vagotomy.

Indirect study
A full blood count and examination of a blood film are useful to screen for hypochromic anaemia, (suggesting blood loss) or megaloblastic anaemia (suggesting possible gastric intrinsic factor deficiency).

Faecal testing for occult blood is particularly important when hypochromic anaemia has been detected.

Sophisticated tests for serum vitamin B_{12} and urinary vitamin B_{12} excretion (Schilling's test) are indicated in megaloblastic anaemia.

Endoscopy

Modern gastroscopes employing fibre optic technology are highly sophisticated yet slender and flexible (*Figure 22.5*). Light is conducted along a bundle of thousands of very fine quartz fibres from a source external to the patient to illuminate

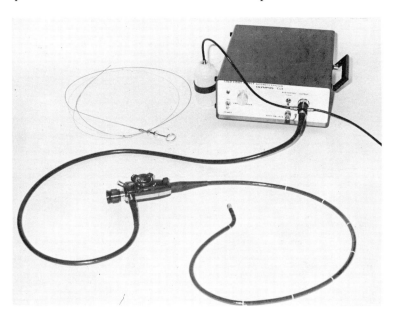

Figure 22.5. Fibre optic endoscope

the inside of the stomach. Another bundle carries the image of the mucosa back to the gastroscopist's eye. There is extreme flexibility which can be controlled to allow inspection in each direction. Furthermore separate channels for air/water infusions and suction biopsy/cannulation may be incorporated while still keeping the gastroscope tube to an overall diameter of 1 cm.

The procedure is carried out on a subject who has fasted overnight. Anaesthesia may be local, with suitable sedation, or general. The whole of the gastric mucosa may be seen and any lesion inspected in detail (*see Figure 22.2b*). This is of the greatest use when a carcinoma is suspected, particularly when the radiological findings have been equivocal.

Duodenoscopy is also possible if the tip of a slender instrument of suitable length is passed through the pylorus into the duodenum. Similarly a postoperative stoma (after gastrectomy, pyloroplasty or gastroenterostomy) may be inspected from the gastric or intestinal side. When stomal ulceration is suspected, such inspection is generally more useful than radiology.

Biopsy

Tissue for histological examination may be obtained from the stomach or duodenum at gastroduodenoscopy. Biopsy under vision with special forceps, introduced through the 'scope, affords accurate removal of tissue from the edge of an ulcer or tumour or the complete removal of a small polyp.

In some instances the microscopic examination of mucosal cells alone may allow a positive diagnosis of cancer. These may be obtained by gastric lavage, but this technique is not in general use.

TREATMENT

Medical treatment

Medical treatment is the first line in uncomplicated gastritis, gastric and duodenal ulcer patients. Until quite recently the following were the staple methods used.

(1) Diet — a bland soft food diet is advised and this may be graded from milk alone through to a normal diet with the exclusion of gastric-stimulating or irritating items such as alcohol, black coffee or pickles. Cigarette smoking has this effect also and is therefore inadvisable. An important point, particularly with duodenal ulcer, is that symptoms are often aggravated by acid flow from the active but empty stomach. Frequent small meals are favoured.

(2) Gastric acid neutralization by alkaline mixtures such as magnesium trisilicate.

(3) Relaxation of smooth muscle spasm as by propantheline bromide (Pro-Banthine).

(4) Symptomatic treatment by sedation — great care must be taken, however, with regard to the ingestion of any gastric erosive agent, such as salicylates.

These measures still have a place but in the last few years chemical agents have been developed which inhibit gastric acid secretion. Cimetidine (Tagamet) is now in clinical use and it has been shown that a 6-week course (cimetidine 200 mg three times a day and 400 mg at night) will result in the healing of 80 per cent of duodenal ulcers. Unfortunately relapse may occur in some 80 per cent of those that heal unless prolonged treatment (cimetidine 400 mg at night) is given but even then relapse may be anticipated in about 20 per cent.

These figures are mentioned to make it clear that at the present time there is still a need for surgery for duodenal ulceration and its complications although there is good reason to expect that further developments will continue to lessen this.

Surgical treatment

When complications of perforation, haemorrhage and stenosis occur, operation is usually mandatory, although the urgency may be a matter of degree. For example, there is a tendency for spontaneous arrest of haemorrhage to occur and it is usually only when this persists or recurs or there are complicating factors that emergency operation is undertaken.

The only chance for a 'cure' in gastric carcinoma lies in early operation in the suitable case. Occasionally if this is not possible, or there is recurrence, regression for a period may follow treatment with cytotoxic agents.

The management of complex postoperative problems must be based on a detailed and accurate assessment of the situation. With a definitive diagnosis, further surgery may be indicated, for example, an inadequate vagotomy may be completed or a stenosis relieved. It is important to appreciate, however, that operations may be expected to have some disadvantages (for example, decrease in stomach size, diarrhoea following vagotomy in some cases and so on) and further operation is not usually the solution.

Preoperative treatment

Preoperative treatment is reasonably standard whatever the operation. It is important that the patient should be, as far as possible, in an optimum condition. This will necessitate a clinical assessment (nutritional and hydration) and radiological (chest radiograph) and laboratory (blood count, electrolyte estimation) studies. Attention will also be paid to dental caries and a predisposition to chest problems. If these give any cause for anxiety, treatment should be undertaken (for example, blood transfusion and calorie and fluid replacement) and, in particular, strict preoperative breathing exercises should be the rule.

The patient should have fasted overnight before the operation and on the morning a nasogastric tube is passed. Some patients find this particularly troublesome and, provided there is no doubt that the stomach is empty (for example, not where there is pyloric stenosis) this may be done after the anaesthetic has been started. The abdomen and pubic area are shaved. Premedication, usually with atropine and sedatives, is given 45 minutes before the operation.

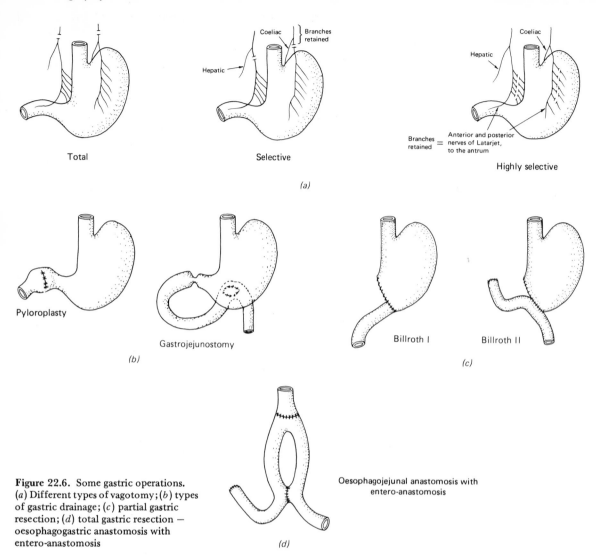

Figure 22.6. Some gastric operations.
(*a*) Different types of vagotomy; (*b*) types
of gastric drainage; (*c*) partial gastric
resection; (*d*) total gastric resection —
oesophagogastric anastomosis with
entero-anastomosis

Operation

Operations are all usually performed under general anaesthesia
and the approach to the upper abdomen is through a vertical
(midline or paramedian) incision. Some gastric operations are
indicated in *Figure 22.6*.

Simple closure of a perforation The edges of the opening are
drawn together with two or three sutures and omentum is
usually tied over. Biopsy at the edge of a gastric ulcer is
advisable if carcinoma is suspected.

Gastrectomy The distal line of resection is usually in the first part of the duodenum and resection should include any ulceration in the duodenum. Gastrectomy is now not commonly done for this disease. The proximal line of resection will either be well clear of a gastric ulcer or very well clear of a carcinoma (to total gastrectomy). Reconstruction depends on the reason for, and degree of, resection. After a partial gastrectomy with a normal duodenum, a reconstruction in continuity (Billroth I) is done. When the disease is in the duodenum or the resection more extensive, the duodenal stump is closed and the gastric remnant anastomosed to the side of the upper jejunum (Billroth II). After total gastric resection a loop of jejunum may be anastomosed to the oesophagus, with a side-to-side jejunal anastomosis to minimize bile reflux into the oesophagus.

Vagotomy with gastric drainage The principle of the operation is the fact that vagal (parasympathetic) section abolishes the nervous phase of gastric acid secretion. 'Drainage' is added because unopposed sympathetic activity will result in pyloric spasm and gastric dilatation in the early stages in some cases. This may be avoided either by a plastic operation to widen the pylorus (pyloroplasty) or by a gastrointestinal short-circuit (gastrojejunostomy).

Vagotomy without gastric drainage Highly selective vagotomy (HSV), which has also been called 'proximal gastric vagotomy' or 'parietal cell vagotomy' (and the latter term is descriptive of the intent: which is to denervate only the bulk of the parietal or acid-secreting cells of the stomach) has now been used for ten years. As the innervation of the pylorus is retained the gastric-emptying mechanism functions satisfactorily after the operation and a 'drainage' procedure is unnecessary. It is attractive because normal mechanisms are interfered with less than in other procedures. It has super-seded selective vagotomy but both are illustrated, alongside total vagotomy, in *Figure 22.6a*.

Gastrotomy The term gastrotomy simply means 'opening the stomach'. Possible indications are to remove a foreign body or to inspect the mucosa for a bleeding point.

Gastrostomy In gastrostomy a passage is established between the stomach and the front of the abdominal wall. It may, as a temporary measure or a last resort, be necessary when a severe or malignant stricture totally obstructs the lower oesophagus.

Postoperative management

The postoperative management will be essentially uneventful in the great majority of cases. The nasogastric tube is retained and aspirated regularly until the patient tolerates oral fluids well; 24 to 48 hours is a usual time. During this period fluid and electrolytes may be given intravenously (2–3 litres of dextrose and saline solutions in 24 hours). Good evidence of the resumption of bowel activity is the passage of gas or faeces, but this may precede adequate gastric emptying and, where there is anxiety, a Gastrografin meal radiograph may be helpful. This is certainly the case following an oesophago-jejunal anastomosis when oral intake should not be recommended until radio-opaque swallow, one week following the operation, has confirmed that the anastomosis is satisfactory.

An upper abdominal drainage tube or wick will commonly be employed in all but the simplest gastroduodenal operations and may usually be removed at 5 days.

Rehabilitation

The patient will leave hospital 7 to 10 days after most gastro-duodenal operations except total gastrectomy. At this time the skin wound should be soundly healed (although the deeper layers will be gaining in strength over the next 3 months) and the drainage site dry. He should be drinking liberally and eating a normal diet. However, some patients will be slow in comfortably managing a normal quantity of food. After partial gastrectomy, this may be related to the size of the retained gastric segment. The patient may be advised to take frequent small meals ('half as much food, twice as often'), but the recuperative capacity of the upper gut is remarkable and even following total gastrectomy patients may return to eating 'normally'. Usually, of course, the relief provided by the operation will encourage them to minimize disabilities.

Effective weight gain may, however, be very slow following partial gastrectomy and nil following total gastrectomy. This may be discouraging to the patient but is not serious providing nutrition, specifically for maintenance of tissues, such as blood or bone, is adequate. Supplementary iron, calcium and vitamins are necessary. A circumstance of particular importance is that total gastrectomy removes the source of intrinsic factor and unless vitamin B_{12} is given regularly by injections megaloblastic anaemia will inevitably develop. This may not occur until a couple of years after the operation, but it is reasonable to start the injections shortly after the patient's return home.

A reasonable period of convalescence after most upper abdominal operations is a month. This is certainly adequate for sedentary workers, but may have to be extended when the patient's job is a heavy one. It is usual for him to be reviewed by the surgeon at about this time. Subsequently it is important that he is seen at least annually by his doctor or the surgeon and a general review with particular reference to his nutritional state (with blood studies as indicated) is carried out.

REFERENCE

Baron, J. H. and Lennard-Jones, J. E. (1971). Gastric secretion in health and disease. *Br. J. hosp. Med.* **6**, 303

23

Surgery of the liver and spleen

Roger Brearley

THE LIVER

In several ways the liver is unique among the organs of the body. It is the largest organ; its known functions are more numerous and varied than those of any other organ; it derives its blood supply from two sources, one venous and one arterial; and it has the extraordinary ability to regenerate after partial loss of substance so as to return to its original weight.

Anatomy

The liver is a firm, solid, red-brown body situated beneath the diaphragm and largely concealed by the lower right ribs. In the adult it weighs around 1.5 kg or 2 per cent of the body weight. It is shaped approximately like a wedge with its base to the right. Its surfaces are smooth and rounded, merging into one another except for the under surface which is separated from the others by sharp borders and marked by grooves created by structures entering and leaving. The areas thus outlined are called anatomical lobes but they bear no relation to internal structure, which follows the distribution of the branches of the portal vein and hepatic artery and the tributaries of the bile duct. The groove through which these pass is called the portal fissure or hilum. *Figures 23.1, 2, and 3* show these features.

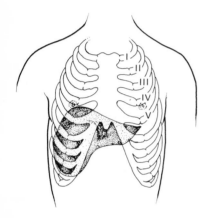

Figure 23.1. Position of the liver

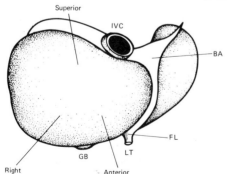

Figure 23.2. Liver seen from in front and above. GB, gall bladder; IVC, inferior vena cava; LT, ligamentum teres; BA, bare area; FL, falciform ligament

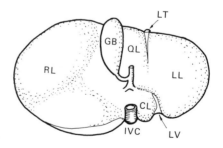

Figure 23.3. Liver seen from below. CL, caudate lobe; GB, gall bladder; IVC, inferior vena cava; LL, left lobe; RL, right lobe; QL, quadrate lobe; PV, portal vein; BA, bare area; LV, ligamentum venosum; LT, ligamentum teres

Structurally the liver is composed of parenchymal cells, reticulo-endothelial cells, vessels for blood lymph and bile and peritoneal covering, with their associated connective tissue (Glisson's capsule).

Physiology

Many of the liver's numerous and varied functions are continuous processes essential for life, and complete removal of the liver (in the dog) is followed by death after about 10 hours. Others are potentialities which may never be exercised, such as the ability to excrete or otherwise dispose of chemical substances artificially introduced into the body. It is the varied pattern of failure or derangement of the liver's functions which accounts for the differing manifestations of liver disease. Many of the activities of the liver lend themselves readily to biochemical testing.

The liver functions may be grouped under five headings:

(1) metabolism of nutrients (carbohydrates, fats, proteins) and the storage of related substances (vitamins, iron);
(2) synthesis of blood constituents including serum albumin and certain clotting factors;
(3) disposal of foreign or noxious substances (for example, drugs) by **conjugation**, excretion, oxidation and so on;
(4) secretion of bile; and
(5) activities of the fetal liver, for example, haemopoiesis (blood formation).

Metabolism of nutrients

Carbohydrate metabolism   The liver glycogen store is used to maintain the blood sugar at an adequate concentration. When this store is exhausted (as by 24-hour fasting) the liver synthesizes glucose from other carbohydrates, amino acids, and fats. Muscle glycogen cannot be mobilized for this purpose and total **hepatectomy** (always) and liver failure (sometimes) lead to hypoglycaemia. Glycogen protects the liver from injury by many poisons, including anaesthetic agents, and copious supplies of glucose are given in the pre-operative preparation of patients with any form of liver damage.

Protein metabolism   Much food and body protein is broken down in the liver and the final stage — deamination — releases ammonia. Ammonia is also formed in the gut, absorbed into the portal vein system and carried to the liver. All this ammonia is converted to urea by the liver which is the sole site of urea formation. In liver disease, the blood urea may be

Conjugation The combination of one compound with another to form a product of biological importance.

Hepatectomy Resection of the liver.

abnormally low and the blood ammonia abnormally high. Both can be measured.

The liver is also concerned with protein synthesis, considered in the section on blood constituents.

Fat metabolism Bile salts aid the digestion and absorption of fats by facilitating emulsification. The fats of lower molecular weight are broken down to glycerol and short-chain fatty acids. These are soluble in water, pass to the liver in the portal vein and are oxidized. The less digestible fats enter the lymphatics in the form of fine droplets (like thin cream) and ultimately reach the veins of the neck, where they enter the bloodstream, to be picked up by the fat stores (adipose tissue) and liver. Such fat is not normally visible in the liver as it is utilized in various ways, but the liver may become fat laden (fatty infiltration) in certain diseases, including alcoholism, starvation and kwashiorkor (a tropical protein-deficiency disease). Fatty infiltration impairs liver function, interfering with the detoxication of barbiturates and making hazardous the use of fat-soluble anaesthetics, such as ether or halothane. It may lead to cirrhosis.

Synthesis of blood constituents

Albumin plays a vital role in maintaining the osmotic pressure of the plasma and hence in preventing oedema. It is also directly available to the cells as a source of cytoplasm protein. Normally the plasma concentration is 45 g per litre and all of it is produced by the liver. In liver disease the concentration may fall below 30 g per litre and this leads to ascites and peripheral oedema.

The **globulins** are mostly produced outside the liver and therefore are not reduced in liver disease. Indeed, gamma globulins (which are the antibody fraction) may be increased, as may some of the other fractions.

A number of the clotting factors including fibrinogen, prothrombin and factors V and VII are formed in the liver, the synthesis especially of factor VII requiring vitamin K. Deficiencies of these factors result in defective coagulation and hence in operative haemorrhage. When liver failure is the cause, the defect cannot be fully corrected by administering vitamin K, but when liver function is good and the trouble has arisen (as in obstructive jaundice) from defective absorption of the vitamin which is fat soluble, parenteral administration restores coagulation to normal.

The diseased liver also may produce increased quantities of fibrinolysins which dissolve formed clots and thereby use up all the normal clotting factors. This increases the bleeding tendency, sometimes even rendering the blood totally

Globulins A class of proteins occurring widely in nature.

incoagulable. The treatment is by antifibrinolytic drugs, such as Epsikapron.

Disposal of foreign or noxious substances

The liver is rich in enzymes and these enable it to dispose of noxious substances, both foreign and endogenous. Some, e.g. alcohol and barbiturates, are destroyed by oxidation; others are rendered inactive by chemical combination with various acids, such as, sulphuric, acetic, glucuronic and some amino acids (conjugation). Oestrogens are dealt with in this way, and liver failure may lead to an increase of circulating oestrogen causing breast enlargement in the male and, in both sexes, **palmar erythema** and **spider naevi**.

The liver also acts, like the kidney, as an organ of excretion and some substances, for example, phenolphthalein, are passed out in the bile. Advantage is taken of this fact to study the excretory capacity of the liver using a related compound — bromsulphalein sodium (BSP). Similar compounds containing iodine (which is opaque to x-rays) are used to outline the bile ducts and gall bladder for radiological examination (cholecystography and cholangiography).

Bile formation

Bile is formed in the liver cells and enters the bile capillaries whence it passes through the cholangioles into the intrahepatic bile ducts and ultimately, via the common hepatic duct and common bile duct, into the duodenum.

About 1000 ml of bile are secreted daily, but the quantity normally entering the duodenum is only 750 ml since, in the fasting state, bile is stored and concentrated in the gall bladder. As secreted by the liver, it is a thin, golden, alkaline liquid. After concentration in the gall bladder it becomes darker, greenish and **viscid**. If the common bile duct is obstructed, the liver continues to secrete bile until the duct pressure reaches 250 to 300 mm of water. After this bile secretion ceases but the secretion of mucus continues. As the pressure rises further, bile pigments are actually reabsorbed leaving the ducts distended with clear mucus known as white bile.

Apart from water, bile has five major constituents: (1) bile pigments (which will be discussed last), (2) bile salts, (3) cholesterol, (4) electrolytes, and (5) mucus.

Bile salts Bile salts (sodium glycocholate and sodium taurocholate) are formed in the liver by the conjugation of cholic acid (a steroid itself formed in the liver) with the amino acids glycine and taurine. Their function in the gut in aiding the absorption of fats and fat-soluble vitamins has already been noted. The bile salts are themselves absorbed in the small

Palmar erythema Redness of the palms due to vasodilation.

Spider naevi These are clusters of blood vessels in the skin radiating from a central red spot. They blanch on pressure and when the pressure is released can be seen to fill up again from the centre outwards.

Viscid Semiliquid; having a glutinous consistency (viscous).

intestine and re-excreted by the liver in a continuous cycle (called enterohepatic circulation). In the presence of an external biliary fistula, bile salts are lost from the body. In obstruction of the bile duct (obstructive jaundice) they are absorbed into the bloodstream, and cause pruritus. In the presence of blind loops of small gut and jejunal diverticula they are broken down by bacteria, releasing cholic acid which has little power of emulsification and is irritant to the small and large intestine, leading to fatty diarrhoea (steatorrhoea).

Cholesterol Cholesterol is a steroid mainly formed in the liver. It is the source of bile acids, adrenal cortical hormones and oestrogens. Partly combined with fatty acids (esters) and partly free, it circulates in the blood. It is excreted by the bile in concentrations above its normal solubility, kept in supersaturated solution by complicated mechanisms involving the bile salts and choline. Inflammation in the wall of the gall bladder (cholecystitis) upsets these mechanisms and so favours the formation of gall-stones. The presence of gall-stones also leads to attacks of cholecystitis.

Electrolytes The main electrolytes (also known as inorganic or mineral salts) are sodium chloride and sodium bicarbonate. The latter is mainly responsible for the alkaline reaction of bile. The bile salts are also sodium salts, alkaline in solution. The total sodium content of bile is high and a biliary fistula may quickly lead to severe sodium losses.

Mucus Mucus, though a constituent of bile, is not secreted by the liver but by the mucous membrane lining the bile ducts and the gall bladder.

Bile pigments Bilirubin imparts a characteristic golden brown colour to the bile in the hepatic ducts. It is mostly derived from haemoglobin released by haemolysis (breakdown) of old red cells in the spleen and bone marrow*. The haemoglobin yields iron and globin which can be used again, and porphyrin which is further changed, first to biliverdin, then to bilirubin. Bilirubin is insoluble in water, but it enters the bloodstream by becoming attached to albumin molecules, and so reaches the liver. Here it is conjugated with glucuronic acid, which renders it water-soluble, and is excreted in the bile. If present in excess, conjugated bilirubin can easily pass through the kidney and appear in the urine, which the insoluble, unconjugated bilirubin cannot do.

In the gall bladder and duodenum, some of the bilirubin is

*Other phases of the metabolism of haem pigments (haemoglobin, myoglobin and cytochromes) account for a smaller part of the daily production.

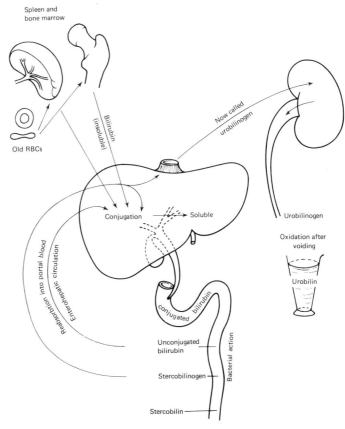

Figure 23.4. The process of formation and distribution of bile pigments

oxidized to biliverdin, giving gall-bladder bile and duodenal juice their characteristic green colour.

In the intestine, a small amount of the bilirubin is deconjugated and recirculated to the liver for re-excretion as the bile salts are. The rest is reduced by bacteria to stercobilinogen (colourless) and then oxidized, yielding a brown pigment, stercobilin, which gives faeces (and the contents of the lower small intestine) their characteristic colour. Some stercobilinogen is absorbed from the gut and excreted in the urine. Here it is called urobilinogen. It is colourless but oxidizes on standing to the brown urobilin. These two pigments are chemically identical with stercobilinogen and stercobilin, the prefixes 'uro' and 'sterco' simply indicating the location of the pigment in urine or faeces. The whole process is summarized in *Figure 23.4.*

The fetal liver Much of the biochemical activity of the liver begins at or after birth. For example, the transient jaundice often seen in normal infants is due to a relative inability to conjugate and excrete bilirubin. On the other hand, at the sixth week of fetal life, the liver is an important site of haemopoiesis (blood formation).

INVESTIGATION OF THE LIVER

Clinical examination

General features of liver disease are mentioned elsewhere.

Palpable enlargement of the liver is a common diagnostic problem. Liver swellings emerge from the costal margin and move freely on respiration. They may present an oblique edge running from upper left to lower right or may occur as rounded bulging swellings. Some of the common causes are summarized below.

(1) Congestion:
    venous — congestive cardiac failure;
    biliary — obstruction of extrahepatic bile ducts.
(2) Abnormal deposits:
    multiple metastatic deposits including melanoma and all forms of carcinoma, especially breast, bronchus, stomach and colon;
    diffuse tumour deposits — Hodgkin's disease;
    storage diseases — Gaucher's disease.
(3) Parenchymal disease: any form of hepatitis; cirrhosis sometimes.
(4) Primary liver tumours and cysts.
(5) Hydatid cysts.
(6) Liver abscesses — pyogenic and amoebic.

Liver function tests

A number of general tests of liver function are routinely performed on any suspected case of liver disease. Many such tests have been developed, but the most important and widely used are those summarized below.

Serum bilirubin Free and conjugated bilirubin are measured separately by the indirect and direct van den Bergh's reactions. Normally there is less than 12 μmol per litre of which less than 3.5 μmol is conjugated.

Serum proteins The fall in albumin content and the possible increase and change of composition of the globulins previously described can be measured quantitatively. The normal values are: total protein 60 to 70 grams per litre, albumin 35 to 45 grams per litre, globulin 25 to 30 grams per litre; albumin/globulin ratio A/G = 1.5/l.

Flocculation tests Addition of certain reagents to serum causes it to become turbid or cloudy. The readiness with which this happens depends on its precise protein composition and, generally speaking, stability is decreased in liver disease.

The results of such tests are expressed in arbitrary units. Commonly used flocculation tests are thymol turbidity test (normal result 0 to 4 units) and zinc sulphate turbidity test (normal result 4 to 8 units).

Serum enzymes Damaged liver cells shed their enzymes which may then be detected in the plasma. Those commonly tested for include aspartate transaminase and alanine transaminase.

Alkaline phosphatase normally excreted in bile is raised by biliary obstruction (also by bone disease).

Dye excretion test Bromsulphalein sodium (BSP) is a dye which can be injected intravenously and is excreted by the liver. Its plasma concentration is easily measured. Normally less than 10 per cent of an injected dose is still present after 30 minutes. Retention of more than 30 per cent after 30 minutes indicates serious impairment of function.

Prothrombin time Prothrombin time (PTT) is prolonged even after an adequate intake of vitamin K if the liver is damaged. Besides its diagnostic significance, a persistently raised PTT is a warning of serious haemorrhage if operation is attempted.

Liver biopsy A small portion of the liver may be removed for microscopic examination by means of a special needle. The most commonly used patterns are the Menghini needle, the Vim—Silverman needle and the Trucut needle. The operation can be done in the patient's bed and only local anaesthesia is required. It should not be attempted if the PTT is raised.

Imaging techniques These include radiography (cholecystography and cholangiography using either biliary excretion of contrast medium or direct injection of it into the ducts) and scanning by ultrasound or radioactive isotopes.

Liver diseases of surgical importance

Liver diseases which are of interest to the surgeon are: (1) injuries of the liver, (2) pylephlebitis and abscesses, (3) hydatid cysts, (4) tumours and other causes of liver enlargement, (5) portal hypertension and (6) jaundice.

Injuries of the liver
The liver may be damaged by penetrating injuries (gun-shot wounds, stab wounds) or blunt trauma (for example, in road traffic accidents). In both cases other organs are often injured (rib fractures, rupture of diaphragm, spleen or other viscera,

X

laceration of lung and so on). Usually the need for surgical exploration is evident and urgent and after securing an adequate supply of blood, starting transfusion and rapidly assessing other injuries, including chest injuries, exploration is undertaken. Adequate exposure is essential and right **thoracolaparotomy** is usually required. Attention is given to other injuries according to priorities as judged at the time. Lacerations of the liver are often more extensive than they may at first seem. Dead and devitalized portions of the liver should be excised according to the principles of the segmental anatomy and the dead spaces drained after securing proper haemostasis. The most lethal injuries are lacerations running round to involve the posterior surface in the region of the hepatic veins and inferior vena cava, and pulping injuries in which the interior of the liver has been extensively disintegrated, often with only a deceptively small laceration extending to the surface.

Pylephlebitis and liver abscesses

Suppurative pylephlebitis means the presence in the portal vein of an infected clot. Portal pyaemia means the passage through the portal vein of septic emboli. Both conditions lead to the formation of multiple abscesses in the liver. They are less common than formerly but still occur, sometimes as complications of abdominal sepsis (gangrenous appendicitis, pericolic abscess) and are highly lethal. Multiple abscesses may also result from septic **cholangitis**.

Solitary liver abscesses occur, too. In tropical countries they are usually due to the *Entamoeba histolytica* and are complications of amoebic dysentery. In Great Britain they are seen occasionally, usually containing sterile pus. Careful search generally reveals a gastrointestinal lesion (often a gastric ulcer). Treatment by aspiration, drainage and appropriate antibiotics gives good results.

Hydatid cysts

Hydatid cysts are larvae of the tapeworm *Echinococcus granulosus (Taenia echinococcus)* which lives in the dog's intestine. The intermediate host which harbours the larval or cyst stage is normally the sheep, and the disease is commonest in sheep-rearing countries such as Australia and New Zealand. In Great Britain, Wales is the most affected area. Sheep are infected by eating grass contaminated by dogs' faeces and dogs are infected by eating offal from the carcasses of affected sheep. In man, infection is also due in the last analysis to eating minute quantities of dog faeces which contain the ova, and most infections probably arise in childhood when hygienic habits are least developed and intimate contact with dogs

Thoracolaparotomy A surgical approach to the peritoneal cavity by a wound through the chest wall and diaphragm with or without an extension of the wound through the abdominal wall.

Cholangitis Inflammation of the bile ducts.

common. After being swallowed, the ova make their way into the liver and develop into cysts, though about 30 per cent pass further, reaching other organs, such as the lungs, brain and bone. The liver often contains a number of cysts and, when mature, these may be several inches in diameter causing palpable irregular enlargement of the liver. The wall is frequently calcified and therefore visible on radiography. The fluid contains foreign protein which is antigenic. As a result it is possible to carry out a specific test (Casoni's test) by intradermal injection of fresh sterile hydatid fluid. Another consequence is that leakage from a cyst may lead to urticarial reactions and **eosinophilia**. On occasion it can cause severe anaphylactic shock.

It is possible to remove the cysts surgically though elaborate techniques are required to prevent rupture and spillage which can lead to widespread development of new cysts. Spontaneous rupture may also occur with the same result. Cysts may also discharge themselves into bile ducts or intestine, evacuating their contents harmlessly but later becoming infected and transformed into badly-draining abscess cavities.

Tumours

The tumours of the liver are generally blood-borne secondary deposits from carcinomas of the gut (arriving via the portal vein) of other organs, such as breast, lung or bladder (arriving via the hepatic artery). They are usually multiple, giving rise to hard irregular palpable swellings of the liver and later jaundice (through pressure on the bile ducts). Their only importance to the surgeon is in the bearing they have on deciding the treatment of the primary tumour and determining ultimate prognosis. On opening the abdomen to perform an operation for any malignant condition, it is invariable practice to palpate the liver for secondary deposits. Though seemingly crude, this is an effective screening test capable of detecting quite early involvement. If the abdomen is not to be opened, probably the best methods are radioactive and ultrasound scanning. Many radioactive substances are available which are taken up by normal liver. After a suitable dose, a detecting instrument will demonstrate the outline and extent of the liver and tumours are demonstrated as areas of absent radioactivity. Ultrasound scanning is an even simpler procedure.

Occasionally a single large secondary deposit is encountered, and this may be worth removing, especially if it first appears long after removal of the primary tumour.

Primary tumours of the liver are not common and some varieties are very rare. Most arise either from liver parenchymal cells or from bile ducts though connective tissues and ectopic cells are sometimes the source. Sometimes (as in cirrhotic

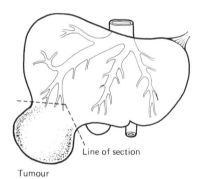

Line of section

Tumour

Figure 23.5. Peripherally placed liver tumours may be removed by wedge excision

Eosinophilia An excessive number of eosinophil cells (a type of white blood cell) in the blood.

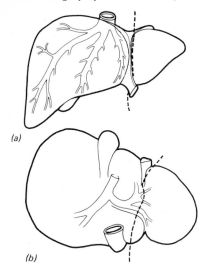

(a)

(b)

Figure 23.6. (*a*) The liver from below showing line of section for left lobectomy and its relation to the arcade of the left branch of the portal vein. (*b*) The liver from in front showing the line of section for left lobectomy and its relation to the left hepatic vein. (Redrawn from Dagradi and Brearley, 1962, by courtesy of the Editor of *Postgraduate Medical Journal*)

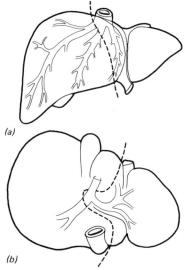

(a)

(b)

Figure 23.7. (*a*) The liver from below showing line of section for extended right hepatic lobectomy and its relation to the branches of the portal vein. (*b*) The liver from in front showing the line of section for extended right lobectomy and its relation to the left hepatic vein. (Redrawn from Dagradi and Brearley, 1962, by courtesy of the Editor of *Postgraduate Medical Journal*)

livers) the tumours are very malignant and arise simultaneously at many points (multicentric origin) but sometimes they are large and solitary and lend themselves to surgical excision by partial hepatectomy, especially benign forms such as adenoma and angioma.

Diagnosis Tumours of the liver are sometimes discovered accidentally during an abdominal operation. Often they present as an upper abdominal swelling, perhaps associated with discomfort, tenderness, fever or jaundice. Angiography, radioactive scanning, peritoneoscopy and laparotomy are the most useful tests.

Partial hepatectomy Small tumours situated near the edge of the liver, or actually growing out of the edge on a pedicle, can be removed locally with a wedge from the liver edge (*Figure 23.5*). The radiating distribution of portal structures nearly always allows this. Larger tumours may require removal of the left or right half, dividing the liver through the principal plane, after isolating and dividing the left or right portal vein, artery and duct in the portal fissure (*Figures 23.6* and *23.7*). The left anatomical lobe may also be removed without damage to the blood supply of the quadrate lobe. As the ducts and vessels are transected they are ligated and mattress sutures may be passed using liver needles (Kuznetsoff needles). Haemorrhage is less of a problem than might be supposed and, when it occurs, may be due to the presence of haemolysins, rendering the blood incoagulable. Air embolism may also occur during operation, respiratory movements sucking air into the larger hepatic vein radicles.

The liver blood flow and portal hypertension

The normal blood flow through the liver is about 1500 ml per minute (about one-third of the cardiac output). Of this about one-third enters through the hepatic artery and two-thirds (1000 ml or slightly more) enter through the portal vein

The hepatic artery is the sole source of blood supply to the connective tissue of the liver and to any tumours, primary or secondary, which may be present, but it provides only about 30 per cent of the flow into the lobules. The remaining 70 per cent is derived from the portal vein. Blood from the two sources enters the sinusoids at the periphery of the lobules where it mixes while passing towards the centrilobular veins.

The pressure in the portal tributaries is normally between 10 and 15 cm of water, while that in the vena cava just below the diaphragm is around 2 cm of water, so there is only a small pressure gradient available to drive the portal blood through the liver. The flow may be impeded by obstruction in the portal vein itself, in the liver, or in the hepatic veins draining the liver. Obstruction at any of these sites leads to an increase of pressure in the portal vein below the blockage, and in all the radicles which drain into it. The condition is known as portal hypertension and the sites of blockage are described as pre- or extrahepatic, intrahepatic, and posthepatic.

The portal vein receives all the blood from the intra-abdominal part of the gut (between the lower oesophagus and the lower rectum) and from the spleen, pancreas, bile ducts and omentum. At the anus and lower oesophagus lies a watershed, on one side of which the network of veins drains into the portal system and on the other, into the caval (or systemic) system. Similar watersheds exist where organs with a portal drainage lie in direct contact or continuity with organs having caval drainage. Examples are the upper surface of the liver (in contact with the diaphragm), the spleen and tail of the pancreas (in contact with the posterior abdominal wall), the root of the mesentery, the falciform ligament, and any inflammatory or postoperative adhesions between omentum and body wall.

Effects of portal hypertension

Collateral vessels In the presence of portal hypertension blood may start to flow across these watersheds from the portal to the systemic drainage beds, and as there are no valves in the portal system blood may be diverted from the main veins (splenic and superior mesenteric) to drain into systemic veins at the points of portal-systemic contact. This is called portal-systemic shunting, and it leads to great dilatation of the small veins which provide the escape channels. Such dilated channels are known as collateral vessels and the blood flow through them as collateral circulation.

Surgical importance of collateral vessels is summarized below.

(1) Oesophageal varices — large veins in the submucous coat of the oesophagus. They have thin walls, are under high pressure and are liable to sudden and catastrophic bleeding.
(2) Dilatation of veins running in the falciform ligament to the umbilicus, which may be followed by dilatation of subcutaneous veins radiating out from the umbilicus. These have been fancifully likened to the Gorgon's head and called Caput Medusae*. Sometimes a venous

---

*Medusa the Gorgon — her hair was composed of snakes standing out from the head.

hum can be heard with a stethoscope and the condition is then known as Cruveilhier—Baumgarten syndrome.

(3) Veins in the retroperitoneal tissues and abdominal wall may cause difficulties at operation but are otherwise silent.

(4) Collaterals in the region of the anal canal are of no clinical importance and do not seem to cause haemorrhoids.

Enlargement of the spleen Because the spleen is distended with blood, it gradually enlarges, becoming also tough and fibrous. This is called congestive splenomegaly and it is accompanied by an increase in the spleen's activity as a destroyer of blood cells, the red cell count, white cell count, and platelet count all falling (anaemia, leucopenia, and thrombocytopenia, or all together, panhaemocytopenia). This increased splenic activity is called hypersplenism.

Pathology

Posthepatic portal hypertension is usually due to tumour deposits compressing the hepatic veins or to thrombus occluding them. It leads to great enlargement of the liver and ascites but is of no importance surgically. It is known as Budd—Chiari syndrome.

Prehepatic portal hypertension usually results from thrombosis within the portal vein or its main branches or tributaries. This may be followed later by recanalization of the clot by narrow tortuous channels and also the development of a dilated network of collateral small vessels in the liver hilum, by-passing the obstruction. The whole forms a mass of small vessels resembling a cavernous angioma and is referred to as cavernoma formation. Thrombosis of the portal vein may follow splenectomy, it may be caused by intra-abdominal disease (abscess, internal strangulation) and it may arise at birth if the obliteration of the umbilical vein extends to affect the left branch of the portal vein. Umbilical sepsis and umbilical vein exchange transfusion may be responsible for some cases. Liver function is in no way impaired and haemorrhage from oesophageal varices is the main danger. Treatment will be discussed later.

Intrahepatic portal hypertension is due to cirrhosis. The name cirrhosis (meaning tawny) was coined by Laënnec, the inventor of the stethoscope. The liver may be smaller, larger or unaltered in size but the surface is nodular (hobnail liver). Microscopically cirrhosis has three features: (1) death of liver cells with collapse of lobules, (2) regeneration of liver cells forming nodules without lobular structure, and (3) involvement of all the liver. Three main forms are recognized, known as portal, postnecrotic and biliary cirrhosis. Portal and postnecrotic cirrhosis may sometimes be due to alcoholism and virus hepatitis respectively, and there are also a number of rare diseases which can be responsible, but in many cases, no cause can be discovered. Biliary cirrhosis may result from repeated attacks of ascending cholangitis (usually due to the presence of stones) but there is also a primary form, commonest in middle-aged women.

Clinical features

The picture is that of portal hypertension combined with liver dysfunction or, ultimately, failure. The spleen is palpably enlarged and the liver may also be enlarged.

The following are some important signs of liver failure (*Figure 23.8*).

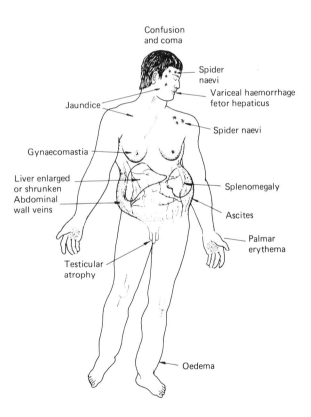

Figure 23.8. Some features of liver failure

Ascites and peripheral oedema   Ascites and peripheral oedema are associated with a low plasma albumin due to defective synthesis. Salt restriction and diuretics usually provide effective control.

Neuropsychiatric symptoms Neuropsychiatric symptoms include flapping tremor of the outstretched hands, confusion, drowsiness and coma. These symptoms are called hepatic encephalopathy and are accompanied by characteristic electroencephalographic changes. They are due to failure of the liver to dispose of toxic substances (including ammonia) produced by protein breakdown in the gut. Both the hepatocellular dysfunction and the collateral shunting enable these substances to enter the peripheral blood. Hepatic fetor, a characteristic smell on the breath, is due to the same phenomenon. High protein diet, gastrointestinal haemorrhage and ammonia-containing medicines make the condition worse. Neomycin (which stops bacterial protein breakdown in the gut), aperients such as Epsom salts, which keep the gut empty, and lactulose (Duphalac), a synthetic sugar which does both, all improve the condition. Enemas may be required in emergency.

Jaundice, fever and malaise Jaundice, fever and malaise are common. The jaundice is due to impairment of all phases of bilirubin metabolism. Fever, especially with worsening neuropsychiatric symptoms, may indicate the onset of septicaemia or peritonitis.

Superficial manifestations Some superficial manifestations are due to disordered oestrogen metabolism (palmar erythema, spider naevi, loss of body hair, testicular atrophy, **gynaecomastia**, infertility and menstrual irregularity). Other manifestations, such as white nails and finger clubbing, are of uncertain cause.

The essential principles in the management of liver failure are to treat its treatable aspects as outlined above, and provide a generous carbohydrate calorie intake. Supplementary vitamins, iron and so on may also be needed. Liver transplantation and perfusion of the patient's blood through an isolated pig liver are still experimental procedures.

Surgical treatment of portal hypertension

There is no surgical treatment which will cure liver failure, though sudden worsening or deterioration may occur following haemorrhage or operation and require vigorous medical treatment. However, both haemorrhage (in the short term) and portal hypertension (its long-term cause) are amenable to surgery.

The most radical and the most effective method is to reduce portal pressure by anastomosing the portal vein direct to the inferior vena cava. This is usually done by dividing the portal

Gynaecomastia Hypertrophy of the male breasts to resemble the female form.

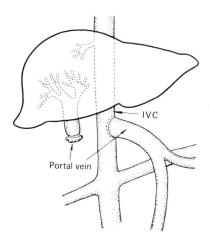

Figure 23.9. Portacaval shunt. (Reproduced from Shields, 1978, by permission of the Author and Publishers)

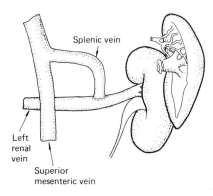

Figure 23.10. Conventional splenorenal shunt. (Reproduced from Shields, 1978, by permission of the Author and Publishers)

vein and implanting it into the side of the cava (*Figure 23.9*). Other possibilities are shown in *Figures 23.10, 23.11* and *23.12*. After a successful operation oesophageal varices disappear and further bleeding is almost unknown. If liver function is good, the operation has no untoward effect, but if it is poor, further deterioration is likely. For this reason, the operation should not be attempted unless the serum bilirubin is below 3 mg per 100 ml, (50 μmol/litre) the BSP retention below 30 per cent at 30 minutes, and the serum albumin above 30 grams per litre. It is also necessary to prove that portal hypertension is present (by measuring venous pressure in the splenic pulp through a needle), that the splenic vein is patent (it may be outlined on a radiograph by injecting contrast medium into the spleen through the same needle — known as a splenoportagram) and that oesophageal varices are the source of the patient's haemorrhages (they can be demonstrated on barium swallow and on endoscopy).

Extrahepatic portal obstruction may be recognized by splenoportagram. Usually there is no portal vein available for anastomosis and surgical treatment must be limited to measures directed against the oesophageal varices, or to the emergency treatment of haemorrhage.

Arrest of the haemorrhage

Bleeding oesophageal varices account for about 5 per cent of all cases of haematemesis and melaena admitted to hospital. The diagnosis is suggested by the finding of a palpable spleen or stigmata of liver dysfunction. The combined effect of haemorrhagic shock on the liver and the presence of large quantities of protein-rich blood in the gut may precipitate acute liver failure with coma. Deficient synthesis of coagulation factors may make the bleeding persist and when liver function is very poor, the patient is likely to die in liver coma and still bleeding, despite all measures. On the other hand, with good liver function and a moderate bleed, spontaneous recovery is usual without any more elaborate treatment than bed-rest and transfusion.

If spontaneous arrest does not occur within a few hours (or sooner if haemorrhage is rapid), an intravenous infusion of Pitressin is given (20 units in 10 minutes or continuous infusion). This lowers portal pressure by reducing arterial blood flow into the gut, and allows natural haemostasis to occur. It also causes violent peristalsis which empties the gut of blood with beneficial effect.

If Pitressin fails, the next step is to pass a Sengstaken tube. This is a long stomach tube with two inflatable balloons. The

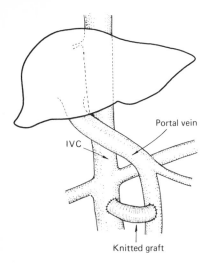

Figure 23.11. Interposition mesocaval shunt. (Reproduced from Shields, 1978, by permission of the Author and Publishers)

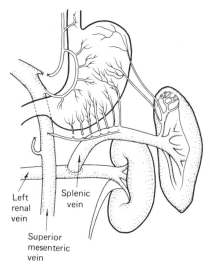

Figure 23.12. Distal splenorenal shunt. (Reproduced from Shields, 1978, by permission of the Author and Publishers)

lower one is large and spherical and, when inflated in the stomach, prevents the tube from being withdrawn. Above it is a long sausage-shaped balloon which lies in the lower oesophagus. When inflated, this fills the lower oesophagus and compresses the varices, arresting the haemorrhage. The tube is passed over a pulley and weights are attached to it to keep the lower balloon drawn up against the cardia. Such tubes may lead to pressure necrosis if used for more than 48 hours. If bleeding persists after this time and liver function is reasonable, a direct surgical attack may be made on the varices or their feeding vessels. Such operations may also be performed as planned procedures in an attempt to stop recurrent haemorrhages in cases of extrahepatic portal hypertension when there is no portal vein available for portal-systemic anastomosis. There are several operative methods for stopping haemorrhage.

(1) Crile—Boerema operation. The lower oesophagus is opened through the left pleural cavity and the varices undersewn with continuous catgut sutures running up and down in three rows.
(2) Milnes Walker's operation is similar to the Crile—Boerema operation but the mucosa and its veins are divided transversely across and resutured after opening the outer layers of the oesophagus longitudinally.
(3) Tanner's operation (gastric transection or porto-azygos disconnection). The stomach is cut completely across just below the cardia and re-anastomosed. Vessels passing up into the mediastinum alongside the oeso-phagus are also divided. This interrupts the flow of blood from the portal radicles up through the oesophageal varices.
(4) In oesophagogastrectomy the lower oesophagus and upper stomach are resected and continuity restored by oesophagogastric anastomosis. This not only stops the flow upwards to the varices but actually removes them, though more may form at a later date as new veins develop across the suture line.

All these operations are effective for a time but bleeding usually recurs ultimately. Oesophagogastrectomy is probably the most effective but is also the biggest operation and liable to be followed by gastro-oesophageal reflux and troublesome oesophagitis. Other methods of little value are splenectomy, which reduces the portal pressure very little and is liable to be followed by splenic vein thrombosis, and the Talma—Morison operation of inducing adhesions between omentum and abdominal wall to provide extra collateral channels.

Jaundice

Jaundice means yellow staining of the tissues of the body by bilirubin. Visible staining does not appear until the serum level exceeds 35 μmol per litre. An increase less than this is sometimes referred to as subclinical jaundice. The tissues most conspicuously stained are those rich in elastic fibres such as the skin and the sclera of the eye (not the conjunctiva as often stated). Secretions may also be stained including even tears. Either conjugated or unconjugated bilirubin or both may be responsible.

There are three ways in which jaundice may arise. It may be due to excessive production of bilirubin, to failure of liver cells to take up, conjugate, and excrete bilirubin, or to obstruction somewhere in the bile duct system. The first kind is known as haemolytic jaundice and the third kind as obstructive jaundice. In the second category there are many different conditions.

Haemolytic jaundice

Excessive production of unconjugated bilirubin resulting from abnormal haemolysis causes only slight increase of the serum bilirubin to 30–50 μmol per litre, since the liver has great functional reserves. Being insoluble in water, unconjugated pigment does not appear in the urine which is therefore normal in colour — whence the name acholuric jaundice (a-chol-uric — no bile in the urine; bile salts, of course, are also absent as the condition does not interfere in any way with normal bile salt metabolism). As the liver is working to full capacity conjugating and excreting bilirubin, there is plenty of pigment in the faeces which may even appear unusually dark.

The causes of excessive haemolysis (which, of course, also produces anaemia) are of interest to the physician. They include hereditary forms (familial spherocytosis), acquired forms (mostly due to auto-immune disturbances) and one well-known congenital form, Rh incompatibility. In some cases benefit follows splenectomy.

Liver cell dysfunction

The liver cells take in bilirubin from the plasma, conjugate it and excrete it into the bile ducts. There are a number of rare familial diseases affecting one or other of these activities but widespread disease of the liver cells is liable to affect all three. Failure to take up and conjugate plasma bilirubin leads to a form of acholuric jaundice. Failure to excrete it into the bile ducts (known as intrahepatic cholestasis) leads to an increase in conjugated bilirubin in the blood, and other features similar to those of obstructive jaundice (*see below*). Generally speaking, defective liver cell function reduces bile salt formation so there is no excess of these at any site. Alkaline phosphatase, however, may have difficulty in passing from cells to bile and may therefore appear in increased amounts in the blood.

Widespread damage to liver cells may result from:

(1) acute conditions — infections (virus hepatitis, Weil's disease); drugs (chlorpromazine, halothane), and poisons (phosphorus, carbon tetrachloride); or

(2) chronic conditions — chronic active hepatitis, chronic alcoholism, and advanced cirrhosis.

Obstructive jaundice

The state of affairs obtaining when the main bile duct is obstructed may be roughly described by saying that a normal liver is secreting normal bile into an obstructed duct and, as it

Table 23.1   Main features of the different types of jaundice

Type	Cause	Blood	Gut	Urine
Haemolytic (acholuric)	Excessive bilirubin production due to haemolysis	Excess unconjugated bilirubin (20–50 μmol/litre) Salts: normal enterohepatic circulation Alkaline phosphatase normal	Plenty of pigment, dark stools	No pigments or salts
Hepatocellular	Failure to conjugate or excrete bilirubin	Findings in blood, gut and urine depend on which function is deficient. Failure to take up bilirubin and to conjugate it produces acholuric picture above. Failure to excrete conjugated bilirubin produces obstructive picture below. Features of both may be present		
Obstructive	Bile duct obstruction	Excess of conjugated pigment and salts, bilirubin may be over 200 μmol/litre High alkaline phosphatase (may be over 30 King–Armstrong units)	No pigment — pale stools No bile salts — fatty stools	Pigment and salts — dark frothing urine

cannot escape normally, it is reabsorbed into the bloodstream and excreted through the kidney. As a result, bile pigment and salts are absent from the gut and present in the blood and urine. Alkaline phosphatase and cholesterol are also re-absorbed into the blood in increased amounts. Absence of bile salts from the intestine increases the fat content of the faeces. Their presence in the bloodstream causes itching of the skin and scratch marks are a tell-tale sign of obstructive jaundice. In the urine they lead to the formation of a frothy head on the specimen and it is notable that the froth shows the yellow-brown colour of bilirubin. The normal tiny drops of urine stain the patient's underclothing a bright yellow.

In long-standing obstructive jaundice, the raised serum cholesterol leads to the appearance of cholesterol deposits in the skin (xanthelasmata).

For the discussion of causes and treatment of extrahepatic biliary obstruction *see* Chapter 24.

There is one form of chronic obstructive jaundice which lies on the frontier between the bile ducts (which are normal) and the liver cells. It is a form of intrahepatic cholestasis known as primary biliary cirrhosis. It is commonest in women over 35 years of age and ultimately proves fatal, the liver becoming markedly cirrhotic. Chronic extrahepatic biliary obstruction when combined with infection (usually due to stones in the common duct) may also lead to a form of cirrhosis known as secondary biliary cirrhosis.

The main features of the three different forms of jaundice are summarized in Table 23.1.

THE SPLEEN

Anatomy and physiology

The spleen is a deep plum-coloured, tongue-shaped organ of firm uniform consistency. It lies beneath the left half of the diaphragm, nestling between the fundus of the stomach, the splenic flexure of the colon, the tail of the pancreas and the left kidney. In health it is 2.5 cm (1 inch) thick, 7.5 cm (3 inches) wide, 12.5 cm (5 inches) long, 198 g (7 ounces) in weight and is situated deeply between the ninth and eleventh ribs, to which its long axis lies parallel. Its anterior end is well behind the costal margin and not accessible to palpation. Its internal structure (a connective tissue framework supporting a pulp of lymphoid tissue, miscellaneous phagocytic cells, blood and lymph vessels and autonomic nerve fibres) is fully described in textbooks of anatomy, physiology and medicine. It is of no practical importance to the surgeon except in so far as it accounts for the spleen's friability and consequent proneness to traumatic rupture and its relative inability when ruptured to stop bleeding. It is also because of its spongy consistency that it is possible after introducing a needle in the spleen first to measure the venous pressure in the portal vessels and then to outline them by injecting contrast material. It is also possible to aspirate splenic pulp for microscopic study.

Its functions are of more importance to the physician than to the surgeon. They include:

(1) removal from the blood of particulate matter including ageing and abnormal red cells and platelets, bacteria and artificially introduced particles;
(2) antibody production;
(3) iron storage;
(4) splenic haemopoiesis, especially erythropoiesis, which is normal in the fetus (it may also occur in adults suffering from haemolytic states or diseases leading to bone marrow destruction; a small proportion of the circulating lymphocytes of healthy adults are splenic in origin).

In some animals the spleen acts as a storage site for red cells which can be released into the circulation when required (for example, following haemorrhage). This is not so for the normal human spleen, though it does appear to store platelets. Pathologically enlarged spleens may also store red cells to a limited degree.

Most splenic disorders lead to enlargement, and when the spleen reaches about three times its normal size, it emerges rather low down from the left costal margin where it may be felt as a firm, smooth mass with a notched anterior border moving on respiration. Further increase carries it down in the line of the left tenth rib towards the right iliac fossa. Enlargement from any cause (so long as it entails an increase in the quantity of splenic tissue and not its replacement by other elements) leads to an increase in functional activity (hypersplenism) shown by reduction of the circulating haemoglobin, red cells, white cells (granulocytes) and platelets (pancytopenia).

Removal of a normal spleen is followed by broadly opposite effects, though after a short initial increase, there is a drop in red cells and haemoglobin lasting several months before normal values are restored. The leucocytes, however, especially the polymorphs, are increased in numbers and remain so for months, later returning gradually to normal values, though sometimes with a permanent eosinophilia or lymphocytosis. The platelet count also increases briskly, reaching a maximum about 10 days after operation when there is a considerably increased danger of venous thrombosis, thereafter falling to normal values. These changes in the peripheral blood are accompanied by proliferation of the red marrow of the bones which extends into areas of yellow marrow, causing mild bone pains. Enlargement of the lymph nodes may also be noted.

Diseases of the spleen

The spleen has many diseases but the treatment of them accounts for but a small fraction of surgical practice, the majority being solely of interest to the physician. The only operation applicable to splenic disease is splenectomy. Enlargement of the spleen may occur in many diseases. These include:

(1) infections: bacterial, viral, spirochaetal, protozoal, and parasitic (for example, typhoid, septicaemia, infectious mononucleosis, syphilis, malaria, hydatid disease);
(2) malignant and related conditions (for example, leukaemia and Hodgkin's disease);
(3) cysts, abscesses, simple tumours (for example, angioma);
(4) abnormal deposits (for example, amyloidosis, Gaucher's disease);
(5) blood cell destructive diseases (for example, haemolytic anaemia, thrombocytopenic purpura);
(6) venous congestion, for example congestive cardiac failure, portal hypertension (the combination of cirrhosis of the liver, portal hypertension, congestive splenomegaly, hypersplenism, anaemia and pancytopenia, and possibly ascites, used to be known, before it was fully understood, as Banti's disease); and
(7) collagen diseases (for example, Still's disease and Felty's syndrome — both forms of rheumatoid arthritis).

The following are splenic diseases and abnormalities not associated with enlargement of the spleen.

(1) Congenital absence which is very rare and always accompanied by other malformations.
(2) Accessory spleens (spleniculi or splenunculi) — small collections of splenic tissue usually located in the posterior abdominal wall and roots of the mesenteries adjacent to the splenic vessels. After splenectomy they enlarge and take over the functions of the excised organ. Therefore, when performing splenectomy for haemolytic anaemia or thrombocytopenia, splenunculi must also be found and removed.
(3) Wandering spleen. Excessive length and mobility of its pedicle may enable the spleen to find its way into any

part of the abdomen or pelvis, even interfering with micturition, defaecation or parturition. The condition may be complicated by twisting of the pedicle to produce torsion.

(4) Torsion of the spleen which, if acute, presents as an abdominal catastrophe, usually with a large tender palpable mass. Intermittent but milder attacks may also occur.

(5) Aneurysm of the splenic artery. It is usually symptom-less until it ruptures, causing signs of intra-abdominal haemorrhage in the left upper quadrant resembling the picture seen in splenic rupture.

(6) Rupture of the spleen.

Rupture of the spleen

Despite its friable consistency, considerable violence is required to rupture a normal spleen on account of its sheltered position. Usually the injury results from a severe fall or kick, or a crushing or run-over accident, and splenic injury is often associated with fractures of lower left ribs and other injuries within the abdomen and chest. Pathologically enlarged spleens are more friable and more exposed and may be ruptured by quite minor blows. This is particularly true in infectious mononucleosis and malaria.

Clinically there are three forms of ruptured spleen: (1) the rapidly fatal rupture, (2) rupture followed by shock, and (3) delayed rupture.

The rapidly fatal variety   The spleen is either torn from its pedicle or pulped into fragments. Profound shock rapidly develops and death ensues either before treatment can be started or rapidly despite attempts at resuscitation.

Rupture by shock   Shock follows the injury but passes off while signs of haemorrhage in the left upper abdomen appear. Diagnosis is usually possible and is suggested by the following phenomena.

(1) History and evidence of a blow over the left hypo-chondrium — bruising, rib fractures.

(2) Signs of haemorrhage — increasing pallor, cold extremities, sweating, rising pulse, falling pulse pressure and later falling systolic blood pressure, sighing respirations.

(3) Signs of haemoperitoneum — generalized tenderness and moderate guarding (Kehr's sign — pain in the left shoulder tip due to irritation of the left diaphragm by blood and clot; Ballance's sign — shifting dullness in

the right flank and fixed dullness of the left. A dull note on percussion in the right flank indicates the presence of blood. On turning the patient right-side uppermost, the blood drains away and gut floats up giving a resonant note (shifting dullness). Percussion of the left flank gives a dull note also and this persists when the patient is turned left-side uppermost because it is due to clotted blood (fixed dullness).

(4) Boggy fullness and tenderness in the rectovesical pouch on rectal examination.

(5) After a few hours, abdominal distension and disappearance of peristaltic sounds occur.

(6) A plain radiograph of chest and abdomen may show rib fractures, elevation of the left diaphragm, displacement or distortion of the stomach gas bubble and loss of soft tissue outlines (spleen, kidney, psoas muscle).

(7) Diagnostic paracentesis with a small syringe and aspirating needle yields blood.

Delayed rupture In delayed rupture initial shock and localizing signs pass off and the patient becomes sign and symptom-free for a period lasting from a few hours to 10 days. Suddenly the signs of internal haemorrhage reappear and progress rapidly, sometimes to a fatal conclusion. This sequence of events may arise from a laceration which is wholly within the spleen and forms an intrasplenic haematoma. As this liquefies it expands by taking up fluid, making its way to the surface and bursting through the capsule. At other times a small surface laceration is covered by adherent omentum enclosing a haematoma which then follows a similar sequence.

Patients suspected of having a splenic injury which could lead to delayed rupture require admission to hospital for observation for a period of not less than 10 days.

Treatment of ruptured spleen

A diagnosis or reasonable suspicion of ruptured spleen call for laparotomy and (if confirmed) splenectomy. Shock should be treated first but not too much time should be lost on preoperative measures. Blood replacement often makes little headway until the bleeding has been stopped and it is better to have plenty of blood available for the actual operation and several infusion points established. Opening the abdomen often leads to torrential haemorrhage for a few moments until the splenic artery and veins have been secured, and this is the time for rapid transfusion. Both before and during the operation, every effort must be made to find and treat other injuries. Loose pieces of pulped spleen should also be sought and removed as it is possible for them to establish themselves as splenic grafts, seeding the upper abdomen with myriads of small spleens embedded in vascular peritoneal adhesions, a condition known as splenosis.

The indications for splenectomy are:

(1) rupture of the spleen or of a splenic aneurysm;
(2) as part of some other operation, e.g. total gastrectomy, either to facilitate access or to allow radical excision of the lymphatic drainage field of a carcinoma, or to perform splenorenal anastomosis;
(3) local splenic disease — cysts, tumours, abscesses;
(4) at the request of a physician, usually for some form of haemolytic anaemia or thrombocytopenia with the aim of reducing the rate of red cell or platelet destruction or for staging in Hodgkin's disease.

The spleen may be approached abdominally either through a left paramedian incision or an oblique incision parallel to the left costal margin similar to Kocher's gall-bladder incision on the right. If there is a likelihood of adhesions between the spleen and diaphragm, a transthoracic approach may be adopted. The posterior part of the spleen is firmly attached to the posterior abdominal wall by the lienorenal ligament. This must be divided before the spleen on its pedicle can be delivered and the splenic artery and vein displayed as they appear from behind the tail of the pancreas. After these have been divided, a second set of vessels must be severed, the vasa brevia which run between the spleen and the greater curvature of the stomach. The spleen is then free and can be removed. It is wise to close the wound with non-absorbable or tension sutures as coincidental injury to the pancreas may lead to effusion of pancreatic juice which digests both fibrin and catgut, predisposing to wound disruption. A drain introduced into the splenic bed through a separate stab is desirable for the same reason. Dilatation of the stomach, ileus, subphrenic abscess, hiccup and thrombosis of splenic, portal and other veins are additional possible postoperative complications.

REFERENCE

Shields, R. (1978). Portal hypertension and bleeding oesophageal varices. In *Current Surgical Practice*, Vol. 2. Eds. J. Hadfield and M. Hobsley. London: Edward Arnold

24 Surgery of the biliary tract and pancreas

John McFarland

ANATOMY AND PHYSIOLOGY

The extrahepatic biliary tract is a duct system conveying bile from the liver to the duodenum. The gall bladder, which lies under the right lobe of the liver, is essentially a pouch connected by a duct to this system near its midpoint. It acts as a place of storage for the bile which may be concentrated five to ten times by absorption of fluid across its mucous membrane lining. The bile duct, which runs behind the first part of the duodenum and the head of the pancreas, usually shares a common opening (papilla of Vater) with the pancreatic duct into the medial wall of the second part of the duodenum (*Figure 24.1*).

The pancreas lies obliquely behind the stomach, separated from it by a peritoneal pouch known as the lesser sac. The head is cradled in the curve of the duodenum, the body lies in front of the spine and the tail stretches upwards laterally towards the spleen. It has a lobulated appearance and is covered with a fine capsule. The main pancreatic duct runs

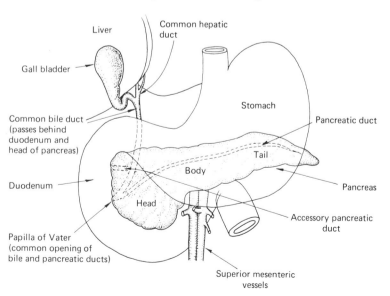

Figure 24.1. Anatomy of the biliary tract and pancreas

through the centre of the gland to its common opening with the bile duct. Usually a small accessory pancreatic duct opens into the duodenum about 2.5 cm above the papilla of Vater. Under the microscope several different cell types are evident. Columnar epithelial cells line the ends of tiny duct systems which connect eventually with the main duct. These are the source of the enzyme-rich pancreatic juice (exocrine secretions). Scattered throughout the gland irregular cell groups (islets of Langerhans) may be seen. These are central to the endocrine system of the pancreas which is concerned with the release of the hormones, insulin and glucagon, into the bloodstream.

The embryological origin of the biliary tract and of half the pancreas is as a bud growing ventrally from the digestive tube. The other half of the pancreas develops from a dorsal bud. Subsequently, following rotation of the gut, the two halves of the pancreas fuse.

Bile is an amber coloured fluid consisting mainly of water but containing small amounts of bile pigments (the end-product of red blood cell breakdown), bile salts, cholesterol, electrolytes (inorganic salts), and mucus. A more complete description of bile is given in Chapter 23. Although bile flow from the liver is virtually continuous (the hormone secretin stimulates this) discharge into the duodenum is intermittent and depends on gall-bladder contraction associated with relaxation of the muscle around the lower end of the common duct (sphincter of Oddi). The stimulus for this is the hormone cholecystokinin liberated from the duodenal mucosa in response to the presence of food in the lumen.

Pancreatic secretion is clear and contains a high concentration of bicarbonate in water which is elaborated following stimulation by secretin. In addition, a series of enzymes, or their precursors (notably trypsin, acting on proteins; amylase, acting on carbohydrates; and lipase, acting on fats), result from pancreatic stimulation by cholecystokinin. Secretion of both inorganic compounds and enzymes is not continuous but is usually in response to the presence of food in the duodenum and is mediated by the release of these hormones (secretin and cholecystokinin) from the duodenal mucosa. The importance of the bicarbonate is that the food, acidified in the stomach, must be rendered alkaline before the enzymes can act on these constituents.

There is also a nervous (vagal) effect on both the biliary system and the pancreas.

The endocrine secretion of the pancreas is concerned with carbohydrate metabolism. Insulin causes a fall in blood sugar level (hypoglycaemia) while glucagon causes this to rise (hyperglycaemia).

PATHOLOGY

Diseases of the biliary tract and the pancreas may reasonably be considered in the same context because of anatomical and functional association and also because of interlocking aetiology (for example, gall-stones as a causative factor in pancreatitis) and sequelae (e.g. stones in the common bile duct and carcinoma of the head of the pancreas both lead to obstructive jaundice).

The commonest problems of the gall bladder and bile ducts are related to gall-stones and to inflammation (cholecystitis). Less commonly, problems arise in connection with developmental anomalies, strictures of the ducts or cancer.

Inflammation and cancer are the major pancreatic diseases of surgical interest. Less commonly pancreatic problems arise because of developmental anomalies, trauma, cysts or rare tumours.

Diseases of the biliary tract

Gall-stones

There are several types of gall-stones: pigment (3 per cent), cholesterol (10 per cent) and mixed (80 per cent). Classification according to type is not completely possible (for example, a mixed stone may surround a central **nidus** of cholesterol) and these percentages are approximate. The remaining 7 per cent includes a large variety of rarities (for example, stones surrounding foreign bodies).

The aetiology of gall-stones is obscure. In rare types some specific factor may be evident; for example, pigment stones have been shown to have an increased incidence in conditions of excessive red cell destruction (haemolytic anaemia). Theories of the general nature of causation centre on consideration of altered constitution of bile, biliary stasis and the effects of inflammation.

Gall-stones may cause symptoms only when complications arise. Hence it is not unusual for them to be first recognized as an incidental finding on abdominal radiography (10 to 15 per cent of gall-stones are radio-opaque). Some possible complications are indicated in *Figure 24.2*. The likelihood that one or more stones will perpetuate mucosal irritation and inflammation is clear. Frank perforation of the gall bladder wall is uncommon (in contradistinction to the high incidence of appendiceal perforation) and is unlikely to spread throughout the peritoneal cavity. Usually omentum will have become attached to the area and, at most, a local abscess will result. If the duodenum lies in contact, a fistula may form with discharge of the stone into the gut. The stone

Nidus Literally — nest; the focus of, for example, an infection or a gall-stone.

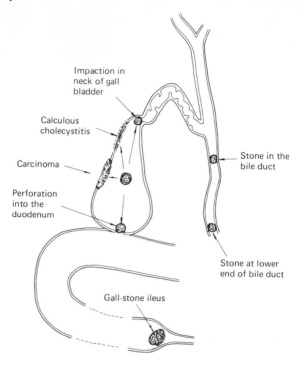

Figure 24.2. Composite diagram of some possible complications of gall-stones. Carcinoma is very rare; in case of perforation into the duodenum, the gall-stone may become impacted in the terminal ileum causing 'gall-stone ileus'. Impaction of the gall-stone in the gall bladder neck leads to mucocoele (if infected — empyema) of gall bladder. Moving gall-stone causes biliary colic. Stone in the bile duct may cause obstructive jaundice. Stone at lower end of bile duct may be a factor in pancreatitis

will be moved on through the small intestine, but if it is large, it may impact near the lower end of the ileum. This type of obstruction is known as gall-stone ileus. Small stones are commonly thought to give more symptoms than large ones as they can more readily be moved from the neck of the gall bladder (Hartmann's pouch) towards the cystic duct and the associated muscle spasm results in severe pain. A stone may pass through the cystic duct or, if large, may become impacted in this area. This will prevent bile or fluid moving through the duct in either way. A mucocoele of the gall bladder will result due to distension by mucus ('white' bile). If there is infection present, this may be pus (empyema of the gall bladder). Larger stones may pass into the common duct through a fistulous tract.

It is clearly possible that under some circumstances (stasis, infection, debris) stones may form in the common duct and it is quite evident that small stones may enlarge. They need not cause trouble immediately. Intermittent hold-up by a stone at the lower end of the common duct may cause the duct to dilate (this does not happen if the obstruction is sudden and complete) and it is possible for the stone to pass (naturally or by fistula) into the duodenum. Commonly, however, obstructive jaundice will develop.

Cholecystitis

Inflammation of the gall bladder may be acute or chronic. In acute cholecystitis the pattern of inflammation of other hollow organs is followed; that is, local inflammatory oedema, distension and exudation with irritation of local viscera. In appendicitis perforation may occur but this is uncommon in cholecystitis in which either resolution or the development of a chronic inflammatory state is more usual.

Chronic cholecystitis runs a less definite course. There may be local inflammation and adhesions are the rule, although they do not usually cause trouble. The gall bladder may become thick-walled, fibrotic and shrunken and will fail to function adequately as a reservoir for concentration and storage of bile.

A particular type of infection, not necessarily with marked inflammation, is when the gall bladder harbours typhoid bacteria. This may make the subject a particularly resistant typhoid carrier.

Congenital defects

Congenital lesions of the biliary tract are rare. The duct system growing from the gut may not fuse with the elements in the liver (congenital biliary atresia) with a resulting jaundice which is particularly difficult to treat. Or there may be a cystic developmental anomaly (choledochal cyst) which may compress and obstruct the duct but which, quite commonly, does not present until adult life.

Stricture

A benign stricture of the bile duct is almost always due to fibrosis following damage sustained at an earlier operation. The most frequent site is near the point of entry of the cystic duct.

Carcinoma

Carcinoma may arise in the gall bladder or at any point in the duct system. Mucosal irritation by gall-stones has been suggested as a possible causative factor. The best chance of a cure is in those cases where the distal part of the duct is involved. Jaundice may lead to early diagnosis and there is a possibility of resection. When the site is the gall bladder, jaundice is likely to be late. A palpable mass may be the first sign and the condition is then usually inoperable.

Diseases of the pancreas

Pancreatitis

Pancreatitis is the term for the situation when the integrity of the pancreatic cell structure is breached and enzymes, usually tracked through the duct system, leak into the retroperitoneum and peritoneum. The initiating factors are unknown although there is a marked association between acute pancreatitis and excessive alcohol consumption or biliary disease (some authorities quote one or other association in over 80 per cent of instances).

The condition may be acute and severe with very considerable extravasation of ferments resulting in depletion of circulatory fluids and shock, both toxic and hypovolaemic. Unless this can be reversed the mortality risk is high. Such an attack (successfully treated) or lesser incidents may recur (relapsing pancreatitis) but are not so likely to be fatal. A state of chronic pancreatitis may develop with resultant subnormal exocrine and (later) endocrine function.

A complication of acute pancreatitis is the development of a pseudocyst — essentially a 'walled-off' collection of fluid exudate eventually presenting as a mass which may press on the upper abdominal viscera and even be visible by distension of the upper abdomen.

Carcinoma of the pancreas

Carcinoma of the pancreas may develop in any part of the gland, but only if it arises in the head is the clinical presentation (by obstructive jaundice) likely to be early enough to give much hope for surgical treatment. The involved pancreas will be enlarged and hard and at operation the surgeon can find this difficult to differentiate from chronic pancreatitis.

Trauma

Traumatic lesions of the pancreas are becoming more common with the increasing number of road traffic accidents. The pancreas is indirectly vulnerable to abdominal injuries. Lying stretched across the spine it can be severely compressed or torn, partially or completely, near its midpoint.

Pancreatic cysts

Pancreatic cysts are rare. Congenital cysts (very rarely), cystadenoma and cystadenocarcinoma may present as upper abdominal swellings. Treatment, especially for the latter two conditions, is operative removal.

Hypovolaemia Diminished blood volume in the body.

Rare tumours

Two rare types of tumour may arise in the pancreas, each apparently originating from a cell type seen in small numbers in the normal pancreas. An **insulinoma** arises from the beta cells of the islets of Langerhans. The histological pattern is similar to that of normal islet tissue. Excessive secretion of insulin is the result and the patient is subject to irregular bouts of hypoglycaemia (low blood sugar) with resultant headaches, dizziness, weakness and fainting.

Equally rare is a pancreatic islet cell tumour secreting excessive amounts of the hormone gastrin, which constantly stimulates the gastric mucosa to secrete large volumes of hydrochloric acid (Zollinger–Ellison syndrome). Severe and persistent duodenojejunal ulceration usually results from this.

In each condition the tumours may be multiple and may also be malignant. A patient with the Zollinger–Ellison syndrome may well have had one or more gastric operations before this is diagnosed and failure to control the massive outpouring of acid may result in the patient's death.

CLINICAL PRESENTATION

There is some overlap in the usual clinical presentation of biliary or pancreatic disease. Major presenting symptoms are pain (usually in one or other of several patterns) and obstructive jaundice.

Symptoms

Pain in biliary disease

Biliary colic is characterized by intermittent upper abdominal pain of extreme severity. It appears to originate in the epigastrium and may spread round (or through) to the back, usually, but not invariably, on the right side. Women commonly volunteer the information that, at its peak, the pain seems more severe than labour pains. The patient is characteristically helpless in his efforts to relieve the pain and usually keeps moving round, as lying still brings no relief and may increase his awareness. The natural course is for the attack to rise to a peak over several hours and then fade. This type of pain appears to be due to extreme muscle spasm as a gall-stone moves from the body of the gall bladder and for a while becomes impacted towards its neck. Relief after injection of strong analgesics (such as morphine or pethidine) is usually dramatic although both of these have the disadvantage of causing spasm of the sphincter of Oddi and must therefore, be given with an antispasmodic drug such as atropine or promethazine hydrochloride.

Insulinoma A tumour which secretes insulin.

Y

In acute cholecystitis pain due to acute inflammation of the gall bladder usually commences as a poorly localized dull ache in the upper abdomen. After several hours, or even after a day or so, it may 'settle' at a point just below the ribs at the right upper abdomen.

The initial pain is caused by the distension of the gall bladder. The localization is due to irritation of the inflamed organ of the overlying peritoneum. Associated with this is relative spasm of the abdominal muscles in the area. There may be modification of this feature if omentum is interposed between the gall bladder and the peritoneum. However, local external pressure (as by the examining doctor) will usually exaggerate the muscle spasm and elicit local tenderness. In chronic cholecystitis pain is quite variable but is usually similar to that described above for the early stage of the acute disease. This rather vague 'indigestion' may be aggravated by gall bladder contractions stimulated by the patient's consumption of food — particularly fats.

The considerable variation of a patient's response to pain must be recognized and other difficulties of interpretation may arise as, for example, when gall-stones coexist with acute inflammation or are associated with other upper abdominal disease, such as peptic ulcer or hiatus hernia. Nonetheless, an accurate diagnosis may be made, in most cases, from the clinical presentation alone.

Pain in pancreatic disease

Pain in pancreatic disease may be due to the effects of chronic inflammation or erosion into the gland by a peptic ulcer or a cancer, either primary or secondary. The pain is usually midabdominal but not well localized and may also be felt in the back at the same level. The pain is usually intermittent but may become persistent and severe.

A more acute pain is that associated with acute pancreatitis when the cellular integrity of the gland is breached and pancreatic ferments spread into the retroperitoneum and peritoneal cavity. This is likely to be felt in the whole abdomen and the patient may be in a seriously shocked state.

Obstructive jaundice

The liver secretes about 1000 ml of bile in 24 hours. This passes through the common bile duct into the duodenum. Jaundice, i.e. tissue staining with bile, will inevitably follow if the flow is blocked (*Figure 24.3*). The blockage may be within the duct, as by a gall-stone, and this may be intermittent if the stone should shift in position and allow bile to flow around it. It may arise from pathology of the duct wall causing a stricture. This may be due to fibrosis originating in most instances from damage to the duct at an operation to remove the gall bladder. Hence the commonest level is at the point of entry of the cystic duct. A stricture may also be caused by a carcinoma which may arise at any point in the biliary system. There may be pressure from outside the duct. Near to the liver this is most commonly enlargement of lymph nodes by metastatic carcinoma. Local oedema associated with cholecystitis may cause a mild and short-lived

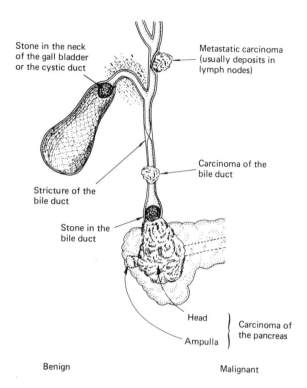

Figure 24.3. Composite diagram of possible causes of obstructive jaundice. Stone in the neck of gall bladder or the cystic duct may cause transient jaundice due to inflammatory oedema

jaundice. At the lower end cancer of the pancreas will initially cause compression and later spread into the duct. If the carcinoma originates at the papilla of Vater (so-called 'ampullary cancer'), ulceration may occur to relieve the obstruction leading to an unexpected alleviation of the jaundice. Carcinoma of the head of the pancreas itself causes unremitting deepening jaundice.

Bile formation and circulation is described quite fully in Chapter 23. With this knowledge the various types of jaundice may be understood and these are discussed later in the same chapter. In the current chapter obstructive jaundice (post-hepatic biliary obstruction) will be dealt with. This condition is likely to present with a typical pattern of bile-stained urine and pale (bile-free) faeces. There is commonly troublesome skin irritation (pruritis) which is thought to be due to bile-salt retention. Differentiation from jaundice due to prehepatic causes (haemolytic/acholuric jaundice) is relatively simple but separation of jaundice due to hepatic and posthepatic causes can be a difficult problem. Some of the complexities may be evident if it is appreciated that interference with bile formation may be effective at different stages of its intrahepatic course and also that continued posthepatic obstruction may lead to hepatic damage due to 'back pressure'. It is in this situation that information from liver function tests may be helpful; these are mentioned briefly later in this chapter and are also discussed in Chapter 23. With regard to obstructive jaundice a key observation is the relationship between the serum alkaline phosphatase level — this is normally 21—100 i.u. per litre (3—13 King— Armstrong units/100 ml) — and other indices of the liver function such as the flocculation tests. These will be abnormal in hepatic disease when the alkaline phosphatase level may also be raised. However, they are likely to be normal in posthepatic obstruction (at least until a late stage) in which situation the alkaline phosphatase level may be increased more than three-fold.

Signs

Biliary disease

If the patient with biliary disease is not jaundiced, physical signs will range from nil to those occasioned by severe upper abdominal inflammation and even gall bladder perforation. Physical findings will be confined to the abdomen.

When recovery has been good following an attack of biliary colic, the abdomen will be soft and non-tender without a palpable swelling. However, following an attack of acute cholecystitis, tenderness may persist in the right hypochondrium. This may be present in some cases of chronic cholecystitis and may be elicited by asking the patient to take a deep breath while the examiner's fingers are pressed quite firmly below the point of the ninth rib (Murphy's sign). A mucocoele of the gall bladder will usually be palpable as a non-tender swelling at this point.

Jaundice, a yellow staining of the skin and other tissues, occurs when the serum bilirubin level is raised (hyperbilirubinaemia). The exact level at which this is observed will depend on several factors, not least the skill of the clinician. The sclera and the gums are useful places to inspect and daylight may be more helpful than artificial light which itself may sometimes impart a yellowish tinge. Clinically detectable jaundice usually indicates a bilirubin level of more than 34 μmol per litre (0.2 mg/100 ml). Normal serum bilirubin level is below 12 μmol per litre (0.7 mg/100 ml); thus hyperbilirubinaemia is not always detectable clinically. The patient may have volunteered, or agreed on direct questioning, that his urine has been dark and his faeces pale. The latter may usually be confirmed by inspection of faeces on the glove after digital examination of the faeces. The former requires inspection and then testing of the urine (it will be appreciated that excessively concentrated urine, as when the patient is feverish, may be dark without having an excess of bile). The confirmation of this triad is strong clinical evidence of obstructive jaundice. The key observation is then whether a distended gall bladder may be detected by palpation. If not, previous calculous cholecystitis may be the factor preventing its distension and jaundice may be due to bile duct obstruction by one or more of the stones. If it is distended, the gall bladder walls must be thin and distensible (that is, not fibrotic as after inflammation) and the obstruction is more likely to be due to a carcinoma at the lower end of the duct or head of pancreas. This is the principle of Courvoisier's law that 'when the common bile duct is obstructed by a stone, dilatation of the gall bladder is rare'. It is a critical point in operative treatment, for, if the growth cannot be removed, it may be possible for it to be by-passed by anastomosing the distended gall bladder to the intestine distal to the obstruction (cholecystenterostomy).

Pancreatic disease

A patient in an attack of acute pancreatitis will be seriously ill. He may be pale and clammy with a racing pulse and, possibly, a low blood pressure (incipient shock). This is the effect of the combination of severe pain, release of toxins and retroperitoneal sequestration of fluid. There may, of course, be lesser degrees and, when the patient has established pancreatitis with acute relapses, these are not likely to be as severe as an initial fulminating incident. Examination of the abdomen will elicit extreme tenderness, usually throughout, but this is variable as is the degree of abdominal wall rigidity.

A late complication of pancreatitis, a pseudocyst, may reach a large size and be readily palpable in the upper abdomen.

Carcinoma of the pancreas is not usually palpable until a late stage. Preoperative suspicion of this condition in the head of the pancreas is by inference in a patient with obstructive jaundice (*see above*).

Special investigations of the biliary tract

Radiology

A considerable amount of information may be obtained from a plain radiograph of the abdomen. About 10 to 15 per cent of gall-stones are radio-opaque. The biliary duct system may be outlined by intestinal gas if there is a fistulous or operative connection between it and the gut. Indeed, when there is evidence of obstructed bowel associated with biliary gas, the intestinal obstruction is almost certainly due to a gall-stone that has passed through such a fistula ('gall-stone ileus').

Methods of outlining the gall bladder and duct system may be indirect or direct. The indirect methods are as follows.

In oral cholecystography (Graham—Cole test) the subject takes an iodine compound which is excreted by the liver and, when concentrated in the gall bladder, becomes radio-opaque. In current practice this is usually done with fractionated dosage, that is the patient takes capsules the evening before the study on the morning of which he swallows a sachet of powder (Solu-Biloptin). If the compound is adequately absorbed, absence of opacification indicates a malfunctioning (or absent) gall bladder. Non-opaque gall-stones may be outlined, showing as radiolucent points in the opacified area. Ingestion of fat will normally result in gall bladder contraction and this may be observed radiologically.

In the normal case an outline of the duct will usually be obtained following gall bladder contraction in the oral method. If this is not the case or the gall bladder is diseased or has been removed, the ducts may be outlined by intravenous cholangiography, that is, by injecting a suitable iodine compound (for example, Biligram) intravenously. This is excreted by the liver in a more concentrated form and usually shows the pattern of the duct system.

This is attractive in principle but in practice the image may be poor and unfortunately this is particularly likely in the jaundiced patient who has a serum bilirubin above 50—70 μmol per litre (3—4 mg/100 ml). Here introduction of radio-opaque fluid (Urografin) directly into the duct system is most valuable and the following methods are available.

(1) Percutaneous transhepatic cholangiography (PTC). The simplicity and safety of this technique of introducing under local anaesthesia, a very fine (outer diameter 0.7 mm) flexible hollow needle has lead to its widespread use at an early stage in the diagnosis of jaundice with an obstructive pattern (*Figure 24.4*).

(2) Endoscopic retrograde cholangiopancreatography (ERCP). Access to the biliary or pancreatic ducts is

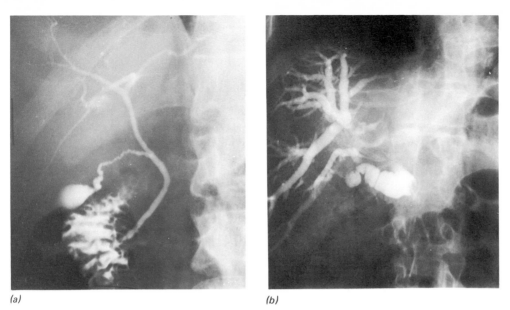

(a)   (b)

Figure 24.4. Percutaneous transhepatic cholangiography (PTC). (*a*) Normal biliary system in a patient with non-obstructive jaundice. When PTC is attempted on a normal duct system it may be successful in about half the cases. (*b*) The bile duct is obstructed by a carcinoma. The whole duct system is distended, particularly the cystic duct and the gall bladder which has just begun to fill. (Radiographs by courtesy of Dr Austin Carty)

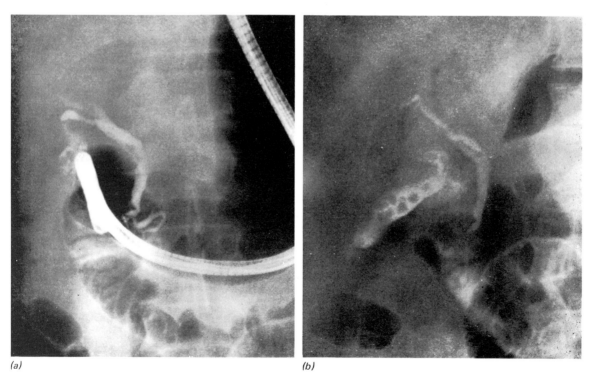

(a)   (b)

Figure 24.5. Cannulation of the papilla of Vater at duodenoscopy in a jaundiced patient. This allows retrograde injection of radio-opaque fluid. (*a*) A radiograph showing the bile duct and the pancreatic duct outlined in this way. (*b*) A radiograph taken 10 minutes later. Gall-stones are outlined in the gall bladder. The pancreatic duct has emptied

gained via a fine tube introduced at duodenoscopy (*Figure 24.5*).

(3) Operative cholangiography. Access to the duct system for needling or intubation is usually easiest at this time.

(4) Postoperative cholangiography. This is done via the T-tube left in the duct for a period of time after this has been explored.

Indirect study of function

One of the most important factors is the serum bilirubin level. The normal level is below 12 μmol per litre (0.7 mg/100 ml). This may be raised in several situations (discussed in Chapter 23). It is usual for the highest levels to be reached in obstructive jaundice, most particularly that due to carcinoma of the head of the pancreas and a figure over 250 μmol per litre (14.6 mg/100 ml) is suggestive of this. Other liver function tests (serum protein levels, flocculation studies, serum enzymes, prothrombin time and dye excretion rate) are described in Chapter 23.

Special investigations of the pancreas

Radiology

A plain radiograph of the abdomen is not directly helpful in pancreatic disease with the one exception that it may reveal areas of calcification in the gland, a sequel to pancreatitis; also gall-stones shown on this may be important.

Valuable information may be obtained by a barium meal examination when encroachment by pancreatic pathology (for example, distortion of the stomach by a pseudocyst (*Figure 24.6*) or of the duodenum by a carcinoma of the head of the pancreas) may be suggested.

Biliary radiology, as already described, is clearly important in the full investigation of the pancreas but may be limited by jaundice. ERCP (*see above*) is the only method of outlining the pancreatic duct short of operation.

Modern arteriographic techniques have made cannulation of the coeliac axis (a branch of the aorta) possible. This selective angiography can give a clear picture of the blood supply of the pancreas.

Indirect radiology (as in cholecystography) is not possible but the nearest in principle to this is the use of radioactive isotope scanning. Selenomethiomine injected intravenously is taken up by the pancreas. If the isotope ^{75}Se is used, gamma rays are emitted which can be detected by a sensitive scanning instrument and a pattern printed on a photographic plate. The outline of the pancreas obtained is not a detailed one but in expert hands the technique can be useful.

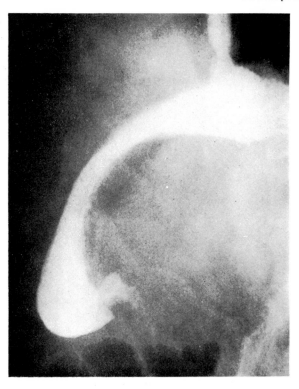

Figure 24.6. A barium meal radiograph. The body of the stomach is pushed forward by a pancreatic pseudocyst

Until very recently it has not been possible for the pancreatic duct to be outlined by contrast medium except at operation when the duct may be cannulated. However, recent improvements in fibreoptic endoscopes have made it possible to inspect and cannulate the papilla of Vater in the conscious patient (*see Figure 22.5*). This advance should result in the better understanding and diagnosis of pancreatic disease.

Direct study of function

The direct study of pancreatic function involves duodenal intubation and collection of the secretions arising following stimulation of the pancreas by an injection of secretin/pancreazymin. Estimation of volume and bicarbonate and enzyme concentration may give useful information.

Indirect study of function

The key test is estimation of the serum amylase level. Normally this is below 340 i.u. per litre (180 Somogyi units/100 ml). A five-fold increase is diagnostic of acute pancreatitis, although this peak may be short-lived. Interpretation of lesser increases must be cautious as other acute conditions may lead to high amylase levels.

New methods of visualization

Ultrasound and CAT (Computerized Axial Tomography) scanning are both non-invasive methods of imaging that have great potential in the diagnosis of biliary and pancreatic disease. Diagnostic ultrasound is relatively inexpensive and widely used. As it gives pictures of cystic dilatation it may help in the diagnosis of jaundice or show up pancreatic cysts. CAT scanning is used to give cross-sectional pictures throughout the body but the very considerable expense of the equipment has limited its availability.

TREATMENT OF BILIARY AND PANCREATIC DISEASE

Medical treatment

Symptomless gall-stones do not require urgent treatment, but a decision regarding operation (cholecystectomy) should be made and will depend on the circumstances in each case.

Biliary colic should be treated initially by powerful analgesics such as pethidine or morphia by injection. This will relieve the acute attack but subsequent cholecystectomy is usually advised.

Acute cholecystitis will usually settle with bed rest, sedation and possibly intravenous fluid replacement and antibiotics. Occasionally this approach is not successful. Deterioration of the situation (such as free perforation or the extension of an abscess) may make operation essential. After an acute attack, an elective operation is usually advised some two months later when the inflammation may reasonably be expected to have settled.

Symptoms arising from chronic cholecystitis may be lessened by the patient's avoidance of possible gall bladder stimulation and a 'fat-free' diet is usually prescribed. Persistence or worsening of symptoms may indicate the need for operative treatment.

Initially, obstructive jaundice may be treated conservatively. A particular point is that vitamin K (an intramuscular injection of 10 mg daily) should be given to support prothrombin production in the liver. With an improving situation, particularly when gall-stones are strongly suspected, avoidance of urgent operation is favoured. Persistent deepening jaundice and a high suspicion of malignancy make operation mandatory.

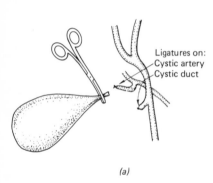

Ligatures on:
Cystic artery
Cystic duct

(a)

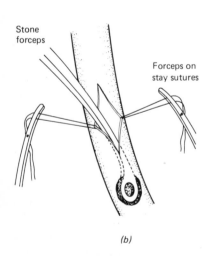

Stone
forceps

Forceps on
stay sutures

(b)

Figure 24.7. Biliary operations most commonly performed. (*a*) Cholecystectomy; (*b*) removal of stone from the bile duct

Surgical treatment

The possible surgical procedures on the biliary system are limited (*Figure 24.7*). In principle, they are: (1) the removal of the diseased gall bladder which may be done for relief of symptoms to which that disease had given rise; (2) the production of a free flow of bile through the ducts by removal of obstructing stones or resection or by-pass of stricture or growth.

The preoperative and operative management will depend considerably on whether or not the patient is jaundiced.

Biliary surgery on the non-jaundiced patient
Before operation the patient is fasted from the previous night and it is usual for a nasogastric tube to be passed before he is taken to theatre. Premedication and abdominal shaving and cleansing are routine.

To remove a diseased gall bladder the surgeon operates using a general anaesthetic. The right upper abdominal incision may be either transverse or vertical. After confirmation of the diagnosis and a general abdominal inspection the surgeon identifies, ligates and divides the cystic duct and artery. The gall bladder is dissected away from its liver bed and removed. The bile duct must also be identified and in no way interfered with unless the surgeon considers that it should be explored. The decision regarding this may be difficult and the surgeon can be greatly helped by operative cholangiography at which radio-opaque fluid is injected into the bile duct usually through a fine cannula introduced through the cystic duct. Radiology of the duct system is then possible and is most usefully demonstrated by immediate viewing on image-intensified television. If the bile duct is explored, this is done formally by incising it and drawing apart the edges of the cut. This allows for the removal of stones and debris, usually with special forceps, and the confirmation of a clear distal passage by slipping a catheter through to the duodenum or by radiology following injection of a radio-opaque dye.

The drain is usually removed at 5 to 8 days following operation. If the common duct has been opened, it is usual to close it round a T-tube. This should be radiologically examined with dye injected before it is removed at 7 to 10 days.

Biliary surgery in the jaundiced patient
The patient may be very ill and the operation a considerable undertaking. The cause of the obstructive jaundice may not be clear before operation. It is essential, therefore, that the patient is as fit as possible. In addition to the possible correction of anaemia and fluid and electrolyte imbalance, vitamin K must be given regularly by injection and prothrombin levels estimated. Other preoperative measures are as already described.

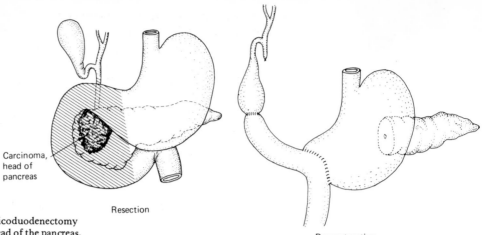

Resection

Reconstruction

Figure 24.8. Pancreaticoduodenectomy for carcinoma of the head of the pancreas. Resected structures are indicated by hatching. One possible method of reconstruction to allow function to be resumed

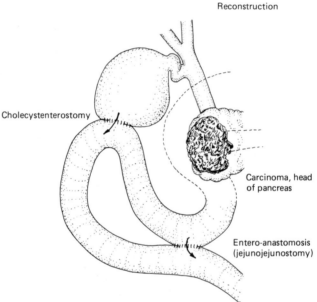

Cholecystenterostomy

Carcinoma, head of pancreas

Entero-anastomosis (jejunojejunostomy)

Figure 24.9. By-pass procedure for inoperable carcinoma of head of pancreas. Entero-anastomosis (jejunojejunostomy) is performed to minimize intestinal reflux

Pancreaticoduodenectomy Surgical removal of the pancreas and duodenum.

Cholecystenterostomy The making of a direct communication between the gall bladder and the intestine.

The surgeon's initial approach is as described, but the anaesthetist will be aware that this patient's liver and kidneys may be more vulnerable to the anaesthetic agents and will take particular precautions. If stones in the duct are found to be the problem, they are removed and the duct is closed with the bile draining through a rubber T-tube. A stricture is best treated by resection and end-to-end anastomosis of the duct but if it is extensive or high, more complex procedures may be necessary. If there is a growth at the papilla of Vater or head of pancreas, an extensive removal (**pancreaticoduodenectomy**) (*Figure 24.8*) may be possible, but a by-pass procedure (**cholecystenterostomy**) (*Figure 24.9*) may be a less hazardous and equally effective way of relieving the jaundice.

Postoperative management will depend to some extent on the procedure but severe jaundice may exaggerate problems, particularly the danger of haemorrhage. These patients are especially vulnerable to postoperative oliguria. This danger may be minimized by liberal intravenous fluid replacement coupled with an infusion of mannitol, an osmotic diuretic (50 g of a 20 per cent solution may be given on one occasion). Peritoneal bile leakage is very serious. Supervision of abdominal drainage must be meticulous. A simple drain may usually be removed at 5 days. With a T-tube in position radio-opaque fluid can be injected and radiographs taken to ensure that there is free flow with no residual stones. The tube is removed about 10 days after the operation and the opening in the common duct will close.

Treatment of pancreatic disease

The management of acute pancreatitis is supportive; that is to say fluid, sometimes in the form of blood or plasma, is given intravenously, antibiotics are administered and the pain is controlled by strong analgesics. Some benefit may be obtained by attempting decompression and relaxation of the upper gut by gastric aspiration and propantheline (Pro-Banthine) given by intramuscular injection. Subsequently operation may be necessary to drain a pancreatic pseudocyst or to remove coexisting gall-stones which may be a causative factor.

Relapsing or chronic pancreatitis is not usually amenable to surgery unless definite obstruction to the pancreatic duct may be demonstrated and relieved. Surgical removal of the pancreas may be a necessary operation in an extreme situation but is likely to result in severe diabetes.

Carcinoma of the body or tail of the pancreas may well have spread too far for surgery to be contemplated, but, occasionally, a local carcinoma in the head of the pancreas may be treated by resection. The reconstruction is complex (*Figure 24.8*). The alternative is a by-pass procedure to relieve the jaundice.

An insulinoma is best dealt with by partial pancreatic resection. A gastrin-secreting tumour (causing massive gastric hyperacidity) may be dealt with in this way but most authorities consider that in this (Zollinger–Ellison syndrome) it is best to remove the target organ – the stomach. Hitherto there had been no medical means of containing this situation but effective control of the hyperacidity has been reported with cimetidine therapy (p. 484).

Pancreatic trauma is usually coincident with other abdominal injuries. The damaged part of the pancreas must be removed or adequately drained.

Postoperative management is along the lines already described for biliary disease. In each instance, gastric aspiration via a nasogastric tube may be necessary for 24 to 48 hours.

Jaundice usually indicates severe disease; initially slower wound healing may be expected. Postoperative haemorrhage is not usually a problem and vitamin K injections may be discontinued.

After total pancreatectomy insulin replacement by injection is necessary straight away.

Rehabilitation and follow-up

Following a straightforward biliary operation, such as cholecystectomy, patients may expect to leave hospital after removal of the stitches at 7 to 10 days. Diet should be normal at that time and the surgeon will usually review his patients at one month by which time they should be back at work.

More complex operations may necessitate a longer stay in hospital. Follow-up review will continue for longer and following operation for carcinoma the patient's doctor or surgeon will arrange to undertake this indefinitely. Special circumstances call for particular supervision (for example, total pancreatectomy, when the need for insulin injections has already been emphasized and oral pancreatic supplements may be helpful).

25 Surgery of the intestines

Robert Shields and John McFarland

ANATOMY

The first part of the small intestine is the duodenum which has been described in Chapter 22. The remainder is made up of the jejunum and ileum, the latter representing two-fifths of the combined length of between 9 and 10 feet (2.7–3 m). The small intestine ends in the right lower side of the abdomen at its junction with the caecum at the ileocaecal valve.

The jejunum and ileum are attached to the posterior abdominal wall by a fan-shaped piece of tissue called the mesentery. This contains blood vessels (in the case of the small bowel the blood vessels belong to the superior mesenteric vascular trunk), lymphatics, lymph nodes, nerves, both sympathetic and parasympathetic and some fat.

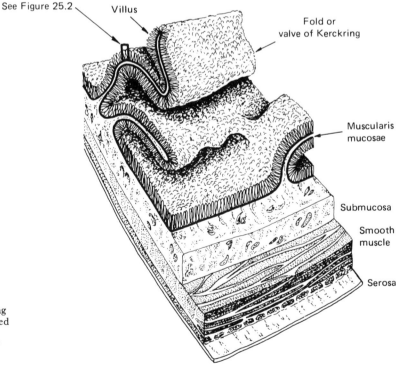

Figure 25.1. The several layers forming the wall of the small intestine. (Adapted from Laster and Ingelfinger, 1961, by courtesy of the Authors and Editor of *New England Journal of Medicine*)

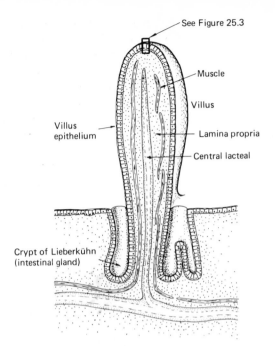

Figure 25.2. The structure of the villi and the crypts of Lieberkühn. (Adapted from Laster and Ingelfinger, 1961, by courtesy of the Authors and Editor of *New England Journal of Medicine*)

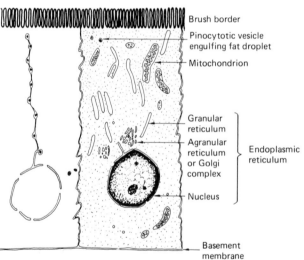

Figure 25.3. Diagram of columnar absorbing cell. (Adapted from Laster and Ingelfinger, 1961, by courtesy of the Authors and Editor of *New England Journal of Medicine*)

Microscopic features of the small intestine

The lining mucous membrane of the small intestine is arranged greatly to increase the epithelial surface area available for absorption (*Figures 25.1, 25.2* and *25.3*). First the mucosa of the small intestine is thrown up into a number of undulating folds (valvulae conniventes or folds of Kerckring) particularly prominent in the upper small bowel. Projecting into the lumen of the intestine from these folds are the long finger-like protrusions (0.5—1.5 mm in length) called villi, between the bases of which are a number of gland-like structures called the crypts of Lieberkühn. Within the core of the villi are strands of smooth muscle responsible for the pumping action of the villi, an important aid to absorption, and blood and lymphatic vessels by which nutrients absorbed from the intestinal tract pass into the body generally. The free borders of the columnar absorbing cells of the mucous membrane show a brush border which is composed of microvilli. By all these means the surface area of the intestine is increased by a factor of nearly 600 times that of a simple cylinder of similar gross dimensions.

Large intestine

The anatomy of the colon which extends from the ileocaecal valve to the pelvirectal junction is comparable in general respects to that of the small intestine, but is strikingly different in detail. It is no more than a quarter of the length of the small intestine, its calibre throughout is wider and the longitudinal muscle coat, lying outside the circular layer, is split into three strips (taenia) which give it a sacculated form. The mucosal lining is of columnar epithelium with a plethora of goblet cells producing a highly mucous secretion. Distal to the caecum there are three main anatomical divisions — the ascending, transverse and descending colon — suspended by mesentery and supplied and drained by branches of both the superior (right side) and inferior (left side) mesenteric arteries and veins. Lymphatic drainage follows the arteries and the nerve supply is both sympathetic and parasympathetic.

PHYSIOLOGY

The primary function of the small intestine is absorption. To perform this function the intestinal muscles act in a rhythmic fashion to give a segmenting movement, which serves to mix the contents of the bowel, and peristalsis which propels the contents of the bowel onwards.

The large intestine is designed for the reception and storage of the intestinal content discharged through the ileocaecal valve. Movement in the large intestine is less vigorous than in the small intestine and the major muscle activity is a mass peristalsis once to twice daily, usually after eating (gastrocolic reflex), by which faeces in the colon enter and distend the rectum giving rise to the desire to defaecate.

Digestion and absorption

The complex molecules of protein, carbohydrate and fat are broken down by appropriate enzymes which are secreted by the stomach, the pancreas and the small intestine. These enzymes along with agents such as bile salts render the foodstuffs simple enough for absorption by the intestinal mucosa. Other substances, for example, vitamins and minerals, water, are also absorbed by several mechanisms — some highly specific and involving active work by the intestinal cell. Other mechanisms are passive and perhaps non-specific by which substances, for example water, are carried across the intestinal cell into the body, secondary to, and influenced by, the movement of other substances.

Absorption of most substances takes place in the upper part of the small intestine, but the lower jejunum and ileum are also capable of absorbing and will do so, either if the intake of food is great, or if the upper jejunum is diseased or has been removed. There are, however, two substances which are specifically absorbed in the terminal ileum — vitamin B_{12} and bile salts. Therefore, if the ileum has been removed, is diseased, or is by-passed, these substances are not absorbed and so there may develop megaloblastic anaemia (due to vitamin B_{12} deficiency) or diarrhoea (due to the irritating action of bile salts on the colonic mucosa).

The absorptive function of the colon is largely confined to the removal of water and salt, thus converting the fluid chyme, received from the ileum, into the semi-solid faeces. However, the colonic mucosa is capable of absorbing other substances, for example drugs, and at one time many medicaments were administered to the patient using the intestinal route by enema.

DISEASES OF THE INTESTINES

Intestinal obstruction

In addition to the food and fluid taken in the diet, up to 8 litres of fluid are secreted into the upper reaches of the intestinal tract by the glands of the stomach and intestine as well as by the liver (bile) and the pancreas. All of this material is reabsorbed in the small and large intestines and only about 100 ml of fluid are lost in the faeces. If there is any obstruction to the onward passage of this fluid, the orderly sequence of secretion and reabsorption is disturbed. Not only will fluid and nutrients be prevented from reaching adequate mucosal surface area, but they will accumulate in the bowel above the obstruction causing it to distend.

Ultimately, the bowel may perforate but more usually the fluid and other intestinal contents are discharged towards the mouth and lost as vomiting.

Types of intestinal obstruction

There are basically two types of intestinal obstruction: those due to (1) mechanical causes, or (2) paralysis of the intestine, called paralytic (adynamic) ileus. Mechanical obstruction may be a simple occlusion of the lumen, for example by a foreign body but, in addition, the blood supply to the bowel may be so impaired that necrosis of the bowel occurs (strangulation obstruction). This latter type of obstruction is seen where a loop of intestine slips into the sac of a hernia so that not only is the lumen of the bowel occluded, but also the venous drainage is obstructed. Arterial blood continues to be pumped into the intestine but no blood can leave. The intestine becomes greatly congested and ultimately will undergo infarction.

Causes of intestinal obstruction

Traditionally the causes of obstruction (*Figure 25.4*) may be:

(1) lesion within the lumen, such as a swallowed foreign body or a gall-stone, impacted faeces;

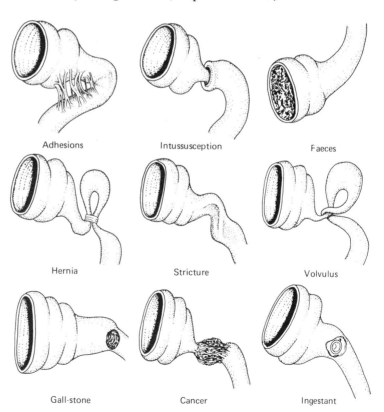

Figure 25.4. Causes of intestinal obstruction. (Modified from Elmslie and Ludbrook, 1971)

Adhesions   Intussusception   Faeces

Hernia   Stricture   Volvulus

Gall-stone   Cancer   Ingestant

(2) disease of the intestinal wall, such as simple or malignant stricture; or

(3) disease from without (pressure on the bowel due to hernia or fibrous band, and so on).

In infants obstruction is usually caused by a congenital atresia or stenosis. In older children the causes are usually a fibrous band related to a Meckel's diverticulum or intussusception; in a middle-aged patient the cause of the obstruction is usually a hernia or adhesion band following operation and in old age the causes are more commonly cancer and mesenteric vascular occlusion.

Clinical features

The features are usually the triad of pain, vomiting and constipation.

The pain is usually colicky in nature, causing the patient to feel very restless and unable to obtain a position of relief. Where the obstruction lies in the upper part of the small intestine, the pain usually comes on frequently and is felt in the upper part of the abdomen. With obstruction lower down the intestine, the pain is usually less frequent, although still severe, and radiates in a vague manner throughout the lower part of the abdomen. There may be more localized pain if the bowel is undergoing strangulation.

The frequency and amount of vomiting depends particularly on the site of the obstruction. With a highly placed obstruction the vomit usually becomes copious with early and marked dehydration of the patient. With lower obstructions vomiting may not be a predominant feature initially but as the disease progresses the vomiting will become more copious and the vomitus, which initially consisted of gastric content and then bile, ultimately has a marked faeculent character. The patient usually empties his rectum at the onset of the disease but thereafter neither flatus nor faeces can be passed and any enemas which are injected into the rectum are returned without faeces.

The patient's general condition depends on the presence or absence of strangulation and the amount of fluid that has been lost. With a high intestinal obstruction, where fluid loss has been great, dehydration rapidly develops and oligaemic shock supervenes with a rapid pulse and falling blood pressure. In strangulation obstruction, the shock is aggravated by bacterial intoxication.

On examination the abdomen may be distended, particularly with lower intestinal obstruction. With higher intestinal obstruction there may be a complete absence of distension. With mechanical obstruction there are usually initially increased bowel sounds which can be heard on auscultation.

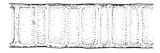

Jejunum

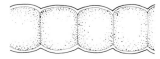

Ileum

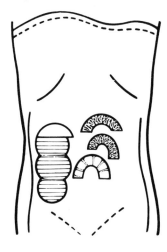

Colon

Figure 25.5. Illustrations of distended bowel. (Reproduced from Meschan, 1962, by courtesy of the Author and Publishers, W. B. Saunders)

Later peristalsis may be visible. Where the small intestine is obstructed the dilated coils of bowel may be seen in the central part of the abdomen forming a step-ladder pattern. A diagnosis of strangulation obstruction will be suggested by persistent pain, localized tenderness and rigidity of the abdominal wall; perhaps a tense irreducible external hernia will be present.

Special investigations

The most important special investigation is a simple radiological examination of the abdomen with the patient both supine and erect. In the erect position fluid with air above can easily be seen in the dilated coils of intestine. The nature of the distended loops may indicate whether they are of small intestine or of the large intestine (*Figure 25.5*). If the caecum is greatly distended, the obstruction is presumed to be in the large intestine (*Figure 25.6*). If the caecum is collapsed, the obstruction is probably in the small intestine (*Figure 25.7*).

Figure 25.6. Schematic diagram of a radiograph in obstruction of the large intestine

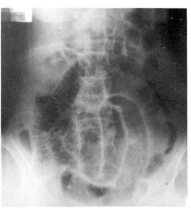
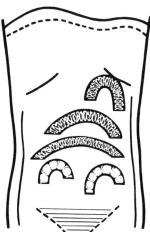

Figure 25.7. Schematic diagram of a radiograph in obstruction of the small intestine

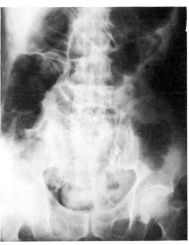

If the large intestine is thought to be obstructed, the obstructing agent may be localized by (1) sigmoidoscopy or colonoscopy; (2) injecting a small quantity of barium into the large bowel to outline the obstruction on radiological examination.

Treatment of the mechanical cause

In the case of mechanical cause of obstruction, operation should be carried out without undue delay, particularly if there is any risk of strangulation. In the preoperative preparation of the patient there are certain steps which must be taken.

(1) Stomach must be emptied and kept empty by inserting a nasogastric tube and applying continuous suction to empty the stomach. This step is particularly necessary immediately before the induction of anaesthesia, because of the grave risk of inhalation of gastric content into the lungs.

(2) A patient, who is greatly shocked due to dehydration, must be resuscitated before anaesthesia and operation are carried out, by the rapid intravenous injection of plasma and electrolyte solution.

(3) Because of the risk of bacterial intoxication antibiotics should be given.

Operative treatment depends upon the nature of the obstruction. Fibrous bands or adhesions should be divided, complicated volvulus should be undone, and external hernia causing obstruction will have to be reduced and repaired. When the obstruction has been relieved the surgeon has to inspect the bowel to see if it is viable. If the intestine is grey or green and flaccid, without any obvious pulsation in its blood vessels, it is probably already dead and will have to be removed. The surgeon may have to wait for a few moments, warming the bowel with wet towels and ensuring that the patient is well oxygenated to see if there is any return of normal colour or blood supply to the bowel. Non-viable or frankly gangrenous bowel must be resected.

In large intestinal obstruction, usually caused by cancer or diverticular disease, a short circuit or colostomy is performed to drain the bowel above the obstruction as a prelude to later radical resection. Such a colostomy is usually constructed by bringing a loop of transverse colon out of the abdominal wall through a small incision. The loop is held in position by passing a glass rod or plastic tube under the loop between its limbs. The lumen of the colon is then opened to allow the discharge of accumulated gas and faeces. Such a loop colostomy is very useful as a temporary procedure (*Figure 25.8*).

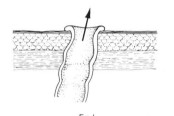

End

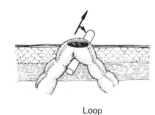

Loop

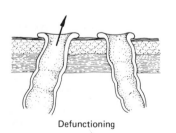

Defunctioning

Figure 25.8. Types of colostomy. (Modified from Elmslie and Ludbrook, 1971)

Treatment of paralytic (adynamic) ileus

In paralytic ileus the bowel is obstructed because of paralysis of its musculature, usually because of peritonitis, for example, rupture of an intra-abdominal abscess, pancreatitis, and occasionally following retroperitoneal disorders, such as a large haematoma. The bowel becomes distended with fluid and gas, vomiting may be copious with the usual general results. In addition, the patient's condition is worsened by the associated bacterial toxaemia. Operation may be indicated to deal with the cause, for example, to drain an abscess or to close a perforation. Apart from this, little can be done about the paralysis except to rest the bowel by stopping all food and fluid by mouth, applying continuous suction through a nasogastric tube, administering antibiotics and to replace, intravenously, fluid and electrolytes. As the peritonitis subsides so the bowel recovers its function and the obstruction is relieved.

Vascular disorders of the intestines

Superior mesenteric vascular occlusion

The superior mesenteric artery which supplies the mid-gut, that is, most of the small intestine and the proximal part of the large intestine, may be occluded suddenly by an embolus, or more slowly, by the clotting of blood (thrombosis) on and around a plaque of atheroma in the wall of the blood vessel.

The patient usually presents with sudden acute pain in the central part of the abdomen which becomes distended. There may be associated vomiting and the passage of blood in soft watery stool. The patient's general condition is usually quite good initially, but the disturbing feature on examination is the marked rigidity and guarding of the abdomen. There is usually marked pallor of the patient. A high **leucocytosis** is another feature.

If operation to deal with the obstructed vessels is not performed urgently the bowel undergoes infarction and it may be necessary to remove an extremely lengthy segment. Such massive resection of the intestine greatly reduces the mucosal surface area available for absorption. Great care may be required to maintain normal nutrition in these patients by judicious use of intravenous and other parenteral therapy.

In other patients the occlusion of the arterial supply to the intestine is more gradual, due to thrombosis occurring on the surface of an atheromatous plaque. This may cause abdominal pain following a meal. Diagnosis may be possible by arteriography of the affected vessel.

Leucocytosis Increased number of circulating white blood cells. The cells are usually polymorphonuclear appearing in response to a bacterial infection.

Occlusion of the inferior mesenteric artery

Less commonly the inferior mesenteric artery or one of its branches may become occluded. The colon may be infarcted particularly on the left side and the patient presents with an acute illness.

Tumours of the intestines

Tumours of the small intestine

Tumours of the small intestine are relatively uncommon. Benign tumours may arise from the mucous membrane, muscle, fibrous tissue or fat. Symptoms are related to the ulceration of the surface giving rise to bleeding, or to obstruction of the lumen causing intestinal obstruction. A tumour may, if it is large enough, be caught up by peristalsis and initiate an intussusception. Usually the diagnosis is difficult and often not made until the operation is performed. On radiological examination, using barium, a rounded defect in the lumen of the small bowel may be evident. More usually the patient undergoes laparotomy for obscure symptoms and the tumour is found on careful inspection of the bowel.

An interesting congenital affliction is the Peutz–Jeghers syndrome, in which multiple adenomata are found throughout the small intestine, associated with pigmentation of the mucosa of the mouth, the face and the fingers. The multiple small tumours of the bowel may cause recurring haemorrhage with or without partial obstruction.

Of particular interest are argentaffin tumours (carcinoid tumours) which arise from silver-staining cells usually found in the appendix, ileum and colon. In these sites, particularly in the appendix, carcinoid tumours are usually small and rarely produce symptoms. Elsewhere the tumours may attain large size. In the ileum the tumour may grow very slowly and become malignant, eventually metastasizing to the liver. A special feature of the tumour is that it may secrete a substance known as serotonin (5-hydroxytryptamine). When this substance is released from hepatic metastases it escapes into the circulation giving rise to a red discolouration of the face, attacks of flushing with dyspnoea and occasionally stenosis of the heart valves. It can often be recognized by identifying, by simple test, its breakdown product, 5-hydroxy-indole-acetic acid, in the urine. Because of the rather slow growth of this tumour both the primary growth and the metastases should be removed if at all possible.

Malignant tumours of the small intestine are rare and will present either because of blood loss or intestinal obstruction. Operation, where possible, consists in the resection of the segment of intestine bearing the tumour.

Benign tumours of the large intestine

The commonest tumour of the colon arises from the epithelium and is called a benign adenoma. Occasionally this may project as a rounded tumour into the lumen of the bowel and is called a polyp. The tumour as it grows may be pulled away from the mucous membrane by intestinal peristaltic action to become suspended by a narrow stalk. Polyps are usually common in the distal part of the colon but are not limited to this part. The tumours may be single or there may be several. The usual presenting clinical feature of a benign adenoma is the discharge of bright red blood from its ulcerated surface.

The importance of these tumours lies in their relationship to malignant disease of the colon. Controversy still exists on whether carcinoma of the bowel arises *de novo* or whether such benign adenomata can themselves undergo malignant change.

In the past it has been possible to visualize them only by double contrast barium enema x-ray in which the bowel is emptied by a simple wash-out, barium is run into the distal colon and then evacuated and the rectum is then filled with air or carbon dioxide. In this way small lesions covered with a thin barium layer can be outlined. However the entire length of the colonic mucosa can be inspected by fibre optic colonoscopy and biopsies may be taken at any level. Indeed small lesions may be excised completely (*Figure 25.9*).

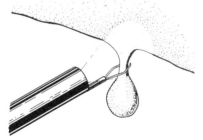

Figure 25.9. Diathermy loop excision of polyp at fibre-optic colonoscopy

Villous tumour A particular type of adenoma is the sessile villous tumour which usually occurs in the rectum. Although these tumours are usually small, they may be quite extensive, as a velvety bleeding tumour on the surface of the rectum. The importance of these tumours is that on occasion they may secrete large quantities of mucinous fluid to such an extent that a patient may present with severe acute water and electrolyte depletion. This tumour is usually regarded as precancerous and, while local resection and **fulguration** may be possible in many cases, formal resection has to be carried out.

Familial polyposis There is a rare familial disorder called familial polyposis, in which the whole of the large intestine is studded with little adenomatoma usually varying in size up to about 1 cm in diameter. These tumours usually appear in childhood or adolescence and the disease can be transmitted either by the father or mother to children of either sex. On average, one-half of the family will be affected. The importance of the tumours lies in the risk of carcinoma which may

Fulguration Tissue destruction by diathermy.

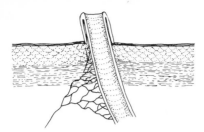

Figure 25.10. Permanent ileostomy

develop in more than one-half of the cases, often at an early age. Operation should always be advised even when there are no symptoms. The most certain method of treatment is to excise the whole colon and rectum, leaving the patient with a permanent ileostomy (*Figure 25.10*). An alternative method of treatment is to remove the colon and anastomose the ileum to the rectum, and then keep the rectum under surveillance by repeated endoscopy. Residual tumours can then be dealt with by fulguration. When a patient is found to have this disease, all other members of the family must be traced, investigated and treated.

Malignant tumours of the large intestine

One of the commonest cancers among peoples of Western civilization is carcinoma of the colon. The cause of this disease is unknown but it may develop as a complication of ulcerative colitis or of familial polyposis. As mentioned above, there is still some discussion about the relationship between carcinoma and polyps of the colon.

The disease tends to be much more common in the left side, particularly in the sigmoid colon, where the tumour usually encircles the wall of the bowel circumferentially to form a ring stricture (*Figure 25.11*). Because of this and because of the semi-solid nature of the intestinal content, obstructive symptoms usually develop early and may be the presenting feature of the disease. Less commonly the tumour, particularly when it occurs in the caecum or in the rectum, may project as a rather luxuriant cauliflower mass into the lumen of the bowel. In this case obstructive symptoms are late because of the capacious volume of this part of the intestine and because of the semi-fluid nature of the intestinal content. At this site the tumour is prone to undergo ulceration and haemorrhage and patients present usually with general ill-health, weight loss and anaemia.

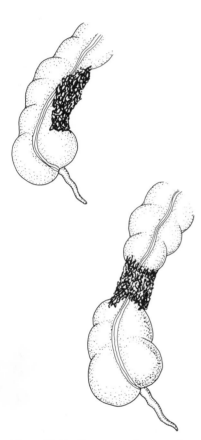

Figure 25.11. Two types of cancer of the colon. (Reproduced from Elmslie and Ludbrook, 1971, by courtesy of the Authors and Heinemann Medical Books)

The spread of the tumour is initially by local invasion through the wall of the bowel and then by lymphatics circumferentially around the bowel and thereafter in the wall of the bowel upwards and downwards. Its further spread is also by the lymphatics, first to the lymph nodes closely related to the tumour, then to others closely related to the veins draining the colon. Ultimately metastases may occur in more distant organs, particularly in the liver. In this way the disease can be divided into four stages: (1) where the tumour is confined to the mucosa, (2) where there is local invasion of the bowel, (3) where the lymph nodes are involved either locally or beyond the limits of surgical removal, and (4) where there are distant metastases.

Where operation can be carried out, the technique depends on the site involved (*Figure 25.12*). Where the tumour involves the caecum, ascending colon or hepatic flexure of the colon, the right half (right hemicolectomy) of the colon is removed in an attempt to remove not only tumour and bowel but the lymph nodes in the territory supplied by the right colic and ileocolic vessels. Continuity of the intestinal tract is re-established by joining the ileum end-to-end with the transverse colon. Where the tumour lies in the transverse colon, the intestine bearing the tumour is resected to include the territory supplied by the mid-colic artery. For a tumour in the descending or sigmoid part of the colon, the affected intestine, 5 cm above and below the tumour, is removed, but the full extent of the resection depends on lymph node involvement. Usually the inferior mesenteric artery below its left colic branch is divided. Continuity is restored by end-to-end anastomosis.

In unresectable cases the tumour may be short-circuited to prevent the late complication of intestinal obstruction. Where the tumour causes obstruction, a preliminary colostomy has to be performed (*see Figure 25.8*). Where a colostomy is to be permanent (for example, a terminal sigmoid colostomy when the rest of the sigmoid colon, rectum and anus have been removed for carcinoma of the rectum) the colon is brought out through an opening in the abdominal wall (*see Figure 25.8*) and cut across, the end of the colon being lightly sutured to the skin and muscles of the abdomen. A light appliance can be worn so that the faecal matter will fall into the bag which can be changed daily. The bag is held in position by a special belt.

Intussusception

In intussusception one part of the bowel becomes invaginated into an adjacent part (*see Figure 25.4*). The portion which enters is then carried distally by the peristaltic action of the bowel. Usually this condition occurs in children below the age of 2 years. For reasons which are not entirely clear, the process begins usually in the distal part of the small bowel and the apex of the entering portion is carried down through the ileocaecal valve into the caecum. As the mesentery and the mesocolon are drawn in, the contained blood vessels become compressed and the intestine may be strangulated.

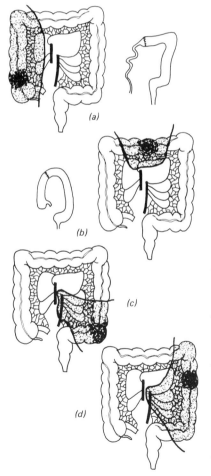

(a)

(b)

(c)

(d)

Figure 25.12. Operations for cancer of the colon. (*a*) Right hemicolectomy and ileotransverse anastomosis for carcinoma of the ascending colon. (*b*) Transverse colectomy for carcinoma of the transverse colon. (*c*) Removal of sigmoid colon and part of descending colon for carcinoma of the sigmoid colon. (*d*) Extended left hemicolectomy for carcinoma of descending colon. (Modified from Scott, 1971)

The child is usually seized with severe colicky pain which causes him to cry out and draw his knees up. Between attacks the child usually lies quietly. Blood may be passed per rectum and on examination it may be possible to feel a mass in the abdomen, initially the right side of the abdomen and later in the epigastrium. Radiological examination of the abdomen after barium is given *per rectum* shows a characteristic cup-shaped filling deformity in the colon. This investigation itself may in favourable cases reduce the intussusception but this is not common and the procedure is not free from danger.

Operation has to be performed without delay. As far as possible the surgeon tries to reduce the intussusception, but great care has to be exercised to avoid tearing the bowel.

In older children and in adults intussusception is usually the result of a tumour of the small intestine acting as a bolus being driven along by peristaltic action so that the intestine is invaginated. Typically, the intussusception complicates a tumour in the caecum and the clinical features are those of recurring partial obstruction. In these patients the treatment consists of not merely the reduction of the intussusception but also the resection of that segment of the intestine which contains the tumour.

Regional enteritis (Crohn's disease)

Regional enteritis is a disease of unknown cause in which the characteristic feature is a non-specific chronic inflammatory reaction, at one time confused with tuberculosis.

From the surgical point of view two forms occur.

Acute form
The acute form runs a rapid course like acute appendicitis. The patient, often a young person, complains of pain in the right iliac fossa of the abdomen associated with nausea and vomiting and on examination there is marked tenderness in this region. Occasionally, a mass may be felt in the right iliac fossa. The diagnosis is usually made only at operation where, instead of an inflamed appendix, the terminal ileum is found to be greatly thickened and congested. No specific treatment is required. The infected piece of intestine should not be excised but the appendix, if not obviously involved in the disease, can be removed. Most patients recover and suffer no further complications or recurrences.

Chronic form
The chronic form of Crohn's disease also tends to occur in young people. The disease may affect any part of the gastrointestinal tract from oesophagus to anus, but characteristically

the terminal ileum is involved, along with the caecum and the ileocaecal valve. The disease may extend by a continuous process to involve other parts of the intestine, or there may be intervening areas of intestine which are seemingly normal. These so-called 'skip' lesions may be scattered in a discontinuous manner throughout the intestine. In addition, the large intestine may be involved, in some cases exclusively so. The involved intestine is thick-walled with a contracted lumen. The mesentery of the affected bowel is thick and oedematous with many prominent lymph nodes evident. The inflammatory process may extend through the intestinal wall to involve the serosal coat which then becomes adherent to other contents of the abdominal cavity and subsequently a **fistula** may develop between segments of intestine, between intestine and bladder or between intestine and abdominal wall.

The characteristic microscopic feature is considerable thickening of the tissues due to oedema and fibrosis of the submucosal layers in which there is an infiltration of lymphocytes and other endothelial cells. Although many giant cells are evident, the characteristic **caseation** of tuberculosis is not present.

Clinical presentation and diagnosis

The clinical features of Crohn's disease are extremely variable. The usual presentation is one of abdominal pain associated with diarrhoea. In addition, the patient may occasionally have attacks of fever and complain of general ill-health with marked weight loss. Another presentation may be that of malabsorption with inability of the affected intestine to absorb fat, protein and other constituents of the diet. Rectal bleeding is uncommon.

On occasion, the complications of the disease may predominate. The thickened bowel may effectively narrow the intestinal lumen and cause obstruction. In other cases a large inflammatory mass of adherent intestinal loops may form, particularly in the right iliac fossa, to be easily palpated as a tender fixed mass. Patients may present with a fistula (occasionally between bladder and bowel) and, if there has been a previous operation, there may be an external fistula between intestine and abdominal wall.

Infections and fissures in the perineum, particularly around the anus, are very common. These lesions tend to be chronic and persisting, and in several cases may precede the manifest intestinal Crohn's disease by several years.

In some cases the colon is also afflicted; indeed there may be no apparent disease in the small intestine. Distinction between Crohn's disease of the colon and ulcerative colitis

Fistula An unnatural communication between the cavity of an organ and the skin or cavity of another organ.

Caseation A form of degeneration or necrosis in which tissues are changed into a cheesy mass.

may be particularly difficult and indeed impossible. Diagnosis often rests on the fact that in Crohn's disease the rectum is relatively spared, abdominal pain is very common, perianal disease is frequent, while frank bleeding from the anus is uncommon. On the other hand, in ulcerative colitis abdominal pain does not usually dominate to the same extent; in most cases there is blood in the stool, and on sigmoidoscopic examination the mucosa shows a uniform reddening, inflammation and granularity.

The diagnosis is usually made on radiological examinations. Barium meal together with follow-through examination of the small intestine is a particularly valuable technique to show the extent of the small-intestinal disease. Barium enema

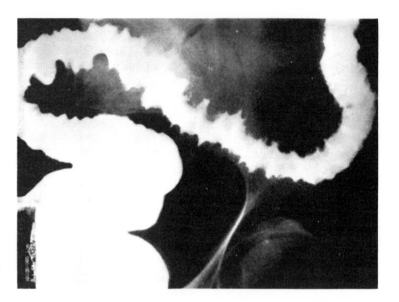

Figure 25.13. Barium enema photograph of a patient with Crohn's disease of the colon

is often the first investigation because of the existence of diarrhoea. A characteristic narrowing and mucosal oedema of the terminal ileum are seen. In the large intestine the appearance is a cobble-stone pattern in which, between deep fissuring due to penetrating ulcers, oedematous mucosa protrudes into the lumen (*Figure 25.13*). The characteristic granulomatous lesions may be seen on histological examination of the rectal biopsy.

Treatment
In most cases medical measures are tried in the first place. These measures are directed to the general improvement of the patient's health by attention to nutrition, vitamins and, in severe cases, to the restoration of fluid deficiencies. The diarrhoea may be controlled by simple palliative measures,

such as, codeine, morphine and kaolin mixtures. In many patients **corticosteroid** drugs are given. In most patients they are of some value in the short-term treatment, but considerable doubt is still expressed about the contribution of these drugs to the long-term management of the patient. These drugs have a number of important side-effects which may detract considerably from the beneficial effects. Recently, there has been an attempt to use azathioprine, an immunosuppressive drug, to treat this disease but its value is still debatable.

If these measures fail and the patient's condition is unimproved or if complications, for example obstruction, abscesses or fistula develop, surgical intervention becomes essential. Surgical treatment is now directed to the excision of the affected portion of bowel. Formerly the diseased intestine was by-passed but there is no evidence that this helped the disease process to subside. The problem about surgical treatment is that the disease may be extensive, or there may be many 'skip' lesions, so that in order to eradicate the disease, the surgeon may have to do a massive resection and the patient will be left with too little bowel for satisfactory absorption of nutrients.

Ulcerative colitis

Ulcerative colitis would be better termed proctocolitis because, almost invariably, the rectum is involved. The mucous membranes of the colon and rectum are inflamed and in places ulcerated. A similar appearance can be found in infective diarrhoea, e.g. dysentery, but in the case of ulcerative colitis (proctocolitis) there is no evidence that organisms play a significant part in its causation. The disease varies both in severity and extent. The inflammation and ulceration may be limited to only one part of the colon, or affect its whole length. In the most severe forms of the disease there are many ulcers, discrete and confluent, throughout the large intestine from the ileocaecal valve distally. The intervening portions of mucosa between ulcers are inflamed and oedematous and project into the lumen as rather swollen tags of tissue known as pseudopolypi.

The cause of this disease is not known. Several types of bacteria have been isolated but these would not appear to be the cause of the disease. Several patients exhibit emotional disturbances but there is no constant psychiatric disorder. Moreover, it is reasonable to expect that a chronic illness characterized by frequent passage of stools could itself lead to considerable emotional disturbance in the patient. The psychological manifestations of this disease are probably a consequence of it.

Corticosteroid Hormones secreted by the cortex of the adrenal glands and connected with carbohydrate and protein metabolism (glucocorticoids, cortisone, etc.); with water and electrolyte balance (mineralocorticoids – aldosterone); male sex hormones (androgens) and female sex hormones (oestrogens).

Clinical presentation and diagnosis

The clinical features of ulcerative colitis vary greatly. At one end of the scale the disease may run a mild course, characterized by the passage several times per day of soft, sometimes watery, stools containing blood. The patient's general health is good and with modifications in the diet the symptoms can be brought under control. Unhappily, in some patients the disease may pursue a rapidly fulminating course and the patient be brought close to death within 2 to 3 days. The colon may dilate ('toxic dilatation') and even perforate to cause peritonitis. Another manifestation of the disease is a long chronic wasting illness characterized by loss of weight, marked ill-health, anaemia and a number of general effects, such as, liver disease, arthritis, **iritis** and infective skin lesions.

An important complication is the development of malignant disease of the colon, which is more likely to occur in those in whom the entire colon is involved and where the disease has been present for a number of years.

The diagnosis of ulcerative colitis is based largely on the exclusion of infective and other specific causes of diarrhoea, and several special investigations. The major investigations are sigmoidoscopy, colonoscopy and barium enema radiology. On sigmoidoscopy the rectum appears very granular and friable and bleeds easily to the touch. Ulceration in the rectum is not common. Histological examination of a rectal biopsy shows a characteristic inflammatory process with crypt abscesses in which polymorphonuclear cells are closely related to the crypts of Lieberkühn. The characteristic granulomatous features of Crohn's disease are not present. In the most severe form of the disease on barium enema radiological examination the colon is seen as a narrow, rigid, foreshortened tube, in which the characteristic **haustrations** are lacking. Ulceration of the colon and pseudopolypi may be seen. By such radiological examination the extent of the disease may be determined.

Treatment

In disease which is limited in extent and not severe the treatment is largely medical and consists of the correction of deficiencies, such as anaemia, the elimination from the diet of any food which may cause diarrhoea and the use of steroids. The steroids may be given by several routes. In mild disease steroids are given topically, either in the form of prednisolone suppositories or, more successfully, hydrocortisone enemas. In more severe disease the steroids should be given orally in the form of prednisolone tablets in doses as high as 60 mg per day. In very severe disease the steroids

Iritis Inflammation of the iris.

Haustration The separation of the colon into saccules.

may have to be given by injection. Occasionally, adrenocortico-trophic hormone (ACTH) is given instead of prednisolone or hydrocortisone. The other drug which can be used is the sulphonamide, sulphasalazine, 1 g 6-hourly, as an alternative, or in addition, to steroids. The two drugs may have to be combined but more usually steroids are used in an attempt to abort an attack of ulcerative colitis and sulphasalazine to maintain a patient in remission and to avoid further attacks.

Operative treatment, however, may have to be considered in a number of occasions. When there is perforation or toxic dilatation of the colon, emergency operation is indicated. Urgent operation may have to be performed if, in acute attacks, there is no response to medical treatment and the patient's condition continues to deteriorate. Operation may have to be carried out in those patients in whom there has been prolonged ill-health with chronic diarrhoea, ill-controlled by conventional medical treatment. The appearance of complications, particularly skin lesions, liver disease and arthritis, is another indication for operation. Occasionally, operation has to be advised as a prophylactic measure in those who have had total colitis for several years, to prevent malignancy. Before operation the patient's condition has to be improved and if the patient is on steroids, or has been on these drugs recently, it is necessary to give increased doses of steroids before and after operation to avoid the possibility of adrenal failure.

Some controversy still exists on the best type of operation. Most surgeons favour a panproctocolectomy in which the rectum and entire colon are excised and the ileum is brought out into the anterior abdominal wall, usually on the right side, as a terminal ileostomy (*Figure 25.10*). A two-piece ileostomy bag can be applied, and once the initial copious discharge from the ileostomy subsides, the patient usually manages very well to cope with the appliance and the ileo-stomy. A relatively new development is the 'continent ileostomy', formed from a valved pouch of the terminal ileum. The patient passes a tube into the ileostomy to empty it about three times a day.

As an alternative to this operation the colon may be removed and the rectum retained. Some surgeons form an ileostomy, in the hope that later the ileum can be anasto-mosed to the rectum to restore intestinal continuity; other surgeons will, at the time of the primary operation, anastomose the ileum to the rectum. In this way the unpleasantness of an ileostomy is avoided but this is achieved at the expense of leaving part of the diseased intestine in place with the possibility of continuing diarrhoea, generalized complications and particularly the later risk of cancer.

Diverticula of the colon

Diverticula of the colon are formed by the herniation of mucous membrane through weak areas in the muscle coat, usually in longitudinal rows beside the taeniae coli where the branches of the colic arteries penetrate the mucosa. Diverticula are extremely common in the elderly and their cause is probably related to the low residue of the diet and to chronic constipation which has become associated with powerful abnormal and irregular colonic contractions. Such diverticula may occur at any part of the colon but are more common in the descending and sigmoid parts. Rarely, single or solitary diverticula may be found in the caecum.

In diverticulosis the colon is studded with thin-walled pouches without any inflammation and without any symptoms. However, these pouches of mucous membrane do not empty completely because of the absence of muscle, and the stagnation of the faecal contents may lead to inflammatory change in the wall of the diverticulum. An entire segment of the intestine may become thickened and fibrosed with marked hypertrophy of the muscles. Several complications may result (*Figure 25.13*). The affected segment becomes so thickened and fibrosed that its lumen is narrowed and

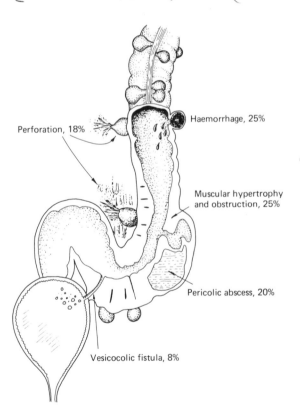

Perforation, 18%

Haemorrhage, 25%

Muscular hypertrophy and obstruction, 25%

Pericolic abscess, 20%

Vesicocolic fistula, 8%

Figure 25.14. The complications of diverticulitis. (Reproduced from Davis, 1968, by courtesy of the Author and Publishers, W. B. Saunders)

(obstructed;) the patient may present with intestinal obstruction. There may be localized perforation of an affected diverticulum so that a pericolic abscess develops. The abscess may penetrate into a neighbouring hollow viscus, for example, another segment of intestine, or the bladder, so that an internal fistula is formed. Free perforation into the peritoneal cavity may take place and a generalized faecal peritonitis develop. Occasionally, massive rectal haemorrhage can occur.

Clinical presentation and diagnosis

The onset of diverticulitis may be characterized by clinical features similar to those of bowel cancer, particularly constipation or diarrhoea, and low left-sided abdominal pain. Differentiation may be difficult even at operation.

When the disease becomes complicated there may be very much more severe pain in the left lower quadrant of the abdomen with spreading peritonitis pyrexia and leucocytosis. These features would suggest the formation of an abscess and if the tenderness becomes more extensive, free perforation into the peritoneal cavity is suggested, with generalized peritonitis.

Barium enema radiological examination of most elderly subjects will show the presence of diverticula. It is, however, the presence of a narrow contracted lumen with marked serration of the barium outline which suggests that secondary inflammatory changes have occurred. Sigmoidoscopy may be of value but it is only rarely that the mouth of a diverticulum can be seen. Its value lies in the possible exclusion of carcinoma.

Treatment

Most mild cases of diverticulitis can be treated by conservative measures including a high-residue diet and the avoidance of constipation. Occasionally, local inflammation can be settled with the use of antibiotics. Operation may be indicated if the pain and constipation become extremely marked but more often operation has to be carried out because of the presence of complications or if cancer is suspected. At operation, if the disease is confined to a segment, the affected segment is removed. This operation may be quite difficult, due to the dense adhesions to the abdominal wall and to the other viscera. If possible, continuity of the intestinal tract is restored by end-to-end anastomosis. If, for technical reasons, it is not possible to resect and re-anastomose the bowel because of very dense adhesions or the presence of a large abscess, a proximal transverse colostomy may be performed. Traditionally, a defunctioning colostomy (*see Figure 25.9*) is carried out in which the transverse colon is divided at a suitable point and the two ends brought out separately with a strip of skin and underlying subcutaneous tissue separating the two ends of the bowel. More recently, the operation of sigmoid myotomy has been advised, in which a longitudinal incision is made along the muscle coat of the affected segment of the bowel. It is hoped that the mucosa is not divided. The value of this operation is debatable.

Where the disease is complicated by abscess formation the abscess should be drained and a defunctioning colostomy established.

Volvulus of the sigmoid colon

A rather redundant loop of the colon, usually loaded with faeces and suspended in a long narrow pedicle, may undergo twisting. This condition, known as volvulus, typically occurs in the elderly and the chronically constipated. In the early stages of this condition it may be possible to pass a tube or sigmoidoscope up through the anus into the affected loop to untwist the volvulus. If volvulus persists, the vasculature of the bowel is compromised and strangulation with gangrene of the intestine may ensue. Usually under these circumstances there is a considerable amount of pain with marked abdominal distension. A straight radiograph of the abdomen is typical, showing an enormously distended sigmoid colon. Under these circumstances the abdomen is opened and it may be necessary to remove the gangrenous bowel, the ends being brought out as a colostomy.

PREPARATION AND SUPPORT OF THE PATIENT UNDERGOING INTESTINAL SURGERY

An important point which has already been mentioned but which should be re-emphasized is that if disease of the bowel has interfered with its function the patient may be dehydrated and/or undernourished. It is essential that the greatest attention is given to promoting a restoration to as near normality as possible for if this is omitted the results of corrective surgery will be prejudiced. Both fluid and calorie replacement must be mainly by the intravenous route and careful monitoring is essential. The principles of fluid balance are described in Chapters 2, 4 and 5 and of intravenous feeding in Chapter 5.

Furthermore one of the first essentials for success in any procedure on the bowel is that it should be satisfactorily prepared — that is to say, it should be as mechanically and bacteriologically clean as possible. Unless the small intestine is grossly diseased (e.g. as in obstructive conditions in which aspiration of fluid and also antibiotic administration may be necessary) little need be done in preparation for surgery. However the large intestine is a different matter for a degree of faecal loading with intense bacterial activity is a norm which may readily be exaggerated in many disease states. For such a procedure as colonoscopy the withholding of a solid diet for a few days associated with bowel wash-outs will usually suffice. When surgery is planned the oral administration of an antibacterial agent such as metranidazole (Flagyl) is usual with the addition of a poorly absorbed antibiotic (e.g. sulphasuccidine) to the bowel wash-out fluid.

Finally it will be evident that there are few situations in surgery that may allow the patient to feel more vulnerable than when he or she is to be left with an ileostomy or colostomy. At this time the sympathetic help of every member of the nursing and surgical team is particularly important and this may be supported by example from someone who has already had a similar operation and by specialized advice from the organizations mentioned on page 24.

REFERENCES

Davis, L. (Ed.) (1968). *Christopher's Textbook of Surgery*. Philadelphia: W. B. Saunders

Elmslie, R. G. and Ludbrook, J. (1971). *An Introduction to Surgery: 100 Topics*. London: Heinemann Medical Books

Laster, L. and Ingelfinger, F. J. (1961). Intestinal absorption: — aspects of structure, function and disease of the small-intestine mucosa. *New Engl. J. Med.* **264**, 1138

Meschan, I. (1962). *Synopsis of Roentgen Signs*. Philadelphia: W. B. Saunders

Scott, P. R. (1971). *An Aid to Clinical Surgery*. London and Edinburgh: Churchill Livingstone

26 Appendicitis and peritonitis

R. B. Crosbie

Acute appendicitis is the most common condition requiring emergency operation. It is a treacherous and potentially fatal illness of rapid onset, where the difference between the quick return to full health or prolonged morbidity and death depends more on prompt diagnosis and expert treatment than in any other disease.

Whilst there are many other causes of peritoneal inflammation, a perforated appendix is in Great Britain the most common cause of peritonitis and so it is convenient to consider these subjects together.

APPENDICITIS

Normal structure and function of the appendix

The vermiform (worm-like) appendix is a narrow, blind-ended tube which arises from the caecum and whilst normally situated in the right lower abdomen, varies considerably in length and position (*Figure 26.1*). It may lie behind the caecum (retrocaecal), along the outer side of the caecum (paracolic), in front or behind the terminal ileum (pre- or postileal), in the pelvis or even within the sac of an inguinal or femoral hernia.

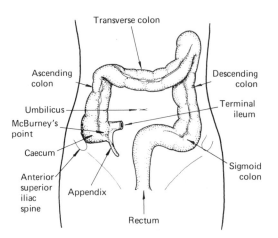

Figure 26.1. The usual situation of the appendix and caecum

When the caecum in the embryo fails to descend to its normal position, the appendix may be found in the upper abdomen close to the liver or stomach or even in the left lower quadrant if there is transposition of the viscera. A knowledge of these variations, of obvious importance to the surgeon, is necessary to understand the different signs and symptoms which occur with an inflamed appendix lying in different positions.

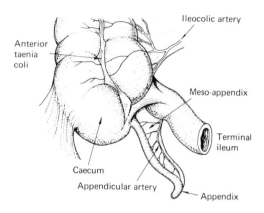

Figure 26.2. The appendix and its blood supply

A fold of peritoneum, the mesentery of the appendix, carries the appendicular artery, a branch of the ileocolic artery, in its free border (*Figure 26.2*). The veins of the appendix drain into the ileocolic vein which in turn drains into the superior mesenteric vein and so to the portal vein. Lymphatics cross the mesentery of the appendix to empty into the ileocaecal nodes.

The appendix is apparently a functionless organ in man though in some animals, such as the rabbit, it is relatively very large and is concerned with the digestion of cellulose.

Aetiology and pathology of appendicitis

Despite being so common, little is known of the underlying aetiological factors of appendicitis. The disease has only been clearly recognized since the end of the last century when it would appear that it became much more common. It is known, however, that although the disease was rare, it has existed since early times, for an acutely inflamed perforated appendix was found in the preserved mummy of a young Egyptian princess. The rise in incidence has been most marked in the more prosperous city dwellers of the highly developed communities of Europe, America and Australia. It is much less common in Asiatics, Africans and Polynesians but individuals of the relatively immune races who migrate to the countries where appendicitis is common, soon acquire the local susceptibility to the disease. This suggests environmental rather than racial factors at play. It seems likely that the characteristic difference between those people who do and those who do not suffer from appendicitis is that the food of the simpler, less sophisticated communities which are relatively immune contains a larger bulk of coarse vegetables containing a lot of cellulose and relatively little meat. That the dietary factors, however, are not the only ones is borne out by the occurrence of appendicitis in breast-fed babies or life-long vegetarians. It is interesting that experimental deprivation of cellulose in the rabbit leads to inflammation of the caecum and one may speculate that cellulose deficiency in man leads to failure of peristaltic movements in the appendix, leading to stagnation within the lumen, blockage and injury to the mucosa initiating an attack of acute secondary bacterial inflammation. About one-third of acutely inflamed appendices contain faecalith (stoney-hard faecal mass) usually about the size of a cherry stone. The popular lay idea of a blocked appendix due to a swallowed foreign body such as an orange pip, grape seeds or pins rarely occurs. Once the lumen has become blocked, the tension of pent-up secretions further damages and impairs the blood supply of the mucosa, delivering the appendix as a prey to its own native bacteria.

Course of acute appendicitis

If the appendix remains unobstructed, the disease may pursue a relatively mild course and resolve spontaneously, the greater omentum wrapping itself protectively around the inflamed organ. This may be palpable in the abdomen (appendix mass). If, however, the lumen blocks, the inflammatory products remain pent-up under great pressure and gangrene with perforation into the peritoneal cavity may speedily occur. Following perforation, a localized abscess may form in the right iliac fossa (appendix abscess) or in the pelvis (pelvic abscess), the abscess being walled off by the omentum, small bowel and caecum. During very severe attacks, especially in children or the aged, the progress of the disease may be so rapid that the peritoneum has no time to prepare its defences and a sudden flood of infective contents leads to a diffuse peritonitis.

Clinical picture and diagnosis

Appendicitis may occur at any age, although it is less common below the age of 5 years and in the elderly, where diagnosis can be treacherously difficult and the disease carries a high mortality. The first symptoms are usually anorexia, nausea and abdominal pain tending to localize in the epigastrium or around the umbilicus. The pain may come in colicky spasms, particularly in obstructive cases, and be accompanied by either nausea or vomiting. After some hours, the pain tends to shift into the right lower quadrant of the abdomen. The bowels are usually constipated, but diarrhoea may occur, especially if the appendix is lying in the pelvis, leading to the dangerous misdiagnosis of enteritis. Urinary symptoms may be prominent if the inflamed appendix lies close to the ureter or bladder and this in turn may lead to delay in operation if the symptoms are misinterpreted as a urinary infection.

Examination

On examination the patient may not appear particularly ill in the early stages. He may be slightly flushed, usually lies quietly in bed with a furred tongue and foul breath. The temperature and pulse rate though normal early on, both tend to rise as the disease progresses, but it is unusual for the temperature to be very high. Inspection of the abdomen may reveal nothing amiss or some lack of respiratory movement in the lower half may be apparent. Bowel sounds are usually normal. Gentle palpation will reveal tenderness with guarding maximal over the site of the appendix, usually in the right lower abdomen. The classical site of maximal tenderness, McBurney's point (one-third of the distance along a line drawn from the right anterior superior iliac spine to the umbilicus), occurs only when the appendix lies immediately below this point, a not invariable position. If peritonitis has supervened, the tenderness and guarding will be diffuse. On rectal examination, definite tenderness anteriorly on the right side may be felt especially if the inflamed appendix lies in the pelvis.

Special diagnostic measures

Special diagnostic measures are secondary to careful clinical appraisal in this disease, but a moderate polymorphonuclear leucocytosis is common and plain abdominal radiographs in the erect and supine positions may show some stasis in loops of terminal ileum revealed by gas and fluid as 'fluid levels'. The disease needs to be differentiated from many others, including mesenteric adenitis, **pyelitis**, **salpingitis**, cholecystitis, basal pneumonia and pleurisy, if dangerous mismanagement is not to occur.

Pyelitis Inflammation of the pelvis of the kidney.

Salpingitis (salpinx) Inflammation of the fallopian tube.

Management

Early diagnosis and prompt surgical treatment is vital if morbidity and mortality from this disease are to be reduced to a minimum. If perforation has not occurred, immediate operation will allow the appendix to be removed neatly and cleanly, with a minimum of postoperative problems. If a localized peritonitis has supervened, in addition to removing the appendix, the infected peritoneal exudate is aspirated and the wound closed without drainage.

If there has been some delay before the patient is first seen by the surgeon, an inflammatory mass consisting of the appendix, adjacent viscera and omentum bound together by adhesions, may be palpable. A conservative approach may be decided upon, the mass either resolving or going on to form an abscess when simple drainage alone may be advisable, although it is more usual these days with powerful antibiotic cover to remove the appendix and the necrotic mass, once the decision to operate has been made. If at operation, when there is a mass or abscess and the appendix cannot be seen on gentle dissection, the wise surgeon may content himself with drainage and leave the appendix to be removed safely at a later date. If diffuse peritonitis is present when the patient is first seen, operation should be carried out only when the patient has been additionally prepared by intravenous fluids, antibiotics and gastric aspiration.

Preoperative preparation

On admission, the patient is examined and as soon as the decision to operate has been made, he can be given pre-anaesthetic medication to allay apprehension and relieve pain. No fluids are given by mouth and enemas are absolutely forbidden. The abdomen is prepared in whatever particular way the surgeon prefers and in patients with advanced disease, an intravenous infusion of saline together with antibiotics is started and gastric aspiration carried out by a Ryle's tube, which has been passed through the nostril into the stomach.

The operation

A general anaesthetic is administered and the patient positioned on the operating table lying on his back. The incision carried out is usually a McBurney's gridiron incision in the right iliac fossa. Each layer of muscle is split in the line of its fibres, so that the openings in each layer lie across one another in gridiron fashion. The peritoneum is opened and retractors inserted. The caecum is identified and the appendix delivered gently into the wound. The meso-appendix with its blood vessels is ligated and divided. A purse-string is placed in the caecum around the base of the appendix which is crushed, ligated and divided, the stump being inverted as the purse-string is drawn tight. The wound is closed in layers, a drain being inserted if the appendix was perforated.

Postoperative treatment

Postoperative care is simple and the convalescence is speedy in the patient who has had an unperforated appendix cleanly removed. If the patient had peritonitis before operation, the postoperative care may demand all the skill which the surgeon and his nurses can muster and put a great strain on the patient's reserves. An analgesic is injected as soon as the patient is fully recovered from the anaesthetic and again every 6 to 8 hours for the first couple of days. Pain arising later may be relieved by administration of simple tablets, such as codeine or paracetamol. The patient is nursed in whatever position he is most comfortable. Deep breathing, leg movements and early ambulation are encouraged. If there is no nausea or vomiting, small amounts of water or fruit juice may be started early in uncomplicated cases. Solid food should not be given until bowel sounds are heard or flatus is passed, usually about the third postoperative day. Should vomiting be troublesome or distension occur, nothing should be given by mouth, a Ryle's tube should be passed and intravenous fluids administered. Retention of urine, if it does not respond to simple measures or the injection of 1 ml of carbachol, may necessitate catheterization. If constipation is troublesome, a Dulcolax or glycerine suppository can be given on the morning of the third postoperative day, but on no account must large volume enemas or colonic wash-outs be given, lest distension blow out the appendix stump. A small enema gently administered is permissible after 4 or 5 days. Ordinary diet may be allowed as soon as the patient has satisfactory bowel actions. If there is a drain present, daily dressings may be necessary until it is removed after several days. As a rule, the patient can return home or to convalescence when the sutures have been removed between the seventh and the tenth day and should be able to return to school or work within the next 3 or 4 weeks.

PERITONITIS

Anatomy of the peritoneum

The peritoneum is a serous membrane which invests the abdominal organs in the same way that the pleura and pericardium invest the lungs and heart. The arrangement of the peritoneum is very complicated. The external (parietal) layer lines the inside of the abdominal cavity investing the back of the abdominal wall muscles and the front of those organs which lie behind the peritoneum on the posterior abdominal wall (retroperitoneal organs, i.e. the kidneys, suprarenals, part of the duodenum, the aorta, the inferior vena cava, the ureters and the true pelvic organs). The

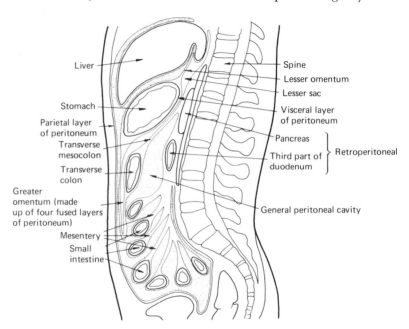

Figure 26.3. Sagittal section of the abdomen

parietal peritoneum is reflected back from its attachment to the posterior abdominal wall to enfold other organs in a complete outer cover, the visceral peritoneum. The lesser omentum is a fold of peritoneum which extends from the lesser curve of the stomach upwards over the liver. The greater omentum, similarly, extends downwards from the greater curve of the stomach like a blanket over the intestines. The mesentery is a double layer of peritoneum which is reflected off the posterior abdominal wall, spreads out like a fan to clothe the intestine in its free edge. The arteries, veins and lymphatics to the intestines lie between the two layers of the mesentery. The viscera and parietal layers of the peritoneum, which are smooth and lubricated by serous fluid, can slide easily over one another as the viscera move (*Figure 26.3*).

Aetiology and pathology of peritonitis

Inflammation of the peritoneum may result from non-bacterial irritants such as blood, bile, urine, gastric or pancreatic juice

(b)

IV B

escaping into the peritoneum, or acute bacterial inflammation secondary to appendicitis, cholecystitis, diverticulitis, pancreatitis, salpingitis and uterine or pelvic sepsis (*Figure 26.4*). Initially, the non-bacterial irritants produce a sterile peritoneal exudate, but sooner or later this becomes infected, producing a frankly septic peritonitis. Very rarely, peritonitis may occur for no apparent reason (primary peritonitis) due to blood-borne infection, usually streptococci. The exudated fluid may contain fibrin, which causes coils of intestine and omentum to stick together, thereby walling off the contaminant area from the rest of the peritoneal cavity. Free

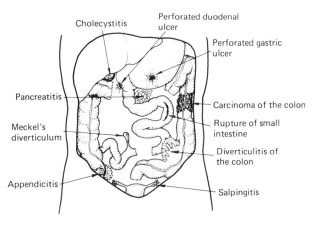

Figure 26.4. Some causes of peritonitis

gas may be present in cases of gastrointestinal perforation. If the peritonitis is not treated, localized abscesses under the diaphragm, in the pelvis or between glued coils of intestine, may occur. If these abscesses are not drained, a fatal result from toxaemia or paralytic ileus with gross fluid and electrolyte disturbance is almost inevitable. Acute perforation of hollow organs, the stomach, duodenum, small bowel, large bowel or gall bladder, may occur as the result of injury or disease giving rise to diffuse peritonitis of rapid onset. Perforated peptic ulcers in the stomach and duodenum rank second only to appendicitis as the cause of peritonitis. Perforated diverticulitis of the colon, or ruptured malignant growths of the stomach or large bowel, give rise to a particularly virulent form of generalized peritonitis. Peritonitis may occur as a complication of any abdominal operation, particularly when the gastrointestinal tract has been opened. Paralytic ileus is the most common complication of diffuse peritonitis; the neuromuscular mechanism responsible for peristalsis is thrown out of action by congestion and oedema in the intestinal wall. Furthermore, the extrinsic sympathetic nerves are irritated and peristaltic inhibition may result from this cause.

Clinical picture

The first stages are marked by the clinical signs of the responsible lesion: appendicitis, peptic ulcer, gall bladder disease, and so on. The pain may be sudden in onset in cases of perforation of a viscus and more gradual and insidious in non-perforative lesions. It may be severe and unremitting or no more than a dull ache. Collapse, especially when a viscus is perforated, is due in the initial stages to peritoneal shock. Vomiting, slight at the start, becomes persistent. The vomitus at first is clear, later becomes bile-stained and eventually foul-smelling and brown in colour — so-called faecal vomiting. The temperature may be normal or even subnormal when there is sudden onset, but tends to rise as sepsis supervenes. A rising pulse rate and falling temperature are of grave significance, whereas a gradually rising temperature and a slightly falling pulse rate suggest that localization is occurring. Respirations are quick and shallow, the tongue is furred and the bowels usually constipated, though in pelvic peritonitis diarrhoea may occur. On examination, diminished or absent abdominal respiratory movements may be observed; the patient lies still, often with the legs drawn up. Tenderness and rigidity of the abdominal muscles occur, possibly, with rebound tenderness (i.e. pain caused by the sudden release of pressure of the examining hand). Intestinal sounds are diminished from the start and later, when ileus supervenes, there is silence. In the terminal stages, the pain is continuous, faecal vomiting profuse and effortless, the pulse becomes weaker and the appearance of the face (facies hippocratica) tells that death is near. The eyes are hollow and bright, the face pale, pinched and blotchy, the lips are blue and the brow and head bathed in cold perspiration. The whole body is cold and the abdomen distended, tympanitic, tender and rigid.

Management

It is often possible to prevent diffuse peritonitis by prompt treatment of the initiating cause, such as appendicitis, gall bladder disease or intestinal obstruction. Once established peritonitis is present, operation should be delayed until the patient has been adequately resuscitated with intravenous fluids, electrolytes, blood or plasma transfusion and antibiotics have been administered. Distension should be reduced by gastrointestinal aspiration by Ryle's tube. Continued conservative treatment may be advisable in certain circumstances, such as moribund patients or when the infection is localizing. Generally speaking, however, early operation should be performed in most cases in which acute diffuse peritonitis is known or suspected to be due to a local cause, such as a perforated viscus.

The operation

The incision varies according to the suspected causative lesion. As always, meticulous gentleness is essential but speed may also be important. The actual procedure depends on the nature of the cause. Perforations are closed, gangrenous appendix is excised or a necrotic loop of bowel removed with end-to-end anastomosis. Pus is aspirated by suction or gently mopped up. Drainage should be provided whenever there is a localized abscess or a necrotic viscus, such as a gall bladder that cannot be safely removed. All unnecessary manipulation should be avoided and left, if necessary, to a second operation when the patient's condition has improved.

Postoperative care

The patient is nursed in whatever position he finds most comfortable. Analgesics are injected as necessary. Ryle's tube aspiration and intravenous infusion of fluids and electrolytes will be needed until intestinal activity returns. Antibiotics are continued by intravenous or intramuscular injection. No enemas or purgatives should be given, though when bowel sounds have been present for a couple of days a small oily enema may be administered. As soon as flatus or faeces are passed, the the patient may take liquid nourishment by mouth and the Ryle's tube is removed.

TUBERCULOUS PERITONITIS

Currently, tuberculous peritonitis is a rare disease in Great Britain. It occurs mainly in children and is due to infection by the bovine type of tuberculous bacilli from infected milk. Spread to the peritoneum may occur from an infected lymph node, a tuberculous ulcer of the ileum or a tuberculous Fallopian tube. The peritoneum is usually studded with small nodules (tubercles) and a large volume of straw-coloured fluid accumulates. This may later resolve, leaving widespread adhesions. The diagnosis is difficult for there is a great variety of presenting signs and symptoms. Treatment is primarily medical with rest in bed, good food and anti-tuberculous drugs. Surgery may be necessary to establish the diagnosis, to relieve intestinal obstruction or to deal with a perforation or localized tuberculous abscess, but as a rule the condition will respond to adequate medical treatment without any need for surgical intervention.

27

Surgery of the rectum and anus

T. R. Preston

RECTAL ANATOMY AND PHYSIOLOGY

The rectum commences as the continuation of the pelvic colon at the level of the third sacral vertebra. It follows the concave contour of the hollow of the sacrum and, on reaching the level of the coccyx, turns acutely backwards and runs for about 2.5 cm as the anus. At a point a little below this angle the mucous membrane lining the gut changes its secretory pattern to something which more nearly resembles perineal skin with which it gradually merges (*Figure 27.1*). This junctional area is also the site where the portal venous system draining the gut joins the systemic venous system draining the remainder of the body, and the site where the insensitive autonomic nerves of the gut give way to the exquisitely sensitive spinal nerves supplying the anus. At the anus there are two sphincters, an internal one and an external one, continence depending on the integrity of the former. The rectum and anus have a plentiful blood supply, derived from the superior, middle and inferior rectal arteries on each side. Venous drainage from the anus is into the external venous plexus and from the rectum into the internal venous plexus. Both plexi lie in the submucosa of the gut and communicate with each other. The internal venous plexus drains superiorly via the rectal veins into the portal system, while the external plexus drains partly into the internal plexus, and partly also into the systemic venous system. The lymphatic vessels of the anorectal region tend to follow the course of the arteries. Lymph from the rectum passes upwards to the glands around the aorta and laterally to the internal iliac vessels. From the anus, drainage occurs to the glands of the groin.

Normal defaecation occurs in response to distension of the rectum by faeces and flatus resulting in the desire to pass a motion. The normal tone of the external and internal sphincters is inhibited, their musculature relaxes and the intra-abdominal pressure is raised by forced expiration against a closed glottis, which aids the intrinsic musculature of the gut to propel the faeces onwards. Control of the bowels is

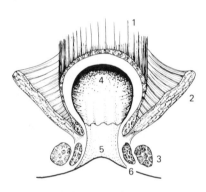

Figure 27.1. Diagram of normal anatomy of the anorectal region. 1, longitudinal muscle; 2, levator ani muscle; 3, external sphincter muscle; 4, rectum; 5, anus; 6, external venous plexus

largely achieved by the action of the internal sphincter, which, when inadvertently damaged at operation, may result in a permanent state of faecal incontinence.

PATHOLOGICAL CONDITIONS AND THEIR MANAGEMENT

Anal fissure

The condition of anal fissure can occur at any age but is usually found in adults. It is thought to be caused by the passage of a hard motion which results in a small longitudinal tear of the anal margin. Once established, it is prevented from healing by the incessant movement of the external anal sphincter and the presence in it of inevitable infection. An acute fissure is characterized by severe sharp pain when the anus is dilated by the passage of a formed motion. The stool, which is thin and nipped off at the ends by the contracting sphincter, may be smeared with traces of bright red blood derived from the granulating base of the stretched fissure. The diagnosis is usually made on the history alone because digital or proctoscopic examination of the anorectal region is impossible due to excessive pain. In patients with long-standing fissures which have become chronic the condition can be better felt than seen. Relief can be obtained from local anaesthetic creams and suppositories, used before and after a motion. If the condition persists, then the external sphincter may be temporarily paralysed by dilating the anus under a short anaesthetic; this allows the fissure to heal. Untreated chronic fissures may not respond to these measures and may require surgical excision.

Proctalgia fugax

The term proctalgia fugax is used to describe an acute boring pain in the rectal region which affects otherwise normal adults of both sexes. The cause of the condition is quite unknown, but it is believed to be due to spasm of the muscles constituting the floor of the pelvis. The patient is often woken at night by the pain, which is of sudden onset and lasts 5 or 10 minutes. Relief can sometimes be obtained by applying pressure to the midpoint of the perineum.

Haemorrhoids

Proctoscope A tubular instrument for the examination of the anus and lower rectum.

Haemorrhoids or piles are of two main types — internal and external.

Internal piles

Internal piles are one of the commonest surgical conditions affecting both sexes. They are found at all ages except during early childhood and are sometimes described as 'varicose veins of the rectum'. Strictly speaking, piles are formed by prolapse of the rectal mucous membrane, carrying with it the internal haemorrhoidal plexus of veins. This prolapse occurs in three main positions around the circumference of the anal ring and it is customary to refer to the piles in these positions as 'primary piles'. The internal haemorrhoidal plexus of veins drains upwards into the pelvis. As a result, anything which causes obstruction to this drainage will predispose to piles, for example, tumours in the pelvis, pregnancy and carcinoma of the rectum. However, in most patients with piles no underlying cause can be found other than gravity — part of the penalty that man, a two-legged animal, pays for the adoption of the erect attitude. Piles can be classified according to their degree of severity, on which treatment depends.

First degree piles The first degree piles bleed and prolapse only slightly; enough, however, to be momentarily gripped by the internal sphincter muscles when the patient is straining at stool (*Figure 27.2*). The mucous membrane over the surface of the pile may be abraided by hard faeces, so breached, sudden venous bleeding occurs and the lavatory pan is spattered with blood. A momentary alteration in sphincter tone allows the congested pile to slip back into the rectum and the bleeding from it ceases. It is important to realize that the only symptom of first degree piles is bleeding.

Second degree piles Second degree piles prolapse on defaecation and are either replaced digitally or reduced spontaneously. Furthermore, the prolapse is more severe, enabling the sphincter to grip the pile at its base. Failure to return the pile to the rectum at the conclusion of defaecation embarrasses its venous return and it becomes heir to a number of complications.

The blood contained in the congested veins of the pile clots and the patient experiences acute pain which continues for 2 or 3 days if the condition is unattended. Immediate relief can be obtained by incising the pile under local anaesthetic and evacuating the clot.

When the grip of the sphincter on the oedematous pile base is sufficient to cut off the arterial supply, the pile is said to be strangulated. The patient experiences acute pain which requires his confinement to bed, the application of cold compresses and the administration of morphia for its

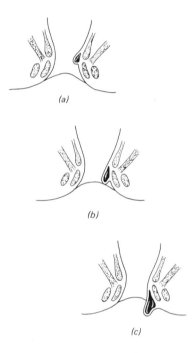

(a)

(b)

(c)

Figure 27.2. Diagram showing position of the pile in relation to the external sphincter in first (*a*), second (*b*), and third (*c*) degree haemorrhoids

relief. Sometimes strangulation is complete and the pile becomes ulcerated, infected, frankly gangrenous and may even slough off completely.

Third degree piles The prolapse of third degree piles is complete and present the whole time. Digital replacement is immediately followed by re-prolapse and the mucous membrane can be seen hanging from a rather open anus.

A patient suffering from piles may go to the doctor complaining of a number of symptoms. When the piles are of first degree type he may be alarmed by the blood found in the pan following defaecation. When the piles are of second degree type he may be troubled by prolapse, discharge, bleeding, pruritus or the pain which heralds the onset of one of the complications, and when the piles are of the third degree type he may complain of prolapse only. Whatever the symptoms, an enquiry should always be made into the patient's bowel habit to find out whether there has been any recent change, and this must be followed by a complete physical examination, together with digital and proctoscopic examination of the rectum. These measures are necessary not only to assess the state and degree of the piles present, but to exclude any other cause for them, such as a carcinoma of the rectum.

Treatment and complications

Conservative treatment in the form of local anaesthetic creams or suppositories is used for the control of minor attacks of piles.

Injection treatment is advocated for first and less severe forms of second degree piles, the object being to introduce a mildly irritant liquid, such as 5 per cent phenol in almond oil, into the submucosa of the pile-bearing area. In this way the mucosa becomes firmly adherent to the submucosa and in the process the plexus of veins becomes obliterated.

Haemorrhoidectomy is advocated for second and third degree piles and consists of dissection, ligature and excision of each of the three primary piles. Proper preoperative and postoperative nursing care does much to mitigate what is otherwise a painful procedure. Two nights before the operation the patient is given a purgative, followed by an enema on the second night, and a rectal wash-out is given on the day of the operation. Postoperatively the patient usually has a motion on the fourth or fifth day and its passage is much eased if the faeces have been rendered soft or even liquid by the administration of liquid paraffin or Milk of Magnesia from the second postoperative day onwards. On the tenth day these medicines are stopped to allow the formed motion to stretch the healing anus. A number of complications can occur after this operation.

Bleeding Bleeding may occur on the return of the patient to the ward from the theatre, as a result of the rise in blood pressure. Bleeding occurs from improperly secured vessels. It usually soon ceases, but may continue and, moreover, be concealed by being contained within the rectum. Secondary haemorrhage can also occur on or about the tenth post-operative day as a result of infection.

Retention of urine Retention of urine is a complication which frequently occurs after haemorrhoidectomy, particularly in males, and may require catheterization.

Stricture formation Stricture formation not infrequently follows haemorrhoidectomy. Before the patient leaves hospital a gloved finger is passed into the rectum to ensure that there is no tendency to stricture formation. If there is, then an anal dilator is supplied and the patient instructed to pass it twice a day until this tendency is overcome.

The use of wide dilatation of the anus in the treatment of all forms of piles has recently become popular. The basis of the method rests on the premise that spasm of the anal sphincter is responsible for the onset of the condition. Wide dilatation of the anus under a general anaesthetic paralyzes its musculature and the piles shrink and disappear. Thereafter the patient combats his tendency to anal spasm by passing a dilator twice daily for the next few months.

External piles External piles are caused by rupture of the tributaries of the inferior haemorrhoidal plexus producing a small haematoma at the anocutaneous verge. These piles are extremely painful and relief can only be obtained by incision and evacuation of the clot.

Pilonidal sinus

The condition of pilonidal sinus is common among dark hirsute males with low standards of personal hygiene. In the main it only affects white races. It consists of the appearance of one or more small openings in the midline of the body in the cleft between the buttocks. Most authorities are now agreed that the complaint is of acquired rather than congenital origin. Loose hairs tend to accumulate in the cleft and some penetrate the skin to form small sinuses lined by granulation tissue. Repeated bouts of infection lead to the formation of side tracks and so the condition progresses, running a chronic course, punctuated at intervals by the development of abscesses. The patient usually presents when he has such an abscess requiring incision. The mere possession of one or more sinuses in a quiescent phase is not in itself sufficient indication for surgery, but repeated bouts of infection drive the patient to seek a definitive cure, other than the mere incision of the abscess.

The definitive treatment consists of wide excision of the lesion. The wound is then stitched together and healing occurs by first intention. However, some surgeons prefer to leave the wound to heal from the bottom. The dressing of such wounds demands a high standard of nursing skill. The object is so to arrange the packing material that the granulation of the wound proceeds evenly and gradually from the deep to the superficial parts without skin bridging occurring. The success of the treatment of this condition depends as much on good nursing as on the surgery.

Rectal prolapse

Rectal prolapse commonly occurs in the elderly and may be due to the loss of supporting fat around the rectum and to the poor tone of the muscles of the pelvic floor. The whole rectum prolapses for several centimetres and all its layers are involved in the process. Occasional prolapse requires replacement by the nurse or doctor but, should this become persistent, more active measures may be required. In the very elderly or those unfit for more extensive procedures, a malleable silver wire or a nylon ligature may be inserted around the anus, to leave an aperture no larger than the size of the base of an index finger. This critical size of aperture prevents prolapse without causing obstruction to the passage of faeces, providing the latter are softened by the use of oral liquid paraffin. Some patients able to withstand a more extensive surgical procedure may benefit by a curative operation. The rectum is hitched up via an abdominal approach and fibrosis between it and the sacrum encouraged, thus effecting a permanent anchorage.

Anal fistula

An anal fistula is a deep track near the anus which may or may not communicate with the interior of the rectum, and in this respect may be referred to as complete or incomplete. Occasionally, such a fistula is the herald of serious intra-abdominal pathology such as Crohn's disease, ulcerative colitis or carcinoma of the rectum, but the commonest cause is an anorectal abscess. An initial history of such an abscess is therefore obtainable, followed by the appearance of a continuous chronic discharge of pus from the mouth of the track. Full examination of a fistula is usually only possible under an anaesthetic, when the track is carefully probed and the presence of a communication with the interior of the rectum established. It is important to note the relationship such a fistula bears to the internal sphincter.

Treatment

From the point of view of treatment the condition can be divided into high and low level types (*Figure 27.3*). Low level fistulas lie below and do not involve the region of the anorectal ring upon which continence depends, thus these tracks can be probed and laid open with impunity without fear of producing incontinence. Such a wound requires the most careful and skilled nursing care. The principle involved is to prevent the superficial parts of the wound uniting until the deeper parts have done so. Unless this is done, an infected space or abscess cavity is produced below the level of the healed skin. This state of affairs invites further fistula formation. Therefore, dressings are so laid that union of the skin and superficial parts of the wound are prevented while the wound heals from the bottom. High level fistulae involve or pass above the level of the anorectal ring, thus only the more superficial parts of these tracks can be laid open. The deeper parts are probed and a stout piece of thread passed through the track and out of the anus, the two ends then being tied together. This circle of thread, called a 'seton', is drawn down and rotated several times a day, the muscle fibres are slowly sawn through and heal again by fibrosis. Thus the cut ends of the muscle do not fall apart, as when the whole muscle is cut completely with a knife, and thus continence is preserved. In a short time the seton comes away entirely and the wound is allowed to heal progressively from the deep parts to the skin surface.

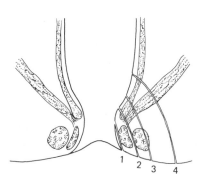

Figure 27.3. Diagram showing various types of anorectal fistula. Numbers 1, 2 and 3 are of the low type, number 4 is of the high type

Pruritus ani

Pruritus ani is a condition in which the patient experiences severe itching in the anal and perianal areas. This itching is continuous and intractable, leading to insomnia and general deterioration of health. Two types are recognized — idiopathic, in which the cause is unknown, and secondary, which develops as a result of existing pathology. Examples of such pathology are persistent vaginal or rectal discharge, poor hygiene, or any fungal or parasitic infection of the perineum. Whatever the underlying cause, the perianal skin becomes wet, soggy and excoriated by constant scratching. Rational treatment rests upon correct diagnosis of the underlying cause and its eradication. If no cause is found, then the pruritus is treated empirically; the skin is cleansed by bathing twice a day and dried by dabbing the area with a towel rather than by vigorous wiping. Scratching is avoided, astringents applied locally and the patient given a hypnotic to help him sleep.

Injuries of the rectum and anus

Injuries of the rectum and anus are rare due to their relatively protected situation. They usually occur when a person becomes impaled upon a stick or other sharp instrument. They can also happen in road traffic accidents when one buttock is suddenly and forcibly distracted from the other or when a fragment from a severely fractured pelvis penetrates the wall of the rectum. If these injuries remain untreated, infection of the perirectal and pelvic tissues occurs and gives rise to a spreading cellulitis which may be fatal. A relieving colostomy is an urgent necessity in such cases, together with prophylactic antibiotic therapy.

Foreign bodies in the rectum

Occasionally foreign bodies are inserted into the rectum. Their removal is sometimes difficult and may require general anaesthesia.

Anorectal abscesses

Abscess formation around the lower rectal and anal regions is common. Infection of the perianal soft tissues occurs from the gut if there is a breach in the mucous membrane, such as is found with a fissure, fistula, ulcer or an infected pile. Infection of these tissues also occurs from the skin of the perineum when a boil or pustule is present in this area, or from above if there is an abscess in the pelvis.

Anorectal abscesses are classified according to their site (*Figure 27.4*) as follows.

(1) Pelvirectal abscess;
(2) ischiorectal abscess;
(3) submucous abscess;
(4) perianal abscess.

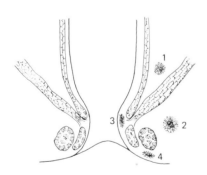

Figure 27.4. Diagram showing different types of anorectal abscess. 1, pelvirectal abscess; 2, ischiorectal abscess; 3, submucous abscess; 4, perianal abscess

The patient with an anorectal abscess goes to his doctor complaining of pain in the posterior part of the perineum which he describes as constant, throbbing and made worse by the passage of a motion. Examination reveals tenderness in a particular area and the exact site of the abscess can be located on rectal examination. The treatment of these abscesses is essentially no different from those found elsewhere. They require antibiotics to localize the infection, and incision and drainage followed by careful dressing to ensure that the mouth of the abscess does not close before the deeper parts have healed. Frequent baths are encouraged. Not only do frequent baths relieve rectal discomfort but, by keeping the perineal area clean, they prevent the spread of infection to other areas of the skin.

Benign tumours of the rectum

Benign tumours are frequently found in the rectum, the two commonest types being the simple and the villous adenomata. The simple adenoma arises from the rectal mucous membrane and is polypoidal in form, looking rather like a raspberry on a stalk. It is a true benign tumour and is not a precancerous condition as was formerly thought. Several of these tumours may be found in one patient. It gives rise to bleeding and the patient may be alarmed by the intermittent passage of small amounts of bright red blood from the rectum. The villous adenoma also arises from the rectal mucous membrane and its surface is less discrete, being said to resemble velvet in appearance and feel. It produces excessive quantities of mucus rich in potassium. The patient may complain of watery diarrhoea and, in addition, suffers the symptoms of potassium deficiency.

These tumours are usually found on rectal examination and subsequent sigmoidoscopy, but it is important also to examine the patient radiologically. A barium enema often shows additional missed adenomata high in the rectum. Benign tumours situated in the lower part of the rectum can be reached directly or through a sigmoidoscope and removed by dissection or with the aid of a loop diathermy snare. Adenoma situated in the higher reaches of the rectum may only be dealt with by exposing the bowel from above through an abdominal incision, opening it, and removing the tumour under direct vision.

Mention should be made of the condition known as 'familial intestinal polyposis' which may affect the entire colon, including the rectum. This condition is inheritable and is recognized by the appearance of myriads of tiny adenomatous polyps all over the surface of the large bowel. The condition is precancerous and sooner or later one or more of the polyps undergoes malignant change. Although families of sufferers exist, they are fortunately rare. In such families where the tendency to early malignant change is marked, preventative total or near total colectomy may be required.

Carcinoma of the rectum

The commonest malignant tumour of the rectum is the carcinoma. This condition affects men and women of all ages, but its highest incidence occurs in the elderly. Carcinoma arises from the cells of the mucous membrane of the rectum as a new growth, or from a pre-existing papilloma or adenoma which is in the process of undergoing malignant change. Initially the lesion spreads locally and invades the deeper layers, spreading circumferentially round the bowel. Not only does the carcinoma spread locally, but also distantly via the lymphatics. At first the glands immediately adjacent to the rectum are involved, then those in the large bowel mesentery, followed by the glands around the aorta. Spread via the bloodstream finally occurs and the liver, lungs and bones may eventually be involved. The success of treatment depends largely on the extent of the growth when the diagnosis is made.

The first symptom is usually a show of bright red blood from the rectum. Unfortunately it is frequently overlooked or disregarded, the cause being mistaken for 'piles'. Sometimes the patient complains of pain, a sense of rectal fullness or the passage of quantities of mucus. As the condition progresses, an element of rectal obstruction may be added, with alternating periods of constipation and diarrhoea accompanied by lower abdominal colicky pain. Examination of such a patient must include a digital and sigmoidoscopy search for the growth, and failure to find the cause of the bleeding must be followed by a barium enema. If the growth can be visualized, a biopsy is taken and submitted to histological examination.

The treatment of a malignant growth of the rectum may be curative or palliative.

Curative treatment
Suitable antibiotics and chemotherapeutic agents, such as neomycin or sulfasuxidine, are given preoperatively by mouth with the object of sterilizing the bowel contents. In addition, the patient is given a purgative 2 nights previously, followed by an enema the night before, and a rectal wash-out on the morning of the operation. Surgery offers the only hope of a complete cure and the objective must be to remove the growth together with the glands and the mesentery through which the draining lymphatics run. This objective can be achieved by a number of different operations. The one selected will depend on the site of the growth.

A carcinoma in the upper part of the rectum can usually be resected and the free ends of bowel joined again; thus the anal sphincter is conserved. This procedure is known as an anterior resection of the rectum (*Figure 27.5*). Growths in the lower part of the rectum which can be felt on digital examination are too close to the anal sphincter for a resection to be accomplished without rendering the patient incontinent of faeces. The rectum, together with its mesentery and the anus, is therefore resected, the remaining bowel being brought out of the abdominal wall to form a colostomy. This procedure is performed by two surgeons, one working from inside the abdomen and one working from the perineum, and is known as combined synchronous excision of the rectum. Post-operatively a watch must be kept on the urine to ensure that damage has not occurred to the ureters, on the perineal wound, blood pressure and pulse for bleeding, and on the colostomy for its viability.

The type of procedure to be done is sometimes unknown before operation, therefore every patient must be warned of the possibility of having to have a permanent colostomy. He must be made to realize that with modern 'stick on' self-applied plastic bags he can lead a full life afterwards.

Palliative treatment

Some rectal growths are so far advanced at the time of presentation that fixation to surrounding structures prevents their removal. Diversion of the faecal stream via a colostomy is sometimes employed to overcome the symptoms of partial obstruction. This form of treatment does not, however, relieve the patient of his rectal pain or the passage of blood and mucus; it may merely mean that to these symptoms are added any problems of a colostomy.

Carcinoma of the anus

Carcinoma of the anus is fortunately uncommon. It arises from the skin of the anus and is therefore histologically a squamous cell carcinoma. The growth commences as a small wart or ulcer and spreads locally to involve adjacent areas of skin. Distant spread occurs via the lymphatics to the groin glands. Owing to the fact that the anal skin is so sensitive, patients with this condition tend to present early, before the glands become involved, complaining of pain, pruritus and slight bleeding. The lesion is readily accessible to examination and its limits can be defined digitally. A biopsy can also be taken.

The treatment of the condition may be of a palliative or a curative nature.

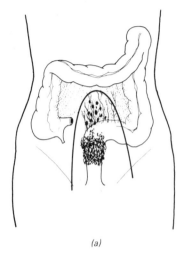

(a)

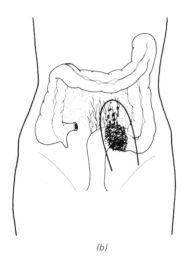

(b)

Figure 27.5. Operative treatment of carcinoma of the rectum. (*a*) Extent of resection for a tumour situated low in the rectum which requires the formation of a colostomy; (*b*) the extent of resection for a tumour situated high in the rectum when end-to-end anastomosis is possible

Palliative treatment

When the growth is inoperable or has recurred after operation, radiotherapy is employed. It may then regress and, in a proportion of such patients, an inoperable growth may be rendered operable.

Curative treatment

Most patients present early for treatment and are amenable to surgery, which offers the best chance of cure. An abdomino-perineal resection of the rectum is performed involving removal of the rectum and anus with a wide area of normal skin around the growth. If spread to the groin glands occurs, then a block dissection is added at a later date.

28

Hernia

John McFarland

GENERAL PRINCIPLES

Hernia is a Latin word meaning a rupture or break in the containing wall of a cavity in the body with the resultant protrusion of the contents.

It occurs most commonly at a natural opening which has become widened or weakened and thus the protruding viscera are still covered by several layers of tissue, although these may be very thin. This situation is clearly different from a separation of the abdominal wall (dehiscence) such as may occur when a surgical wound has healed inadequately (*Figure 28.1*). It follows that bowel or other viscera normally contained within the body wall may, as it protrudes into the hernia, become irreducible (impaction) (*Figure 28.2a*) and this may lead to obstruction of the flow of its contents.

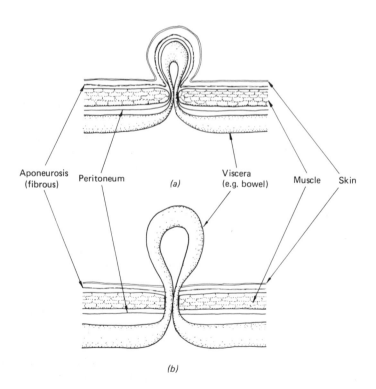

Aponeurosis (fibrous) Peritoneum *(a)* Viscera (e.g. bowel) Muscle Skin

(b)

Figure 28.1. Highly diagrammatic representation of the situation in (*a*) a hernia and (*b*) postoperative wound separation (dehiscence)

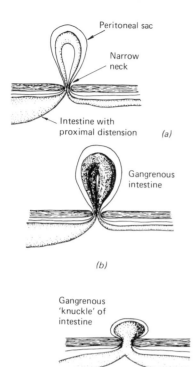

Figure 28.2. Diagrammatic representations of (*a*) intestine impacted in a hernia with obstruction; (*b*) intestine strangulated in a hernia; (*c*) Richter's hernia

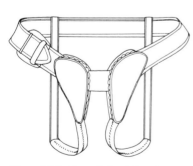

Figure 28.3. Scrotal elastic band truss. This may be single or double, as illustrated here, and is useful particularly to control direct inguinal hernia in the elderly and infirm when operation is contra-indicated

Furthermore, bowel may be damaged either directly or more usually by interference with its blood supply (strangulation, *Figure 28.2b*) and herein lies the greatest danger. A special situation occurs when the hernia contains only a 'knuckle' of bowel (*Figure 28.2c*). This is called a Richter's hernia and is particularly dangerous, for here obstruction, giving some warning of the gravity of the situation, does not precede strangulation, but an ischaemic necrosis (gangrene) of the bowel wall with perforation and resultant peritonitis may be the first major incident. Clearly this is especially a danger in an obese person in whom a small hernia may hitherto have been unnoticed.

Treatment may also be considered in principle and there are three possibilities.

(1) Disregard

Occasionally there is a reason for doing nothing, usually either in the elderly infirm patient in whom operation could be hazardous, or in the very young child with an umbilical hernia in which spontaneous improvement, in whole or degree, is likely. In either case this approach should only be adopted if the nature of the hernia is such that strangulation will not occur. It is clearly not advisable when the neck of the hernia is narrow.

(2) External control

For a groin hernia this means a truss, and for an incisional hernia, a surgical corset; and each must be fitted when the hernia has been reduced. Again the situation must be such that strangulation is not a danger, whether or not the truss or corset is in place. This type of control is widely used in the elderly and infirm when operation itself may be hazardous or when technical difficulties may make effective repair unlikely (*Figure 28.3*).

(3) Operation

It is convenient and logical to describe this in terms of the suffixes —otomy, —orraphy and —oplasty (except, that is, to the linguaphile who might reasonably shudder at this miscegenation of Latin and Greek derivations).

(a) *Herniotomy* – cutting the hernia, that is dissection and excision of the sac which, in inguinal hernia in children with otherwise completely normal anatomy, may suffice on its own. Herniotomy is the simplest operation resulting in the least disturbance of the anatomy. Otherwise, it is the necessary first stage of most groin hernia operations.

(b) *Herniorraphy* — repair by suture. The material used is almost invariably non-absorbable and non-reactive; a monofilament polymer such as nylon or prolene is popular. The precise technique, especially in inguinal hernia, is variable — one approach seeks to strengthen the inguinal canal while retaining some semblance of normality (Bassini). In another, any pretence at normality is abandoned and the area is refashioned to leave a single laterally-placed inguinal ring with the spermatic cord lying anteriorly to the sutured apo-neurotic layer. In these, as in hernia repair of every type, a cardinal principle is that the sutured tissue should not be under tension.

(c) *Hernioplasty* — reshaping of the area. For this many techniques, varied and ingenious, have been devised. The principal aim is to strengthen the posterior wall of the inguinal canal and most methods involve either use of the body's own tissues, such as fascia lata, or the implantation of foreign material which may be inert (e.g. stainless steel mesh) or, conversely, which may stimulate a vigorous fibrous reaction, e.g. polyvinyl sponge.

In all these methods it will be evident that in the inguinal area the problem is to strengthen the canal while keeping it open for the spermatic cord, something that becomes more difficult the weaker are the involved tissues. In the female this problem does not arise, for the round ligament (the vestigial equivalent to the spermatic cord) may be divided with impunity and the canal obliterated by sutures. This is also possible with regard to the spermatic cord in the male if the resultant testicular damage can be accepted, as for example in an elderly male with a recurrent hernia, with the advantage that the repair can then be made very secure.

TYPES OF HERNIA

From this simple consideration of general principles it will be evident that, broadly speaking, there are two sorts of hernia — those that follow abdominal surgery when the healing of the wound has been inadequate (incisional hernia); and those that occur through a structurally weak point somewhere in the containing walls of the abdominal cavity.

This latter type of hernia may be subdivided further and labelled as either *congenital* or *acquired*, but, where the former is categorized as any hernia which has been present from birth, the latter term is correct only in degree. It is

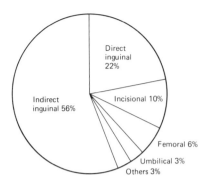

Figure 28.4. Relative frequency of types of hernia. (Modified from Harkins, 1965)

used, of course, to describe any hernia which occurs later in life apparently as a result of strain or stress, but this is only half the story for this is almost always in a vulnerable area, in over three-quarters of cases in the groin (*Figure 28.4*). Such herniae are inguinal or femoral and, because of their frequency, will be considered in most detail. Recurrent hernia — a sort of incisional hernia, after operative repair — is best considered with other groin herniae. Umbilical hernia and other much rarer types will be discussed more briefly, as will internal hernia, including hiatus hernia, which is a particularly special case and is discussed in Chapter 21.

Inguinal hernia

Anatomy

The key to the understanding of this is an appreciation of the anatomy of the area immediately above the medial half of the inguinal ligament which stretches from the anterior superior iliac spine to the pubic tubercle (*Figure 28.5*). This ligament is, in fact, the rolled-over lower border of the external oblique muscle of the abdominal wall which here is aponeurotic (fibrous). The gap between the ligament and the bony pelvis accommodates the femoral vessels and the iliopsoas muscle as these pass into the leg. The aponeurosis of this anterior layer, the external oblique muscle, is split at the medial end to form the superficial inguinal ring. The two other muscles which form the abdominal wall at this point are the transversus abdominis (continued inferiorly as the transversalis fascia), which lies most deeply and gives strength at the medial end of the canal; and the internal oblique which arches across from its lateral end, where it takes part in the

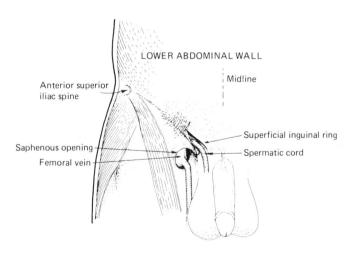

Figure 28.5. Diagram of the right groin in the male. An inguinal hernia, whether indirect or direct, will protrude through the superficial inguinal ring. A femoral hernia will protrude through the saphenous opening below and lateral to this

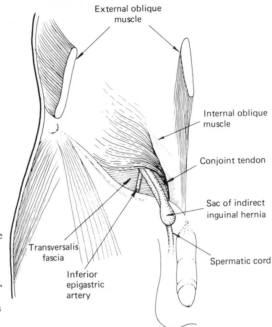

Figure 28.6. Diagram of the anatomy deep to the external oblique muscle. The internal oblique muscle arches over the inguinal canal which contains the spermatic cord and is the channel down which an indirect inguinal hernia enlarges. A protrusion medial to the inferior epigastric artery is a direct inguinal hernia

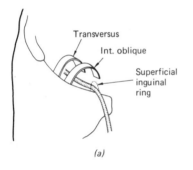

(a)

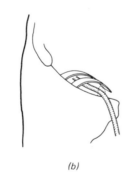

(b)

Figure 28.7. Diagram of the relationship of the lower border of the internal oblique and transversus muscles to the spermatic cord. (Parry, 1966; modified from Grant, *Method of Anatomy*, Bailliere, Tindall and Cox)

anterior wall of the deep inguinal ring, to its medial end, which is largely aponeurotic and which joins the transversus abdominis to form the conjoint tendon lying directly behind the superficial inguinal ring (*Figure 28.6*). The potential space between these two rings is the inguinal canal; in the male it contains the spermatic cord (in the female, the round ligament) which passes obliquely over the medial end of the inguinal ligament so that, in effect, it lifts the two posterior muscles off the ligament at this point. The lower border of these two muscles makes a contractile arch over the cord and is attached to the pubic tubercle behind the cord. This is shown in *Figure 28.7*.

The inguinal canal is inevitably a weak point in the abdominal wall, and man, with his upright posture and particular muscle action, is prone to develop a hernia in this area.

Indirect inguinal hernia

In this the sac of the hernia arises either from the opened-up processus vaginalis, a peritoneal vestige carried down as the testis descends during development, or from the bulging peritoneum along the same line. It thus follows an oblique course down the canal to the testis, and this course gives an indirect inguinal hernia its physical characteristics, particularly the fact that it may be controlled by firm pressure over the midpoint of the inguinal canal.

Direct inguinal hernia

This is a protrusion of the medial part (conjoint tendon) of the posterior wall of the inguinal canal. As with an indirect hernia, it may be felt as a bulge forwards through the external ring, but its course is not oblique and it does not extend as far as the testis. Nor may it be controlled by pressure so far laterally as may the indirect type. However, although in theory the differentiation of these two types of inguinal hernia is clear, in practice it may sometimes be difficult, at least, that is, until operation when the inferior epigastric artery is an absolute landmark (*Figure 28.6*).

Recurrent inguinal hernia

Following most operations, the anatomy is disturbed. This recurrence which, if it occurs, is usually early rather than late, does not follow a definite pattern, although it is most often related to the medial or lateral end of the repair.

Femoral hernia

The femoral canal lies in the corner between the medial end of the inguinal ligament and the pectineal line of the pelvis from which arises the pectineus muscle; laterally is the femoral vein which is the sole non-rigid border (*Figure 28.8*). This canal is occupied by a lymph node which is pushed aside when a femoral hernia occurs and the peritoneal sac of the hernia is usually nipped tightly at the narrow point of the canal, that is the femoral ring (bounded by the inguinal

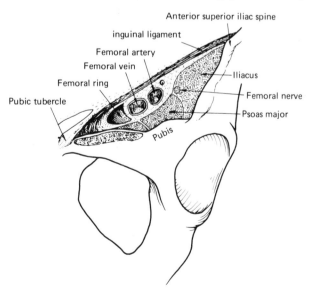

Figure 28.8. Diagram of the structures that fill the gap between the inguinal ligament and the pubis on the right side. This is the view from below and is the same in the male and female

ligament in front, the edge of the lacunar ligament medially, the pectineal continuation of that ligament posteriorly and the femoral vein laterally). The hernia then bulges through the saphenous opening in the fascia of the thigh (*Figure 28.5*) and subsequently *may* roll upwards superficial to the inguinal ligament and may contain fluid, omentum or bowel. The last of these is the critical situation for the reasons discussed in the section on General Principles. If bowel is caught in the hernia, reduction is usually impossible, and may be dangerous if any part of the bowel wall is ischaemic. Operation is urgently necessary and should be through an incision above the inguinal ligament in case bowel resection is necessary.

For elective operation, there is a choice between this route and the low approach which is simpler. In either case the sac is removed or turned in, and the defect is closed with non-absorbable sutures. For the reasons outlined it is imperative that there should be no delay between diagnosis and operative treatment.

Epigastric and umbilical hernia

Tiny defects in the linea alba (the midline fusion of the layers of the rectus sheath) may allow the protrusion of a lump of fat, possibly followed by a small peritoneal sac. Almost invariably these occur between the umbilicus and the xiphisternum, but similar defects may be related to the umbilicus. Strictly speaking, these are para-umbilical herniae. A narrow neck is the rule and strangulation or a Richter's hernia is a definite possibility if such a hernia is left untreated. At operation it is usual to effect a repair by overlapping the aponeurotic layer.

True umbilical herniae are mainly seen in babies and are due to a failure of closure at the umbilical opening by the time of birth. There is a natural tendency for this to close subsequently and only rarely is operation necessary. Exomphalus is a particular type of congenital umbilical hernia and is discussed in Chapter 7.

Rare abdominal wall hernia

These are many and varied and are too numerous to describe individually here. Nor is this important, for they are all rare and most surgeons have encountered but one or two in a lifetime. As is often the way with surgical curiosities, many are identified eponymously, usually after their discoverer, such as a Spigelian hernia which occurs at the lateral border of the sheath of the rectus abdominis.

All the main complications of hernia are possible but operative repair is usually simple.

Diaphragmatic hernia

There are two main types, the lateral congenital diaphragmatic hernia which is very rare, and the central hiatus hernia, usually diagnosed in adults.

(1) *Congenital hernia.* The development of the diaphragm is complex and failure of fusion at one or other point will leave a gap through which abdominal viscera may protrude into the chest. Treatment is by operation.

(2) *Hiatus hernia.* The hiatus in question is the naturally occurring opening in the diaphragm through which the oesophagus passes. If there is a weakness here, the lower oesophagus and upper part of the stomach may slide up into the chest ('sliding' hiatus hernia); or, much less commonly, the lower oesophagus may stay in place and the upper stomach roll up alongside it ('rolling' hiatus hernia). In the latter, impaction of this part of the stomach in the chest may occur and operation may be necessary for this. In the 'sliding' hiatus hernia the main problems of inflammation, ulceration and subsequent stricture arise from reflux of gastric contents into the oesophagus. Conservative treatment (antacids and postural care) should be given a prolonged trial as the place of operation in the uncomplicated case is controversial. This subject is considered further in Chapter 21.

Internal hernia

Of great rarity are herniae that may occur in relation to a peritoneal pouch arising as a minor developmental anomaly. These may occur in the area of the mesentery of the small or large bowel and their interest lies in the possibility of impaction or strangulation of a loop of bowel. Far more commonly, however, this is related to an adhesion following an earlier operation which will be evident from the abdominal scar.

Incisional hernia

This is the second most frequent type of hernia (inguinal hernia is the commonest and femoral the third in incidence, *Figure 28.4*). Some abdominal wounds are more prone to this complication than others; in particular, midline incisions are the most vulnerable. These are made through fibrous tissues which has a blood supply relatively less than the more muscular lateral abdominal wall. This may be one predisposing factor; others are poor surgical technique, infection and the susceptibility of a patient who is obese or, conversely, malnourished. Factors such as excessive coughing or other straining may be disruptive to the healing wound. The extreme situation, of course, is when a complete separation, or dehiscence, of the abdominal wound occurs in the postoperative period. Emergency resuturing is necessary and this must usually be done without reconstitution of individual layers. It is not surprising that this may be followed later by the development of an incisional hernia.

Such a hernia is usually wide-necked and impaction or strangulation of bowel is not a common problem. However, there are exceptions if the defect is a complex one or is complicated by associated adhesions.

If nothing is done, an incisional hernia usually becomes progressively larger. Therefore, the abdominal wall must either be supported by a surgical corset made to measure for the individual, or operative repair must be undertaken. This may simply involve suturing of the body's tissues, or foreign material may be implanted to give greater strength. In either situation the principles are those already outlined, and, of course, complete avoidance of tension at the healing suture line is essential.

PRACTICAL POINTS IN CONNECTION WITH OPERATION

Preparation of patients for all groin hernia operations requires meticulous shaving and washing of the abdomen, groin and scrotum or vulva. Complete bladder and bowel evacuation immediately preoperatively is very important; catheterization is not usually done but sometimes an enema is necessary.

In the early postoperative period the wound is usually quite painful and analgesics are prescribed. Initial micturition is uncomfortable and patience is required. Some degree of scrotal swelling may be encountered and a support is helpful. Although it is the usual practice for the patient to start to be up and about within forty-eight hours and to have the stitches removed about a week later, he should avoid any strain to the area of the operation for a couple of months.

REFERENCES

Harkins, H. N. (1965). *Hernia in Surgery, Principles and Practice.*
   Ed. C. A. Moyer, J. E. Rhoads, J. G. Allen and H. N. Harkins. p. 1155.
   Philadelphia: J. B. Lippincott
Parry, E. (1966). The influence of rotation of the trunk on the
   anatomy of the inguinal canal. *Br. J. Surg.* 53, 205

29

Surgery of the kidney and ureter

R. M. Jameson

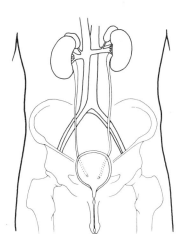

Figure 29.1. Diagram showing the kidneys and ureters. Renal vessels enter hilum in front of renal pelvis. The three sites of ureteric narrowing are: pelvi-ureteric junction, pelvic brim crossing iliac vessels and the vesico-ureteric valve

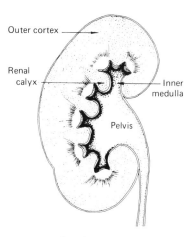

Figure 29.2. Renal anatomy

INTRODUCTION

The kidneys are paired organs situated at the back of the upper abdomen behind the peritoneal cavity and in front of the lowermost two ribs and lumbar muscles. Rarely, one kidney may be absent or in an abnormal position. Each kidney lies in a pouch of fat and the ureter conducts the urine from the renal pelvis to the bladder (*Figures 29.1* and *29.2*). The blood supply to each kidney comes directly from the aorta by the renal arteries which may be multiple. Each renal artery on reaching the kidney divides into branches which end in the glomeruli. The renal artery is an end artery; its branches do not communicate with other arteries so that blockage of a branch will give rise to tissue death of the segment of the kidney it supplies. The venous drainage, however, is multiple into the inferior vena cava. Nerves reach the kidney from the autonomic nervous system by running along the walls of the arteries. These nerves are unable to register pain; loin pain in kidney disease occurs when the disease spreads outside the kidney. However, distension is felt in the collecting system when spasm of the muscles (to overcome any obstruction or spasm during a severe infection) is felt as ureteric colic. This severe pain is referred down the nerves of the abdominal wall which supply the groin, hence the 'loin-to-groin' distribution of ureteric colic. The upper lumbar ureter lies in front of the back muscles at the tips of the transverse processes of the vertebrae aiding its identification on radiography. At operation it is lightly adherent to the peritoneum in front of it, and enters the bony pelvis by running in front of the iliac vessels towards the ischial spine turning inwards and forwards to enter the bladder by a valvular opening. In the pelvis the lower ureter can be damaged by disease or during surgery. It runs on the left under the pelvic colon and alongside the rectum and may be damaged in the abdominoperineal operation for rectal cancer. In the female it runs along the cervix and lateral fornix of the vagina crossing the uterine artery and may be blocked by an advanced cervical or rectal cancer or damaged by radiotherapy to the pelvis. In its course from the kidney to the bladder the ureter is narrowed in three

589

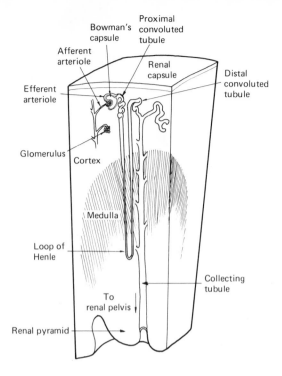

Figure 29.3. The nephron

places, common sites for impaction of stones: the pelviureteric junction, the pelvic brim where it crosses the iliac vessels and the vesico-ureteric junction (*Figure 29.1*).

The junction of the ureter with the bladder is important as there is a muscular valve to prevent reflux of urine up the ureter to the kidney. Temporary reflux is found after the passage of a ureteric stone or during a bladder infection (cystitis); permanent reflux occurs when the valve is damaged. Reflux of infected urine is dangerous; in children it prevents growth of the kidney and at any age it will produce permanent renal damage with scarring and loss of function. Duplication of the ureter is common; it predisposes to reflux and infection.

The functioning unit of the kidney is the nephron (*Figure 29.3*) which consists of the capillary knot, the glomerulus, which is surrounded by the beginning of the renal tubule, Bowman's capsule; the nephron then continues in the renal cortex as two convoluted tubules separated by the loop of Henle which dips into the medulla. The glomerulus acts as a filter and the convoluted tubules and the loop of Henle concentrate and alter the filtrate to form the urine. The functions of the kidney are to maintain normal volume and composition of the body fluids, to eliminate waste products, to aid in red blood cell production and assist in the regulation of the blood pressure. This is done in the following ways.

(1) Excretion of urea and other waste products.
(2) Water and electrolyte balance.
(3) Erythropoietin secretion to stimulate the bone marrow to form red blood cells. In uraemia loss of functioning cells leads to an anaemia; excess secretion is sometimes found in renal cancer, polycystic disease and intrarenal haemangioma.
(4) Blood pressure regulation. If an area of the kidney near the glomerulus becomes ischaemic, a renin is secreted which will raise the blood pressure. Many patients with pyelonephritis develop hypertension; and unilateral kidney disease, with ischaemia of the affected kidney, will produce hypertension.

Damage to different parts of the nephron accounts for the various signs of kidney disease: for example glomerular damage produces an excess of protein and blood in the urine (glomerulonephritis); failure of the proximal tubule to remove glucose from the filtrate gives rise to glycosuria (a harmless condition); in diabetes insipidus the antidiuretic pituitary hormone (ADH) is absent so that the loop of Henle does not concentrate the urine. Ascending infection and obstruction to the flow of urine damages the distal tubules so that the kidney excretes dilute urine with a high salt content. In renal failure the tubular damage results in acidosis which makes the patient have slow sighing respiration, 'air hunger', in an attempt to correct the abnormal blood bio-chemistry. The working of the kidneys is impaired by ischaemia, infection and obstruction.

Principles of nursing and surgery

In urinary tract disease the aims of the treatment are:

(1) to ensure free urine flow without obstruction;
(2) to eliminate infection and protect the urinary tract from further infection;
(3) to restore and improve renal function;
(4) to prevent or cure any urinary leak;
(5) to remove completely any growth rising in or involving the urinary tract; and
(6) to remove any stones in the urinary tract and to prevent their recurrence.

The outstanding features of a good nurse are kindness and reliability. The day-to-day teamwork involved in urological work needs reliable and accurate recording of observations about fluid intake and urinary output, pulse, blood pressure and any of the patient's symptoms. Such nursing observations must be recorded so that they are readily available to other team members. Many patients with urological disorders are chronically ill, depressed, incontinent and frightened. The condition of a uraemic patient can change from hour to hour and the kindness and reliability of nursing care do much to improve morale and lead to an uncomplicated recovery. Routine observations enable complications to be avoided; the hallmark of a good urological unit is not the speed and drama with which complications are treated, but the fact that they are prevented from happening.

INVESTIGATION OF THE URINARY TRACT

The structure and function of the urinary tract may be shown by various investigations. The nurse plays an important part by allaying any fears a patient may have and by conscientious and accurate collection of urine and blood samples. The purpose of all investigations is to show the site and nature of the disease and to find out that the rest of the urinary tract is working satisfactorily. Renal investigations are only complete when the answers to the following questions have been obtained.

(1) Are both kidneys present and of normal site, shape and size?
(2) Are the collecting systems of the renal pelvis, ureters, bladder and urethra normal and by their muscular action capable of freely propelling urine without any reflux or obstruction?
(3) Are both kidneys working well and is it possible to improve their function rather than remove one unnecessarily?
(4) Having found disease in the urinary tract, is the rest of the tract normal?
(5) As a last resort, having decided to remove a diseased kidney, is the other capable of supporting life?

Ward urine tests

Although extensive biochemical tests are of help in reaching an accurate diagnosis, it must not be forgotten that success in treatment depends upon teamwork between medical, radiological and laboratory staff as well as physiotherapists and the hospital dietician. Valuable help can be obtained by the nurse's care in, for example, examination of the urine and the recording of its volume. Admission specimens of the urine and those obtained during out-patient attendances are always examined by the nurse and if anything abnormal is found in its appearance or by testing, the medical staff must be informed. Each urine specimen must be clearly labelled with the patient's name, date and the time it was obtained. When a patient is in hospital, the hurried emptying of bedpans and urinal must not stop the nurse from noting any abnormality of the urine and keeping any abnormal specimens and reporting her findings to the medical staff.

Table 29.1 Coloured urine and its possible causes

Colour	Cause	Remarks
Black	Old haemoglobin in acid urine Phenol poisoning Melanin in patients with malignant melanoma Prophyrin (brown urine which blackens on standing)	Note that concentrated blood may appear black but comes red on dilution This metabolic condition can mimic the acute abdomen and barbiturates may precipitate an attack
Blue-green	Methylene blue (De Witt's pills)	
Green-black	Severe jaundice	
Brown	Myohaemoglobin	
Orange-red	Haemoglobin in fresh alkaline urine Vegetable dyes (beetroot, carrots, berries) Eosin (boiled sweets) Drugs (Pyridium, vitamin B, rifampicin, Furadantin)	

For ward urine testing the urine is collected in a clean container. Normal urine is clear and has an amber colour. The causes of coloured urine are shown in Table 29.1. Chemical tests are performed by using reagent strips made by the Ames Company (Table 29.2). The only test which requires heating the urine is that for Bence-Jones protein. This is a paraprotein (found in multiple **myelomatosis**) which appears as a coagulated deposit on heating acidified urine (like the white of an egg) and it disappears on boiling the urine.

Specific gravity

The urine is placed in a wide-mouthed container. A glass float, the hydrometer, is used to measure the specific gravity (SG). The reading on the instrument varies with the urine

Myelomatosis A malignant disease in which the bone marrow is infiltrated with myeloma or plasma cells (these may also appear in the blood).

Table 29.2   **Significance of urine reagent strip test ('Multistix')**

Substance	Significance of positive result
Urobilinogen	Formed in gut by breakdown of bilirubin, reabsorbed and excreted by kidney. Present in haemolytic jaundice because bile pigments are derived from red cell breakdown.
Blood	Cancer, sever infections, stone, glomerulonephritis and hypertension. *Haematuria always needs urgent investigation.*
Bilirubin	Water soluble conjugated bile pigment which is excreted in urine if bile duct obstructed. Present in hepatitis.
Ketones	Starvation, vomiting and diabetic pre-coma.
Glucose	Diabetes, pregnancy glycosuria due to low renal threshold.
Protein	Nephritis, hypertension, pregnancy toxaemia, severe infections and amyloidosis
pH	Low pH = Acid. High pH = Alkaline. Calcium stones do not form if pH low. Urate and cystine stones do not form if pH high. High pH found in *Bacillus proteus* and *Pseudomonas pyocyanea* infections. In renal failure low pH = acute tubular necrosis, pH high in glomerular disease.

temperature; each instrument is marked to be accurate at a certain temperature. If the urine temperature is known and differs from that used in calibrating the hydrometer (usually 18°C) for each difference of 3°C add or subtract 0.001 to the hydrometer reading. The normal range of specific gravity of urine is 1.001–1.040.

Renal biopsy

The diagnosis of a renal disease can be made by examining the kidney tissue under the microscope. A needle is passed under local anaesthetic through the loin into the kidney to obtain a sample of kidney tissue for examination. Nursing after-care entails bed rest, observations of the pulse, blood pressure and urinary output. Haematuria is common and a high fluid intake is needed.

Pyelography (urography); the intravenous urogram (IVU)

Whatever type of renal radiograph is taken, a preliminary film is taken to see if there is any stone or other abnormality in the abdomen or pelvis. Any spinal abnormality which may influence the function of the urinary tract will also be shown, for example, spina bifida. To demonstrate the kidney, an injection of a radio-opaque iodine dye is given; the kidney concentrates the dye in the urine so that views of the renal pelvis, ureters and bladder are obtained. When renal function is poor an outline of the kidney tissue may be revealed (the nephrogram). Films taken which focus at different depths, tomograms, may give further detail.

Retrograde pyelography

Under an anaesthetic in the operating theatre a cystoscope is passed into the bladder and a fine graduated opaque ureteric catheter is passed up the ureter. The contrast medium is injected into the catheter and radiographs of the renal pelvis and ureter taken.

Cystogram

A catheter is passed and the bladder filled with contrast medium, radiographs are taken to see if there is ureteric reflux and the bladder outlet is studied. Any abnormal leakage will be shown. It may be combined with pressure flow studies (urodynamics) in patients with incontinence, e.g. video cineradiography with urodynamics, the pressure/flow records and the film of the patient voiding are simultaneously recorded on a TV monitor and stored in a cassette for later study.

Urethrogram

A radio-opaque water-soluble jelly is introduced into the urethra and radiographs taken.

Renal angiograms

A fine catheter is passed into the renal artery, contrast medium is injected and radiographs are taken to show the blood circulation of the kidneys. The arterial catheter is commonly introduced through a puncture in the groin and passed along the femoral artery up the aorta to the renal vessels. Nursing after-care includes regular observation of the pressure dressing in the groin and pulse and blood pressure recordings. The medical staff must be called at the first sign of bleeding.

Urodynamics

Pressure flow studies, urodynamics, provide valuable information. In the renal pelvis and ureter, urodynamic studies show if dilatation is caused by obstruction, e.g. pelviureteric junction obstruction and hydronephrosis. In incontinence and in neurological disorders urodynamics are essential. Incontinence is caused by either bladder muscle (detrusor) overactivity or sphincter weakness; urodynamic studies can differentiate and prevent unnecessary and unsuccessful surgery, e.g. pelvic floor repair. The bladder is a poor witness and on history-taking it is not possible to determine the cause of incontinence; this is why many pelvic operations in the past were unsuccessful as urodynamic studies were not available.

Isotope studies

Most isotope studies are performed in departments of nuclear medicine; any studies that are performed on the wards are safe as the radiation to patients and staff is much less than that emitted during ordinary radiographs. For isotope

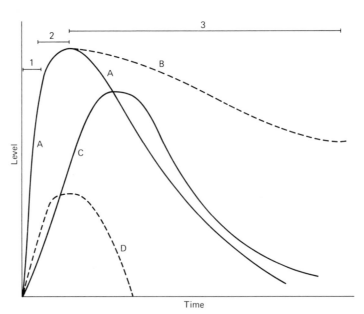

Figure 29.4. Isotope renograms. A, normal; B, obstruction; C, ischaemic D, atrophic; 1, vascular phase; 2, tubular phase; 3, excretory phase

renograms and renal scans a radioactive substance is injected intravenously; it is concentrated in the kidney and its uptake recorded. Isotope renograms are tracings, over a period of time, of the concentration of the isotope by the kidney. Renograms give information about renal blood flow, tubular function and show if an obstruction is present (*Figure 29.4*).

Using various isotopes, renograms can scan the kidney to show its function in various parts and detect cysts or tumours.

Isotope studies may be used to detect deep vein thrombosis (DVT) using ^{125}I fibrinogen. The patient is given sodium bromide to block iodine uptake by the thyroid. If a DVT occurs there will be a localized concentration of isotope in the clot in the calf muscles. It can be simply detected by using a scanner. Prompt treatment of DVT is life-saving.

Bone metastases can be detected by isotopes months before they are shown on ordinary x-rays. Isotopes are also used to treat various forms of cancer.

Ultrasound

Ultrasound is a safe, non-invasive investigation using sound waves. Echos are reflected at the margins of solids and fluids, and with experience a map of underlying structures can be obtained, e.g. fetal parts and placenta, renal cysts, bladder tumours.

Renal function tests

Before surgery it is necessary to know the state of the renal function. The value of the blood urea depends upon diet and will also be altered if the patient is dehydrated. A more accurate test is the serum creatinine. Clearance tests measure the rate of excretion of a substance by the kidney. They involve taking a blood sample and accurate timing and collection of urine samples. If the nurse permits an incomplete or inaccurate urine sample over the period of time for the tests, the results are worthless. The medical staff are dependent upon the nursing staff for painstaking and accurate collection of urine samples. The normal value of the endogenous creatinine clearance test is 80 to 130 ml per minute. A 24-hour urine collection may also be needed to find out the calcium excretion in patients with renal stones. An excessive excretion of calcium is found in many patients with urinary tract stones; it is called hypercalcuria. Normal biochemical values are shown in Table 29.3.

Urine cytology

The urine may be examined for the presence of cancer cells; cytological tests are regularly performed in patients whose occupation puts them at risk, for example, rubber workers. Cytological tests are only of value in patients with bladder cancer as it is rare for renal tumours to be detected in this way. A clean freshly voided urine sample is added to an equal

Table 29.3   Some important biochemical findings in blood and urine and the range of normal values

Biochemical values in normal patients		*SI units*	*Old units*
Serum creatinine in adults and infants	below:	110 μmol/l	1.3 mg %
Blood urea in babies and infants under 2 years	below:	3 mmol/l	20 mg %
Blood urea in late pregnancy/puerperium	below:	3 mmol/l	20 mg %
Blood urea in adults, normal diet	below:	5–7 mmol/l	30–40 mg %
Blood urea in adults, high protein diet	below:	12 mmol/l	70 mg %
Any adult with a blood urea above 8 mmol/l (50 mg %) needs investigation. The average rise of the urea is 8 mmol/l (50 mg %) after surgery or injury for 3–4 days.			
Sodium		136–145 mmol/l	136–145 mEq/%
Potassium		3.5–4.5 mmol/l	3.5–4.5 mEq/%
Chloride		95–107 mmol/l	65–107 mEq/%
Carbon dioxide as bicarbonate		24–32 mmol/l	24–32 mEq/%
Calcium		2.2–2.5 mmol/l	9–10 mg %
Phosphate		0.8–1.4 mmol/l	2.5–4.5 mg %
Uric acid (urate)		0.12–0.42 mmol/l	2–7 mg %
Blood gases			
Pco_2 – Carbon dioxide		4.1–5.6 kPa	31–42 mmHg
Po_2 – Oxygen		10.5–14.5 kPa	80–110 mmHg
Bicarbonate		24–32 mmol/l	24–32 mEq/l
Base excess	+/–	3 mmol/l	3 mEq/l
Urine biochemistry — normal values 24-hour collection			
Creatinine		9–17 mmol/l	1–2 g/24 h
Calcium		2.5–7.5 mmol/l	300 mg/24 h
Urate		30–120 mmol/24 h	1.5–3 g
Protein	less than:	0.05 g/l	50 mg %
VMA	less than:	3 mmol/l	3.5 μg
Sodium	less than:	200 mmol/l	200 mEq/l

volume of preservative and the urine passed through an ultra-filter which is examined under a microscope. The test is of no value in the presence of an obvious haematuria (when investigation is urgently indicated in any case) or during menstruation as too many red blood cells are present. In women, contamination of the urine by talcum powder or vaginal cells may occur and the test will have to be repeated preferably by using a catheter specimen. Urinary stones may cause false positive results.

Bacteriological investigations

For urine culture and bacteriological examination the urine must be obtained without contamination and collected in a sterile container and promptly sent to the laboratory. The urine specimen must not be placed in the sun or over a radiator to ferment but be sent immediately to the laboratory. If the laboratory is closed, it can be placed in a refrigerator to delay bacterial multiplication and then sent to the laboratory as soon as it opens. Every specimen must be clearly labelled with the patient's name, ward, record number and time and date of collection.

Midstream and early morning samples

The midstream urine is a clean catch sample of the middle of the voiding stream which avoids contamination from the external genitalia. To identify the site of infection, a three-glass test is sometimes used, urine specimens at the beginning, middle and end of voiding being collected for examination. In men with prostatic infection a urine sample collected after rectal massage may be examined. In all these samples the number and type of organisms are noted together with the sensitivities to various antibiotics. In patients with suspected tuberculosis an early morning sample is collected on 3 consecutive days, for the tubercle bacilli collected in the bladder overnight are found in the highest numbers in the early morning urine obtained on rising. The samples must be examined on the day they are obtained, otherwise the delay may result in the decomposition of the bacilli in the stale urine and the chances of detecting tuberculosis will be lessened.

Catheter samples

Catheter samples of urine provide uncontaminated bladder urine specimens and are obtained during the course of treatment. Catheter specimens must never be obtained just to gain a sample for the bacteriologist. At one time it was the custom to take catheter urine specimens to avoid contamination but it has been proved to be a dangerous practice as some healthy patients will develop pyelonephritis as a result of catheterization. Not only is unnecessary catheterization dangerous, it is just as dangerous to disconnect a urine drainage tube from a catheter drainage system to obtain a urine sample. To obtain a urine sample for culture from a patient with an indwelling catheter, needle aspiration of urine from the catheter or drainage tube is required. Other methods of urine sampling may be used by medical staff, for example, suprapubic needle aspiration of the bladder, particularly valuable in antenatal work, or ureteric urine samples in the diagnosis of renal tuberculosis.

PATHOLOGICAL CONDITIONS AND THEIR MANAGEMENT

Bacteriuria and renal infections

Microscopy of urine samples is performed in the laboratory to detect blood cells, and in order to distinguish between infection and contamination of the urine the number of organisms in the specimen is counted. Hence delay in sending specimens to the laboratory encourages bacterial multiplication and it may not be possible to tell if the urine is either infected (significant bacteriuria is more than 10^5 organisms/ml) or contaminated. If white cells (pus cells) are found in sterile urine, the condition is called abacterial pyuria; this may be found in analgesic nephropathy, tubercle, stone or tumour of the urinary tract. Bacteriuria of pregnancy is important for, if treated, the risks of pyelonephritis, toxaemia and small babies are reduced.

Pyelonephritis and vesico-ureteric reflux

Pyelonephritis is an infection of the kidneys; the pathogenic organisms originate from the bowel and enter the urinary tract from below by the bowel lymphatics, perianal skin, urethra and bladder to the kidney. In babies the infection may be blood-borne. The patient may have a fever and the urine contain blood and protein. If the condition is caused by reflux of infected urine up the ureters, pain or rigors may develop when the bladder is full or during voiding. Many cases of long-standing pyelonephritis have generalized ill health without urinary symptoms. The urine will grow the infecting organisms and an excess of white cells will be found in the urine and the blood may contain antibodies to the infecting organisms. The urogram will show clubbed dilated calyces, a scarred cortex and in chronic cases shrinkage of the kidney. If extensive bilateral damage is present, there will be renal failure present as shown by a raised blood urea and serum creatinine. Hypertension is common. Certain conditions, such as an anatomical abnormality or stone, predispose to recurrence of the condition. Medical treatment involves administration of antibiotics and the management of the complications, such as hypertension, renal failure, correction of abnormalities and so on. The nursing care entails bed rest while a fever is present and the encouragement of a high fluid intake of at least 3 litres daily. The most important task of the nurse is to ensure that the patient takes the antibiotic treatment, particularly when it is necessary to continue for many months. Incomplete courses of treatment lead to the development of bacterial resistance to treatment and if patients hoard antibiotics in anticipation of another attack, the antibiotics may become dangerous as they deteriorate.

During pregnancy the kidney is more sensitive to harm and if infection and toxaemia develop, there is a risk of hypertension in later life.

Amyloidosis

Amyloidosis is a condition in which a starch-like substance is deposited in the kidney causing enlargement and loss of function. There is a gross proteinuria. It is found in patients who are paraplegic or arthritic and occasionally in ulcerative colitis or long-standing suppuration.

Analgesic nephropathy and renal hypertension

Analgesic nephropathy deserves mention, for the nurse may make the diagnosis on finding out that the patient has a long-standing history of taking analgesics.

Rarely a kidney with an impaired blood supply (e.g. in unilateral pyelonephritis or renal artery stenosis) can cause hypertension. Provided that the condition is diagnosed before irreversible damage to the arteries has occurred, it may be cured by removal of the ischaemic kidney or less commonly by vascular surgery.

Renal and genital tuberculosis

Renal and genital tuberculosis results from blood-borne infection. The onset is insidious but can present as bleeding from the urinary tract. Later, severe frequency of micturition and sterility develop as the bladder contracts and the sexual organs are affected. The earliest finding is that of abacterial pyuria and an irregular calyx on pyelography. Management is three-fold: the strict adherence to a regimen to ensure that the treatment is taken and the prompt treatment of any complications; chemotherapy with at least two antituberculous drugs to minimize the risk of drug-resistant tubercle; and surgical management of complications or removal of localized disease. For example a contracted bladder may be enlarged by using the caecum or colon as a graft on a vascular pedicle. Treatment can be given on an out-patient basis using two of the following oral drugs in rotation: rifampicin, isoniazid (INH), pyrazinamide. At first these drugs are given daily for two months, later twice weekly for six months, and are all given with large doses of vitamin C. International long-term multicentre trials demonstrate that this out-patient treatment is more effective than the traditional sanatorium regimen of triple therapy with streptomycin INH and PAS. However if the patients are not co-operative or cannot be supervised easily sanatorium management is best.

Renal and ureteric injuries

A blow in the loin may tear the kidney (*Figure 29.5*). An emergency urogram will show the extent of damage. The treatment is by sedation, administration of antibiotics to prevent infection and bed rest until the urine no longer appears blood-stained. Ureteric colic may occur due to a blood clot. Nursing observations will show if the condition

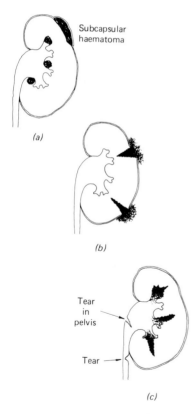

Subcapsular haematoma

(a)

(b)

Tear in pelvis

Tear

(c)

Figure 29.5. Renal injuries. (*a*) Bruising; (*b*) renal tear; (*c*) pelvic and ureteric tears

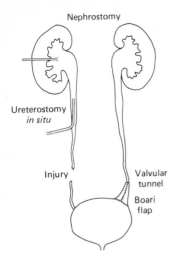

Nephrostomy

Ureterostomy
in situ

Injury

Valvular
tunnel

Boari
flap

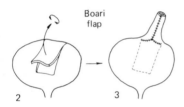

Boari
flap

2   3

Ureter
reimplanted

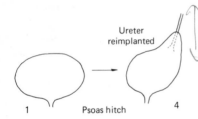

1   Psoas hitch   4

Figure 29.6. Management of ureteric injuries. In psoas hitch the mobilized bladder is sutured to psoas muscle

worsens; for example, rising pulse rate and falling blood pressure indicate further internal bleeding. By saving each specimen of urine and labelling them with the time each specimen was obtained, one can tell at a glance from the appearance of the urine if it is more blood-stained or not. Sometimes abdominal distension occurs; this is treated by gastric aspirations using a Ryle's tube. Rarely, hypertension, perinephric abscess and ureteric damage may occur.

Ureteric damage may result from extensive and difficult pelvic surgery. The patient may complain of loin pain, abdominal swelling and leak of urine from the wound. After any pelvic operation the nurse must record the time and volume of urine passed and report any unexpected findings. If the ureter is damaged, the kidney function must be saved by a temporary nephrostomy; later the ureter can be repaired or reimplanted into the bladder (*Figure 29.6*).

Diseases of the upper urinary tract

Complete obstruction of the urinary outflow from the kidneys by mechanical blockage of the ureters will show itself by a sudden stoppage of the urinary output without bladder distension. Sudden one-sided obstruction produces loin pain and swelling and a fall in urine output. Nursing observations, which include daily records of the urine output, are invaluable, for example a widely fluctuating urine output suggests an incomplete obstruction; a gradual fall in urine output suggests a medical cause in the kidney itself.

Hydronephrosis

Obstruction to the kidney outflow at the junction of the renal pelvis and ureter causes hydronephrosis; the kidney enlarges to become a distended bag. To restore urine flow and prevent kidney damage, the obstruction must be overcome. Hydronephrosis due to pelviureteric obstruction is due to fibrous obstruction and may later develop also in the other kidney. The treatment is surgical, the kidney outlet being enlarged by plastic surgery, as the condition may occur on the opposite side, a hydronephrotic kidney is preserved whenever possible. Outflow obstruction may be caused by a ureteric stone or the ureter narrowed by scar tissue or compressed by tumour. Ureteric reflux produces similar damage to the kidney if the urine is infected. Reflux acts like intermittent high pressure obstruction; if the urine is infected there will be forceful reinfection of the kidney with progressive renal damage. It can be prevented by reconstructing the valve between the ureter and bladder.

Congenital disorders

Rarely, one kidney may be absent at birth or be in an abnormal position, for example, in the pelvis. The other kidney increases in size to compensate for that absence. A common abnormality is ureteric duplication, a kidney emptying by two ureters; this condition is wrongly termed 'double kidney' by the public. Occasionally one of the double ureters will open in an abnormal site producing incontinence. Cysts also are found in the kidney; some types of these are inherited. Polycystic disease of the kidneys is one type of inherited and progressive cause of renal impairment. Usually both kidneys can be seen and felt; there is hypertension, anaemia and renal failure in severe cases. Although it can be detected in childhood it usually presents in middle age, but a few survive to a ripe old age without treatment.

Tumours

At any age haematuria, loin pain and kidney enlargement suggest renal tumour. *All patients with haematuria need urgent investigation.* A urogram will show a mass in the kidney. Ultrasound, isotope studies and a renal angiogram can differentiate between cyst and tumour. Some tumours in adults have hormone-like effects (polycythaemia, pseudo-hyperparathyroidism). In adults the kidney is removed with the perinephric fat and lymph nodes (radical nephrectomy) through a loin incision. In children an abdominal approach is better. Whichever technique is chosen the renal vein is first tied off to stop tumour spread before the kidney is handled. Nephrectomy is the method of choice; metastases, if present, may need radiotherapy or excision. Bilateral renal tumours may be treated surgically by partial nephrectomy using regional hypothermia to protect the remaining renal tissue. In children the nephroblastoma (Wilms' tumour) is found and is best treated by a combination of radiotherapy, surgery and antimitotic drugs (cancer chemotherapy). In specialized centres the results of treatment (with earlier diagnosis) are very good.

Urinary tract stones

Stones may be found in the kidneys and ureters. Where the stone causes harm by obstruction and infection, it needs removal. More important, the recurrence of a stone must be prevented. Any stone removed is analysed. The nurse plays an important part in the collection of blood and urine samples to determine the cause of the stone. Estimations of the blood calcium and phosphorus are taken from a fasting patient whenever possible and to avoid falsely high values the blood is collected without using a tourniquet.

Nursing care plays an important part in the management of patients with stone; every patient who has had a stone must drink at least 3 litres of fluid daily. If the stone contained calcium, acidification of the urine with oral vitamin C (2 g daily) hinders further stone formation. If the stone is made of uric acid or cystine, the urine can be kept alkaline with sodium bicarbonate to minimize stone recurrence. As 70 per cent of patients with stone in the urinary tract develop further stones within 5 years, the nurse in ward or clinic must make certain that the patient has continued to keep to the high fluid intake. Some patients have an excess of calcium in the urine (hypercalcuria) and need medical treatment. About 1 out of every 300 patients with urinary tract stone will be found to have an overactive parathyroid gland as the cause of the stone formation and will need parathyroidectomy. Thus the nurse's role is to check that a fluid intake of 3 litres daily is maintained, to instruct the patient to test the pH of the urine so that it is kept at the correct value to minimize recurrence, and to ensure that the patient adheres to the medical and dietary treatment to prevent stone recurrence. These principles apply to all patients with urinary tract stones. When urinary infection (usually with *B. proteus*) is the cause of the stone, all will have pyelonephritis and need a nightly antibiotic (nitrofurantoin, sulphonamide) for many months to control infection and prevent recurrence. This method of treatment is often forgotten.

Stones in the upper urinary tract may cause infections and ureteric colic; in the bladder severe cystitis and retention may occur. Stones which on radiography are less than 6 mm in diameter may pass spontaneously. Larger stones will need operative removal if they cause obstruction, infection or renal impairment. Once more the aim is to conserve renal tissue rather than needlessly remove the kidney. Stag-horn calculi are large kidney stones which fit the renal pelvis and calyces like fingers inside a glove. At one time they were an indication for nephrectomy, but modern techniques, which may include cooling the kidney to prevent vascular damage if the pedicle needs temporary clamping, enable most kidneys to be saved. In removing stag-horn calculi the aim is to keep the kidney intact, if necessary crushing the stone during its removal, and not to remove the stone intact leaving behind a battered and bruised kidney. A radiograph taken of the kidney, using a small film, which is slipped inside the wound will confirm that all stone fragments have been removed before completion of the operation. Alternatively an image intensifier in the operating theatre will confirm that all the debris has been

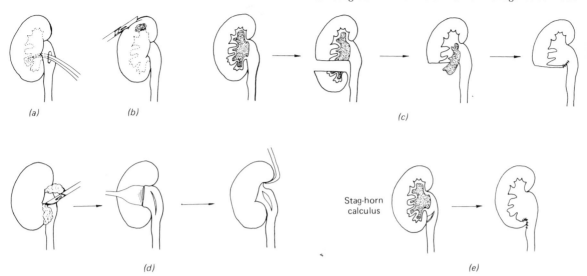

Figure 29.7. Various operations for renal stone. (*a*) Pyelolithotomy with Randall's forceps; (*b*) nephrolithotomy; (*c*) partial (polar) nephrectomy for stag-horn calculus; (*d*) Gil–Vernet pyelolithotomy – fat is dissected from pelvis, renal tissue is retracted to reveal intrarenal pelvis; (*e*) ureterocalycystostomy – lower calyx is joined to ureter to avoid need for partial nephrectomy

removed. The operation of splitting the kidney is old fashioned and damages the kidney and should no longer be used without regional renal hypothermia. Various operations on the kidneys and ureters for stone are shown in *Figure 29.7.*

Ureteric stones Most stones in the ureter will be passed if a high fluid intake is maintained. If the urine is strained through a gauze, any small stones can be saved for analysis. Larger stones (larger than 6 mm on radiography) will impact at the narrowest parts of the ureter, the pelviureteric junction, where the ureter crosses the iliac vessels to enter the pelvis and at the vesico-ureteric junction. An impacted stone must be removed as soon as possible; a stone blocking a solitary ureter is an emergency. Stone in the lowest part of the ureter may be removed by endoscopic surgery using a ureteric stone dislodger (*Figure 29.8*). Obstruction by sloughed renal papillae occurs. Like urate stones they are non-opaque on x-ray. They occur in analgesic abusers, diabetics and in severe pyelonephritis. They too may be removed with the endoscopic ureteric stone basket after location by contrast radiology.

Renal failure

Renal failure is fatal if facilities for treatment are not available. There are three forms of renal failure.

(1) Acute: rapid onset of uraemia in a patient with no known renal disease;

(2) acute-on-chronic: rapid increase in renal failure in patient with previous kidney damage; and

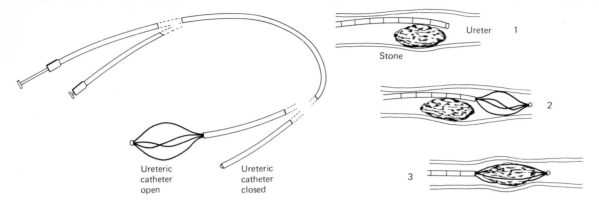

Figure 29.8. Endoscopic Dormia ureteric stone basket

(3) chronic renal failure: uraemia of several weeks' duration with a gradual deterioration of the general condition of the patient.

No patient can be diagnosed as suffering from chronic irreversible renal failure until observations have been made over a period of several months. All patients with renal failure deserve investigation to see if there is a treatable cause of their condition. Nursing care of patients with renal conditions involves accuracy of fluid intake and urinary output observations, prevention of infection and dietary management. Anuria is defined as cessation of urine production, whereas retention means that urine has not been passed. Oliguria is defined as the excretion of too small a volume of urine to support life, e.g. less than 400 ml per day. Wide fluctuations in the urinary output indicate an intermittent incomplete obstruction.

The treatment of acute and acute-on-chronic uraemia is straightforward. Obstructive causes can be dealt with by surgery and the patient kept alive by dialysis until the kidney recovers. Chronic renal failure has received much publicity in recent years as treatment by dialysis and transplantation has proved to be effective. Dialysis is of two types: haemodialysis where the patient's blood is purified by passage through an artificial kidney machine, and peritoneal dialysis which utilizes the abdominal cavity. When haemodialysis is used the patient connects his blood supply to the machine either by using an indwelling plastic cannula inserted into vessels in the leg or arm (Scribner shunt – *Figure 29.9*), or by introducing needles into forearm veins which have become enlarged by the surgical formation of an arteriovenous fistula. Whatever method of connection to a haemodialysing machine is used, any clotting or infection in the limb vessels must be treated in a specialized centre. The basic features of haemodialysis are shown in

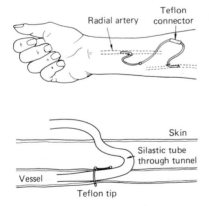

Figure 29.9. Scribner shunt

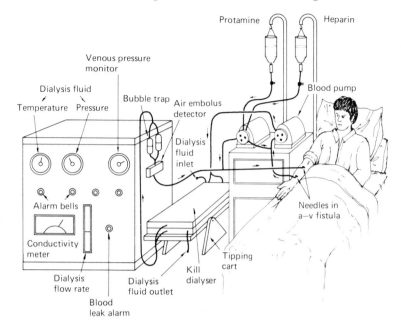

Figure 29.10. Diagram of haemodialysis using Cimino–Brescia arteriovenous fistula. Tipping cart is tipped at the end of dialysis to empty blood back into patient. Note that heparin is introduced into arterial blood to prevent clotting. Protamine solution introduced at the same rate by blood pump counteracts anticoagulant before blood is returned to patient

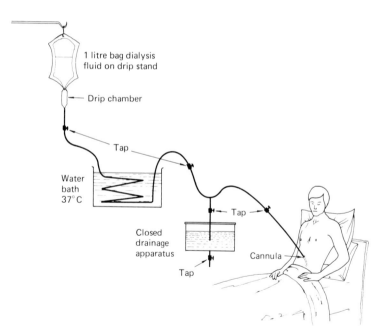

Figure 29.11. Peritoneal dialysis

Figure 29.10. In peritoneal dialysis a cannula is inserted into the abdominal cavity and irrigating fluid run in and out of the abdomen at intervals (*Figure 29.11*). The peritoneum acts as a dialysing membrane. At present this treatment is mainly used for acute cases. Nursing observations include recording of the pulse and blood pressure; if fluid is removed too rapidly from a patient with renal failure, hypotension results. To prevent a rise in the blood urea, patients need a diet low in protein and high in calories. If they are overhydrated, restrictions of the fluid and salt intake are necessary.

Dialysis facilities are combined with renal transplantation in many units. The success of kidney transplantation is high, but the transplantation centres are few.

Renal operations

Before any form of surgery is carried out, the general condition of the patient is improved as much as possible and the operation is then performed at the optimum time. General measures such as stopping smoking and preoperative physiotherapy are of value.

Nephrectomy is a relatively easy operation but the surgeon should always consider alternative procedures which, although more difficult, may save the kidney. However, a kidney which is destroyed by tumour, back-pressure or infection or causes severe hypertension must be removed.

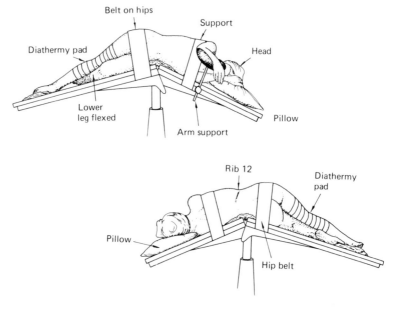

Figure 29.12. Diagram showing the position of patient on an operating table for right kidney operation

The difficulties of surgery are the difficulties of access. The anaesthetized patient is positioned on the operating table as shown in *Figure 29.12,* to obtain an easy access to the kidney through a loin incision. Care must be taken to see that the patient is not in contact with metal in order to prevent burns due to earthing of the diathermy current. Many surgeons remove the lowermost rib to approach the kidney. Cutting through the loin muscles below the rib may cause damage to the nerves of the abdominal wall and access to the kidney is poor. The author prefers Turner–Warwick's incision which cuts through the eleventh intercostal space; the diaphragm is freed upwards and the twelfth rib displaced downwards. Pleural damage is less common with this incision than with the twelfth rib removal and the renal pedicle is more easily accessible. In dealing with renal cancer it is important to tie off the renal vessels before handling the kidney to prevent the tumour spreading in the bloodstream. Very large tumours can best be removed by an incision in the ninth or tenth intercostal space. In children an anterior abdominal approach is better.

Various conservative renal operations are shown in *Figure 29.13*.

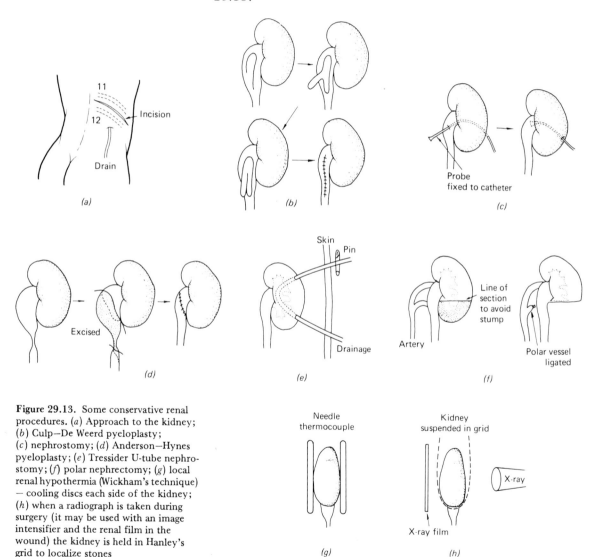

Figure 29.13. Some conservative renal procedures. (*a*) Approach to the kidney; (*b*) Culp–De Weerd pyeloplasty; (*c*) nephrostomy; (*d*) Anderson–Hynes pyeloplasty; (*e*) Tressider U-tube nephrostomy; (*f*) polar nephrectomy; (*g*) local renal hypothermia (Wickham's technique) – cooling discs each side of the kidney; (*h*) when a radiograph is taken during surgery (it may be used with an image intensifier and the renal film in the wound) the kidney is held in Hanley's grid to localize stones

Where renal drainage by nephrostomy is needed, the tube is led out through a stab incision in such a way that it lies in a direct line from the renal pelvis to the skin to facilitate changing of the nephrostomy tube.

In incisions tube drainage is better than the old-fashioned corrugated rubber. Using a tube, any fluids can be collected in a sterile drainage bottle. Drains from wounds should not be led out through the operative incision but through a separate stab incision, thus the wound dressings are left undisturbed when the drain is shortened.

SUMMARY OF PRINCIPLES OF NURSING CARE IN RENAL PATIENTS

In both medical and surgical conditions knowledge of the fluid intake/output is important. In oliguric and oedematous patients the fluids must be restricted. In patients with infections and stone or after surgery daily intake of 3 litres of fluid is needed. Uraemic and oedematous patients need a diet low in protein and salt but high in carbohydrate and calories. Ill patients need more calories.

Uraemic patients are prone to infections. Oral fungicides (nystatin) are used to prevent thrush. The dosage of other antibiotics may need modification in renal failure.

Urine is an excellent breeding ground for bacteria and a high urinary output flushes out the organisms. A closed drainage bag system is essential. Connecting tubes must not be disconnected without firstly clamping off the tube near the patient. All connections or taps must be wiped with antiseptic and emptying of the bags must be done without contamination.

REFERENCES

Jameson, R. M., Burrows, K. and Large, B. (1976). *Management of the Urological Patient.* Edinburgh and London: Churchill Livingstone
Uldall, R. (1977). *Renal Nursing.* Oxford: Blackwell

30

Surgery of the bladder and male genitalia

R. M. Jameson

THE BLADDER AND URETHRA

Introduction

The bladder is a muscular reservoir situated in front of the peritoneal cavity. The normal bladder holds about 500 ml of urine. Urine enters the bladder by the ureterovesical valves which are situated on each side of the trigone (*Figure 30.1*). The trigone is an important muscular area concerned with control of the bladder outlet and ureteric orifices. It is recognized by its triangular shape, its mucosa is adherent and pale in colour. The bladder receives its blood supply from adjacent vessels. The nervous control of the bladder is discussed later in the chapter.

Congenital anomalies

Ectopia vesicae
Ectopia vesicae is a congenital abnormality; the pubic bones fail to join in the midline anteriorly, there is a defect in the anterior abdominal wall, the bladder mucosa lies flat open on

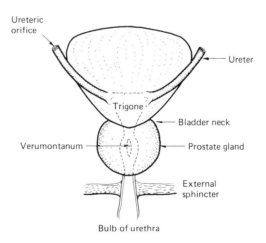

Figure 30.1. Anatomy of the bladder in the male, viewed from behind

611

the lower abdominal wall and the urine continuously dribbles out of the exposed ureteric orifices. The exposed bladder becomes inflamed and may also become cancerous. The abdominal wall muscles are weak, rectal prolapse and herniae are common.

Babies with this condition are irritable as the uncontrollable urinary leakage makes the skin sodden and infected. Vaseline gauze inside the napkins prevents excessive skin damage. Major surgery is delayed until the child is 6 to 9 months old. In the meantime the baby is nursed in the normal way, care being taken to keep the skin as dry as possible. Major surgery involves either ureteric transplantation into the colon or bladder reconstruction. Bladder reconstruction involves forming a bladder reservoir including sphincters, joining the pubic bones anteriorly and correcting major deformities of the penis. It is not always possible to achieve urinary control either by ureteric transplant or bladder reconstruction. Even after surgery the child may have recurrent urinary infections and renal stones.

Posterior urethral valves

Posterior urethral valves are due to abnormal mucosal folds found in the urethra of male infants producing a partial obstruction to the flow of urine. If severe, the baby may be born with uraemia and with hydronephrotic kidneys, due to back pressure. The bladder is always distended. Treatment is by resection of the valves through a perineal urethrostomy. A temporary nephrostomy or cutaneous ureterostomy may be necessary initially if the baby's condition is precarious when first seen.

LOWER URINARY TRACT INFECTION

Cystitis and the urethral syndrome

The term cystitis means inflammation of the bladder but is loosely used by patients to describe any symptoms of painful or frequent micturition (*Figure 30.2*). Urinary tract infections are caused by the bowel type of organisms (Gram-negative bacteria, *Escherichia coli*, *Bacillus proteus*, *Pseudomonas pyocyanea*) which are present on the perianal and genital skin and are found in the urinary meatus. When the body defences are lowered, the organisms enter the urethra and bladder and cause infection. In women true cystitis is rare and only found in severe infections. The condition which many women call 'cystitis' is an inflammation of the urethra and its surrounding glands.

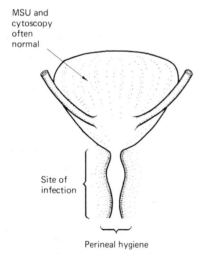

MSU and cytoscopy often normal

Site of infection

Perineal hygiene

Figure 30.2. The urethral syndrome (cystitis in women). Scarring may develop at either end of urethra producing residual urine. Urethral tissues are inflamed and high pus cells and bacterial counts are observed in the first and last urine specimens. Perineal hygiene prevents recurrence

If the site of infection is in the urethra, midstream urine specimens and cystoscopy will often be reported as normal. However, if a urethral swab or an initial urethral sample of the urinary stream is examined, pus cells and bacteria will be found, and if the urethra is examined with an endoscope, it will appear inflamed.

The basis of all treatment of lower urinary tract infections is to enable the bladder to empty completely and to free the urine of pathogens. The emphasis is upon complete bladder emptying rather than indiscriminate use of antibiotics which only leads to the development of resistant strains of bacteria.

Treatment

The treatment of acute lower urinary tract infections is as follows.

High fluid intake is needed to wash out the organisms. Before antibiotics were used many patients were cured by a high fluid intake alone, for example, the traditional lemon and barley water remedies.

Complete bladder emptying is also of great importance and patients with recurrent cystitis should be investigated. If urethritis and stenosis prevent complete emptying, the urethra needs widening. In men incomplete bladder emptying is caused by prostatic enlargement or fibrosis at the bladder neck.

Antibiotics are the least important part of the treatment of cystitis. With antibiotic treatment symptomatic relief occurs within a few days if the organisms are sensitive. Because the pain and frequency of micturition disappear, patients stop the treatment and fail to complete the course of therapy, hoarding the tablets in anticipation of future urinary symptoms. Personal experience has shown that over half of patients referred with recurrent urinary infections had failed to complete courses of treatment supplied by their family doctor. An experienced nurse can obtain information about treatment from patients and instruct them about the need to complete the treatment. Failure to complete therapy has the following dangers.

(1) Bacteria are reduced in numbers, not eradicated, and the disease can continue without symptoms.
(2) Inadequate therapy encourages the emergence of resistant strains of bacteria until in the end after many courses of antibiotics totally resistant strains are encountered.
(3) Repeated antibiotic treatment alters the **bowel flora** and encourages not only resistant strains but fungous (monilial) infections and malabsorption syndromes such as vitamin B deficiencies.

Bowel flora The naturally occurring bacterial content of the lumen of the bowel.

(4) Hoarded antibiotics deteriorate and are not only ineffective but also harmful. For example, old tetracycline may damage the kidneys and liver.

Recurrent cystitis

Cystitis only recurs if there is an abnormality in the urine or urinary tract. The causes of recurrent cystitis are:

(1) inadequate treatment — commonly an incomplete course or the wrong antibiotic as the organisms are resistant; new infection;

(2) incomplete bladder emptying — a residual infected urine is present;

(3) infection from above — pyelonephritis or renal stone; and

(4) incorrect diagnosis — perhaps a yeast or Trichomonas infection, less commonly tuberculosis or bladder cancer.

In tuberculosis the bladder becomes congested with ulceration of the mucosa; later shrinkage and scarring results, the capacity is greatly reduced and intractable frequency of micturition develops, the bladder being reduced to thimble size. The treatment of genito-urinary tuberculosis is discussed in Chapter 29. In the early stages of tuberculous cystitis, chemotherapy is sufficient. A contracted bladder can be enlarged by surgery, using bowel transplanted on its vascular pedicle.

Hunner's ulcer is a rare form of cystitis starting at the fundus of the bladder. It is almost always found in women and causes severe frequency of micturition and suprapubic pain with terminal haematuria.

If patients with the urethral syndrome do not improve on treatment, a fungous or gonococcal infection should be excluded.

Urethral **caruncle** is an inflammatory reaction to *Trichomonas vaginalis.* Treatment with metronidazole (Flagyl) or painting with povidone-iodine is effective. True neoplasms of the urethra are rare (carcinoma, melanoma) and carry a bad prognosis.

Gonococcal urethritis in the male produces a watery white discharge 7 to 14 days after intercourse. Untreated gonorrhoea can produce urethral strictures, **epididymitis** and arthritis. The diagnosis must be demonstrated in the laboratory before treatment is begun. In the female the diagnosis of gonorrhoea may be difficult. Swabs from the urethra immediately cultured in Stewart's medium and Gram staining of the urethral and vaginal secretions for the Gram-negative intracellular diplococci of gonorrhoea are more reliable than serological

Caruncle A small fleshy excrescence.

Epididymitis Inflammation of the epididymis which lies along the testis.

tests. Urethral stricture may develop many years after the urethritis. Syphilis must be looked for in every patient suspected of acquiring venereal infection. Non-specific urethritis is the commonest cause of urethral discharge in men. It too can produce a stricture. Treatment with tetracyclines is effective. Prostatitis is common. Fungous urethritis can occur in both sexes after prolonged antibiotic therapy.

OBSTRUCTION OF THE LOWER URINARY TRACT

Obstruction of the lower urinary tract (*Figure 30.3*) causes incomplete bladder emptying, urinary infection and back-pressure effects upon the kidneys and ureters. The obstruction may be functional, resulting from nervous disease, or structural, such as a urethral stricture or narrowing of the bladder neck. If the obstruction is of sudden onset, a painful acute retention of urine occurs. Where it is of gradual onset, the bladder muscle hypertrophies to provide the necessary strength to overcome the obstruction and empty completely the bladder. In this state the bladder is compensated. Later the muscle is not powerful enough to empty the bladder fully, a residual urine occurs and increases in volume, and the bladder is then decompensated. The distended bladder muscle, the detrusor, becomes overstretched and replaced by fibrous scar. Thus weaknesses appear in the bladder wall and these pouches are called diverticula. As they have no muscle in their walls they cannot empty and will become infected and the site of stone and cancer formation. This state of insidious chronic retention is painless. At any time the decompensated bladder may suddenly obstruct producing a painful acute retention. Patients with chronic retention may be unaware of the seriousness of their condition as they are pain-free and may not notice the abdominal swelling due to gross distension of the bladder. However, they may complain of dribbling (retention with overflow).

Acute urinary retention and catheterization

The first duty of the doctor and nurse is to relieve pain. The agony of an acute retention is only relieved by catheterization of the bladder. This has a risk of introducing infection from the anterior urethra which normally contains pathogens which in this situation, however, do little harm. To avoid introducing infection during catheterization, a water-soluble antiseptic/anaesthetic jelly is introduced into the urethra a few minutes before catheterization. The catheter is then passed gently with sterile precautions. In some centres a suprapubic needle

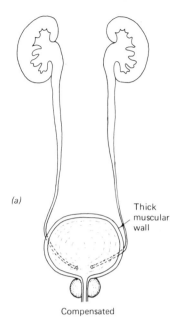

(a)

Thick muscular wall

Compensated

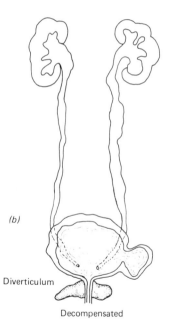

(b)

Diverticulum

Decompensated

Figure 30.3. Lower urinary tract obstruction. (*a*) Bladder empties fully, upper urinary tract is found to be normal and the muscular wall of the bladder is thick. (*b*) Dilated kidneys and ureters are observed together with failing function of the renal cortex. Muscle in bladder wall is replaced by fibrous scar which stretches to form a diverticulum

is introduced into the bladder and a special cannula threaded along it into the bladder. Whatever means of bladder emptying is used, the drainage system must be closed to the atmosphere and kept sterile (*Figure 30.4*).

Choice of urethral catheter

The only place for red rubber catheters is the dustbin or museum as they cause a chemical urethritis and strictures.

Latex catheters are less irritant and are soft and pliable which makes introduction in some patients uneasy and aspiration of clot can be difficult as the catheter walls collapse together on suction. Plastic (polyvinyl chloride — PVC) catheters are best. They are firm at room temperature yet soften at body temperature and are well tolerated by the tissues.

Various designs of catheters are used for different purposes. The catheter size should be the smallest compatible with good urinary drainage, for example 8 to 12 French gauge (F) for bladder drainage for retention, 20 to 24 F for postoperative bladder and prostate operations. The calibre of the catheter must be small to allow the normal urethral secretions to drain and not block or become encrusted at the meatus. Women are particularly prone to damage by prolonged catheterization; the mucosa becomes ulcerated and the meatus patulous with leakage around the catheter. Use of a larger catheter makes matters worse. A small Gibbon catheter and the frequent use of urethral antiseptic jelly will cure most cases in a few days.

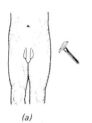

(a)

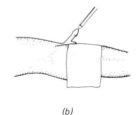

(b)

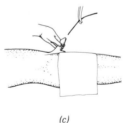

(c)

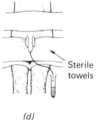

Sterile towels

(d)

Figure 30.4. Catheterization in the male. (*a*) Pubic hair is shaved; (*b*) thighs and perineum are draped and antiseptic gel injected into urethra; (*c*) 'no touch' technique is used, sterile gloves or forceps hold catheter, penis is held straight in other hand; (*d*) sterile towels are placed on abdomen, thighs and between legs, catheter sample urine sent for culture; (*e*) Gibbon catheter fixed with strapping, strapping fixing wings to catheter prevents slipping; (*f*) catheter strapped to thigh and wing tips strapped to abdomen

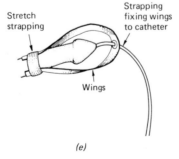

Stretch strapping

Strapping fixing wings to catheter

Wings

(e)

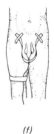

(f)

In men, too large a catheter will produce a postmeatal stricture in the distal 5 cm of the urethra; this develops after a few months when the patient will have been sent home. The urinary stream will become narrowed and cure is by dilatation. A plastic golf tee kept in antiseptic is suitable for the patient's own use after instruction. The postmeatal stricture is dilated twice weekly for a fortnight then once weekly for a month. This treatment prevents recurrence of the stricture.

Types of urethral catheter

Gibbon catheter The Gibbon catheter is a fine plastic non-irritant catheter. Because of its design it causes little upset to the delicate urethral mucosa. Various modifications have been devised: a balloon to assist its retention in the bladder or the addition of an irrigating channel to a larger size for postoperative use (Gow–Gibbon). The method of fixation has already been described (*Figure 30.5a*).

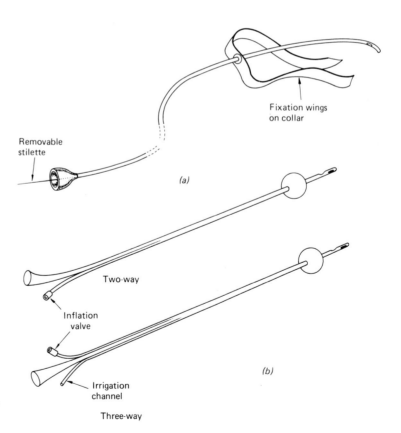

Figure 30.5. Types of catheters. (*a*) Gibbon catheter; (*b*) two-way and three-way Foley catheters

Foley catheter The Foley catheter also is a useful and versatile catheter. Near its tip there is an inflatable balloon behind the catheter eyes. The inflated balloon holds the catheter in the bladder without any other need of fixation although it is wise to fix the connection tubing to stop tugging on the catheter. The balloon is inflated with sterile saline. For postoperative use the catheter can be fitted with an irrigating channel. The catheter can be obtained either in latex rubber or plastic (*Figure 30.5b*).

The care of patients with an indwelling catheter

After the catheter has been introduced, the urine sample obtained and the catheter connected to the sterile drainage system (*Figure 30.6*), care begins with fixing the connecting tubing so that it does not become kinked or tug on the catheter. Twice daily the meatus is cleaned with saline or an aqueous antiseptic (povidone-iodine). In females foam sponge pad soaked in povidone-iodine several times daily is kept between the labia. This is comfortable, reduces infection and prevents tugging. Prophylactic antibiotics must not be used as they increase the chance of infection and produce resistant organisms.

Any outlet from the drainage apparatus must be kept clean and not drag on the floor. The drainage system must be kept closed to the ward air and its sterility kept intact. When changing the bag, the connection tube is first clamped off, then the connection between the tube and bag is wiped with spirit and the full bag removed, a fresh bag being immediately placed in such a way that the connections remain sterile. Finally, the clamp is removed from the drainage tube. By this technique infected air or urine from the bag does not enter the bladder.

If the urine collection apparatus is of better design so that the bag can be emptied, the emptying valve is opened after it has been cleansed in spirit. If a bung is used, it must not be placed on the floor but put in a gallipot of iodine or spirit while the bag is being emptied.

If it is essential to obtain a urine sample, needle aspiration of a rubber ensheathed drainage tube near the patient or from the catheter, if of rubber, is the only reliable method. Note that bag samples of urine for bacteriological examination are valueless. Urine should be cultured when the catheter is first introduced and the day after catheterization is discontinued.

Immediately before removal of the catheter, 50 ml of 1/5000 pure chlorhexidine (Hibitane) are instilled into the bladder and left *in situ* for the patient to void later. The fixation of the catheter is undone or the Foley balloon deflated and the catheter gently removed.

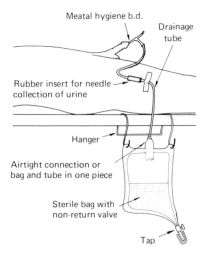

Meatal hygiene b.d.

Drainage tube

Rubber insert for needle collection of urine

Hanger

Airtight connection or bag and tube in one piece

Sterile bag with non-return valve

Tap

Figure 30.6. Closed drainage system. If the bag at the airtight connection needs changing, the tube is clamped off and joint wiped with spirit. Tap is emptied, cover on spout is replaced. Drainage tube is strapped to leg to avoid tugging. The tap is kept covered when not in use

Urethral stricture

A urethral stricture may follow infection or injury or the misuse of an indwelling catheter (that is, too large and left in for too long); it occurs behind the meatus. The treatment and prevention of postmeatal stricture have been discussed earlier. Strictures take many years to develop and cause obstruction and infection. Initial management is to determine the cause, site and size of the stricture. Urethrography is most helpful. Initially the stricture will need a frequent dilatation but if the response to treatment is satisfactory, the period between each bougienage will increase. Sometimes the bougies will not enter the bladder or may penetrate the wall of the urethra (false passage). If a stricture is impassible, a suprapubic cystostomy should be performed and the patient referred for urethroplasty.

Gram-negative septicaemia may follow urethral dilation. Some strictures are vascular and pathogens from the urethra are easily introduced into the bloodstream after dilatation, inducing a rigor in the patient. The use of urethral antiseptic jelly and systemic antibiotics makes urethral dilatation safe. Urethral antisepsis must be used on every patient needing an insertion of a bougie or catheter.

At one time it was thought that life-long dilatation was needed in the treatment of stricture. This is no longer the case and the stricture may be removed and the urethra reconstructed. The principle upon which these repairs work is that a strip of skin or mucosa will tend to form a tube.

Most of these operations are done in two stages. In the first stage the stricture is removed and the inflammatory reaction is allowed to settle. In the second stage several months later the urethra is reconstructed. Between the stages the patient voids through a perineal urethrostomy.

Bladder irrigation and bladder wash-outs

In patients with severe infections with purulent urine or in postoperative cases where bleeding is anticipated, bladder irrigation is used. An irrigating catheter (Gow–Gibbon or 'three-way' Foley) is used. In infected cases a 1/5000 chlorhexidine (Hibitane) solution is run into the bladder slowly, about 1 litre in 8 hours. Note that whenever Hibitane is used in the urinary tract it must be in its pure form as an aqueous solution. Ward stock solutions of Hibitane must never be used as they contain a wetting additive to help in cleansing; if used in error, the solution will cause pain and delay or prevent healing.

Clot retention is a serious complication of any operation on the urinary tract. The bladder fills with blood clot and urine and the draining urethral catheter will not work if it is blocked by clot. The patient becomes restless and has all the signs of internal bleeding (rising pulse, falling blood pressure and pallor); later there is severe abdominal pain and a visible mass, the distended bladder. After any bladder operation a regular check must be made by the nurse to see that the urine flow is satisfactory. It can be helped by squeezing the drainage tube at intervals and increasing the rate of bladder irrigation if the urine is thickly blood-stained. Milking the blood clot along the tubing should always be tried before carrying out bladder wash-out. Whenever a bladder wash-out is done the sterility of the drainage system is broken. Therefore every bladder wash-out must be performed with due aseptic precautions. If repeated suction does not free the clot, 50 ml of saline or citrate solution are gently injected along the catheter to free the clot and repeated suction applied. When it is clear a final wash-out is given and a sterile drainage system reconnected, using a fresh one if needed. Bladder wash-outs must only be done by experienced staff.

Examination of the bladder and urethra

Panendoscopy and cystoscopy

Panendoscopy and cystoscopy should be performed under a general anaesthetic. In women and in ill patients the examination may be performed using a local urethral antiseptic (*see* catheterization) and sedation. Whenever bladder tumour is suspected, i.e. with patients with haematuria at a check cystoscopy, a general anaesthetic must be given. Patients need to be reassured that cystoscopy is a minor procedure.

As with catheterization so also with urethral instrumentation, after preparing the skin of the genitalia and lower abdomen with antiseptic, a urethral antiseptic/anaesthetic jelly is introduced into the urethra and 3 to 5 minutes allowed to pass before any instrument is inserted. If the patient has an infection proven by urine culture or is known to have had rigors indicating a Gram-negative septicaemia after previous instrumentation, antibiotic cover must be given. The intramuscular dose of antibiotic is conveniently given at the time of premedication.

The instrument is assembled, the lighting system and moving parts tested and the instrument with its attached obdurator (which prevents urethral damage) passed gently so that it glides into the bladder. The best fluid for filling the bladder is 1 per cent glycine but sterile water may also be used. Saline or any other electrolyte solution cannot be used if any diathermy apparatus is needed. Whatever type of fluid is used it is run into the bladder from a sterile apparatus, its flow being controlled by a tap on the endoscope. The height of the fluid reservoir must not exceed 100 cm for fear of bursting the bladder, nor must the bladder be filled beyond its capacity. Finally, under the anaesthetic a bimanual examination of the pelvic organs is performed.

Stones and foreign bodies in the bladder or urethra

Bladder stones are related to infection in a residual urine. In children they may be related to malnutrition, especially to vitamin A deficiency. In adults stones in the bladder develop after prolonged catheterization for several months and where the nursing standards of catheter care are poor. They are preventable by good nursing and a high fluid intake (3 litres daily). Thus, patients immobilized for long periods, e.g. paraplegics and patients with severe head injuries, must have a high fluid intake to prevent stone formation. Small and soft stones can be crushed by a **lithotrite** passed down the urethra to the distended bladder. Large and hard stones need removal by a suprapubic cystostomy. In each case any stenosis of the bladder outlet must be dealt with.

Foreign bodies in the bladder are inserted by the psychopathic patient for erotic reasons; rarely they are accidental as, for example, women inserting a thermometer into the bladder instead of recording the vaginal temperature to determine the date of ovulation. The same principles apply to urethral foreign bodies; if the object can be removed with a panendoscope, this is preferable to open operation.

Rupture of the urethra

Intrapelvic rupture of the membranous urethra occurs after major injuries, for example, fractured pelvis. The bladder and prostate are torn off the pelvic floor, urine may leak into either the peritoneum or soft tissues. Suprapubic drainage, administration of antibiotics and repair by suture of the urethra are needed. An ascending cystourethrogram will reveal the site of injury. An indwelling catheter will act as a splint. It must be small and not put on heavy traction. Impotence is common after this injury.

Rupture of the penile bulbar urethra is a result of direct trauma; there is often urethral bleeding and marked bruising of the perineum. Again ascending urethrography confirms the diagnosis. Under anaesthesia a urethral catheter is introduced into the bladder. If it passes freely, it is left indwelling for several days. If it will not enter the bladder, suprapubic drainage is performed and the haematoma drained.

Lithotrite An instrument (shaped like jaws on the end of a cystoscope) for crushing stones in the bladder.

Both forms of urethral injury may develop a stricture (scarring) at the site of injury. This urethral narrowing may take years to develop.

BLADDER NECK OBSTRUCTION

The causes of bladder neck obstruction are:

(1) benign hypertrophy of the prostate in men;
(2) chronic urethritis in women — usually postmenopausal (senile stenosing urethritis);
(3) acute inflammations of the prostate and urethra;
(4) fibromuscular disease of the bladder neck (Marion's disease);
(5) cancer of the prostate.

Benign prostatic hypertrophy

The prostate gland develops at puberty and gradually enlarges with advancing years. The size of the gland is of no importance as huge glands may give rise to no symptoms at all. The important factor is the compression of the urethra which produces obstruction; sometimes even very small glands can produce obstruction to the urinary outflow. As acute retention is often found during other illnesses which force the elderly to retire to bed, for example, bronchitis, the mortality of prostatectomy and its complications is three times as high in patients with acute retention. The symptoms of any bladder neck obstruction are urgency and frequency of voiding due to the bladder neck disease and residual urine. At first the stream is poor; the patient has to wait until sufficient pressure has been built up in the bladder to overcome the obstruction (hesitancy). The flow of urine may then be good but later poor in force with an after-dribble. Cystitis may occur and the congested gland may bleed. The general condition of the patient will decline with advancing renal failure. Therefore, prostatectomy is advised before retention and decompensation of the bladder develop. Before operation the patient's general condition is assessed; if retention occurs, the bladder is drained with due sterile precautions. The exception is in patients with chronic retention and overflow with sterile urine and a blood urea level below 25 mmol per litre; here it is safer to avoid infection by not draining the bladder. Sudden decompression (i.e. complete emptying) of a chronically distended bladder may cause renal and bladder bleeding; rarely, it is fatal. Slow emptying in retention is advised. There is no place for emergency prostatectomy, as the mortality is high. Before

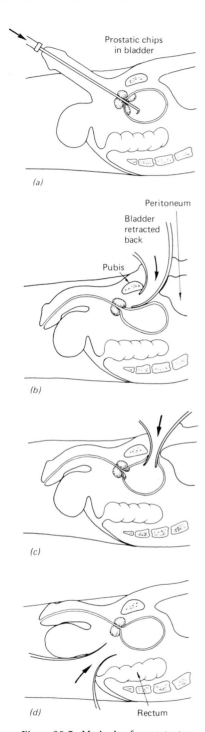

(a)

Prostatic chips
in bladder

(b)

Peritoneum

Bladder
retracted
back

Pubis

(c)

(d)

Rectum

Figure 30.7. Methods of prostatectomy.
(a) Transurethral resection (TUR);
(b) retropubic Millin's prostatectomy;
(c) transvesical prostatectomy (Wilson—
Hey); (d) perineal prostatectomy

operation a pyelogram, blood urea, haemoglobin and urine culture must be done. The type of prostatectomy chosen (*Figure 30.7*) depends on the size of the gland and the calibre of the urethra. However, few general surgeons have the training to carry out endoscopic resections.

Prostatectomy

Transurethral resection of the prostate Transurethral resection of the prostate is the safest operation but it requires much experience to do it well. The whole gland is removed by an instrument passed along the urethra. If the gland is very big or the urethra narrowed, for example by stricture, or if the surgeon is not trained in the technique, this method of prostatectomy is unsuitable and an alternative operation must be chosen.

Retropubic prostatectomy (Millin's operation) After the patient is anaesthetized, cystoscopy is performed to detect any bladder abnormality which may make this operation impracticable. The operative incision is usually a Pfannensteil's incision in the lower abdomen. This exposes the previously emptied bladder which is retracted upwards to expose the prostatic capsule. Stay sutures are placed in the capsule which is incised to reveal the gland. The prostate gland is removed under direct vision, its junction with the distal urethra divided with scissors and the gland turned upwards and lifted out of its bed.

Transvesical prostatectomy Through a similar operative incision in the abdomen, the bladder, which has been distended following previous cystoscopy, is exposed. Note that preliminary cystoscopy is necessary even though the intent is to open the bladder later. If a tumour, undetected by pyelography, is found, it could influence the course of treatment. If it was situated on the anterior wall and cystoscopy omitted and the incision was made through the tumour, the outlook will be bad. Previously unsuspected bladder growths are found in 2 per cent of men at cystoscopy before prostatectomy. The exposed bladder is held in stay sutures, the bladder opened and the prostate removed. The prostate is dissected out, usually with a diathermy needle, the distal apex of the gland is cut off from the urethra and the gland removed. Bleeding vessels are either cauterized by diathermy or under-run with sutures. No foreign bodies to cause stone or infection (that is, packs or absorbable sponges) are left in the prostatic cavity at the end of the operation. A catheter is introduced along the urethra, the operator's gloves changed and the incisions closed. A bladder wash-out is performed and the drainage system connected.

Perineal prostatectomy   In perineal prostatectomy the patient is placed in the lithotomy position and an incision made in the perineum between the urethra and rectum. This operation runs the risk of causing incontinence and impotence and is generally reserved for patients with prostatic cancer. It is more popular in the United States of America than in Great Britain.

Nursing care

The dangers of prostatectomy result from bleeding and infection. Even temporary blockage of a catheter with clot retention will be harmful. Therefore, nurses should make sure that the urine drains freely as well as note the pulse and blood pressure. Postoperative infection may be due to tampering with the closed drainage system; the correct method of care has already been described. Haemorrhage during surgery and in the postoperative period may be dramatically reduced with ϵ-aminocaproic acid (EACA — Epsikapron). It is given orally, 3 g thrice a day for 2 days before operation and intravenously afterwards. Bladder irrigation or, as the author prefers, a diuretic regimen using mannitol and frusemide (Lasix), prevents clot retention. The catheter is removed as soon as the urine is clear — on the third day for transurethral resection, on the fifth day after other operations.

The dangers of operation are trebled in patients with acute retention and the mortality is increased in frail and elderly patients. However, previous strokes or coronary thromboses or old age (i.e. over 80 years) are in themselves no contra-indication to operation.

Chronic urethritis, senile stenosing urethritis and acute prostatitis

The above conditions may produce retention and after catheterization the patient's symptoms will be relieved. Occasionally urethral dilatation does not relieve symptoms and resection may be needed.

Fibromuscular disease of the bladder neck

Fibromuscular disease of the bladder neck (Marion's disease) occurs in young men well below the age of benign hypertrophy. The symptoms are similar but on rectal examination the gland is not enlarged leading to the description of the disease as *prostatism sans prostate*. The treatment is by resection of the bladder neck tissue.

Cancer of the prostate

Cancer of the prostate is commoner in the elderly. The presentation may resemble that of benign prostatic obstruction, or bone pains and anaemia resulting from bone metastases, or the growth may be silent and account for malaise and weight loss — 'occult' carcinoma. On rectal examination the gland is irregular and hard. Prostatic stones or certain rare allergic conditions of the gland may feel the same on rectal examination so treatment for prostatic cancer must not be started without histological proof of the diagnosis of malignant disease. The bone deposits are very dense (osteosclerotic) and produce a raised enzyme level in the blood, the serum acid phosphatase. The serum acid phosphatase will be raised after rectal examination or in retention and therefore blood must not be collected for its estimation after a rectal examination. Proof of the diagnosis of prostatic malignancy may be made by needle biopsy of the prostate (or bone marrow if widespread deposits are present), by radiographs of the pelvis and lumbar spine to show metastases and by a very high serum acid phosphatase content. Most cancers of the prostate regress if female hormones (oestrogens) are given. They are fat-soluble so liquid paraffin must not be given if the patient is constipated. Oestrogens cause breast enlargement, impotence and skin pigmentation of the nipples and genitalia and prevent the testes from forming male hormones. Hence the importance of precision in the diagnosis before treatment. However, a transurethral resection will remove the obstructing tissue and provide material for a histological diagnosis. Sometimes patients with prostatic cancer have a tendency to bleeding. If painful bone metastases are present, castration (bilateral orchidectomy) will relieve symptoms; less commonly adrenalectomy or yttrium radioactive implants will be inserted into the pituitary to destroy androgenic tissue. The hormone therapy will need to be continued for life; doubling the dosage of oestrogens does not improve its effect but increases the dangers of the side-effects (salt retention, cardiovascular disturbances and so on). If there is a failure to respond to oestrogen therapy alone, the methods outlined above should be tried.

BLADDER CANCER

All bladder tumours are malignant. The term 'papilloma' is outdated but the word is still used for industrial tumours as it is written into the Industrial Injuries Act as 'prescribed disease No. 39 — papilloma of the bladder'. Workers at risk are those in the rubber industry and certain chemical industries. The carcinogenic chemical was barred in 1949 but there is a delay of many years from exposure to tumour development. Cigarette smoking causes bladder cancer and recurrent tumours form more often in cigarette smokers. Staff must advise patients to stop smoking. Cancer of the bladder, renal pelvis and ureter is due to a disorder of the lining of the urinary tract, the urothelium, and therefore the disease is multicentric and tumours can arise at different sites. The bladder growths may be of low-grade malignancy or highly malignant. The more malignant tumours are solid and often appear calcified by the deposition of urinary salts on their surface. Treatment of the cancer depends on the staging of the tumour. Stage 0 is carcinoma *in situ*, whilst, at the other extreme, stage 4 has spread outside the bladder (*Figure 30.8*).

Haematuria, whether painless or not, is the characteristic symptom. Sometimes the patient presents with recurrent urinary infections or in tropical regions there is a history of schistosomiasis (bilharzia). Haematuria is a symptom that must always be taken seriously; it is never due to old age. *Every patient with painless haematuria is assumed to have malignant disease in the urinary tract until proved otherwise.*

The basic investigations include pyelography, urine cytology — which is not possible if the bleeding is obvious — and cystoscopy. Patients suspected of having malignancy must not be put on the waiting list for pyelography and cystoscopy, but must be admitted for investigation without delay. It has been shown that where there is a delay of more than 6 weeks from the onset of the first symptoms to the start of treatment, the chances of the average patient living for more than 3 years is halved. However, if the diagnosis and treatment are prompt patients can live a normal life with an expected 10-year cure rate of about 80 per cent.

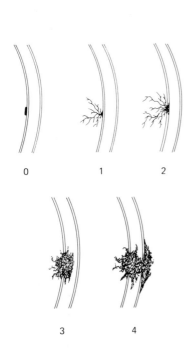

Figure 30.8. Staging of bladder cancer. Stage 0, carcinoma *in situ*; stage 1, only mucosa invaded; stage 2, mucosa breached and a little muscle invasion; stage 3, more than half of bladder muscle thickness invaded but no spread outside bladder; stage 4, whole thickness of bladder wall invaded with either pelvic spread or distant metastases

Treatment

Stages 0–2

In the first stages of the disease endoscopic treatment affords better results. The malignant cells may be found in the urine many months before the visible appearance of a tumour at cystoscopy. At the first cystoscopy biopsy, bimanual examination and measurement of the bladder capacity must be noted. The tumour may be cauterized by diathermy with an electrode or, better still, resected. Suprapubic removal of the bladder tumour is dangerous and rarely necessary; if tumour cells implant into the abdominal wall the patient will not live a year.

Stages 3—4

In later stages radiation therapy (local or external megavoltage) and radical cystectomy have good results. In carefully selected cases radical cystectomy combined with pelvic lymph node dissection and a urinary diversion offers an excellent hope of cure. Megavoltage therapy is not to be despised and many patients are symptom-free and tumour-free even after palliative courses of radiation. Occasionally after irradiation to the pelvic organs the patient will have a temporary bowel cramp and diarrhoea. Such a rectal reaction is treated by a bland low-residue diet and prednisone suppositories. Other methods of treatment include instillation of cytotoxic drugs into the bladder. Watch must be kept on the patient's blood count or absorption of cytotoxic drugs will produce a fall in the platelet and white cell count. The drug commonly used is 45 mg of thiotepa in 100 ml normal saline. Such treatment is only suitable for carcinoma *in situ* and multiple tumours no larger than a few millimetres in size. The hydrostatic pressure technique (Helmstein) is effective in advanced tumours associated with severe haemorrhage.

Schistosomiasis (Bilharzia)

This condition is found in Egypt, East Africa, around Lake Chad and in the Far East. It is caused by a parasite which burrows into the skin and migrates to the pelvic veins. It lays its eggs within the bladder or rectum. The body reacts by intense inflammation and multiple strictures of the ureters and a contracted bladder may result. The chronic irritation may form a squamous cell cancer of the bladder, a type of tumour that carries a poor prognosis.

Vesico-ureteric reflux

Vesico-ureteric reflux has been dealt with in Chapter 29.

URINARY DIVERSION

When there is an obstruction to the urinary tract with renal failure, free flow of urine must be established and a temporary diversion performed, further surgery being deferred until the patient is fit. Temporary diversion is sometimes used after various plastic procedures on the lower urinary tract. If the bladder is removed, diversion is needed. Rarely, urinary diversion is indicated if the patient is incontinent, for example spina bifida patients may need an ileal conduit. The various forms of diversion are illustrated in *Figure 30.9*.

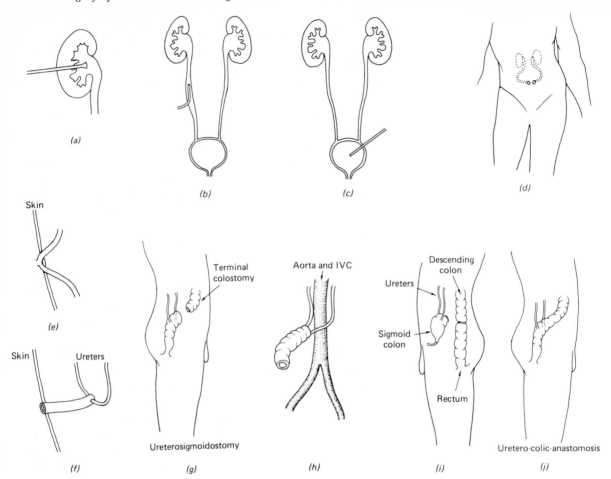

Figure 30.9. Methods of urinary diversion. (*a*) Nephrostomy; (*b*) ureterostomy; (*c*) cystostomy; (*d*) double-barrelled ureterostomy; (*e*) loop ureterostomy; (*f*) ileal conduit; (*g*) terminal colostomy and ureterosigmoidostomy; (*h*) Wallace ureteroileostomy — ureters joined together in midline and anastomosed to ileal loop behind peritoneum in front of great vessels; (*i*) colon joined to rectum, sigmoid colon isolated as ileal conduit

Different types of diversion

Nephrostomy

The track of the tube must lie in a direct line to the skin to ease changing of the tube at fortnightly intervals. For permanent use a Tressider U-tube nephrostomy is useful; the replacement tube is fitted onto one end of the U-tube which is withdrawn until the new tube is in a satisfactory position (*Figure 29.13e*). If the nephrostomy is temporary, radio-opaque dye may be injected down the urinary tract to confirm that there is no obstruction before removal. Changing of a nephrostomy tube must be done promptly; the new tube must be ready as the old one is being removed. Before discontinuing nephrostomy drainage, the tube is clamped off for 24 hours; if there is a fever or leakage of fluid in the loin, the patient is not ready to have the tube removed. After removal the hole will close very quickly.

Pyelostomy

Pyelostomy is only used as a temporary measure as tube changing is rarely possible. The tube passes directly from the renal pelvis to the skin. It is used after conservative renal surgery as a safety valve and is usually taken out after a week.

Ureterostomy

Ureterostomy is a useful diversion after pelvic surgery. The author uses a special tube for this purpose, an incision is made into the ureter which is left undisturbed. In the child ureterostomy is a useful means of diversion as the ureters are tortuous and dilated following congenital obstruction. They are mobilized as a temporary loop and brought to the skin surface or anastomosed together in the midline as a double-barrelled cutaneous ureterostomy (*see Figure 30.9*).

Ileal conduit

Ileal conduit is sometimes misnamed as ileal bladder; but the isolated segment of ileum does not act as a reservoir, it conducts the urine to the skin surface where it is collected in an appliance which is emptied periodically (*Figure 30.10*). The ileum can also be used to form a new ureter or enlarge the bladder. Appendicectomy is always performed after an ileal loop is formed. In theatre an ileostomy appliance may be fitted, its site having been determined by trying the appliance and skin marking beforehand. Better still is the transparent wound drainage bag (Down Bros) which can be glued directly onto the skin. It has a tap fitting on the lower end so that the ureteric splints can be coiled into the bag and the urine drained into the bladder drainage set without disturbing the patient.

The ileal conduit may reabsorb urine and produce biochemical imbalance or produce a tendency to uric acid stones. Once weekly the patient should dilate the stoma with a soapy little finger to prevent stenosis. Stoma disorders are very uncommon and usually result from a lack of proper care; sometimes the stoma may need surgery.

Patients with an ileal conduit may benefit from joining the local branch of the Urinary Conduit Association. Many urological units have a stoma therapist. The Institute of Urology, St. Peter's Hospitals, Shaftesbury Avenue, London WC2 will give postal advice about stomatal care.

Ureterocolostomy (ureterosigmoidostomy)

The ureters are transplanted into the pelvic colon by a valvular technique. The urine mingles with the faeces and is voided when the patient empties the bowels. As the function of the colon is to absorb water, salt from the urine is absorbed from

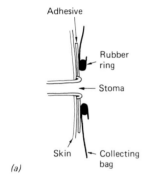

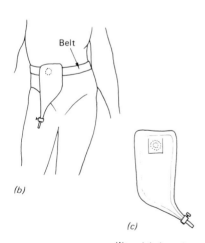

Figure 30.10. Ileostomy device and wound drainage bag. (*a*) Detail diagram of the stoma; (*b*) position of ileostomy device; (*c*) wound drainage bag

the colon and in many patients hyperchloraemic acidosis results. If a pyelogram is performed, the dye can be seen as far as the ileocaecal valve and sometimes the urine may be found in the terminal ileum. Urinary control after this form of diversion may be poor for a few weeks but may improve rapidly. Reflux of bowel content may occur and cause pyelonephritis. To reduce the bowel pressure and prevent reflux, the muscle of the bowel wall may be divided down to the mucosa (sigmoidmyotomy). When either pyelonephritis or hyperchloraemic acidosis occurs the patient will become drowsy but urinary drainage with a rectal tube will produce a rapid improvement. Patients with hyperchloraemic acidosis are drowsy and dry and need intravenous sodium lactate or bicarbonate to correct the biochemical disturbance. The biochemical abnormality may be prevented by proprietary mixtures such as Citralka liquid (sodium acid citrate) or sodium bicarbonate (1 teaspoonful baking soda twice a day). An isolated loop of pelvic colon may be used in a similar manner to an ileal conduit.

Suprapubic cystostomy

Suprapubic cystostomy is usually a temporary form of diversion; if permanent, the tube will need changing weekly. A solution of Renacidin may prevent phosphate encrustation if used as a bladder wash-out at the time of tube change.

URINARY INCONTINENCE

Patients are vague about urinary symptoms and may confuse urgency with incontinence. It is important to find out what type of incontinence affects the patient as this decides the course of treatment.

Incontinence is caused either by an overactive detrusor or sphincter weakness. The investigation of incontinence by urodynamics is discussed in the previous chapter.

Types of incontinence

Urge incontinence

The patient has an infection usually in the urethra which produces bladder irritation together with frequency of micturition and, if the patient is unable to reach the toilet in time, incontinence follows. In women this may be confused with stress incontinence and if a colporrhaphy is performed on patients with urge incontinence, their symptoms will be no better, in fact usually worse. Treatment as for urethritis in women with drugs to reduce bladder irritability (Tryptizol,

10 mg thrice a day or Pyridium, 1 tablet thrice a day) is effective.

Stress incontinence

When the intra-abdominal pressure is raised by coughing or lifting a heavy weight, there is a urinary leakage. Sometimes there is an associated urinary infection (urethritis). This condition is commoner in women who have borne children or after the menopause. In women there is a loss of the posterior vesico-urethral angle, widening of the internal urinary meatus and a foreshortening of the urethra with sagging of the pelvic floor. This can be demonstrated radiologically. Whatever type of operation is performed in women with stress incontinence the aim is to restore the vesico-urethral angle to normal and to elongate the urethra. Not all women with stress incontinence need surgery. Menopausal women benefit from synthetic oestrogens which are believed to act on the pelvic floor. Electrical stimulation of the pelvic floor muscles by a rectal plug or a vaginal pessary is of value and the device may prove unnecessary after several months' use as the urinary control returns to normal.

Complete incontinence

Complete incontinence means that the patient is always wet, day and night. An ectopic ureter or bladder injury must be considered and any defect repaired surgically. In men a condom appliance or catheter is used, but in women no satisfactory appliance has been devised. Avoidance of skin damage by the urine (pressure sores), pelvic floor exercises and surgery are the basis of treatment. The problems of the neurogenic bladder will be reviewed later. In men a penile clamp worn in the day is useful but the clamp must not be worn all the time. Rarely, urinary diversion is needed if other means of treatment fail.

Senile incontinence

For discussion of senile incontinence *see below*.

The neurogenic bladder

In the elderly, inhibition of the desire to void is imperfect and frequency and urge incontinence result, for example, in cerebral arteriosclerosis. Drugs with an atropine-like action (Tryptizol, imipramine) inhibit the bladder and improve control. Children suffer from enuresis which has the same basis, but children normally are continent by the age of 4 years. The true enuretic has day-time frequency and wets the bed at night and similar drug treatment will relieve symptoms.

Regular bladder emptying to avoid over-distension of the bladder is also valuable in dealing with geriatric patients. Diseases of the spinal cord, for example, multiple sclerosis, will affect bladder control. The most important factor is avoidance of bladder over-distension, particularly in the patient unconscious from strokes, head injuries, postoperative reaction etc. Bladder over-distension can damage the bladder and control of micturition may take months to return to normal. Therefore the nurse in geriatric wards or on intensive care units must palpate the abdomen to anticipate the possibility of a retention of urine. This must be promptly dealt with by catheterization with due sterile care. Any obstruction to the urinary outflow is dealt with by endoscopic surgery. Paraplegics need regular surveillance and are best looked after on a specialized unit. Patients with lower cord lesions are dealt with in a similar manner. Endoscopic division of the external sphincter and the use of non-irritant (Gibbon) small lumen catheters have revolutionized the care of the neurogenic bladder.

MALE GENITALIA

Hypospadias

Hypospadias is a congenital penile abnormality; the urethra fails to develop fully, the meatal opening being underneath the penis. Operation is best done before the child reaches school age. Boys with hypospadias must never be circumcised as the foreskin can be used to form the new urethra. The principles of repair are similar to the Swinney urethroplasty.

Circumcision

Medical indications for this ancient operation are few, for example, phimosis, balanitis and, rarely, tumour. Parents may demand circumcision of their children unnecessarily, and it must be remembered that the operation has a low but definite mortality. The operation is unnecessary if there are no religious or medical indications. The foreskin does not fully develop until after the first year of life. Boys, if uncircumcised, must be shown how to retract the foreskin when bathing to clean away the secretion (smegma) on the glans; the retracted foreskin must be replaced. Repeated attacks of infection may cause narrowing of the foreskin over the glans preventing retraction; sometimes a pin-hole opening will develop and the patient will be unable to void freely. This condition is called phimosis and, if long-standing, the glans underneath becomes infected and may become cancerous.

When the foreskin is retracted and a tight band is present preventing its replacement over the glans, the condition is called paraphimosis. In uncircumcised men the retracted foreskin after catheterization must always be replaced, otherwise a swelling of the foreskin will result. In the early stages paraphimosis can be reduced; if the infection and swelling are great, a dorsal slit of the prepuce is performed and circumcision effected when the infection has settled.

Cancer of the penis

Cancer of the penis is found in uncircumcised men whose standard of personal cleanliness is poor. Radical amputation is needed in most cases but small tumours can be treated by radiotherapy.

Diseases of the testes and scrotum

Undescended testes

The testes form in the abdominal cavity and migrate into the scrotum. In neonates, particularly if premature, the testes may not have descended. About 5 adult men per 1000 have an undescended testis. An undescended testis should be brought into the scrotum (orchiopexy) before the age of 12 years, otherwise the testes will be unable to produce sperm although the hormone production will be unaffected. Undescended testes are prone to torsion, injury or malignancy and should be treated surgically. Torsion of the testis is common in infants and adolescents. In case of doubt the scrotum should be explored and the testis fixed on each side as the condition is potentially bilateral; if epididymitis is present, the operation will do no harm.

Epididymitis

Epididymitis is a result of a prostatic and urethral infection, but if tuberculous in origin, it may be blood-borne. Tuberculosis must be excluded by examination of an early morning specimen of urine. Treatment of the painful swollen testis is by bed-rest until the fever has settled, copious intake of fluids, a scrotal support and antibiotics. The thickening of the epididymis may take months to disappear.

Varicocele

Varicocele is a condition which causes infertility by overheating the scrotum and preventing both testes from manufacturing sperm. A varicocele is varicosity of the veins to the testicle. Surgery will restore fertility in most men, but any testicular atrophy will not improve. The veins are ligated at the internal inguinal ring through a small inguinal incision; direct ligation through the scrotum risks damaging the testicular blood supply.

Hydrocele and epididymal cysts

Hydrocele and epididymal cysts (spermatocele) cause large scrotal swellings which may be mistaken for hernia. Although the fluid can be aspirated by tapping, the modern radical operation (Lord's operation) will cure the condition without unsightly and uncomfortable scrotal swelling. Older operations (excision of the hydrocele or turning it inside out) are not as satisfactory and often produce a scrotal haematoma.

Scrotal haematoma

Scrotal haematoma is uncomfortable but usually settles with bed-rest and elevation of the scrotum between the thighs. Drainage of the haematoma is not advisable. Injury to the scrotum or penile skin is uncommon; such lesions heal quickly and skin grafting is rarely needed.

Tumours of the testes

Tumours of the testes (seminoma, teratoma) are all malignant. Biopsy of the testis must never be done, the spermatic cord should be clamped off, the testis delivered into the inguinal incision and removed if it is abnormal. Any scrotal incision will fungate. Metastases may be treated by chemotherapy and radiotherapy.

REFERENCES

Jameson, R. M., Burrows, K. and Large, B. (1976). *Management of the Urological Patient.* Edinburgh and London: Churchill Livingstone

Spraggon, E. M. (1975). *Urinary Diversion Stomas.* Edinburgh and London: Churchill Livingstone

Blandy, J. P. (1976). *Lecture Notes on Urology.* Oxford: Blackwell

31

Surgery of the arteries

Averil O. Mansfield

The arterial system plays a vital role in supplying essential nutrients to the tissues. When the arteries are interrupted by either disease or injury, ischaemia of the organ or limbs supplied may occur and, if unrelieved, death of the tissues results.

When there is acute interruption of flow as, for example, in accidental division of a vessel, or blockage by an embolus, the effect is usually severe. When the onset is gradual, there is time for the development of a collateral circulation and the effect may be less marked.

ANATOMY

The left ventricle of the heart pumps blood into the aorta, and from the aorta all the major organs and limbs are supplied. The first branch of the aorta is the innominate artery or brachiocephalic artery, which divides to form the right carotid artery and the right subclavian artery, and subsequently supplies the head and neck and the arms. The next branch of the aorta is the left common carotid artery and then the left subclavian artery. These are all branches from the arch of the aorta itself. The arteries of the head and neck are principally the common carotid artery which divides into the internal carotid artery to supply the brain and the external carotid artery which supplies the superficial structures of the face and neck.

The subclavian artery goes on to supply the arm and becomes, in turn, the axillary and brachial arteries. In the arm, the peripheral pulses which are palpable at the wrist, are the radial and the ulnar arteries which are the terminal branches of the brachial artery.

Smaller branches are given off as the aorta passes down the posterior wall of the chest. The next major branches are in the abdomen below the diaphragm. These can be divided into single and paired branches. The most important paired arteries are the renal arteries coming off, one from each side of the aorta, to supply the kidneys. The first single branch is the coeliac axis which divides almost immediately after its commencement into the left gastric artery, the splenic artery and the hepatic artery. The next single branch from the anterior surface of the aorta is the superior mesenteric artery which supplies most of the small bowel, and below that, the inferior mesenteric artery, which supplies most of the large bowel. There are several small branches coming from the aorta during its passage through the abdomen.

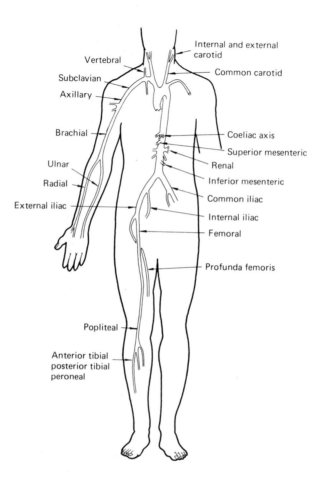

Figure 31.1. Diagram illustrating the anatomy of arteries

The aorta finally divides into the right and left common iliac arteries, and these ultimately pass behind the inguinal ligament to become the femoral artery in the leg. During the course of the iliac artery through the pelvis, it gives off a major branch, the internal iliac artery, and the parent trunk from then on is known as the external iliac artery.

In the legs, below the inguinal ligament, the common femoral artery gives off a major branch, known as the profunda femoris artery, and the parent trunk continues as the superficial femoral artery. These two divisions are frequently of almost equal calibre. The superficial femoral artery continues down the leg through the adductor canal and enters the popliteal fossa to become the popliteal artery. It terminates by dividing into three branches.

Two of these terminal branches can be palpated in the foot and are commonly sought during examination of the peripheral vascular system. They are the dorsalis pedis artery on the dorsum of the foot, and the posterior tibial artery, behind the medial malleolus at the ankle (*see Figure 31.3*).

The distributing arteries break up into arterioles and then into capillaries.

The wall of an artery has three layers. The intima lines the lumen and is in contact with the blood. The media is the next layer and contains muscle and elastic tissue. The outer layer is the adventitia.

PATHOLOGY

Arteriosclerosis

The commonest name applied to degenerative diseases of arteries is arteriosclerosis or hardening of the arteries. It is a broad term which covers several types of change. In the large arteries the main features are:

(1) fatty streaks — these may be seen in quite young subjects;
(2) plaques of a waxy consistency containing a porridge-like material (atheroma);
(3) ulcers which are the further development of the above;
(4) thrombosis — clots are often found on the irregular wall of the vessel; and
(5) calcification — calcium is deposited in the vessel wall which then becomes hard and brittle.

Many of the features are due to the deposition of fats including cholesterol in the wall of the vessel. In small vessels a relatively small plaque can markedly narrow the lumen and in a short time may block the vessel completely. The coronary arteries are examples of such small vessels and they may become blocked as the result of arteriosclerosis. As the coronary arteries supply the muscle of the wall of the heart itself, the effect of blockage can be serious or even fatal.

When an artery becomes narrowed or blocked by disease, the effect is seen in the part supplied by that vessel. For example, if it is the heart muscle or myocardium, then infarction (death) of part of the muscle occurs and the patient experiences a heart attack (that is, coronary thrombosis, myocardial infarction); if it is the brain that is affected, then a stroke results, and if it is a hand or foot, then gangrene may be seen.

The following factors may be involved in the development of arterial disease of this type:

(1) raised blood pressure;
(2) raised serum cholesterol and other lipids; and
(3) tobacco smoking.

Aneurysm

Aneurysm is a localized ballooning of the wall of the artery when the wall of the vessel has been weakened by disease. Arteriosclerosis is the commonest cause now, although, formerly, syphilis was frequently responsible.

The commonest site for an aneurysm formation due to arteriosclerosis is the abdominal aorta. It usually arises below the origin of the renal arteries. As the aneurysm enlarges, the wall becomes thinner and there is an increased danger of rupture.

Dissecting aneurysm

The diseased wall of the artery involved becomes split and this allows blood to flow within the wall of the vessel in addition to within the lumen. As a result the split tends to be extended and may pass from the heart to the lower part of the abdominal aorta and even into the iliac arteries. The branches of the vessel so involved are depleted of blood and the blood supply to the brain or kidneys may be cut off (*Figure 31.2*).

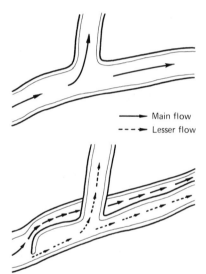

Main flow
Lesser flow

Figure 31.2. Dissecting aneurysm. As the wall of the main vessel splits, the bloodflow in the subsidiary vessel is diminished

Arteriovenous fistula

The arteriovenous fistula is an abnormal connection between an artery and a vein, and may be a congenital abnormality. It may also be formed as a result of an injury, or may be created surgically as part of the management of renal failure (Cimino—Brescia fistula) for haemodialysis.

Buerger's disease

Buerger's disease is an inflammatory change in the vessel wall, as a result of which the vessel becomes thickened and may be occluded. It occurs predominantly in young male tobacco smokers, although these are not the only sufferers. It affects the peripheral vessels mainly and may result in gangrene of fingers or toes.

Arteritis

Arteritis is an inflammation of the wall of a vessel and may result from several causes including the following.

(1) Infections:
(a) pyogenic, local or carried from a distance;
(b) syphilitic, most commonly affecting the cerebral vessels and the aorta;
(c) tuberculous.
(2) Non-specific causes:
(a) disseminated lupus erythematosus affecting the small vessels of young women;
(b) polyarteritis nodosa which may present with widespread and variable symptoms;
(c) rheumatoid disease;
(d) temporal (giant-cell) arteritis affecting older age group. Vessels in the head and neck are mainly affected, with a high risk of blindness;
(e) pulseless (Takayasu's) disease affecting young women especially from the Far East; there is absence of some pulses in the upper body and evidence of deficiency of blood supply to the head or arms.

Thromboembolism

At the site of arteriosclerotic disease, a thrombus may form on the artery wall and in time may enlarge sufficiently to occlude the lumen. This clot will usually spread along the artery to its next major branch.

When an arterial thrombus becomes detached, it is then called an embolus. This embolus will in turn lodge in a smaller vessel and may block it.

In addition to emboli which arise from diseased arteries, there are a far larger group of emboli which arise from the heart. These arise from either a diseased valve or from the thrombus which may form on the ischaemic heart muscle after a myocardial infarction. Many of these patients show a disorder of heart rhythm known as **atrial fibrillation**.

CLINICAL PICTURE OF ARTERIAL DISEASE

Symptoms

Exercise pain or claudication

Exercise pain is the most important symptom in arterial disease. During the exercise of a limb, a rapid increase in its blood supply normally occurs. When there is narrowing or

Atrial fibrillation A quivering uncoordinated movement of the atrium of the heart. This gives an irregular pulse and a characteristic electrocardiograph pattern.

obstruction of vessels, this increase in blood supply cannot occur and pain results. When pain occurs in the calf muscles during exercise it is known as intermittent claudication. It is intermittent because it causes the patient to rest and the pain is thereby relieved. He is then able to walk a similar distance again before pain recurs. The patient often comments that the pain begins after a shorter distance when he is walking uphill or hurrying.

Although exercise pain is most common in the calf it also occurs in the thighs and buttocks when the iliac arteries are involved, and in the arm when the subclavian artery is involved.

Rest pain
When the blood supply to a limb becomes severely limited, the normal metabolism of the tissues is interfered with and pain at rest ensues. The pain is most troublesome at night and disturbs the patient's sleep. In order to minimize the pain the patient frequently hangs the affected limb out of bed.

Temperature change
The patient may complain that the involved extremity is cold and this is particularly troublesome during the winter months. In diseases affecting the hands this may be a particularly incapacitating symptom and is often followed by pain.

Colour change
The extremity may appear white or blue and the patient may be concerned by this. Rubor (red-purple discolouration) is also a feature of arterial insufficiency. It is only in the very late stages that a black colour appears which signifies the occurrence of gangrene.

Sensory changes
Numbness of the foot may be a symptom of arterial insufficiency. Other causes of numbness have first to be excluded, in particular, diabetes.

Cerebral symptoms
There is a wide variety of cerebral symptoms in relation to diseases of the arteries which supply the brain. They range from attacks of unconsciousness and blindness to headache and dizziness.

Impotence
Impotence is an occasional symptom when there is a block at the bifurcation of the aorta.

Signs

The following signs of arterial disease can be observed.

(1) Pallor — this is particularly evident on elevation of the limb.

(2) Cold — the feet or hands feel cold on palpation by comparison with the rest of the patient's skin.

(3) Wasting of muscles is often seen in the area supplied by the blocked artery.

(4) Absence of pulses — palpation of the pulses is the most important single examination. When an artery is blocked it is unlikely that the pulses will be palpable below the block (unless there is an exceptionally good collateral circulation) and so it is usually possible to localize the block fairly accurately by examination of the pulses. In the leg the main arterial pulses which can normally be palpated are the femoral pulse in the groin, the popliteal pulse behind the knee, the dorsalis pedis on the dorsum of the foot, and the posterior tibial pulse behind the medial malleolus. There are of course long gaps between these pulses and it is only possible to state that the block is below the lowest pulse which can be felt.

(5) Bruit — when there is a localized area of narrowing in an artery there is a change in the blood flow at that point, and the resulting turbulence can be heard by a stethoscope applied to the area. It may also be possible to palpate a thrill in the vessel.

(6) Gangrene may occasionally be present when the patient is seen for the first time although patients usually seek advice earlier than after death of tissues has already occurred.

Clinical examination

Arterial disease may manifest itself in one vessel but it must always be remembered that it is frequently a generalized disease and each patient will require a full examination of the cardiovascular system.

In addition, there is one disease above all others which may present itself as arterial disease. This disease is diabetes mellitus and it is therefore of the utmost importance to test the urine.

In each case the patient has to undergo:

(1) general examination;

(2) heart and chest examination — full clinical examination and auscultation, chest radiograph, electrocardiograph, and measurement of blood pressure;

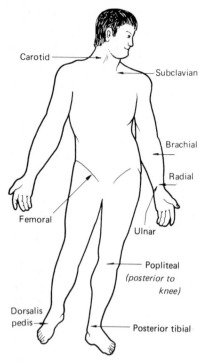

Figure 31.3. Sites of arterial pulses

(3) abdominal palpation;

(4) examination of all accessible major arteries (*Figure 31.3*) by palpation and auscultation (that is, carotid, subclavian, brachial, radial and ulnar, abdominal aorta, femoral, popliteal, posterior tibial, and dorsalis pedis);

(5) special examination of the affected area;

(6) urine examination; and

(7) haemoglobin and haematocrit and other appropriate haematological investigations. It may be appropriate also to measure the cholesterol and other blood lipids.

Special investigations

Arteriography

The most important special investigation which is frequently required in the examination of patients with arterial disease is arteriography. In brief, this consists of the injection of a radio-opaque fluid into the vessel to be examined so that it can be visualized on a series of radiographs of the vessel. The films are taken in quick succession over a short period of time because the flow rate in arteries is so rapid. Two methods of injection can be used.

(1) Direct needle puncture and injection either by hand or with the aid of a pressure injector. This method is mainly employed for femoral, carotid and aortic injections (*Figure 31.4*).

(2) Injection via the Seldinger catheter (needle is inserted into an artery, for example the femoral artery, guide wire passed through the needle and sited in the desired area, catheter threaded over the guide wire and the guide wire withdrawn and radio-opaque material is then injected through the catheter into the blood vessel at the selected site).

When required the tip of the catheter can be manoeuvred into the orifice of a branch of the aorta and a special radiograph of that branch taken, for example renal or superior mesenteric arteries. More commonly the vessels below the catheter tip in the aorta are serially visualized, i.e. iliac, femoral, popliteal arteries, and so on.

Arteriographic findings

Normal vessels are fairly straight tubes. When they are diseased they become tortuous and narrowed. Sometimes, however, the diseased vessel becomes widened and forms an aneurysm.

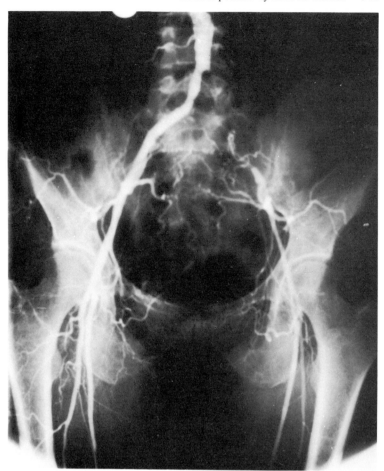

Figure 31.4. Translumbar aortogram showing disease of the aorta and occlusion of the left common iliac artery

The most important abnormality is the occurrence of a complete block in the artery. The length of the block is extremely variable. A number of small vessels will sometimes be seen around the block in the main vessel. These are the collateral vessels which allow a certain amount of blood to get into the area previously supplied by the blocked vessel.

In assessing the arteriogram in respect to possible operative correction, it is important to look at the vessels beyond the block. If these are very narrow and distorted, then removal or by-pass of the block may produce little benefit, or the benefit may be short-lived.

Common sites of narrowing in arteries are at the division or branching of the vessel. In addition, in the leg, the artery is commonly obstructed where it passes through a fibrous tunnel known as the adductor canal (in mid-thigh).

MANAGEMENT

Non-surgical management

The patient is instructed in the care of the ischaemic limb, i.e. prevention of injury, professional chiropody, suitable clothing in winter and so on. Exercise within the limits of pain is encouraged and the patient is advised to stop smoking. Various drugs can be administered, such as vasodilators which are of limited value, although alcohol may be helpful, or drugs to alter blood lipids (their value in established disease is not yet known), and so on. Anticoagulants are sometimes employed to prevent extension of thrombosis, but are more commonly prescribed after surgery. Streptokinase may be used to lyse recent thrombi (*see* Chapter 32).

Surgical management

There are certain features which are common to many arterial operations and these will be dealt with first.

Arteriotomy

Arteriotomy is an opening made into the lumen of an artery. It may be either longitudinal or transverse.

Patch

In order to widen the lumen of an artery an oval patch can be sutured into the artery at the site of the arteriotomy. The patch is usually constructed from a small superficial vein, or a piece of Dacron.

Endarterectomy

In mechanical terms thromboendarterectomy (disobliteration) is the equivalent of the rebore. The narrowed or blocked artery is cored out so that it is once again wide and patent. Part of the wall of the artery is removed along with the plaques of atheroma. The vessel left behind is thin and pliable.

The advantages of this operation are that the patient's own vessels are still used and branches of the vessel may continue to receive a blood supply. The operation may, however, be a very lengthy one. Sometimes the inner wall of the artery is left slightly irregular which results in a tendency to clot formation in narrow vessels.

Various methods of performing an endarterectomy are as follows.

(1) The vessel is opened in the area of the disease and the plaques are removed under direct vision.

(2) The vessel is opened at intervals and the plaques are removed with the aid of a stripper. This is a metal instrument which can be passed up and down the vessel. It often has a sharp ring-shaped end which cores out the vessel as it progresses.

(3) The outer layer of the vessel is punctured with a fine needle and a jet of gas (CO_2) is allowed to enter and this splits the plaque off from the normal outer layers. Following this, longer instruments are passed up the vessel and a jet of gas is emitted from the end, thus extending the separation of the plaque from the vessel wall. The plaque can then be removed and the remaining vessel is usually quite smooth on its inner aspect.

Graft

When it is necessary to by-pass a blocked vessel or to replace an aneurysm, a graft must be employed. Two types of graft are in common use at the present time: a vein obtained from the patient (usually the long saphenous vein), or a Dacron graft (woven or knitted). Other materials may occasionally be used and these include bovine carotid artery, umbilical vein and Gortex.

SPECIFIC DISEASES OF ARTERIES AND THEIR SURGICAL CORRECTION

Embolus

Embolus is the commonest arterial emergency. A clot of blood from the heart, or occasionally the large vessels, becomes loose in the circulation. Its progress is arrested when it reaches a vessel that is too small for it to pass through.

When a large clot lodges at the bifurcation of the aorta (in the lower part of the abdomen) this is known as a saddle embolus because it sits astride the bifurcation.

Wherever the embolus is arrested, there will be either complete or partial obstruction of the blood supply to the area. With a saddle embolus, both legs are affected. At first the patient experiences pain in the limb, the foot becomes blue and, with the passage of time, movement and sensation are both diminished. Eventually part of the limb will die unless an operation is undertaken to remove the clot.

Operation is a matter of urgency, because the longer the delay the greater the possibility of permanent damage. It is frequently carried out under local anaesthetic.

Operation

The affected artery is exposed or, in the case of a saddle embolus (*Figure 31.5*), both femoral arteries are exposed.

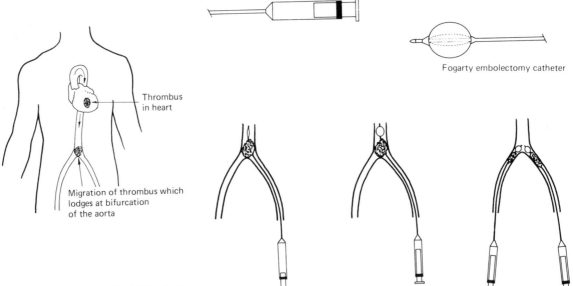

Fogarty embolectomy catheter

Stages in removal of a 'saddle' embolus

Figure 31.5. Diagram of 'saddle' embolus and its removal using a Fogarty catheter

The vessel is controlled with tapes and an arteriotomy is made.

A Fogarty catheter which is a long, fine tube, with an inflatable balloon at the end, is passed along the artery to beyond the limit of the clot. The balloon is then inflated and the catheter is withdrawn bringing the embolus with it. This is repeated both up and down the artery until no further clot can be obtained. The arteriotomy is repaired and the wound closed with drainage. After a successful operation there is a good pulsatile flow of blood down the artery and pulses are restored.

Postoperative care

The foot (or hand) should be closely observed. This should become normal in colour, sensation and movement if the operation has succeeded. If the foot is initially satisfactory and then deteriorates, there may be a need for further treatment.

Peripheral pulses should be palpated to confirm that the blood flow is satisfactory. Anticoagulants may be administered. Heparin therapy is usually prescribed and careful observation for haemorrhage is necessary.

Most of the emboli arise from the heart and therefore treatment for the heart condition may also be needed.

Chronic arterial obstructions

Almost any artery can become obstructed by arteriosclerosis. The effects which have already been described are: exercise pain, changes in skin and muscle, pain at rest (later), and gangrene (also later).

Most patients with exercise pain do not need an operation unless they are unable to work because of it. However, when pain occurs at rest, or there is evidence that the blood supply is becoming so poor that there is danger of developing gangrene, then an operation will be necessary.

In most cases the operation performed will be either a by-pass using a graft, or an endarterectomy.

Aortoiliac obstruction

In aortoiliac obstruction either type of procedure is possible. When a graft is employed, it is commonly of the Dacron type. The graft is usually attached to the aorta above and to the external iliac arteries or femoral arteries below, by-passing the obstruction. Therefore a special type of graft is needed. It has a main limb to replace the aorta and two divisions to replace the iliac arteries. This type of graft is colloquially known as the 'trouser graft'.

Endarterectomy may be used to remove the obstructions in the aorta rather than to by-pass them. This must be continued down both iliac arteries and possibly both femoral arteries until relatively normal vessels are reached.

Following operation frequent pulse and blood pressure recordings are necessary to give timely warning of bleeding which may occasionally occur after either procedure. Measurement of urine output should be carried out usually at hourly intervals because the blood flow along the renal arteries may have been disturbed during aortic clamping. Intravenous fluids will have been prescribed, and sometimes further transfusion will be necessary. Nasogastric tube should be aspirated at regular intervals because the patient will almost always develop an ileus after an operation on the aorta. Prevention of chest complications by physiotherapy and breathing exercises is important. Prophylactic antibiotics are often employed when a Dacron graft has been used, because infection of the graft is a very serious complication. Examination of the legs, as after embolectomy, is also necessary.

Femoropopliteal obstruction

The commonest site of obstruction is in the adductor canal. The best operation in the leg is the by-pass graft, using the patient's own long saphenous vein (*Figure 31.6*). Endarterectomy can also be employed. Dacron grafts are used only occasionally.

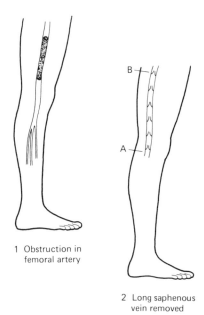

1 Obstruction in femoral artery

2 Long saphenous vein removed

3 Vein inverted

4 Saphenous vein by-passes obstruction in artery

Figure 31.6. Femoropopliteal by-pass

During the operation the popliteal artery is exposed behind the knee and assessed for its suitability for grafting. Then the femoral artery is exposed in the groin. The long saphenous vein is exposed at intervals between the groin and the knee, and all its tributaries are ligated (in order to make it leak-proof when it is acting as an artery). The vein is then removed and turned upside down. This reversal is necessary because the venous valves would otherwise prevent flow along the 'artery'.

One end of the vein is sutured to the side of the femoral artery and the other end to the side of the popliteal artery. A wide anastomosis is made at each end to allow free flow of blood. When the clamps are removed, arterial blood flows from the femoral artery into the vein graft, and finally re-enters the popliteal artery, thus by-passing the block in the femoral artery and re-establishing a blood supply to the leg.

The principle of postoperative care is the same as that following an arterial embolectomy.

Subclavian artery obstruction

The subclavian artery may be narrowed by a plaque or may become completely obstructed. In either case the blood supply to the arm is reduced and exercise pain may occur. When the obstruction is incomplete, there may be clot formation on the arteriosclerotic plaque. This clot may send off emboli down the arm, and sometimes the fingertips may become gangrenous from such emboli which block the small (e.g. digital) arteries.

This type of obstruction can be overcome by means of a graft or endarterectomy.

Subclavian steal syndrome

When the subclavian artery is blocked before it has given off its vertebral branch, the blood supply to the arm may occasionally be obtained by reversal of blood flow in the vertebral artery (*Figure 31.7*).

Thus the blood is 'stolen' from the brain in order to supply the arm. When the arm is exercised, symptoms of cerebral ischaemia (for example loss of consciousness, visual disturbances and so on) may occur.

Carotid artery obstruction

In common with other arteries, the carotid artery tends to become narrowed where it divides into the internal and external branches in the neck. When a plaque forms at this point, it may produce symptoms in the central nervous system (e.g. a transient stroke). A careful evaluation of these

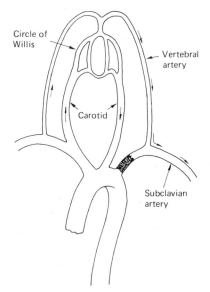

Figure 31.7. Subclavian steal syndrome. Diagram showing reversal of flow in vertebral artery on the affected side

Circle of Willis

Vertebral artery

Carotid

Subclavian artery

symptoms is required, but if it is decided that the plaque in the carotid artery is the cause of the symptoms, then this plaque can be removed. Carotid endarterectomy is usually carried out under general anaesthesia and various techniques may be employed for the protection of the cerebral circulation during the period of arterial clamping.

Aneurysms

The commonest site for an aneurysm is in the abdominal aorta, although many other major vessels may be similarly affected.

The diameter of the arteriosclerotic vessel increases in this condition, and it usually is a progressive abnormality. Ultimately the enlargement of the aorta is so great that there may be a visible swelling in the abdomen. This enlargement of the aorta will eventually produce symptoms such as back pain, abdominal pain, gastrointestinal symptoms, or urinary tract symptoms.

The complications of an abdominal aortic aneurysm are embolism from the wall of the artery and rupture.

Rupture is the most serious complication of all and, if untreated, is invariably fatal. The patient usually presents with severe abdominal pain and signs of blood loss. The shock may be profound when the patient is first seen if the rupture has been directly into the peritoneal cavity. Fortunately in most cases the leak is into the retroperitoneal space, and the posterior wall of the peritoneum limits further bleeding for a variable length of time.

Increase in size of an aneurysm and the development of pain from it should warn that there is a danger of rupture.

Operation for abdominal aortic aneurysm
The aorta is cross-clamped above the upper limit of the aneurysm and further clamps are placed on both iliac arteries. This may have to be done rapidly in the case of the ruptured aneurysm in order to control bleeding.

The aneurysm is opened and in some cases removed. More commonly, however, the posterior wall of the aneurysm is left *in situ*. The bifurcation ('trouser') graft is then sutured to the non-aneurysmal aorta above, and to the common iliac arteries below (*Figure 31.8*). If the common iliac arteries are extensively involved, it may be necessary to attach the graft to the external iliac arteries. When the clamps are removed, blood flow is restored to the legs.

Postoperative care is the same as for operations for aorto-iliac block. However, when the operation has been for a ruptured aneurysm, the postoperative course may be difficult.

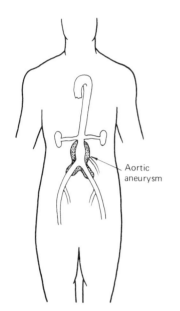

Aortic aneurysm

Dacron graft

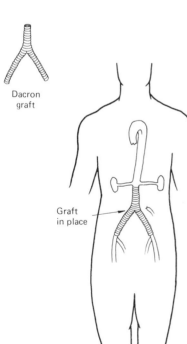

Graft in place

Figure 31.8. Resection and graft of aortic aneurysm

Many of these patients are best cared for in an intensive care unit, where facilities for cardiac monitoring, positive pressure respiration, blood gas analysis and so on are readily available.

The particular postoperative problems may include ileus, thrombosis or embolism in the legs, renal failure, and colon necrosis (because the inferior mesenteric artery has to be ligated).

Other operations

Amputation

When there is irreversible destruction of part of a limb from obstruction of blood supply, injury or infection, surgical removal becomes necessary. Until fairly recently, the common operation was mid-thigh amputation, but it is now possible to preserve more of the limb in many cases.

Indications for amputation are: (1) gangrene, (2) severe rest pain in a patient who is unfit for major arterial surgery, (3) infection (especially with anaerobic organisms, e.g. gas gangrene), (4) severe injuries, (5) failed arterial reconstruction, and also (6) certain malignancies.

Amputation can be carried out at different levels (*Figure 31.9*) summarized below.

(*a*) Above-knee (mid-thigh) amputation is employed when there is extensive disease and it can usually be relied upon to heal well.

(*b*) Through-knee amputation. Useful movement is retained, and this may be particularly important when the patient is not wearing the artificial limb (e.g. in bed).

(*c*) Below-knee amputation which can be useful in arterial disease, especially in the younger age group. It allows knee movement which makes walking easier.

(*d*) Syme's amputation, i.e. the removal of most of the foot, but retaining the heel.

(*e*) Transmetatarsal amputation, i.e. the removal of the forefoot.

(*f*) Toes (or fingers) — for example, in diabetic gangrene.

Limb fitting is an extremely important step in the recovery from an amputation. An attempt should be made to fit every patient with an artificial limb (prosthesis) and to educate him in its use. In some centres a temporary pylon is fitted before the patient leaves the operating theatre so that walking training can begin early. The limb-fitters often visit the patient prior to operation, and when time is available, the patient can be given some training before the amputation takes place.

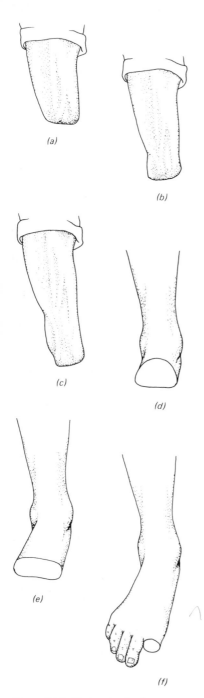

(a)

(b)

(c)

(d)

(e)

(f)

Figure 31.9. Various levels of amputation of leg. (*a*) Above the knee; (*b*) through the knee; (*c*) below the knee; (*d*) Syme's; (*e*) transmetatarsal; (*f*) digital

The nurse and the physiotherapist have a particularly important role at this point in ensuring that the joint above the amputation remains mobile and active, and that the amputation stump is bandaged carefully and frequently so that it is 'shaped' for the prosthetic limb.

Highly satisfactory replacement limbs are now available and are constantly improving. Light-weight materials increase the patient's mobility. The weight is usually taken away from the suture line and this increases the patient's comfort.

Sympathectomy

The sympathetic nervous system is a series of ganglia and their connections, which are situated close to the bodies of the vertebrae. The upper and lower limbs each have their own sympathetic nerve supply, the effect of which is to constrict the blood vessels and to increase sweating. Consequently surgical division of the sympathetic chain will reverse these effects, that is, induce relaxation of blood vessels (vasodilatation) and stop sweating.

Two operations on the sympathetic nervous system are commonly undertaken.

Cervico-dorsal sympathectomy interrupts the sympathetic nerve supply to the arm. The sympathetic chain is usually exposed via the neck or the axilla.

Lumbar sympathectomy interrupts the sympathetic nerve supply to the leg and it is usually exposed via an incision in the lateral part of the abdomen, dissecting behind the peritoneum until the chain is found on the vertebral bodies. Chemical injection is an alternative to operation.

The following conditions can be indications for sympathectomy.

(1) Raynaud's syndrome. When the fingers are exposed to cold they become extremely pale and later turn blue. In some patients these two colour changes are followed by redness and burning of the fingers. These events are common in mild degree especially in women, but when severe they can be very incapacitating. This phenomenon may also be seen in association with other more serious conditions, such as, scleroderma, disseminated lupus erythematosus, and so on.
(2) Hyperhidrosis, i.e. excessive sweating.
(3) Rest pain from chronic arterial obstruction.

Arterial injuries

Arterial injuries are a particularly important aspect of the surgery of the arterial system. Road traffic accidents are resulting in an increasing number of arterial injuries. In addition, many arterial injuries occur as a result of war wounds. One important feature of these injuries is that the vessels involved were frequently normal before the injury and are capable, in many cases, of restoration to normal.

Awareness of the possibility of arterial injury, early diagnosis and rapid treatment are the essentials of success.

Arterial injuries can be caused by either trauma (laceration, e.g. knife wound, or crush, e.g. fracture, direct blow), or iatrogenic injury, e.g. cardiac catheterization, angiography, operation and so on.

Effect on the artery

An artery can be damaged in the following ways.

(1) Division. Laceration results usually in clean vessel ends; traction or crush injury usually results in damaged vessel ends.

(2) Haematoma in the wall of the vessel. Bleeding occurring within the layers of the wall of the vessel may cause obstruction of the vessel.

(3) Tear in the intimal lining of the blood vessel. As a result there may be a dissection (i.e. blood flowing within the vessel) or the intima may roll up causing an obstruction (*Figure 31.2*).

(4) Partial division. This usually produces haemorrhage but may not obstruct the flow.

(5) Thrombosis.

Effect on the patient

Arterial injuries produce haemorrhage which can be very severe when a major vessel is injured. Interruption of the arterial supply will result in death of the tissues supplied by that artery if the injury is not recognized and corrected quickly.

When a major injury has occurred, the effect on the patient is the combined effect of the vascular and the other injuries, e.g. head injury, thoracic and abdominal injuries, and so on.

Investigations

A general examination of the patient for other injuries is essential. Not uncommonly one major and obvious abnormality distracts attention from other injuries. It is wise to make control of haemorrhage the first priority after the airway. Whenever possible, it is safest to stop bleeding by means of direct pressure. When this is impossible a tourniquet can occasionally be of value, but usually an emergency operation is necessary.

The periphery of the limbs and the pulses should be examined in order to detect interruption of arterial supply. This is particularly important when the patient has a fracture, for example, supracondylar fracture in the arm, or shaft of femur in the leg. Occasionally arteriography will be needed in order to establish the site of the injury.

Treatment

When airway obstruction is present, it requires immediate correction. Priorities of treatment are then established and the most urgent is usually the control of haemorrhage and the replacement of blood loss.

The aim of treatment must be to restore the arterial flow to normal. Circumstances will dictate the type of operation necessary and the following procedures may be used.

(1) End-to-end suture of the divided vessel, when the ends are normal.
(2) End-to-end suture after excision of a damaged segment.
(3) Replacement of a damaged segment by a graft. In the limbs this is usually by means of a vein graft.
(4) Removal of a thrombus by means of an arteriotomy and the use of the Fogarty catheter.
(5) When the arterial injury complicates a fracture, it will be necessary to immobilize the fracture first.

Postoperative care consists of:

(1) examination of peripheral pulses;
(2) prevention of local infection, especially with gas-forming organisms, e.g. *Clostridium welchii*;
(3) prevention of tetanus;
(4) passive movements of the foot or hand, when this will not interfere with arterial repair.

Other arterial diseases

Diabetes

There is a common association between diabetes and arterial disease. Chronic arterial obstruction in a diabetic carries a much worse prognosis than in normal patients. In addition, there are the added effects of a peripheral neuropathy with loss of sensation in the foot leading to injury and infection. The importance of testing the urine in a patient with arterial disease must therefore be stressed.

Cervical rib

A partial or complete rib arising from the last cervical vertebra can produce narrowing of the closely related subclavian artery. Operation consists of removal of the rib and, when necessary, correction of the arterial abnormality.

Dissecting aneurysm (*Figure 31.2*)

The layers of the arterial wall in patients with hypertension may split and blood flow within the layers of the vessel. The patients usually present with pain which is sometimes described as tearing and tends to move from the chest to the abdomen. The blood supply of a limb may be cut off or, more seriously, also the blood supply to the brain or kidneys.

The mainstay of treatment is the lowering of blood pressure and early operation is reserved for the rare cases where life or limb are in danger.

Mesenteric ischaemia

Mesenteric ischaemia results from the acute or chronic obstruction of the coeliac axis, the superior mesenteric artery or the inferior mesenteric artery. In acute obstruction the bowel supplied by the artery may become gangrenous unless an adequate blood supply can be rapidly restored.

32

Surgery of the veins and lymphatics

Averil O. Mansfield

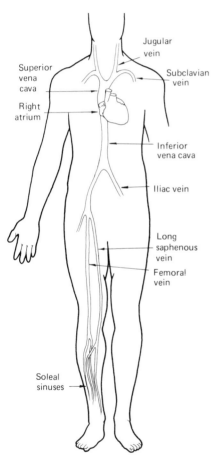

Figure 32.1. Diagram of anatomy of veins

THE VEINS

Anatomy

The return of blood to the heart from the limbs, the organs and the lungs is the responsibility of the venous system which differs in a large measure from the arterial system. There is no pulse to propel the blood and venous return is therefore dependent on the peripheral muscle pump, mainly the calf muscles, and on the negative intrathoracic pressure. The returning column of blood has to be prevented from reversing its direction of flow, and this is accomplished by the venous valves. These consist of delicate webs which allow free forward flow, but when the flow is reversed they open out and support the column of blood. Not surprisingly, this is the part of the venous system which so frequently becomes incompetent.

The veins themselves differ from arteries in their construction. The walls are much thinner and are collapsible. This is an advantage for the transmission of pressure from the muscle pump, but a disadvantage during operations when the veins in the calf may compress and consequently thrombose.

In the legs there are two systems of veins, the superficial and the deep veins. The long and short saphenous veins drain blood from the superficial layers into the deep veins (soleal, popliteal and femoral veins) (*see Figure 32.1*). The two systems communicate at the perforating veins and the direction of flow in these veins is from superficial to deep. While the valves remain competent, this is the normal direction of flow.

The highest communication between superficial and deep veins in the leg is at the groin, at the saphenofemoral junction, and there is a valve at this point.

In the femoral triangle, most of the blood is directed into the femoral vein which passes under the inguinal ligament to become the iliac vein. Above this level venous valves are infrequent or absent. The iliac veins from each leg, after receiving the internal iliac veins from the pelvis, unite to form the inferior vena cava. This is a wide, thin-walled structure in the posterior abdominal wall. It receives blood from both legs, the kidneys and the liver (and therefore indirectly also from the alimentary canal), and finally passes through the diaphragm and enters the right atrium of the heart.

Blood from the upper part of the body enters the heart (right atrium) via the superior vena cava, which is formed by the two brachiocephalic (innominate) veins. The brachiocephalic veins are formed from the union of the subclavian vein draining the arm, and the internal jugular vein draining the head. Both veins receive tributaries from the vertebrae, thorax and the thyroid gland. In addition, the left brachiocephalic vein receives the thoracic duct, which is the route through which lymph returns to the blood.

As in the leg, there are superficial and deep veins in the arm. The superficial veins are the cephalic and basilic veins, and are the vessels commonly employed for intravenous therapy. The deep veins accompany the artery, and the superficial and deep vessels unite to form the axillary vein. This is continued as the subclavian vein to the brachiocephalic vein.

Also draining into the right atrium is the coronary sinus which is the main venous return of the heart. In summary the following vessels drain into the right atrium:

(1) the superior vena cava from the head and arms;
(2) the inferior vena cava from the abdomen and legs; and
(3) the coronary sinus from the myocardium.

The portal vein carries blood from the alimentary canal (via the superior and inferior mesenteric veins), pancreas and spleen to the liver.

Pulmonary veins differ from the other veins in that they carry oxygenated blood. They return blood from the lungs to the heart and enter the left atrium (unlike the superior and inferior venae cavae which enter the right atrium).

The azygos vein connects the superior and inferior venae cavae and receives several tributaries from the thorax.

Veins of the brain drain blood from the brain into the venous sinuses. There are no valves in these veins. One of the sinuses (cavernous) communicates with the facial vein, and because there are no valves here this is one route through which infection may reach the brain.

Physiology

During exercise, the veins in the muscles are compressed as the muscle contracts, and flow in the veins is instituted in the direction of the heart. The valves within the venous system permit flow in the direction of the heart only and blood

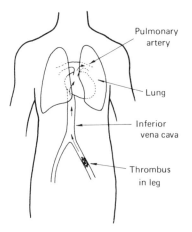

Pulmonary
artery

Lung

Inferior
vena cava

Thrombus
in leg

Figure 32.2. Mechanism of pulmonary embolus

moves from segment to segment in the venous system. At rest, the pressure in a vein at the ankle is over 100 cm of blood, but during contraction of the muscle, this is reduced to about 20 cm of blood.

In addition to muscle contraction, alteration in the intra-thoracic pressure assists venous return when it is in the negative phase.

Pathology

There are two important diseases of the veins: thrombosis and varicose veins.

Thrombosis

Thrombosis is a common abnormality in the venous system. There are two main types of thrombosis.

Phlebitis Phlebitis is an inflammation in the vein wall where the vein becomes thrombosed as a secondary phenomenon. This commonly affects the long and short saphenous veins in the legs and also the superficial veins in the arm. This inflammation is not usually associated with a bacterial infection, but if intravenous injections or infusions have been carried out without sterile precautions, or the vein passes through an abscess cavity, then organisms may be found in the vein wall and in the thrombus within its lumen.

In thrombophlebitis migrans recurrent attacks of phlebitis affect several segments of vein which may be widely separated. It may be associated with a carcinoma, e.g. carcinoma of the head of the pancreas.

Deep vein thrombosis In deep vein thrombosis one or more of the main veins becomes thrombosed. It commonly affects the soleal veins in the calf and sometimes also the femoral and iliac veins. Occasionally the axillary and subclavian veins are similarly affected. The thrombosed vessel may become permanently blocked, or may partly recanalize with damage or destruction of the valves.

The main complication of the disease is the dislodgement of clots which may become pulmonary emboli.

Varicose veins

Varicose veins are the result of failure of the valves within the vein. The long and the short saphenous systems in the leg are most commonly affected. An increase in pressure in the vein may be due to various factors, including prolonged standing, obstruction to the return of venous blood to the heart (e.g.

mitral valve disease), and pressure from without, for example from a pregnant uterus.

As a result the valve fails to function and is no longer able to support the column of blood. The vein below this valve is distended and tortuous.

Clinical presentation and diagnosis of venous disorders

Many of the superficial veins are visible through the skin, for example the cephalic and basilic veins in the arms, and often the long and short saphenous veins in the leg. When the valves are incompetent, the familiar picture of varicose veins in the leg results. The patient observes distended, tortuous veins in the legs. It is possible by examination to determine the site where the incompetent valve is to be found.

When one of the deep veins is obstructed, congestion of the limb will occur because insufficient blood is draining out of it and fluid will collect in the tissues, resulting in oedema. When a major vein is occluded, swelling of the whole limb occurs. In addition to swelling, because of the stasis in the circulation, the affected limb appears warmer than the normal limb. In the presence of acute venous thrombosis examination of the leg may produce pain and there will be localized tenderness over the vein itself.

Special investigations of the venous system

Ultrasonic flow detector Instruments are available which employ ultrasound and the Doppler principle to detect flow in vessels. This technique can be applied both to the arterial and to the venous systems. It is particularly useful in the examination of the venous system because there is no palpable pulse in the vein. For example, flow in the femoral vein can be demonstrated and with experience abnormalities of flow can be detected.

Radioactive fibrinogen Radioactive fibrinogen (^{125}I) can be used to detect clots in veins. A small dose of radioactive fibrinogen is given to the patient and any clots which the patient forms thereafter will contain a small, detectable quantity of radioactivity.

Radiology Radiological investigations are particularly important in the detection of venous obstruction and thrombosis. Radio-opaque material is injected into a vein in the periphery of the limb, usually the leg, and radiographs are obtained at intervals after the injection. The presence of filling defects in the vein suggests that a thrombosis is present. Employing this method, it is also possible to detect the presence of incompetent perforating veins.

When major vessels, such as iliac veins and the vena cava, are to be investigated, it is sometimes necessary to inject radio-opaque material into either the greater trochanter of the femur, or the femoral vein when this is normal. Serial radiographs are obtained of the pelvic veins and vena cava.

Varicose veins

The veins usually affected are the long and short saphenous systems in the legs. A varicose vein is a vein dilated as the result of incompetence of the valves. When the column of blood is no longer supported by the valve, back pressure on the peripheral veins occurs, and the vein becomes dilated and saccular. The tributaries of the main vein may also be affected. A common site of valve incompetence is in the long saphenous vein where it enters the femoral vein. The second commonest site is in the short saphenous vein where it enters the popliteal vein. In addition to these two sites, incompetence of valves between the superficial and the deep systems, i.e. the perforating veins, may allow blood to reverse its direction of flow and pass out from the deep system into the superficial.

In addition to the visible varicosities in the veins, changes may be present in the skin of the region.

Symptoms
The patient is usually concerned by the appearance of the veins, but in addition the leg is frequently uncomfortable and there is a tendency to ache towards the end of the day. Patients whose occupations involve standing are particularly affected by aching and often by swelling of the ankles.

Detection of the site of valve incompetence
The patient's foot is elevated and the veins are emptied. Under normal conditions when the patient then stands up, the veins should fill gradually from below. When a valve is incompetent, there is a rapid reversal of flow and the vein fills from above. By applying a rubber tourniquet to the leg when the foot is elevated, it is possible by repeated examination, to find the level at which filling from above will occur. The tourniquet, acting as a substitute valve, is gradually moved up the leg until such reverse filling is controlled. At this level valve incompetence is present. This incompetence may be in the superficial system or in the communicating (perforating) veins between the superficial and deep veins.

Complications
Phlebitis Superficial varicose veins occasionally develop inflammatory lesions. The vessel wall becomes tender on palpation and is frequently thrombosed.

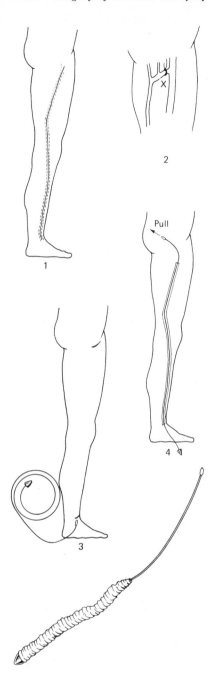

1 Mark veins with waterproof ink
2 Ligate long saphenous vein in groin X
3 Insert stripper into saphenous vein at ankle
4 Remove the vein

Figure 32.3. Ligation and stripping of varicose veins.

Bleeding When a varicose vein is perforated, heavy bleeding may result, because the vein wall does not contract as would an artery. Treatment of this complication is application of direct pressure over the site of bleeding and elevation of the whole limb.

Skin changes The patient may develop eczema, pigmentation and later also ulceration.

Treatment
Conservative Supportive measures may be sufficient; that is, bandaging the leg or wearing an elastic stocking.

Operation Operation involves ligation of the affected vein and frequently its removal. High ligation and stripping of the long saphenous vein is the commonest operation for varicose veins (*Figure 32.3*). When perforating veins are incompetent, it may be necessary to ligate these, in an operation usually known as the Cockett's procedure. Initially following the operation, the patient's leg is kept elevated, but as soon as possible the patient is mobilized so that venous return is stimulated, and blood in the deep veins is prevented from stagnating.

Injection Compression sclerotherapy is a common treatment for varicose veins. A compound is injected into the vein which, when the vein is compressed, will cause the walls to adhere to one another, thus obliterating the lumen. Following injection of the sclerosant solution, pressure bandaging is placed on the leg for a minimum period of 2 weeks. Skilful injection of the perforating veins can sclerose them and prevent the reversal of flow which is present when the valves are incompetent. A course of injections is usually required in order to treat the whole limb, and this may take 4 to 6 weeks to complete.

At the completion of either operation or injection, the patient's leg is firmly bandaged. After injection sclerotherapy, the bandage compresses the vein wall, but after operation the aim of bandaging is to minimize the amount of bruising which would otherwise be inevitable after the vein had been stripped out from the leg.

Venous thrombosis

In venous thrombosis the veins of the limb become blocked when a thrombus is formed within the lumen. This event can occur in either the superficial vein or in the deep veins. Whenever the superficial veins are involved, the vein itself is

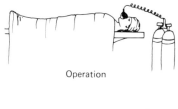

Operation

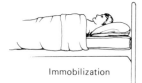

Immobilization

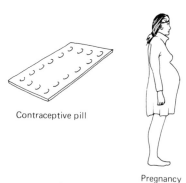

Contraceptive pill

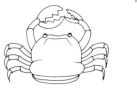

Pregnancy

Cancer

Figure 32.4. Causes of deep venous thrombosis

tender and the patient experiences considerable pain. However, the condition is not a serious one as the major venous return of the leg is not impaired.

When the deep veins of a limb are involved, a deep vein thrombosis exists. This may occur within the veins of the calf muscle (so interfering with the calf muscle pump) or in the femoral or iliac veins. Less commonly, venous thrombosis may occur in the axillary vein, causing venous obstruction in the arm. In the more extreme forms, the vena cava may become thrombosed.

Causes
Causes of venous thrombosis (*Figure 32.4*) are as follows:

(1) surgical operations;
(2) a period of bed rest, after a serious illness;
(3) hormone treatment, e.g. the contraceptive pill;
(4) pregnancy;
(5) malignant disease.

Occasionally patients present who do not have any of the above causes for their venous thrombosis, but in each case some cause should be sought.

Prevention of deep venous thrombosis
There is no certain means of preventing deep vein thrombosis at the present time, but the following measures may help to reduce the postoperative incidence (*Figure 32.5*).

(1) Mobilization of patients after operations. This does not include sitting in a chair with the feet dependent.
(2) Minimization of pressure on veins during operation. A pad is placed under the heels so that the calf muscles are lifted off the operating table.
(3) Prevention of dehydration during and after operation.
(4) Breathing exercises and leg exercises after operations to encourage the return of venous blood to the heart.

2 POSTOPERATIVE PHYSIOTHERAPY

1 OPERATING TABLE

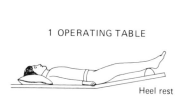

Heel rest

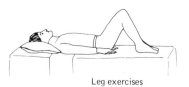

Leg exercises

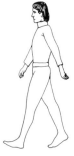

Breathing exercises

Walking

Figure 32.5. Prevention of deep venous thrombosis

(5) Anticoagulants may sometimes be prescribed. The commonest anticoagulant regimen now widely employed is subcutaneous heparin in the following doses: 5000 units (0.2 ml of 25 000 units/ml) heparin subcutaneously 2 hours preoperatively and then 8 hourly for 5 days.

(6) Mechanical compression or stimulation of the calf muscles.

Symptoms of deep vein thrombosis

The patient usually complains because the leg is painful and swollen, and as a result it may be difficult for him to walk. However, it is possible for a venous thrombosis to develop in the total absence of signs and symptoms.

Sometimes the patient develops pain in the chest and coughs up blood (haemoptysis). This may be the first sign of a venous thrombosis and it usually means that a part of the clot has broken off and has become an embolus to the lung.

Clinical appearance of the limb

Examination reveals that the limb, when a major venous obstruction is present, is swollen throughout. When only the calf veins are involved the lower part of the leg is swollen and the calf muscles are tender. When the foot is dorsiflexed, pain in the calf is felt (positive Homans' sign which is not necessarily reliable).

In addition to swelling and tenderness, there may be some visible dilatation of the superficial veins, caused by blood being diverted from the blocked deep veins to the open superficial veins to aid venous return from the leg.

Colour changes may also be present. Frequently in the early stages of a major venous thrombosis, the leg appears pale, so-called 'white leg'. In the most severe forms, the leg may become blue in colour, due to the gross swelling with stasis of the blood in the leg, and to some extent, limitation of the amount of arterial blood entering the leg.

Diagnosis

Clinical diagnosis is notoriously difficult and unreliable and must frequently be confirmed by venography.

Treatment

It is important to prevent the clot from extending up or down the vein. Consequently the main treatment for this disease is the anticoagulant treatment. Anticoagulants may be given intravenously, for example heparin, or orally, for example warfarin. Heparin produces a rapid effect which can, when necessary, be just as rapidly reversed. It is given in

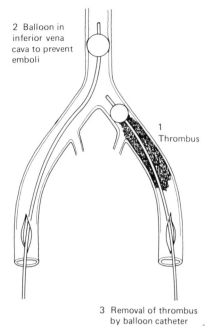

2 Balloon in inferior vena cava to prevent emboli

1 Thrombus

3 Removal of thrombus by balloon catheter

Figure 32.6. Diagrammatic representation of thrombectomy

much larger doses for treatment of the established thrombosis than for prevention and often about 40 000 units may be prescribed over a 24-hour period. When oral anticoagulants are given, the effect takes longer to produce and longer to reverse, and therefore they are usually employed for long-term maintenance treatment.

Thrombolytic therapy may be employed when it is hoped to remove a thrombus from the vein. Intravenous administration of streptokinase (Kabikinase, Streptase) may be employed, which will activate the fibrinolytic system (the opposite to the coagulation system) and produce lysis (breakdown) of the thrombus.

When thrombolytic therapy is employed, there is a danger of bleeding and consequently the patient must be carefully monitored throughout the treatment so that early signs of haemorrhage can be detected. In addition, there may be some reaction to the injected foreign material in the form of a pyrexial illness. Administration of this drug must be continuous and in a regulated dose. It is important that the rate of administration should be constant.

Because of the danger of haemorrhage, streptokinase cannot be employed in the immediate postoperative period, or when there is any potential bleeding site, such as a peptic ulcer.

Operative removal of the thrombus The operative removal of the thrombus is known as thrombectomy. A balloon catheter (Fogarty catheter) is inserted into the femoral vein at the groin and threaded through the iliac vein until it is beyond the thrombus. The clots are withdrawn by inflating the balloon and removing the catheter (*Figure 32.6*).

Complications of venous thrombosis – pulmonary embolus
The major complication of venous thrombosis is the occurrence of a pulmonary embolus. When an extending thrombus in the leg becomes detached, it is then free to migrate into the right atrium of the heart, and from the right atrium of the heart into the right ventricle, from whence it will pass into the pulmonary artery (*Figure 32.7*).

If the clot lodges in the pulmonary artery, its effect will depend to some extent on the size of the clot. A large clot may produce complete obstruction of the arteries and immediate death. The patient usually has a cardiac arrest, often after getting out of bed or going to the toilet. When a major embolus is not fatal, severe dyspnoea will be produced, and there may be pain in the chest. The patient may become cyanosed and be in a state of circulatory collapse. This situation requires urgent treatment to remove the clot either by surgery or by thrombolytic therapy.

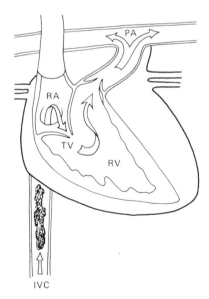

Figure 32.7. Diagram of the course followed by a dislodged thrombus (here shown in the inferior vena cava). It is finally impacted in the pulmonary artery

Smaller pulmonary emboli may produce less serious effects. The patient may complain of shortness of breath, chest pain and may cough up blood. When these symptoms occur it is important to look carefully at the legs of the patient in order to detect the possibility of further clot formation. A number of patients who have had a small pulmonary embolus will later have a much larger one, which can prove to be fatal.

Diagnosis The following investigations may be of help when the diagnosis is uncertain.

(1) Chest radiograph.
(2) Electrocardiogram (ECG).
(3) Pulmonary angiogram.
(4) Radioisotope lung scan.
(5) Venograms of the peripheral veins to detect further clots.

Treatment Supportive measures for the dyspnoea and shock may include the administration of oxygen and intravenous infusions. When the patient is severely shocked, he should be transferred to an intensive care unit, or sometimes directly to the operating theatre for removal of the embolism.

Anticoagulant treatment is almost invariably used in order to prevent further clot formation.

In some hospitals, the vena cava may be ligated, or plicated (that is, divided into channels) in an attempt to prevent any further possibility of emboli reaching the lungs. An umbrella filter can be placed in the inferior vena cava to trap further emboli.

Long-term complications of venous thrombosis

Long-term complications are related to the obstruction of venous return and to the destruction of valves which may follow a venous thrombosis.

In the calf venous thrombosis may result in incompetent perforating veins, skin ulceration and varicose veins.

In major veins there may be permanent obstruction to venous return and consequently permanent swelling of the leg, pain, and frequently ulceration. This is known as the postphlebitic syndrome, and can sometimes be prevented by early removal of the obstructing thrombus.

Treatment of the postphlebitic syndrome The control of swelling is particularly important and can be achieved in two ways; either by firm bandaging of the limb with a crêpe or an elastic bandage, or alternatively with made-to-measure elastic stockings or elastic tights. When ulceration has occurred, healing of the skin can frequently be aided by elevation of the patient's legs, preferably in hospital, to reduce swelling. The ulcer can be dressed in a variety of ways but frequently a topical steroid and a coal tar paste are applied to the ulcer which is then left undisturbed for 1 or 2 weeks.

When the ulcer fails to heal with conservative measures, surgery may be necessary either to assist venous return or to ligate the incompetent perforating veins. At the same time, the ulcer may be excised and a skin graft placed over the area.

Rehabilitation after venous thrombosis

Venous stasis should be prevented whenever possible. The patient is advised to wear a supporting stocking at all times, and to avoid standing. If the patient must stand in one place, he is taught to contract his calf muscles to aid venous return. Walking is advantageous, but when the patient is sitting down, the leg should be elevated. Any signs of skin ulceration should be treated vigorously from the first to prevent extension of the ulcer.

Any possible cause of the venous thrombosis should then be treated. For instance, if the patient has been taking an oral contraceptive, it is generally advisable to discontinue this. When the patient has had an operation, resumption of activity is advised as soon as possible. Venous thrombosis in the presence of carcinoma requires treatment of the tumour whenever this is possible.

The patient is frequently prescribed anticoagulant treatment for some time after the initial episode. This will require regular blood tests to determine the prothrombin level, the coagulation factor altered by oral anticoagulants. The prothrombin index or level is determined at frequent intervals initially, but once a stable dose of anticoagulant agent has been determined then longer intervals between blood tests are acceptable. The patient is given a card warning him of the drugs which may interact with anticoagulant therapy, and of the hazards of this treatment.

THE LYMPHATICS

Anatomy and physiology

The lymphatics are responsible for the return of lymph, a protein-rich fluid, from the tissues into the circulation. The lymphatic channels are small vessels which are about 1 mm in diameter and possess numerous valves. The vessels run both in the superficial and in the deep layers of the skin. In addition to the skin, the organs also have a lymphatic drainage and intestines are particularly well supplied with lymphatics.

The course of the lymphatic vessels leads them to lymph nodes, and after reaching a lymph node the vessels continue and form lymphatic trunks which ultimately enter into the circulation at either the thoracic duct in the left side of the neck or a similar, but smaller duct in the right side. The lymph nodes are found in groups and are generally deeply placed. They consist of a capsule within which there is an outer and an inner part of the node. The lymph drains into the node, and lymphocytes, produced in the lymph node, are added to the fluid as it passes through the node. Many lymphocytes are thus added to the lymph every day and so acquire access to the bloodstream.

Pathology

When failure of this normal flow of protein-containing fluid occurs fluid will accumulate in the skin; this condition is known as lymphoedema.

The failure of the lymphatic drainage may occur because the lymphatics themselves are abnormal or even absent, and this abnormality produces primary lymphoedema. Secondary lymphoedema is most commonly caused by the destructive effect of either surgery or radiotherapy. Either the lymph nodes themselves or the lymphatics may have been damaged or removed, and consequently lymph cannot be returned to the circulation.

Lymphangitis

This disease consists of inflammation of lymphatics usually resulting from an infection in a hand or foot. The appearance of the limb is characteristic in that there are red streaks in the skin which may be tender on palpation. The regional lymph nodes are enlarged and frequently tender, and at a later stage they may discharge pus. Treatment of this condition consists of the treatment of the source of the infection. The patient often requires antibiotics and drainage of the pus.

Lymphoedema

In primary lymphoedema (Milroy's disease) where the lymphatics are abnormal, the oedema is usually progressive, and although it frequently begins in one leg, it may later involve the other limb. The oedema usually begins in the ankles and advances up the leg. Later the skin becomes thickened and horny. The principal complaints of the patient are the ugly appearance of the limb and its heaviness.

Secondary lymphoedema resulting from damage to or removal of lymph nodes may affect either an arm or a leg. Where radical mastectomy is employed in the treatment of carcinoma of the breast, a percentage of patients can be expected to develop serious arm swelling. In the leg, secondary lymphoedema may be related to the removal of the inguinal lymph nodes or radiotherapy to these nodes or to the pelvis.

Diagnosis

Usually the clinical appearance of the limb involved is diagnostic and no further investigation is required. However, for more careful evaluation, lymphangiography may be employed. A tiny needle or cannula is inserted into a peripheral lymphatic, and a radio-opaque fluid is injected into it. This can only be injected extremely slowly and it may take 2 or 3 hours before all the lymphatics are outlined. The lymphatics of the limbs can be seen and also the regional lymph nodes. Beyond the lymph nodes, the lymphatic trunks can often be visualized.

In primary lymphoedema there are usually very few vessels seen and occasionally it may not be possible to find any at all. In secondary lymphoedema they are usually dilated and tortuous because of the obstruction.

Treatment

Conservative

Lymphoedema is usually managed conservatively, i.e. the swelling is controlled by elastic supports and bandages. Elevation of the foot of the bed reduces the amount of oedema and massage may help the return of fluid. In addition, general weight loss is usually helpful and care of the skin may minimize the damage to it.

Operative

Operative treatment is reserved for the more serious cases with severe incapacity. There are two principal operations used.

In Charles' operation the thickened skin and subcutaneous tissues are removed and the skin is excised and replaced as a graft. In Thompson's operation a flap of skin is buried in continuity beneath the deep fascia. This enables the fluid from the superficial tissues to drain into the deeper parts of the leg and a very satisfactory relief of swelling may occur.

Lymph nodes

The determination of the cause of enlargement of the lymph nodes is a frequent diagnostic problem. Lymph nodes may be enlarged because of an infection which may be acute, e.g.

a staphylococcal infection, or chronic, e.g. a tuberculous infection.

The lymph nodes may be involved in a reticulosis which is a type of neoplastic change occurring in the reticulo-endothelial system. An example of this type of disease is Hodgkin's disease.

In addition, lymph nodes may be enlarged when they are in the drainage area from a carcinoma. The removal of one lymph node may enable the diagnosis of the type of tumour which is involved.

Biopsy of a lymph node consists of the formal exposure of the lymph node and its removal in its entirety. Damage to the lymph node must be carefully avoided. The lymph node, once removed, is sent to the pathologist who will make a histological diagnosis.

33 Gynaecology

Charles de Boer

The gynaecologist is concerned with conditions, disturbances and abnormalities of the female genital tract together with its natural function, which is reproduction.

The problems that arise may require medical or surgical resolution but there are almost always emotional or psychological associations, which must not be overlooked.

DEVELOPMENT

The sex of an individual is primarily determined by the sex chromosomes. Two X chromosomes dictate that an ovary shall develop. A chromosome content XY dictates the development of a testis.

The genital tract develops in early embryonic life as a pair of cell cords at the back of the general body cavity; these are known as the Mullerian ridges. These grow tailwards, come to the midline and fuse together. As the fused cord approaches the surface it is met by a column of surface cells growing inwards. Canalization of these cords gives rise to the uterine tubes (Fallopian tubes), the uterus and the upper two-thirds of the vagina. The lowermost third is derived from the surface column of cells.

Adjacent to the developing Mullerian system is a forerunner of the renal excretory system (the mesonephros). This does no more than appear; it does not function. It remains as a vestigial remnant, a few tubules and a duct (Gaertner's duct).

If the sex gland should be a testis, chemical organizing substances from the testis alter the plan profoundly. The whole of the Mullerian system is suppressed and virtually no part of the uterovaginal system develops. The testis links up with the primitive renal excretory duct and takes it over for its own use as the vas deferens. At the same time an action on the hypothalamic control centre abolishes the monthly biorhythm so that subsequent testicular activity and male fertility is relatively constant. At a later stage in development testosterone from the testis stimulates the external fusions necessary to form the male external genitals, the penis and the scrotum.

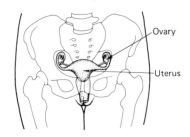

Anterior view of pelvic
cavity and genital organs
(a)

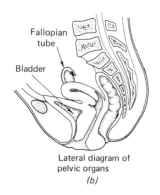

Lateral diagram of
pelvic organs
(b)

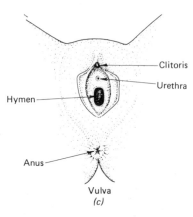

Vulva
(c)

Figure 33.1. (*a*) Oblique view of pelvic cavity and genital organs; (*b*) lateral diagram of pelvic organs; (*c*) vulva

In the female the Mullerian system develops without relation to the ovary. One or other side may fail to develop and different degrees of failure of fusion and canalization lead to the many variations of genital anatomy that are found. Because of the close embryological relationship of the renal and genital tracts, any congenital abnormality in one warns of abnormality in the other.

Abnormalities tend to be negative, i.e. a failure at some stage in a progressive plan of development. Very occasionally the female fetus (the developing baby in the uterus) becomes subjected to a male type hormone. This may result in a positive abnormality; fusions take place in the external genitalia to give a male appearance though the internal organs are female.

ANATOMY AND PHYSIOLOGY

The female genital organs lie deep in the pelvic cavity between the bladder in front and the rectum behind. They are well protected from external injuries as befits their important function (*Figure 33.1a*).

The ovaries

The ovaries are on each side. As well as producing eggs they have a very important role in the production of the female sex hormones. They are oval in shape with a longest diameter of about 3 cm. They are attached to the back of the broad ligament by folds of peritoneum (the mesovarium), but these do not envelop them, otherwise the eggs could not be released into the peritoneal cavity. They are also suspended from the brim of the pelvic cavity by their blood vessels. The ovarian arteries come directly from the abdominal aorta.

During childhood the ovaries are inactive. Once the general development of the body has reached a certain level, the controlling mechanisms in the hypothalamus begin to activate the reproductive apparatus. As childhood nutrition has improved over the years, so has the age of this activation been lowered. It is now not uncommon for breast development to begin at the age of nine years and menstruation about two years later. The whole process of puberty is of slow development; the control mechanisms react to tissue response in a very subtle way. The hypothalamus, influenced both by higher centres and by other endocrine glands, releases gonadotrophin-releasing factor (GRF), a relatively simple polypeptide (available as a synthesized pharmaceutical). This stimulates certain cells in the anterior part of the pituitary gland to elaborate and release follicle-stimulating hormone (FSH), the first of the pituitary gonadotrophic hormones. FSH is a complex molecule as yet only available as a purified extract from human urine. FSH acts upon the ovary to cause it to manufacture and release oestrogen. The whole of the ovary can do this but it is actively produced by the 'granulosa cells' that surround the ova.

Oestrogen, (a group term for a number of different steroid substances) is the first of the female sex hormones. It has its main action on the secondary sex organs such as the genital tract and the breasts, causing growth and activation of sexuality. As the oestrogen level rises so there will be growth; if the level falls there will be regression.

When a certain stimulation: response ratio has been reached the ovarian granulosa cells around one or more ova progress to form a cyst or follicle. One cyst becomes predominant and moves towards the surface of the ovary. The fluid in the follicle is particularly rich in oestrogen and the blood level of that hormone rises appreciably. This alters the function of the hypothalamus and pituitary gland and there is a relatively sudden release of the second pituitary gonadotrophic hormone. Luteinizing hormone (LH) acts on the ovary and the particular follicle that has been enlarging. The ovum inside it commences the chromosomal reduction division (meiosis) and 37 hours later is released from the follicle to be wafted in some way into the opening of the adjacent uterine tube. The remains of the follicle continue to respond to the surge of LH by intense cellular activity and the production of the second of the female sex hormones, progesterone, together with further amounts of oestrogen. Over the next 3 days the progesterone output is steadily increased as the remains of the follicle develop into a fully functioning corpus luteum. Without any further stimulation this will continue to function for about 10 days after which it begins to degenerate.

The uterine tubes (fallopian tubes)

The uterine tubes are about 10 cm long and are suspended from the broad ligament by a fold of peritoneum. The outer **fimbriated** end is relatively free and mobile, is trumpet-shaped and opens into the peritoneal cavity. The lumen steadily narrows down to the uterine end which leads into the cavity of the uterus.

The function of the tube is to receive the ovum when it is released from the ovary. Fertilization takes place in the outer part and then over the next two or three days the developing egg passes slowly down the tube. Though there is rapid cell division of the fertilized egg or zygote, there is little increase in total volume until it reaches the uterus.

Fimbriated Having an extremity or border bearing fringe-like processes or hairs.

Nutrition is maintained by the tubal fluid and the downward passage by a current of secretion activated by the cilia of the epithelium. The main flow through the tubes is however in an upward direction as the powerful contractions of the uterine muscle push uterine secretion in that direction. It is this activity that helped the sperms to reach the site of fertilization.

The uterus

The uterus is a pear-shaped muscular organ about 7½ × 6 × 2½ cm in size. It is flattened from front to back, bent forwards on itself and usually turned forwards in relation to the vagina into which its lower part is projecting. The upper part of the uterus is known as the body or corpus and the lower part as the neck or cervix. Within the body is a flat triangular cavity lined by a glandular epithelium known as endometrium. The upper angles of the triangle connect with the uterine tubes, the lower with the cervical canal which ends in the vagina at the cervical os or opening. The cervical canal is lined by a mucus-secreting epithelium.

The uterus is supported in the pelvic cavity by condensations of fibroelastic fascia round its main blood vessels and nerves. These are given the title of ligaments though they are only condensations in lines of strain. The main condensations around the uterine arteries are known variously as the transverse, lateral, cardinal or Mackenrodt's ligaments. The uterine arteries which are branches of the internal iliac arteries cross to the upper cervix from the side of the pelvis. The uterus is thus supported and has its main blood supply at its lower end, while its upper end is free to expand and to grow into the abdominal cavity, as in pregnancy, without any great vascular disturbance. The upper end is, however, linked to the anterior abdominal wall on each side and to the internal inguinal ring by the round ligament. It is these structures that hold up the peritoneal fold known as the broad ligament. They do not support the uterus.

In the midline the peritoneum leaves the front of the uterus to clothe the top of the bladder. Behind the uterus the peritoneum continues downwards over the back of the upper cervix and on to the posterior vaginal wall to form a deep peritoneal pouch before it sweeps backwards on to the rectum. This is also known as the pouch, or cul-de-sac, of Douglas. The lymphatic drainage of the uterus is to the iliac glands which lie along the vessels deep in the pelvis.

The function of the uterus is twofold. In the cavity the egg implants, the baby is grown (*Figure 33.2*) and in due course it is expelled by the process of labour. The cervix has to

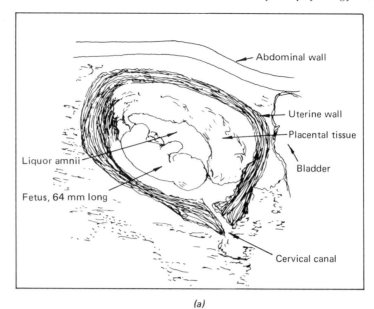

(a)

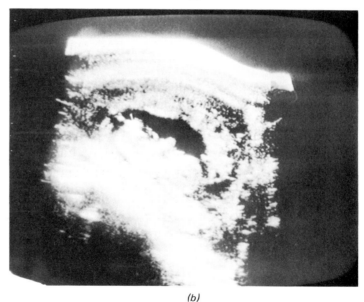

(b)

Figure 33.2. (*a*) Longitudinal section of an ultrasound picture of a 12-week pregnancy *in utero*; (*b*) ultrasound picture of a pregnancy showing a fork of crown rump length 64 which is equivalent to a pregnancy of 12 weeks and 4 days

permit the passage of the sperm that is to fertilize the egg yet keep out any infection and retain the growing baby until the time is right. The lining of the uterus, the endometrium, responds to oestrogen by thickening with glandular proliferation. The cervical glands respond by producing a thin clear mucus, through which active sperms have no difficulty in swimming. Dead or damaged sperms and organisms cannot normally negotiate this barrier. The egg which is fertilized just after ovulation takes three days to reach the uterus at which time the corpus luteum is fully functional. Progesterone has been circulating in increasing amounts since ovulation and the endometrium has responded by entering its secretory phase and releasing nutritious materials into the cavity. The cervical mucus, becoming thick and viscid, flows slowly out of the cervix effectively sealing off the cavity from the outside world.

Once in the uterine cavity the developing egg grows in volume and its surface sprouts projections known as chorionic villi. These, by enzymatic action, help to embed the egg into the endometrial lining of the uterus, which responds by further thickening and is henceforward known as 'the decidua'.

As the egg implants it opens up small maternal vessels so that the chorionic villi can project directly into the mother's bloodstream and more easily obtain the nutriments necessary for development; this is the beginning of the formation of the placenta or afterbirth. Occasionally the villi open up rather larger vessels and the egg may be displaced and lost as an early miscarriage or occasionally flushed from the uterus back into the uterine tube.

By the time the egg has implanted, the corpus luteum is reaching the end of its natural activity. If it is not to fail and allow a sudden fall in the levels of the ovarian hormones and subsequent uterine bleeding, it will need further encouragement. The chorionic epithelium provides the necessary stimulus by elaborating large quantities of a luteinizing gonadotrophin, 'Human Chorionic Gonadotrophin' (HCG), and it continues to do this until the placenta is fully established. The hormone is excreted in the mother's urine where its presence is the basis of laboratory tests for pregnancy.

If the egg is not fertilized it does not develop or implant, and it does not produce HCG. The corpus luteum fails and both of the ovarian hormone levels fall quite suddenly. The blood vessels in the endometrium go into a sudden and profound spasm. This is sufficiently prolonged to lead to the death of the superficial layers, which are then shed together with some blood which escapes when the vascular spasm relaxes. Clotting takes place and the bleeding is brought under control. The shed tissue liberates enzymes which bring about lysis of the clots so that the menstrual flow is fluid and not clotted. It is also believed that this tissue liberates prostoglandins which cause the uterus to contract strongly and possibly act on the ovary to reactivate oestrogen production.

A normal menstrual flow comes from an endometrium that has been stimulated by both oestrogen and progesterone. When the stimulation has been by oestrogen alone, its shedding may not be well ordered and the flow may be unduly prolonged and heavy.

Cyclical hypothalamic → pituitary → ovarian → uterine activity continues more or less regularly throughout the years of sexual maturity. Regular fertility and menstruation is only interrupted by pregnancy, but an end must come. No new ova are developed; the remaining eggs are as old as the individual. In time they are all used up and also gradually the ovarian tissue fails to respond to the command of the pituitary gonadotrophins. Ovulation does not occur and hormonal irregularity may develop. Menstruation may cease suddenly or gradually with decreasing loss and/or increasing intervals between periods. This constitutes the menopause, rarely later than 55, most commonly at 50 but frequently earlier than this. The failure of oestrogen production leads to an increase of pituitary stimulation, and the physiological changes that result constitute the 'climacteric'. Genital and breast atrophy, loss of tissue elasticity, alterations of vasomotor control leading to hot flushes, and a general reduction of physical and emotional drive manifest as depression can all occur. Hormone replacement therapy (HRT) has a dramatic effect on these symptoms, but cannot halt the march of time. It must be appreciated that HRT is prolonging the stimulation of the genital organs, especially the breasts and the uterus, and therefore medical supervision is required by these patients.

The vagina

The vagina is a simple passage. The cervix protrudes into its upper end, the lower end opens on the surface of the body into the vulval vestibule. Its lower limit is marked by the hymenal membrane or its remnant tags.

The vagina has no glands, such secretions as are found in the vagina coming either from the uterus or the cervical glands, or by transudation through its wall. The cells of the epithelium which contain quantities of the carbohydrate material glycogen, are shed and are acted upon by bacteria to liberate lactic acid.

The vaginal walls are supported by attachment above to the cervix and the pelvic fascia, especially where it is condensed as the supporting ligaments of the uterus; also by a general investing fascia. The vagina and other pelvic organs gain further support from the voluntary muscles which form the floor of the pelvic cavity. Deeply the levator ani muscles and certain small superficial muscles unite in a muscular complex which lies behind and below the lowermost third of the vagina separating it from the anal canal.

The vulva

This consists of the vestibule which lies between the labia minora; into the vestibule open the vagina, the urethra and the ducts of the Bartholin's glands. (*See Figure 33.1c.*) These glands have a lubricating function. The labia minora pass forward to meet and partially cover the clitoris which is suspended just under the pubic arch. Laterally lie the labia majora, fat-containing folds, hair-bearing on the outer surface and continuing forwards to blend with the hair-bearing area of the lower abdomen known as the mons veneris.

The vulva and lower third of the vagina are embryologically derived from surface tissues; they have a common blood supply and a lymphatic drainage to the lymphatic glands in the groins.

GYNAECOLOGICAL INVESTIGATION

All patients attending hospital are not unnaturally somewhat nervous. Kindness and reassurance will help. All members of staff can assist in this respect. A history of the condition is necessary and it is often important to relate subsequent findings to the phase of the menstrual cycle; therefore the date and nature of the last menstrual period should be recorded. The examination will be both general and particular, and the patient should be prepared for an examination of the breasts, the abdomen and the internal pelvic organs. A light which can be suitably directed, examining gloves, lubricant and swabs will be required, as well as speculae, sponge-holding forceps, culture swabs and cytological spatulae with glass slides and fixative. Vaginal bimanual examination of the pelvic organs may be made with the patient in the dorsal position (lying on her back) or lying on her side away from the examiner or in a special gynaecological chair. As well as a vaginal examination, a rectal examination may be made. A speculum is required in order to inspect the vaginal walls and the vaginal aspect of the cervix. It is usual to consider the taking of a cervical smear as part of the examination: a scrape biopsy is taken from the cervical os with a cytological spatula. This is immediately spread thinly on to a glass slide, fixed with a few drops of an alcohol—ether—wax mixture, labelled, and allowed to dry, before being sent to the laboratory for examination.

By such means the lower part of the genital tract can be adequately examined. The uterus and ovaries may be felt and assessed by the bimanual examination, but at this time adequate examination of the inside of the uterus cannot be made. For this reason it is frequently necessary for the patient to be admitted for examination under anaesthesia when the cervical os can be dilated to allow the introduction of instruments such as a curette to feel and take samples from the endometrium. Anaesthesia is not always required and small curettes can sometimes be introduced without preliminary dilatation.

The procedure of examination under anaesthesia, dilatation and curettage (EUA, D & C) should not be looked on as 'an operation' though it may be curative. It is a diagnostic examination procedure. Such patients are frequently dealt with on a 'Day Case' basis. Combined with the examination other diagnostic procedures may be carried out, biopsies may be taken, and minor operations performed.

SUBFERTILITY

About 10 per cent of couples are subfertile. The wives may come to the gynaecologist for help but it must be remembered that the husband bears an equal responsibility and must be investigated as well; it is not uncommon to find some degree of subfertility in each partner. Investigation is really a consideration of normal anatomy and physiology. To establish that the male is normal primarily requires the examination of a semen sample. The volume should be around 4 ml with a sperm count of around 50 million per ml (below 20 million per ml it must be considered as subfertile) and the majority must be normal in shape and activity. The sperm require to be taken up into the mucus secreted by the uterine cervical glands. If the mucus is examined microscopically at the time of fertility, usually about the middle of the monthly cycle and within 4 hours after normal intercourse (a post-coital test), many motile sperm should be present.

The simplest way of demonstrating that the cycles are ovulatory is by asking the patient to prepare a basal temperature chart (*Figure 33.3*). She must take her temperature in the mouth first thing each morning, and it should be as near to a sleeping temperature as is possible. For a trained nurse this is no problem but a lay person can have great difficulty and require detailed instruction both in taking and reading the thermometer and in charting the results. The chart is really demonstrating the development and function of the corpus luteum, for progesterone raises the basal body temperature by 0.5°C. Ovulation is thought to be related to the low point on the temperature chart and if the subsequent rise is delayed or inadequate, it is likely that the corpus luteum is insufficiently active. Extra stimulation by the

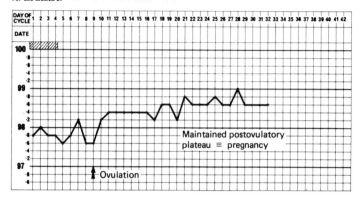

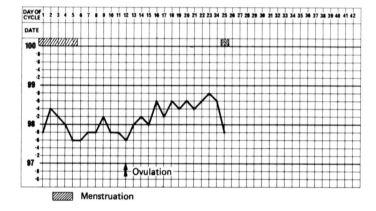

Figure 33.3. Simple infertility temperature charts

Insufflation The blowing of air or gas (either of which may carry powder) into a body cavity.

Hysterosalpingography The x-ray imaging of the cavity of the uterus and the fallopian tubes following the injection via the cervix of a radio-opaque material.

injection of Gonadotrophin LH (Pregnyl) at the time of fertility may effect an improvement.

Patients who have been pregnant previously and are subsequently unable to start again, suffer from secondary infertility. Especially in these, but also in cases of primary infertility, it is necessary to demonstrate that the female passages are patent. **Insufflation** with air or carbon dioxide will demonstrate patency, yea or nay, but to obtain a more exact picture **hysterosalpingography** is required (*Figure 33.4*). Further than this the uterine tubes may be inspected directly by laparoscopy while a dye is injected through the cervix to demonstrate patency.

Obstruction due to adhesions round the ends of the tubes can be treated by salpingolysis but adhesions are liable to reform. Closure of the outer end usually results in the tube becoming distended with fluid, a hydrosalpinx. When the

For the Month of

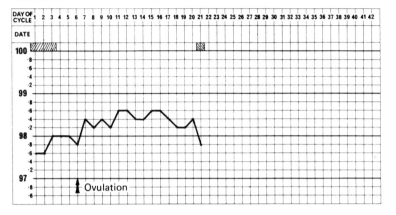

For the Month of

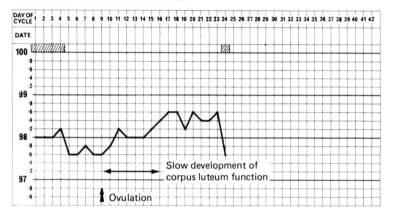

whole tube is affected the results of surgery are poor. Modern microsurgical techniques have improved the results but except for reversal of previous surgical sterilization they are not encouraging. The collection of an egg from the ovary, its fertilization outside the body and subsequent placement in the uterus via the cervix, as described by Steptoe, gives some hope for the future.

Failure of ovulation may be associated with an absence of menstruation, though not invariably so. If the levels of the pituitary hormones are high an ovarian failure, as at the menopause, is indicated and there is little that can be done. Low levels are associated with hypothalamic depression and drugs such as clomiphene and tamoxifen may help. Very low levels indicate a pituitary failure as may be found in Sheehan's syndrome. Pituitary hormone replacements in the form of Pergonal (FSH) and Pregnyl (LH) are available, but if

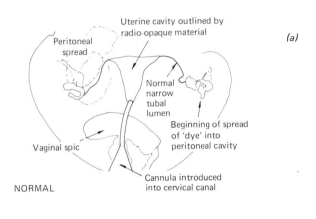

Uterine cavity outlined by
radio-opaque material

Peritoneal
spread

Normal
narrow
tubal
lumen

Beginning of spread
of 'dye' into
peritoneal cavity

Vaginal spic

Cannula introduced
into cervical canal

NORMAL

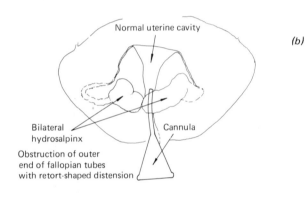

Normal uterine cavity

Bilateral
hydrosalpinx

Cannula

Obstruction of outer
end of fallopian tubes
with retort-shaped distension

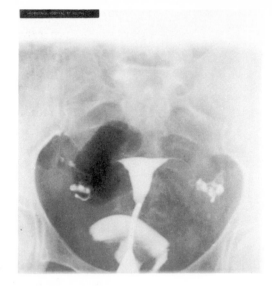

(a)

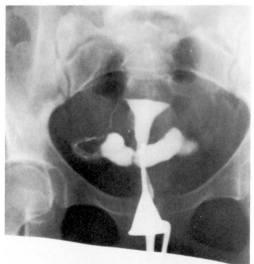

(b)

Figure 33.4. Hysterosalpingograms: (*a*)
normal; (*b*) abnormal

given in excess there may be profound overstimulation of the
ovary with serious general consequences as well as a risk of
multiple pregnancy.

Occasionally ovulation failure may be related to a pseudo-
lactational state, when serum prolactin levels are high. This
can be corrected with bromocriptine (Parlodel) when the
pituitary function will return to normal.

It must not be forgotten that some subfertility is in fact
a failure of implantation as is the situation when the patient
is using an intrauterine contraceptive device. Chronic
endometrial infections such as tuberculosis should be excluded
by the culture of premenstrual endometrial curettings. These

must be sent to the laboratory in an unfixed state. Treatment of tubercular infertility is effective provided that deep tissue damage has not occurred.

PREGNANCY WASTAGE

Abortion

Some 20 per cent of known pregnancies fail to proceed to a stage of viability and terminate as a miscarriage. The commonest cause for this is a genetic abnormality of the pregnancy; in other words 'a bad egg'. Practically all of these are aborted within the first three months of the pregnancy. Occasionally a good egg is miscarried and therefore any threat to miscarry or any bleeding in early pregnancy should be treated initially in a conservative way. Any vaginal bleeding should be considered as significant and the patient put to rest in bed; sedatives may help in this, but there is no specific treatment. Vitamins such as folic acid may be prescribed. Anything that may be passed should be kept for medical inspection.

Pregnancy tests give evidence of the production of chorionic gonadotrophin but this does not necessarily mean that the pregnancy is in a satisfactory state; only an ultrasonic scan can give direct evidence of the state of the developing fetus.

From a state of 'threatening to miscarry' the situation may become 'inevitable'. The uterus contracts to expel its contents. Recurrent bleeding, even amounting to recurrent floodings, will continue until the uterus has emptied itself. It is usual to speed up the process by giving oxytocic drugs or performing a dilatation and curettage under a general anaesthetic.

Infected abortion

If retained products of conception become infected, the patient may become very ill indeed with the development of an anaemic and shocked state to which is added a toxaemia from the absorption of materials derived from the invading bacteria as well as the bacteria themselves.

Symptoms are worsened if the uterus is unable to drain by reason of obstruction in the cervix. Simple dislodgement will have a rapid and beneficial effect but the patient may need blood transfusion, broad spectrum antibiotics, antitoxic sera and hydrocortisone before the uterus is safe to be evacuated surgically. Such patients may be desperately ill and feature in the maternal mortality statistics.

Missed abortion

A missed abortion is present when the pregnancy has died and has not yet been expelled. Sometimes the contents of the uterus are absorbed; alternatively, it is slowly discharged. In the process there can be an alteration of the blood-clotting mechanism. A test for the fibrinogen level (a Fibrindex) should be instituted before the uterus is subjected to curettage.

When the pregnancy has finally come to an end and the abortion concluded, it is important to enquire the future intention of the patient. If she regretted the loss of the pregnancy she should be advised to wait for at least one menstrual cycle before attempting to start a further pregnancy which is more likely than not to be perfectly normal. Alternatively she should be given adequate contraceptive advice and instruction for the future.

Mole

Hydatidiform or vesicular mole must be thought of as a new growth of chorionic tissue with all grades of malignancy from nil to chorioncarcinoma. This is a rare condition though less so in women of mongolian origin. It is in the nature of chorionic epithelium to invade and to produce chorionic gonadotrophin (HCG). Almost invariably a mole is associated with bleeding and vesicles of the mole may be expelled. The ovary responds to the excessive HCG by excessive luteinization and the formation of multiple cysts. The usual treatment is to encourage the expulsion of the mole with Pitocin (now available as a synthetic hormone, but naturally derived from the posterior part of the pituitary) to be followed by curettage. Subsequently a very careful follow-up is instituted in order to discover recurrent or persistent molar activity in the uterus or elsewhere at the earliest possible moment. Treatment is then by antimetabolic cytostatic drugs such as Methyltrexate and 7-Mercaptopurine. These halt the activity of the mole until such time as the natural foreign tissue rejection mechanisms of the body can be activated, for molar tissue is foreign to the mother. In an older woman a hysterectomy may be performed.

Recurrent abortion

Advice and treatment may be requested by the woman if she has had a number of miscarriages previously, in order to avoid a recurrence. The endometrium should be in an ideal state at the time of implantation. Luteinizing hormone (Pregnyl) given just prior to ovulation improves the production of progesterone by the corpus luteum without altering the subsequent menstrual cycle should fertilization and implantation fail to take place. The general nutritional and hormonal state of the patient must be considered and once a pregnancy has been established **depot injections** of progesterone and oestrogen supplements may be prescribed until such time as the placenta is fully formed and functioning.

Ectopic pregnancy

In a normal pregnancy the egg implants in the body of the uterus; a low implantation or an implantation in one of the angles leads to obstetric troubles. More dramatic are the results of implantation in the uterine tubes which may be due either to a hold up of the ovum in its passage down the tube by some obstruction or by a reflux from the uterus of an egg which has failed to implant in the correct site, possibly due to the presence of an intrauterine contraceptive device.

The lining of the uterine tube does not thicken in response to the implantation. Usually, local bleeding leads to the developing egg being aborted into the lumen; it may then be pushed out into the abdominal cavity. Alternatively the tube may rupture either dramatically with sudden intraperitoneal bleeding or more slowly with the chorionic villi obtaining a secondary implantation into any adjacent organ with subsequent fetal growth free in the abdominal cavity. Any sudden bleeding will be appreciated by the patient as sudden and severe abdominal pain which develops characteristically in a matter of seconds. Depending on the amount of the bleeding will be the ultimate degree of shock. Disturbance of the implantation leads to a reduction in the production of HCG and then oestrogen and progesterone, and the uterine lining will begin to shed. Abdominal pain is therefore followed later by vaginal bleeding.

When the tubal rupture occurs the patient experiences peritoneal shock and then the effects of internal bleeding. This is a surgical emergency. The sooner the bleeding can be arrested the better. Resuscitative measures will increase the bleeding, so must be combined with the surgical opening of the abdomen and the clamping of the bleeding site. It is more usual in the gynaecological wards to meet patients who present in a less dramatic way with a pelvic haematoma. Surgical treatment is then not so imperative but it is usual.

Though many patients who have suffered an ectopic pregnancy subsequently have a normal pregnancy, there is 10 per cent risk of recurrence.

Depot injection An injection into the tissues of a drug in such a form (often dissolved in oil) that it is slowly absorbed and thus exerts a prolonged effect

Midtrimester absortion

Pregnancies that persist and progress normally to the middle three months (midtrimester) are usually considered to be established but there is a small group which still come to grief. These are due to a defect in the capacity of the uterus to hold its contents. If the cervix is weak the pregnancy is expelled; if suspected then encircling sutures of non-absorbable material are inserted in order to support the incompetent cervix. Such patients should be warned that should the stitch start to fail in its purpose, it must be cut as soon as possible, otherwise it will be torn out causing damage. If the pregnancy arises in part of a double uterus or if the uterine wall is encumbered with inert fibroids, a midtrimester abortion or a premature labour may result. In between pregnancies these abnormalities can be corrected by surgical means. If the difficulty is due to a congenitally small uterus the failing pregnancy may stimulate sufficient growth to correct the deficiency and the next one may go to term without any treatment, though not uncommonly a supportive cervical suture is used.

FAMILY PLANNING

Advice on family planning is frequently sought by members of both sexes and not only in gynaecological wards and clinics. Coitus interruptus or 'pulling away' cannot be considered as reliable or satisfactory though it is practised by many couples; others, ethically, are required to rely on the so called 'safe period' by restricting intercourse to the less fertile time of the menstrual cycle. This method can be made more reliable by a study of the basal temperature chart as made out by the infertility patient. It is rare to find a second ovulation in any one menstrual cycle and the patient can consider herself safe once the postovulatory plateau of temperature has been reached.

Barrier methods such as the diaphragm or cap for the female and the sheath or condom for the male are reliable, especially if used with a spermicidal cream or pessary, and they have the great merit that they do not alter the physiology of the body. The diaphragm needs to be fitted accurately and training in insertion is required.

The modern contraceptive pill, a combination of oestrogen and progestogen works in three ways. The oestrogen content by feedback to the hypothalamus suppresses ovulation, the progestogen thickens the cervical mucus so that sperms cannot penetrate and, by an exhausting action on the endometrium, impedes implantation. When the 21-day course of tablets comes to an end there is 'withdrawal bleeding', a relatively scanty pseudoperiod. The hormone combination is necessary for a proper control of the endometrium though the progestogen alone, taken every day, is an equally effective contraceptive. Patients must be warned that intestinal upsets including 'mal de mer' and 'traveller's tummy' may lead to non-absorption and therefore risk, and also that they should never discontinue a course of the Pill without first seeking medical advice.

The disadvantages of the Pill are related to the state of pseudopregnancy that is induced. Any condition aggravated by pregnancy may be aggravated by the Pill: for example, in pregnancy there is a threefold increase in the natural risk of thrombosis — the same is true for the person on the Pill. The Pill acts mainly by suppressing the hypothalamus; when discontinued the restoration of fertility may be unduly delayed. Therefore patients who have infrequent periods should perhaps avoid the Pill for contraception or to obtain regular periods.

The intrauterine device (IUCD) is a foreign body introduced through the cervix. It lies in the cavity and prevents implantation of the fertilized ovum. This effect can be intensified by the presence of copper wire around the device. A failure rate of 1 to 2 per cent and an almost invariable increase in the menstrual flow must be accepted. There is also the danger of exacerbating any infection that might arise and of incurring ectopic pregnancy.

Sterilization of either the male or the female is becoming more popular than it used to be. In the female the uterine tubes can be obstructed or partially excised by either an abdominal or a transvaginal approach and whatever the procedure, it is often called 'tubal ligation' or TL. If the abdomen is opened only enough to introduce a laparoscope, the disturbance to the patient is minimal. Under laparoscopic control the tubes may be cauterized or clipped. No method of sterilization can be considered perfect and patients must be so warned though without causing undue alarm.

For male sterilization the operation required is vasectomy. This is a relatively simple and superficial procedure often carried out under a local anaesthetic. The peritoneal cavity does not have to be opened as in the female. After the operation fertility may remain for several weeks whilst sperm stored in the vas below the point of ligation are eliminated. The operation cannot be pronounced a success until two successive seminal fluid tests are reported as sperm-free.

The termination of pregnancy under the terms of the Abortion Act of 1968 should not be looked on as an alternative method of family planning; it is possibly a 'back-up'. When two medical practitioners, in good faith, consider that the risks to the mother or her existing children incurred by the continuation of the pregnancy are greater than if it is terminated, or there is a substantial risk that the baby is abnormal, then the termination before the 28th week is legal.

The great majority of fetal abnormalities are miscarried in early pregnancy. Only in such conditions as mongolism (Down's syndrome), spina bifida, and certain inborn metabolic defects, is the baby born alive. These, if suspected, may be identifiable by obtaining fetal material for laboratory examination by amniocentesis. This technique carries some risk so, as a rule, only mothers over the age of 35 or those with a previous or family history of trouble are tested. Preliminary placental localization by an ultrasound scan is usually carried out.

No doctor or nurse is obliged to take part in a termination procedure though a declaration of an ethical objection is expected if that is in fact the case. Before the 12th week of pregnancy a curettage of the uterus is carried out; often a suction curette is used. After 12 weeks the uterus is stimulated to empty itself by the use of an intrauterine prostaglandin injection together with intravenous Pitocin. The later the termination the greater the risks.

The request for termination is, amongst other things, a cry for help. Careful and considerate counselling is required and the patient should be helped to know her own mind at the time and for the future.

VAGINAL DISCHARGE

Physiological

Discharge is a frequent gynaecological complaint. Since all internal passages require lubrication a certain amount must be considered as normal. The natural secretion is produced by the mucus-secreting glands of the cervix; this is thin and fluid at the time of fertility but thick and viscid when the glands are influenced by progesterone. There is also a continuous oozing through the vaginal wall with a shedding of its superficial cells. These cells contain quantities of glycogen, a variety of starch, which encourages the growth of particular bacteria, the Lactobacilli, which convert the starch into lactic acid. It also encourages the growth of the yeast-type organism *Monilia albicans* (thrush). This may induce the symptom of soreness and irritation. Thrush is hardly an infection, more the flourishing of an organism, commonly present, in relation to the physiological alterations of pregnancy, the Pill, diabetes, and following treatments with antibiotics — a response to a change in the 'balance of nature'.

Thrush may require treatment, pessaries and creams containing antifungals such as nystatin and Miconozole, or painting with 0.5 per cent aqueous gentian violet.

Cervical erosion

'Cervical erosion' is a commonly diagnosed cause of vaginal discharge. This is a misnomer, for though the cervix looks red and raw it is because that is the appearance of normal columnar epithelium, especially when compared with the squamous epithelium of the vagina. Columnar epithelium may be visible due to a persistence of the prenatal state or, by reason of laceration, the cervix has been opened up to expose the epithelium of the canal, a state of ectropion. Columnar epithelium exposed to the acidity of the vagina slowly changes to squamous epithelium, but in the process deep cervical glands may become obstructed, become distended and form small cysts (Nabothian follicles). Treatment of a cervical erosion may be required. Cauterization, by heat, cold, or caustic chemicals is the usual technique.

Foreign bodies

Foreign bodies in the vagina cause discharge. Small girls lose buttons, beads and other small objects. More mature women lose tampons and surgeons and nurses fail to remove dressings or swabs. Small children are best examined under anaesthesia with the assistance of instruments borrowed from the ENT Department.

Infections

Vaginitis may be of venereal origin. The commonest infection is with a unicellular flagellated **protozoon**, *Trichomonas vaginalis*. There are complaints of irritation, soreness and a thin offensive discharge. The discharge is greenish in colour and may be slightly frothy; there is diffuse redness of the whole of the vagina. As with thrush, swabs should be sent to the laboratory in special transport media but direct microscopic examination of the discharge will reveal the organism. Treatment with metronidazole (Flagyl) should be given to both husband and wife.

Gonococcal infection and infection with *Chlamydia* has to be suspected. Investigation, including the tracing of contacts, and treatment is best carried out by a venereologist.

Protozoon An organism consisting of one cell.

Ascending infection

Infection may be introduced to higher levels in the genital tract soon after the birth of a baby or after an abortion, at the time of surgical intervention, and possibly at the time of mentruation by organisms such as gonococcus. Occasionally the infection may come from other abdominal organs such as the appendix or by a bloodstream spread. Chronic infection of the endometrium rarely gives clinical trouble because each month the infection is shed with the endometrium. The rare condition of tuberculous **endometritis** presents as an infertility problem.

Infection in the uterine tubes may present in an acute manner. Ruptured ectopic pregnancy, torsion of an ovarian cyst and appendicitis must be distinguished because surgical intervention is to be avoided in salpingitis. Chronic tubal infection often associated with tubal obstruction and **hydrosalpinx** can give rise to a great deal of pelvic disability. Surgical treatment may be required especially if a tender swelling is found, otherwise antibiotics and local heat in the form of pelvic shortwave diathermy are given.

Atrophic vaginitis

After the menopause the reduction of oestrogen leads to a general pelvic tissue atrophy and a reduction in the acidity of the vagina. Non-specific organisms may set up a low grade state of atrophic vaginitis. Oestrogens by mouth rapidly correct this situation.

Pyometra

Occasionally, as part of the atrophy, the cervix may become stenosed. A collection of fluid in the uterus is almost certain to become infected and every so often an offensive pyometra (pus in the uterus) bursts forth. Dilatation of the cervix is required but at the same time it is necessary to exclude other and less benign causes of stenosis.

OVARIAN TUMOURS

Endometritis Inflammation of the lining of the uterus.

Hydrosalpinx A fallopian tube distended with fluid.

The ovary lies deep in the pelvis and, without a surrounding capsule, is able to enlarge to a considerable size before it produces any symptoms. Some enlargements are indeed physiological. All ovarian tumours are potentially malignant.

Physiological

The follicular cyst

The follicular cyst in which an ovum is brought to maturity may fail to rupture. This is particularly liable to happen at the time of puberty and the menopause, both times of ovarian—hypothalamic imbalance. While a follicle persists, oestrogen production is maintained; this results in excessive endometrial hyperplasia. After a while this endometrium is shed in a prolonged and heavy period. The situation constitutes the syndrome of metropathia. The hormone that is missing is progesterone — if this is prescribed in a cyclical manner adequate control can be obtained.

A somewhat similar, though potentially more serious situation can arise when a patient is treated with FSH in order to induce follicular development. Overdosage can lead to profound hyperoestrogenism.

Luteal cyst

Excess stimulation of the corpus luteum can lead to multiple cyst formation. Rarely seen under normal physiological conditions, it is not uncommon in association with a **hydatidiform** molar pregnancy.

New growth cysts of the ovary

New growth cysts of the ovary are of three general types.

(1) Serous cysts which may or may not have papillae inside them. They contain serous fluid.
(2) Mucinous cysts which are usually multilocular and may even feel solid. They contain mucinous material.
(3) Dermoid cysts in which the contents are sebaceous material (dermoid butter) mixed with hair. The hair usually arises from a node in the wall of the cyst and in this node many other types of tissue may be found.

There is always a danger that any one of these cysts may undergo a malignant change if it is not primarily malignant. Other than this any ovarian tumour can undergo torsion both suddenly and recurrently: episodes of severe abdominal pain develop in a matter of minutes as vascular strangulation occurs.

Cysts may rupture or suffer internal haemorrhage either spontaneously or as a result of trauma. If dermoid butter gets spilt into the peritoneal cavity it excites an intense inflammatory response.

Tumours of the ovary may also be due to a secondary spread of cancer from a primary growth elsewhere; uterus,

Hydatidiform Having a cystic appearance.

breast and the colon are particularly suspect. Because of the absence of a capsule there is little resistance to growth and such secondary growths may be very large and present even before the primary has given symptoms. If the primary is from a mucus-secreting epithelium the secondary has a characteristic microscopic signet ring appearance (a Krukenberg's tumour).

Solid tumours of the ovary are relatively rare. These may secrete oestrogens (granulosa cell tumour) or even androgens which will have a virilizing effect, but usually they are functionless. They are all potentially malignant and because of this any ovarian tumour or any lump that could be an ovarian tumour must be explored as soon as possible.

Congenital cysts

Structures adjacent to the ovary may be responsible for the swelling. Cysts can arise from congenital mesonephric remnants which lie in the broad ligament or at the sides of the vagina.

Tubo-ovarian cysts

Distension of the uterine tube after inflammatory obstruction of the fimbriated end gives rise to a retort-shaped swelling (a hydrosalpinx). When the infection is more acute an abscess involving both the tube and the ovary may be found (tubo-ovarian abscess).

The chocolate cyst

An inflammatory response in the pelvic tissues arises in the condition of endometriosis. Women with few or no children in their middle thirties develop endometrial deposits in areas related to the peritoneum. The mechanism is uncertain: either endometrial cells reach the abnormal site by menstrual reflux along the uterine tube, by lymphatic or venous spread or by a process of cell change (metaplasia). The ectopic endometrium will bleed each month as the normal endometrium is shed and there will be a local dense fibrotic response except on the ovary where this response is so minimal that the blood collects to form a cyst of clinically appreciable size. This blood undergoes change to a material with the colour and consistency of melted chocolate, hence the name 'a chocolate cyst'.

The symptoms that result from endometriosis will relate not only to the position of the endometrial patch but also to the menstrual flow. There is always a degree of discomfort related to the whole duration of the menstrual flow, a concurrent dysmenorrhoea.

Operative exploration

The investigation of the majority of ovarian tumours is by laparotomy. Until they have been inspected they must be considered to be malignant. The incision may have to be a large one to avoid any risk of rupture of the cyst while it is being extracted. If it is benign, a simple excision (ovarian cystectomy) is carried out. The tumour may be obviously malignant with multiple peritoneal secondary deposits and ascites. If possible the main mass is removed and then the patient is treated with cytostatic drugs. These are quite effective in controlling the recurrence of ascites but the ultimate prognosis is poor.

A chocolate cyst or a large area of endometriosis is usually excised. If the bowel is involved resection may be required. Small areas are treated by diathermy cauterization but if they are not generating symptoms they may be ignored. A respite from menstruation either from a pregnancy or medical treatment, or by the natural menopause will allow the natural fibrotic tissue response to obliterate the endometrium. Medical treatment is to suppress the normal menstrual cycle for 6 to 9 months either by a combination of oestrogen and progesterone, simulating pregnancy, or by hypothalamic suppressant drugs such as Danazol.

DYSMENORRHOEA

Pain associated with menstruation is a common complaint. Endometriosis gives rise to tension and pain during the course of the flow. Inflammatory conditions increase the natural congestion of the pelvic tissues and in the premenstrual phase this congestion may be appreciated as pain which will be eased or changed by the onset of the flow. At the same time associated with this congestion there may be a profound disturbance of emotional response. Depending on which symptom predominates, the condition is one of premenstrual tension or congestive dysmenorrhoea.

If a causative pelvic condition can be discovered and treated, well and good; but often there is no local lesion. If the main symptom is one of congestion, diuretics may be helpful.

Mental tensions respond to psychotropic drugs (tranquilizers) or to vitamin B$_6$ (pyridoxine). Alteration of the hormone balance by giving extra progesterone or a modified progestogen such as Duphaston is sometimes effective. Complete suppression of hypothalamic activity by Danazol will be effective but rarely justified.

Much more commonly, especially in younger patients, the dysmenorrhoea is 'spasmodic'. Characteristically this first presents some 3 to 4 years after the start of menstrual cycles in association with the development of fertility. Pain of variable severity is experienced just before or on the first day of the flow. Usually it is of a continuous nature with momentary spasms of increased severity. The pain may be sufficiently severe to generate vasovagal disturbances such as diarrhoea, vomiting, headaches and faintness, and there is often an element of misery and depression. The passage of years usually brings some relief but the development of full sexual maturity with the delivery of the first child usually leads to the disappearance of the pain.

It is believed that the pain is ischaemic in origin, the strength of the uterine contractions which are related to the preceding balance between oestrogen and progestogen, being sufficient to reduce the uterine blood flow. Possibly prostoglandins play a part in initiating the contractions. Simple analgesics may be insufficient to control the pain. Altering the balance of oestrogen and progestogen by prescribing the Pill is usually effective but if this is contra-indicated then antiprostoglandin drugs such as flufenamic acid (Arlef) may be valuable. Nerve-blocking techniques which include the use of counter-irritants, acupuncture and presacral neurectomy are occasionally used and may give relief in selected cases.

UTERINE TUMOURS

Fibroids, or more correctly fibromyomata, consist of a mixture of muscle tissue and fibrous tissue. They arise in the wall of the uterus and under the influence of the ovarian hormones slowly increase in size, compressing the surrounding tissues to form a false capsule around each one. Since the blood supply to a fibroid is from the compressed capsule, in all but the smaller fibroids degenerative changes are found. In pregnancy when there is a particular stimulus to growth there may be the sudden development of necrosis, a state known as Red Degeneration, the fibroid becoming tender and painful. Otherwise fibroids cause symptoms by their position. An abdominal mass may be discovered as a chance finding. Involvement of the uterine cavity will disturb menstruation, the loss being increased with the rhythm of the cycle unchanged. Only if the fibroid projects into the cavity as a polyp will intermenstrual bleeding occur. Occasionally the presence of fibroids may be associated with infertility or mid-trimester abortion. Pressure effects on adjacent organs are rare and it is doubtful if malignant change ever occurs.

The commonest reason for surgical intervention is the uncertainty of the diagnosis. Any pelvic mass could be of ovarian origin and therefore malignant potential. Simple removal of the fibroids (myomectomy) preserves the possibility of childbearing without any significant risk though more frequently, as a safer procedure, a hysterectomy will be performed. Patients worry that this will precipitate the change of life (or climacteric) and reduce their femininity, but this is not so unless the ovaries are removed at the same time. If required, symptoms such as hot flushes and loss of tissue elasticity can be cured or retarded by giving hormone replacement therapy (HRT), though this is inadvisable when there has been malignant disease of the genital tract. If HRT is given for menopausal symptoms if the uterus is present, there is a risk that bleeding may be induced. To avoid this, it is usual to give a progestogen as well as the oestrogen and to give it in a 3-weeks-in-4 cyclical fashion. Bleeding during therapy requires investigation.

Menorrhagia means excessive menstrual loss. The amount must be subjective and personal though the number of sanitary tampons or towels used is an index of volume. Abnormal flow should not interfere with social activities or lead to anaemia though any blood **dyscrasia** and even anaemia itself can cause menorrhagia. Local disturbance of the endometrium by an IUCD not infrequently leads to excessive loss. The behaviour of the endometrium as it is shed is related to the preceding oestrogen—progestogen balance. Near puberty and near the menopause there is often a deficiency of progesterone and this leads to excessive and prolonged loss with the endometrium in a state of cystic hyperplasia, the syndrome of metropathia. This is treated by giving the patient progestogens by mouth. At other ages the commonest cause of a single upset period is an upset pregnancy, an abortion, and may need treatment as such.

Major hormone disturbances may stop the periods (amenorrhoea) but myxoedema, the state of thyroid deficiency, is associated with menorrhagia. At the highest levels the emotions have a part to play; mediated through the hypothalamus which is also in control of the rhythm of the cycle.

Dyscrasia A developmental or metabolic disorder

MALIGNANT DISEASE OF THE UTERUS

Carcinoma of the body of the uterus

A carcinoma may arise in the endometrium. Overstimulation by oestrogen is thought to be an aetiological factor. Women between the ages of 40 and 60 who have had few or no children are often obese; and if they are postmenopausal, have been late in finishing their periods and have suffered excess loss (metropathia), at that time they are predisposed to carcinoma. The woman presents with postmenopausal bleeding (PMB) or discharge and such symptoms must be considered as malignant until proved otherwise. Before the menopause, intermenstrual bleeding will occur.

A diagnostic curettage is almost mandatory. Confirmed malignancy is treated by a hysterectomy and since spread to the ovaries is relatively early, the ovaries and uterine tubes are removed as well (total hysterectomy and bilateral salpingo-oöphorectomy). Patients unfit for surgery can be treated with radiotherapy. Progesterone in high dose slows down the rate of growth of endometrial tissue and, as a weekly depot injection, it is useful in extensive or recurrent growths. Because many of the patients are in poor general health, the 10-year survival rate is low even if removal of the growth has been adequate.

Carcinoma of the cervix

Carcinoma of the cervix arises in the 30 to 50 age group. This tumour, usually of squamous cells, produces either a fungating mass or an ulcer. There is irregular bleeding, often precipitated by coitus or clinical examination, and an offensive discharge. In younger women the growth may have been present for a number of years in a pre-invasive, symptomless state, and be relatively slow to extend. In older women the malignant process seems to be more rapid. It is hoped that the cervical smear campaign will bring the young and early cases to treatment before invasion has taken place.

The cancer is 'staged' on clinical examination according to its degree of spread.

Stage 0:   Pre-invasive.
Stage I: Limited to the cervix.
Stage II: Just involving adjacent tissues.
Stage III: Spreading to the lateral pelvic wall or lower vagina.
Stage IV: Spreading to other organs such as the bladder or outside the confines of the pelvis.

The close relationship of the ureters to the cervix means that ureteric obstruction is likely to occur and urinary assessment (intravenous pyelogram (IVP) and cystoscopy) is an important part of the general assessment.

As a rule, treatment is by radiotherapy. Radium almost always cures the local lesion. The pelvic lymphatic field must be treated with some form of irradiation (e.g. x-rays) but dosage is limited to the sensitivity of the adjacent organs.

Early cases can expect an 80 per cent chance of a 5-year survival, but the overall figure is under 50 per cent.

An early growth in a young woman is sometimes treated by radical surgical excision (Wertheim's hysterectomy) in order to avoid the delayed effects that radiotherapy has on the remaining pelvic tissues.

The cervical smear

A cervical smear can be considered as a 'scrape biopsy' of the cervix. Cells are collected with an Ayre's spatula, immediately spread on to a glass slide and fixed with an alcohol–ether–wax mixture. After staining in the laboratory the cells are examined by a cytologist who reports on the appearances of individual cells. It is like looking at the faces in a crowded street. Usually they are normal and happy, but if some of the faces are scowling, or worse, have knives between their teeth, suspicions must be aroused — trouble is brewing. The only way of discovering what these ruffians are about is by direct examination and histological examination of a biopsy. Either a whole cone of tissue is removed or selected pieces are removed. Examination with a surface microscope called the colposcope may help in this selection.

The removal of a cone may cure this condition but the histological report of an incomplete removal of a pre-invasive lesion may lead to a hysterectomy. At this stage the cure is almost 100 per cent.

There is some evidence that early and promiscuous sexual intercourse is a predisposing factor in the development of cervical cancer. Women at risk are advised to have a smear test every 2 or 3 years, but it is important that they should realize that the test is directed at cervical cancer alone.

Carcinoma of the vulva

Carcinoma of the vulva is a condition seen in older women in the 55 to 85 age group. It usually presents as an ulcer on the vulva but is not infrequently associated with irritation due to leucoplakia. This is characterized by areas of whiteness and thickening of the skin and this is possibly precancerous.

Excision of the whole of the vulva together with the lymphatic glands from both groins appears at first sight to be a very radical operation. The area has to heal by granulation, which is a slow process, but the end result is excellent and the prognosis is good.

UTERINE DISPLACEMENTS

Retroversion

The cervix is suspended in the centre of the pelvis by its 'ligaments'; from this the vagina hangs, passing downwards and forwards to the surface. The uterine body leans forward over the top of the bladder in some 80 per cent of women but in 20 per cent it leans backwards, a congenital retroversion. Occasionally an anteverted uterus acquires a retroverted position. Symptoms then arise, some from the abnormal position and some because of its causation. Almost every gynaecological symptom, excluding stress incontinence, can be implicated. Manipulation of the uterus and encouragement of it to stay forwards by the insertion of a Hodge pessary, which is designed for this purpose, should relieve the symptoms. If the condition recurs when the pessary is removed, then some form of ventrosuspension operation will be required.

Should a pregnancy arise in a retroverted uterus, the position is usually corrected spontaneously. Should this fail to occur, the enlarging uterus becomes trapped in the pelvis, generates tensions, and around the 13th week causes retention of urine. Catheterization will be required until the tensions are resolved by the anterior uterine wall becoming sacculated.

Prolapse

For many reasons the supports of the uterus may stretch: age weakens elastic tissue, some of which may be of poor quality, and also stresses and strains, either long-standing (e.g. from tight corsetting) or acute (e.g. in childbirth) are sometimes too great. If there is muscle weakness or paralysis, these tendencies are exaggerated. The uterus will hang lower in the pelvis than it should, possibly partially outside the body and even completely outside (procidentia). As it descends, it will drag out the vagina and allow displacement of adjacent organs.

As an alternative the vagina may have been stretched and it then sags in folds. Traction by the vaginal wall on the cervix may cause cervical elongation.

The symptoms that result are those of a lump appearing, backache, lower abdominal ache and interference in the functions of the rectum and the bladder. If the cervix comes outside, it may become ulcerated due to trauma and congestion.

Depending on which particular parts of the genital tract come down, the descriptive term urethrocele, cystocele, uterine prolapse, hernia of the pouch of Douglas and rectocele will be applied.

The treatment advised will depend on a number of factors, particularly the age and condition of the patient. Young women, especially those who have just had a baby, will improve with time. Exercises to strengthen the pelvic muscles and pelvic **faradic** stimulation may be combined with a temporary mechanical support (a pessary). For frail and elderly patients it may be wise to avoid operative treatment and for these pessaries may give a control or even a cure, for increasing age reduces the physical strains and stresses.

If a pessary is used, the patient must be seen at regular intervals, not because the pessary deteriorates — modern plastic ones do not — but because vaginal ulceration due to pressure from the pessary is liable to occur. At each visit the pessary must be removed and the vagina carefully inspected; if all is well the pessary may be reinserted. The insertion of a flexible pessary can be made much more comfortable and easy if it is first compressed by wrapping a piece of tape around its waist and securing it with a Spencer Wells clip; once inserted the clip is undone and the tape unravelled.

The operative treatment for prolapse will be related to the particular deficiency that is present. If the uterus is descending because its ligaments have stretched, it is usual to combine a vaginal hysterectomy with a repair operation (a colporrhaphy). If the uterus is well supported but the cervix elongated, amputation of the cervix will be combined with the repair (the Manchester operation).

Any form of repair attempts to replace 'perished' elastic tissue with scar tissue. Scar tissue takes time to consolidate so patients must be warned of the importance of convalescence.

BLADDER PROBLEMS IN GYNAECOLOGY

In association with an anterior vaginal wall prolapse there will be a sagging of the posterior wall of the bladder. Urine may stagnate in this pouch and then infection is liable to develop. Irritation of the bladder leads to frequency of micturition both by night as well as by day and the desire to pass urine may be so strong that the normal voluntary

Faradic Electricity produced by a rapidly alternating current.

inhibition is overcome and the patient may then complain of urgency incontinence.

This is a different symptom from that of stress incontinence which arises when the natural urethral closing mechanism is impaired. The patient complains that she leaks a small quantity of urine whenever she strains. Laughing and coughing generate quite severe rises in the intra-abdominal pressure and leaking may occur then.

Urgency has to be distinguished from stress, but not infrequently they occur together and very careful assessment is required. Stress incontinence may be helped by physiotherapy, but if severe will need some form of bladder neck (the urethrovesical junction) operation. The bladder neck can be approached either through the vagina or from in front through the space between the bladder and the back of the pubic symphysis (e.g. the Marshall Marchetti procedure). Occasionally a dual approach is used.

Incontinence or leaking of urine is also to be encountered when a fistula is present, between either the bladder or the ureter and the vagina. A fistula may be present as a congenital abnormality or arise as a complication of a difficult obstetric delivery or of a surgical procedure such as a hysterectomy.

Incontinence may also develop if there is a functional obstruction of the urethra, a state of overflow incontinence. It must not be forgotten that after any operation and especially a gynaecological one, the patient may find great difficulty in passing urine and while the introduction of infection is to be feared, the risks of retention may be worse. Aseptic catheterization and the use of techniques for preventing ascending infection are very important nursing duties.

Glossary

Achalasia Failure of relaxation, for example, of a sphincter.

Achlorhydria Absence of free hydrochloric acid in the gastric juice.

Acholuria Absence of bile pigments in the urine.

Achondroplasia A hereditary condition of dwarfism due to early fusion of the epiphyses and diaphyses of the long bones.

Acidosis Increased acidity of the blood.

Acinus The basic unit of any glandular structure. It consists of secreting cells gathered round a small central tubule, which ultimately drains into a large collecting duct.

Acromegaly A disease characterized by progressive enlargement of the bones of the head, chest, hands and feet.

Actinomycosis A chronic inflammatory disease due to infection with a fungus, *Actinomyces israelii.*

Adenocarcinoma A carcinoma of gland-like structure.

Adenoma Benign tumour of glandular tissue.

Adrenalectomy Excision of an adrenal gland.

Adrenaline A hormone produced by the adrenal medulla.

Adrenocorticotrophic hormone (ACTH) A hormone which stimulates the cortex of the adrenal gland.

Aerobic bacteria Bacteria growing only in the presence of oxygen.

Aetiology The science of investigation of the cause of disease.

Agranulocytosis Relative or total lack of the neutrophil leucocytes (white blood cells) rendering the patient incapable of resisting infection.

Albumin Important type of protein in body fluids, tissues and blood plasma.

Alkalotic A state in which the body fluids and tissues are more alkaline than normally.

Allograft (homograft) A tissue graft between two unrelated members of the same species.

Alveolus The smallest type of air space in the lung.

Amelanitis Without black pigment.

Amenorrhoea Pathological absence of the menstrual discharge (i.e. due to a cause other than pregnancy, lactation or the menopause).

Amniocentesis Puncture of the amniotic sac, which contains the fetus, to remove amniotic fluid.

Amniotic fluid The fluid which surrounds the fetus.

Amoebic dysentery An inflammatory disease of the bowel due to infection with the organism, *Entamoeba histolytica.*

Anaerobic bacteria Bacteria which grow in the absence of oxygen.

Analgesic A drug or technique which reduces pain without inducing unconsciousness.

Anaphylaxis A violent reaction usually to a foreign protein to which the subject is sensitive.

Anaplastic Characterized by imperfect development or a change back to a more primitive form of cell.

Anastomosis Joining together. May refer to a surgical procedure such as the joining of two blood vessels.

699

Androgen A general name for the male sex hormones.

Androgenic Productive of male characteristics.

Anencephalic Characterized by having no brain.

Aneurysm Dilatation of an artery due to disease of its wall or to escape of blood from the artery to beneath its outermost coat.

Angiography Radiology of blood vessels by injection of a radio-opaque contrast.

Anoplasty Plastic repair of the anus.

Anorexia Lack of appetite.

Antacid Preparation taken by mouth which neutralizes the acid in the stomach, for example, sodium bicarbonate.

Antemetic A remedy to arrest or prevent vomiting.

Anthrax A very serious pustular, or more widespread, infection derived from cattle and sheep.

Antibiotic Drug obtained from moulds which prevents the growth of, or destroys, bacteria.

Antibody A specific protein (immunoglobulin) produced in response to stimulation by antigen and capable of reacting specifically with it.

Anticoagulant A drug retarding or preventing the clotting of blood (for example, heparin).

Antigen A substance which, under suitable circumstances, can stimulate a specific immune response.

Anti-oestrogen Will usually act by blocking the effect of an oestrogen at the site of its action.

Antitetanus serum A serum produced by the body as a reaction to the introduction of tetanus bacteria. It neutralizes the toxin.

Aphthous ulcers Shallow painful erosions, usually of the mouth.

Aplastic anaemia A type of anaemia in which there is failure of proper development of red blood cells.

Apnoea Temporary cessation of breathing.

Appendicectomy The surgical removal of the appendix. By convention this always refers to the vermiform appendix (opening off the caecum) rather than any of the other numerous appendices in the body. 'Appendectomy' is the American term for the same operation. The suffix '-ectomy' is derived from the Greek *ectome* = a cutting out, hence it is used with the appropriate prefix to indicate, in a word, the removal of an organ (e.g. mastectomy − of the breast; gastrectomy − of the stomach etc.).

Arrhythmia Irregular heartbeat.

Ascites An accumulation of fluid in the peritoneal cavity.

Asphyxia Death by obstruction of the respiratory passages.

Aspiration (1) Removal of fluid or air from a body cavity by needle and syringe, or suction apparatus. (2) The breathing in of fluid into small air passages (leading to, for example, aspiration pneumonia).

Ataxia Loss of control over movements and balance.

Atelectasis Local collapse of a segment of lung.

Atheroma Fatty degeneration of the walls of arteries.

Atresia Failure of development, for example, of an organ.

Atrial fibrillation A quivering unco-ordinated movement of the atrium of the heart. This gives an irregular pulse and a characteristic electro-cardiograph pattern.

Atrophy Wasting of a tissue or organ.

Auscultation Listening to sounds produced in any part of the body, usually with a stethoscope.

Auto-immunity A disorder of the body's immune system, whereby antibodies are formed to the patient's own tissue, which is then slowly destroyed.

Autosome An ordinary paired chromosome as distinguished from an extra chromosome found in some abnormal conditions.

Avulsion Forcible separation of a part or structure.

Balanitis Inflammation of the glans penis.

Basophil A tissue which takes the stain of basic (alkaline) dyes.

Bassinet A type of cradle for babies.

Bilirubin A red bile pigment.

Biopsy Inspection during life (from the Greek *bios* = life, *opsis* = view; cf. necropsy = inspection after death), usually relating to small pieces removed from the body for a tissue diagnosis.

Bolus A rounded mass.

Bougie Tapered, often flexible, surgical instrument for passing into and dilating body passages, especially if narrowed by stricture.

Bowel flora The naturally occurring bacterial content of the lumen of the bowel.

Bradycardia Slow heart rate.

Bronchial asthma A disease characterized by difficulty in breathing out, which shows itself as a wheeze and breathlessness. It is due to contraction of the muscles in the small air passages.

Bronchiectasis Severe infection and cavitation of lung tissue.

Bronchoscopy Operation of inserting a long metal viewing tube into the bronchus for diagnostic purposes or to remove obstruction.

Bronchospasm Constriction of the muscle of the bronchial tree, usually giving rise to an audible wheeze, as in bronchial asthma.

Bruit Sound originating from an irregularity in a blood vessel.

Bulla A blister.

Cachexia Extreme generalized wasting due to disease or gross malnutrition.

Caecum A pouch of the gut forming the first part of the large bowel. Usually situated in the lower right abdomen.

Calculus A stone.

Calorie A unit of energy. In nutritional studies this refers to a 'large' Calorie or kilocalorie. In SI units this has been replaced by the joule so that one 'large' Calorie = 4.2 kJ (kilojoules).

Cannula A tube to be inserted into a body cavity, duct or blood vessel to effect a communication with the exterior.

Carbuncle An infection of the skin and subcutaneous tissue by *Staphylococcus aureus* in which there is diffuse necrosis of the subcutaneous tissue.

Carcinoma A malignant tumour arising from epithelial cells; a more precise term than 'cancer' which may also be used, more loosely, to describe any malignant growth.

Caruncle A small fleshy excrescence.

Caseation A form of degeneration or necrosis in which tissues are changed into a cheesy mass.

Celestin tube A type of tube that can be passed through a cancer obstructing the oesophagus to allow fluids and semi-solid food to pass.

Cellulitis A diffuse inflammation (usually bacterial) of connective tissues.

Chancre The primary ulcer of syphilis.

Cholangitis Inflammation of the bile ducts.

Cholecystenterostomy The making of a direct communication between the gall bladder and the intestine.

Chordotomy Surgical division of a nerve tract, or tracts, of the spinal cord.

Chromosome One of several rod-shaped bodies evident in a cell nucleus at the time of cell division.

Chyle Milky-white emulsified fat in the lymph vessels of the small intestine.

Chyme Partly digested food in a liquid state.

Cilia Fine processes on the surface of cells which act together to propel particles of fluid.

Cirrhosis Progressive fibrosis throughout an organ, usually referring to the liver.

Colectomy Surgical removal of the colon.

Colitis Inflammation of the colon.

Collateral A by-pass circulation circumventing a blocked blood vessel.

Colostomy An opening made through the abdominal wall into the colon. The suffix 'ostomy' is derived from the Greek *stoma* = mouth, hence it is used with a single prefix to indicate a surgically made external opening (e.g. ileostomy; ureterostomy etc.) or with a double prefix to indicate an opening fashioned between one internal cavity and another (e.g. gastrojejunostomy, choledochoduodenostomy (*choledochus* = bile duct) etc.).

Colporrhaphy Repair of a vaginal prolapse. In this condition the uterus sags down into the vagina.

Coma depasse Massive irretrievable brain damage.

Comminuted Fragmented.

Compatibility Two individuals whose cells carry different HLA (q.v.) and ABO blood groups may be compatible although not identical. In other words, grafts and blood transfusions may be given by one to the other without rejection taking place.

Complement A substance comprising a system of immunologically non-specific proteins, present in fresh serum and which are necessary for the lysis of cellular antigens in the presence of antibody.

Compound fracture A fracture exposed because of a cut or a tear of the overlying tissues.

Concussion Invisible state of injury of the nerve cells producing an alteration of the state of consciousness.

Conjugation The combination of one compound with another to form a product of biological importance.

Contusion Bruising.

Coronal Plane from side to side of the skull.

Coronary thrombosis The obstruction of a coronary artery by a thrombus; this may cause death of the area of the heart muscle that becomes deprived of blood (a myocardial infarct).

Corticosteroid Hormones secreted by the cortex of the adrenal glands and connected with carbohydrate and protein metabolism (glucocorticoids, cortisone, etc.); with water and electrolyte balance (mineralocorticoids — aldosterone); male sex hormones (androgens) and female sex hormones (oestrogens).

Craniectomy Operation of removing parts of bone of the skull.

Craniotomy Operation of cutting a flap of skull bone which is replaced at the end of the operation.

Crepitus A grating noise produced when two rough surfaces are rubbed together.

Cretinism Hypothyroidism in infancy.

Crohn's disease A non-specific inflammation of an area of the intestine.

Cushing's syndrome A disease produced by excess production of steroids from the adrenal cortex characterized by obesity of the face and trunk, abdominal striae, hypertension and the presence of glucose in urine.

Cyanosis A blue appearance of the skin and mucous membranes due to deficient oxygenation of the blood.

Cystostomy Operation to make an opening in the bladder.

Cystoscopy The inspection of the interior of the fluid filled urinary bladder through an instrument. The suffix 'oscopy' is derived from the Greek *skopein* = to watch, hence it is used with a suitable prefix to denote inspection of various body cavities or internal chambers (e.g. ophthalmoscopy — of the eye; arthroscopy — of a joint, etc.).

Cytotoxic agent A substance acting as a cellular poison.

De-aeration Removal of air, especially from the lung.

Debridement Clearing a wound of foreign matter and dead tissue.

Decerebrate posture Abnormal posture of the body in which the lower limbs are extended with the feet flexed, the trunk and neck are straight or extended, the upper limbs are extended at the shoulder and elbows with the wrists and hands flexed and pronated.

Defibrillate To return a heart which is in ventricular fibrillation (a type of cardiac arrest in which the ventricles are in fibrillation (q.v.)) to its normal rhythm.

Dehiscence Gaping: usually applied to an operational wound that has come apart.

Depot injection An injection into the tissues of a drug in such a form (often dissolved in oil) that it is slowly absorbed and thus exerts a prolonged effect.

Dextran A carbohydrate substance a solution of which can be given intravenously as a substitute for plasma.

Dextrose Glucose or grape sugar. Commonly used for intravenous infusion in 5 per cent solution.

Diabetes mellitus A common disease associated with a pathologically high blood sugar and a tendency to acidosis. It is caused by a relative or absolute failure to secrete enough insulin.

Dialysis A procedure to remove the (unwanted) soluble substances from the body; used in renal failure when either the blood is passed through a machine (haemodialysis q.v.) or fluid is passed through the peritoneal cavity (peritoneal dialysis).

Diathermy Intense local heat, generated in a blade or needle by a high frequency electric current, which may be used to seal bleeding vessels or cut tissues.

Digitalis A drug produced from the foxglove. It is widely used in the treatment of cardiac disorders.

Diplococcus A type of bacteria appearing in pairs.

Diuretic Drug used to increase the secretion of urine in such conditions as cardiac failure (i.e. frusemide/Lasix).

Diverticulitis Inflammation in one or more diverticula (referring usually to the colon).

Diverticulum A pouch or cavity leading off a main cavity or tube.

Dorsiflexion Bending the foot upwards.

Dorsum The back (also applied to the top of the foot).

Dowel A pin fixed to the base of something (e.g. a tooth) to plug it in.

Dupuytren's contracture A progressive flexion deformity of the fingers due to a thickening and contracture of the palmar fascia (a tough membrane under the skin of the palm).

Dyscrasia A developmental or metabolic disorder.
Dysphagia Difficulty in swallowing.
Dyspnoea Shortness of breath.
Dysraphism Defective fusion.

Ectoderm The outermost of the three germinal layers in the embryo, from which is derived the skin and its related structures and the nervous system.
Ectopic Out of normal position.
Eczema A non-contagious inflammatory skin condition.
Electrocardiography The recording of the electrical potentials generated by the activity of the heart.
Electrode A medium used between an electric conductor and the object to which the current is to be applied.
Electrolyte Any substance which in solution dissociates into electrically charged particles. Refers in the blood to the ionized salts of sodium, potassium, chloride and bicarbonate.
Embolus A blood clot (or air, fat, tumour) carried in the blood until it lodges in a blood vessel which it blocks.
Emphysema (1) A common chronic disease of the lungs characterized by breathlessness due mainly to difficulty in breathing out; it is associated with distension of the small air passages and air sacs in the lung, or (2) the presence of air in the body tissues (surgical emphysema).
Empyema Pus in the pleural cavity.
Empyema of the gall bladder Acute cholecystitis with distension of the gall bladder with pus.
Endemic Referring to disease prevalent in a particular area.
Endoderm (entoderm) The innermost of the three germinal layers in the embryo; gives rise to the lining of the respiratory and alimentary systems.
Endometritis Inflammation of the lining of the uterus.
Engorgement Congestion of a blood vessel or vessels.
Enteritis Inflammation of the small intestine.
Enterotomy Incision, division or dissection of the intestine.
Enucleation The separating of an organ from its capsule, or a tumour cleanly from the surrounding tissue.
Enuresis Involuntary passing of urine.
Eosinophilia An excessive number of eosinophil cells (a type of white blood cell) in the blood.
Epididymitis Inflammation of the epididymis which lies along the testis.
Epistaxis A nose-bleed.
Epithelium Term applied to skin or to the lining membrane of the respiratory organs, the alimentary tract and its associated viscera and ducts, and of the orifices and cavities of the genito-urinary tract. Epithelium other than skin is called mucosa.
Eschar The dry scab that forms on an area of skin that has been burned or the superficial layer otherwise destroyed.
Exomphalos A condition in which part of the abdominal viscera protrudes into the umbilical cord.
Extravasation Fluid escaping from its containing vessel (e.g. blood) or cavity (e.g. urine).

Faradic Electricity produced by a rapidly alternating current.
Fibre-optic endoscopy Endoscopy is a general term for internal inspection of a part of the body with an instrument; fibre-optic means

that light, usually for illumination as well as to carry the image, is conducted by numerous very fine glass fibres.

Fibrillation A quivering, unco-ordinated movement of muscle, usually the heart.

Fibrin A protein, the formation of which is an essential part of the blood clotting process.

Fibrinolysis Process of dissolving a deposit of fibrin, for example, in a blood clot.

Fibroadenoma Tumour of mixed fibrous and glandular structures.

Fibrosis The development of fibrous tissue in a part or an organ.

Fimbriated Having an extremity or border bearing fringe-like processes or hairs.

Fistula An unnatural communication between the cavity of an organ and the skin or the cavity of another organ.

Flocculation The aggregation of very fine particles into visible clumps.

Fulguration Tissue destruction by diathermy.

Furuncle A localized infection of the skin and subcutaneous tissue by *Staphylococcus aureus*.

Gamma rays Electromagnetic waves produced by radioactive substances, similar to x-rays but of much shorter wave length.

Gangrene Tissue necrosis and putrefaction due to cutting off of the blood supply; usually either in the bowel or in a limb, in which case the gangrene may be 'dry' or 'wet'.

Gas gangrene An infection with tissue necrosis and gas formation due to an organism of the Clostridia group.

Gastrografin Water soluble radiographic contrast medium containing iodine and especially formulated for gastrointestinal use.

Gastroplasty An operation for reforming the lower segment of the oesophagus from part of the stomach and using it to prevent reflux of gastric juice (in cases of hiatus hernia with stricture of the oesophagus).

Gastrostomy Surgical opening through the abdominal wall into the stomach, usually for feeding through a tube.

Gene A unit of hereditary material incorporated in the chromosomes.

Gigli saw A very flexible wire saw.

Globulins A class of proteins occurring widely in nature.

Gonadotrophin A substance having a stimulating effect on the gonads.

Gram-positive (negative) bacteria A basic classification according to the colour resulting when staining is done by Gram's method.

Granulation tissue Immature fibrous tissue and blood vessels, more or less red in colour and tending to bleed easily, and forming during the phase of healing after inflammation or injury.

Graves' disease Thyrotoxicosis.

Gumma A degenerating mass characteristic of tertiary syphilis.

Gynaecomastia Hypertrophy of the male breasts to resemble the female form.

Haemangioma A tumour of vascular tissue.

Haematemesis Vomiting blood.

Haematoma A collection of blood in the tissues.

Haematuria The presence of blood in the urine.

Haemoconcentration Removal of fluid from the blood resulting in a greater concentration of the more solid constituents, especially red blood cells.

Haemodialysis A process whereby the blood of a patient in renal failure is extracted from the artery or vein, circulated through a machine which equilibrates it with dialysis fluid and pumps it back to the patient. Waste products diffuse out into the dialysis fluid.

Haemoglobinuria The presence of haemoglobin (from the breakdown of red blood cells) in the urine.

Haemolysis The destruction of red blood cells with the release of haemoglobin.

Haemolytic streptococcus A type of streptococcus (bacteria) classified according to its ability to discolour the surrounding area on a blood-agar culture plate due to its ability to break down blood pigment.

Haemoptysis The coughing up of blood.

Haemostasis Arrest of bleeding.

Haemostat Small arterial clip.

Haemothorax Blood in the pleural cavity.

Hartmann's solution A solution for intravenous transfusion with an electrolyte content approximating to that of blood plasma. It contains sodium chloride, sodium lactate, and small amounts of potassium, calcium and magnesium chloride and is sometimes referred to as Ringer-lactate solution.

Haustration The separation of the colon into saccules.

Hemicolectomy Surgical excision of a portion of the colon.

Hemiplegia Paralysis of one side of the body.

Heparin A naturally occurring substance which when injected intravenously prevents the blood from clotting.

Hepatectomy Surgical removal of all (total) or part (partial) of the liver. Total hepatectomy, unless for transplantation, is performed only in animals.

Heterograft (xenograft) A graft between two members of different species.

Hiatus A gap or opening in a structure (especially of the diaphragm where penetrated by the aorta, inferior vena cava and the oesophagus).

Hirsutism Excessive bodily growth of hair.

Histology The study of anatomy through the microscope.

HLA (human leucocyte antigen) A system of lipoprotein substances located on human cell membrane but named leucocyte antigen because the peripheral white blood cell is used in this method of HLA detection.

Hodgkin's disease A malignant disease of the reticuloendothelial system (lymph nodes, spleen, bone marrow).

Hormone A chemical substance produced in an organ of the body which is capable of producing a specific effect on some other organ.

Hyaluronidase An enzyme which, by decomposing a constituent of the intercellular spaces, allows a more rapid spread of solutions through tissues.

Hydatidiform Having a cystic appearance.

Hydramnios Excessive amniotic fluid which surrounds the fetus *in utero*.

Hydrocephalus An abnormal increase of cerebrospinal fluid within the skull.

Hydrosalpinx A fallopian tube distended with fluid.

Hygroma A benign cystic tumour of lymphatic tissue.

Hyperacute rejection The destruction of tissue grafts within minutes or hours of introduction into the host's circulation.

Hyperalimentation Excessive feeding: either by mouth in excess of the demands of the appetite, in which case it may be forced; or intra-venously.

Hyperglycaemia An excessive blood sugar concentration.

Hyperparathyroidism Oversecretion of parathormone which is pro-duced by the parathyroid glands and is concerned with the regulation of calcium and phosphorus metabolism.

Hyperplasia Increase in the number of cells in a tissue.

Hyperthermia High temperature for the given species. In the human, $37°C$ and above.

Hyperthyroidism Overactive thyroid.

Hypertonic Solution stronger than normal for any given soluble chemical.

Hypertrophy Increase in the size or number of cells in a tissue.

Hypochromic anaemia Anaemia with decreased haemoglobin due to iron deficiency.

Hypogammaglobulinaemia Low level of a serum protein fraction, the gamma globulins, and usually, therefore, a low antibody level.

Hypoglycaemia A decrease in the blood sugar associated with such symptoms as sweating, anxiety, clouding of consciousness and eventually coma.

Hypoparathyroidism Undersecretion of parathormone.

Hypophysectomy Removal of the pituitary gland.

Hypopotassaemia A decrease below normal of the plasma concen-tration potassium.

Hypoprothrombinaemia A decrease in the amount of prothrombin in the blood giving rise to a defect in clotting.

Hypothermia Low temperature for the given species. In the human, in current clinical usage, temperatures down to $28°C$ are called moderate hypothermia. Below that, profound hypothermia — a temperature of $15°C$ is the lowest that has been occasionally induced for operations on the blood vessels of the brain.

Hypothyroidism Underactive thyroid.

Hypovolaemia Diminished blood volume in the body.

Hypoxia The condition of inadequate oxygenation.

Hysterectomy Removal of the whole, or the body, of the uterus.

Hysterosalpingography The x-ray imaging of the cavity of the uterus and the fallopian tubes following the injection via the cervix of a radio-opaque material.

Iatrogenic Produced by treatment. Used especially of harmful com-plication of treatment, obviously unintentional.

Ileitis Inflammation of the ileum, or, more usually, a part of it.

Ileus Intestinal obstruction from loss of the muscular activity of the bowel.

Immunocyte Cells concerned in immunity especially antibody for-mation, that is, reticulo-endothelial cells, lymphocytes and plasma cells.

Incontinence Inability to control the flow of urine or faeces.

Induration The hardening of a tissue or organ due to disease.

Infarct Death of tissue resulting from interruption of blood supply.

Insufflation The blowing of air or gas (either of which may carry powder) into a body cavity.

Insulinoma A tumour which secretes insulin.

Intercostal drainage Drainage of pleural cavity by tube inserted between two ribs.

Intrinsic factor A factor which is produced in the stomach wall and is necessary for red blood cell formation.

Intussusception The invagination of one segment of the gut into the next.

Ion A positively or negatively charged particle in solution.

Iritis Inflammation of the iris.

Ischaemia Localized tissue hypoxia (q.v.) due to inadequate blood supply.

Ischaemic necrosis Death of tissue from lack of blood supply.

Isograft A graft between two genetically identical members of the same species (for example, identical twins, members of an inbred strain).

Isotonic solution A solution in equal pressure balance (due to chemical concentration with another solution so that fluid transference does not occur (usually with reference to normal body fluids).

Jejunostomy Surgical operation producing communication between the exterior and the jejunum through the abdominal wall. Used for feeding if it is not possible to utilize the stomach.

Keratin A protein forming the horny superficial layer of the skin, nails and hair.

Ketoacidosis Increased acidity of the blood due to acids derived from ketones.

Ketones Organic compounds (e.g. acetone) produced by an oxidation process.

Ketosis The presence of excessive quantities of ketones in the blood.

Klinefelter's syndrome A congenital condition resulting from a sex chromosome abnormality. Subjects look like males but also have female characteristics and gynaecomastia (q.v.).

Kyphosis Excessive forward spinal curvature.

Laceration Tearing of tissue.

Laminectomy An operation to remove the laminae of a vertebral arch. Done to expose the spinal cord.

Laparotomy An incision made through the abdominal wall to explore the abdominal cavity.

Laryngocoele An air-containing pouch connected with the cavity of the larynx.

Lavage Irrigation or washout of an organ.

Leiomyoma Benign neoplasm arising from smooth (involuntary) muscle cells.

Leucocytosis Increased number of circulating white blood cells. The cells are usually polymorphonuclear appearing in response to a bacterial infection.

Leukaemia An eventually fatal disease of the blood-forming tissues marked by a massive increase in circulating white blood cells.

Leukopenia A diminished number of white cells in the peripheral blood which may arise from bone marrow depression following the administration of cytotoxic drugs, associated with decreased resistance to infection.

Ligation The tying off (with a ligature) of a blood vessel or other hollow structure.

Linear accelerator A machine which produces beams of penetrating (high energy) radiation, usually x-rays.

Lipoma A benign fatty tumour.

Lithotomy position The patient is on his back with his legs raised and spread out.

Lithotrite An instrument (shaped like jaws on the end of a cystoscope) for crushing stones in the bladder.

Litmus Blue dye obtained from lichens. It turns bright red when exposed to acids, and back to blue in contact with alkalis. Hence litmus paper — blotting paper strip impregnated with litmus and used to test fluids for acidity and alkalinity.

Loculus A small cavity without an opening.

Loop colostomy A temporary artificial opening made between the skin and the colon which is brought out as a loop.

Lumen The space inside a tube.

Lymph Interstitial fluid.

Lymphadenitis Inflammation of the lymph nodes.

Lymphangitis Red streaks running up a limb and representing inflammation in lymphatic vessels.

Lymphocyte A cell produced in lymphoid tissue and found also in lymph and blood.

Lymphoedema Retention of fluid in the tissues because of lymphatic malfunction.

Lysis The breakdown of cellular material into a fluid state.

Macerated Moist and soggy.

Malecot catheter A type of self-retaining catheter.

Mastectomy Surgical removal of the breast.

Meatus A passage or opening.

Meconium The contents of an infant's intestines at the time of birth.

Megaloblastic anaemia Anaemia characterized by the presence of megaloblasts (large primitive red cells) in the blood.

Melaena The passage of blood in the faeces which has been changed (blackened) during its passage through the gut.

Meningitis Inflammation of the membranes of the brain or spinal cord.

Menorrhagia Excessive menstrual bleeding.

Mesoderm The middle germinal layer of the embryo, the origin of connective tissue and the locomotor and genito-urinary systems.

Mesothelioma A tumour arising from the pleura, pericardium or peritoneum due to the presence of asbestos.

Metabolic acidosis A condition of increased blood activity (lowered pH) due to the accumulation of non-volatile acids (e.g. lactic acid).

Metabolism The chemical processes essential for life.

Metastasis Secondary deposit of malignant neoplasm occurring at a site distant from the primary growth.

Methaemoglobinaemia The presence of methaemoglobin in the blood. Methaemoglobin is a pigment formed by the oxidation of haemoglobin.

Micro-aerophilic Organisms which grow in an atmosphere of reduced oxygen.

Mitral stenosis A partial closing down of the mitral valve, on the left side of the heart between the left atrium and ventricle, due to the effects of rheumatic fever. Heart failure eventually results.

Morbidity State of illness.

Mucocoele A distended cavity containing mucus.

Myelomatosis A malignant disease in which the bone marrow is infiltrated with myeloma or plasma cells (these may also appear in the blood).

Myxoedema Hypothyroidism in adults associated with swelling of face and limbs, and mental changes.

Myxofibroma Benign neoplasm arising from connective and fibrous tissue cells.

Naevus Birth mark.

Necrosis Tissue death.

Neoplasm New growth or tumour.

Nephrectomy Excision of a kidney.

Nephroblastoma (Wilms' tumour) A malignant renal tumour of children.

Nephrostomy A technique of renal drainage by opening the pelvis of the kidney to the outside.

Neurilemmoma A benign tumour arising from a nerve sheath.

Neurofibroma A benign tumour composed of nervous and fibrous tissue.

Neurones Nerve cells.

Nidus Literally — nest; the focus of, for example, an infection or a gall-stone.

Normotensive Having a normal blood pressure.

Normothermic Temperature normal for a given species. In the human, 36–37°C.

Nuclear reactor An assembly of fissile material (e.g. uranium) leading to the continuous controlled release of energy.

Nulliparous Never having given birth.

Nystagmus A condition in which there is repetitive rhythmical movement of the eyeballs, usually laterally.

Oesophagogastrectomy Operation of removing part of the oesophagus and stomach, for example, for cancer. The remaining portions of the oesophagus and the stomach are then joined together.

Oesophagostomy Surgical opening through the neck into the oesophagus.

Oestrogen General name for certain types of female sex hormones.

Oligaemia A circulating blood volume below normal.

Oliguria Urine output below the normal level.

Omentum A double fold of peritoneum in the abdominal cavity which contains blood vessels and fat.

Oöphorectomy Surgical removal of an ovary or ovaries.

Ophthalmoscope An instrument for inspecting the interior of the eye.

Orchidectomy Surgical removal of a testis.

Orthopnoea Condition in which comfortable breathing is only possible in the sitting or standing position often associated with heart failure.

Osteomyelitis Infection of bone.

Pacemaker Electrical means of stimulating the heart to beat at a set rate when the normal rhythm has been affected by disease.

Palliation Treatment aimed toward relief of symptoms rather than complete cure.

Palmar erythema Redness of the palms due to vasodilatation.

Pancoast's tumour A tumour of the apex of the lung which involves the brachial plexus and the cervical sympathetic chain and so produces a characteristic syndrome of neurological changes affecting the arm and the eye in the involved.

Pancreaticoduodenectomy Surgical removal of the pancreas and duodenum.

Papilloma A benign epithelial tumour usually with a stalk.

Paracentesis Tapping or needling of a cavity to remove fluid. May be therapeutic or diagnostic.

Paraesthesia Abnormal sensation in a part of the body.

Paraparesis Incomplete paralysis of the legs and the lower part of the body.

Paraplegia Paralysis of both legs and the lower part of the body.

Paresis Incomplete paralysis.

Parietal Relating to the walls of a cavity, hence parietal peritoneum means that part lining the inside of the abdominal wall.

Parotitis Inflammation of the parotid salivery gland.

Pathogen A micro-organism or other agent which causes disease.

Pathogenesis The origin and development of disease.

Percussion Process of tapping the body, usually the trunk, and usually with the finger, to determine the nature of the resultant note. A resonant note indicates air, a dull one fluid.

Perforating veins Veins which connect superficial and deep veins by passing through the deep fascia (layer of fibrous tissue).

Perfusion The passage of fluid through an organ or tissue.

Peripheral neuropathy Disease of peripheral nerves.

Peristalsis The process by which solids are carried along any of the hollow tubes of the body — the oesophagus, intestines, and so on. The muscles of the tube in front of the solid relax, while those behind it contract, and hence push the mass along.

Peritoneoscopy Inspection of the peritoneal cavity with an optical instrument.

Peritonitis Inflammation of the peritoneum.

Pernicious anaemia A macrocytic hyperchromic anaemia (larger than normal red blood cells, each containing excess haemoglobin).

Petechial Small spots, pin-point to pinhead in size.

Phimosis A narrowing of the opening of the foreskin.

Photophobia Severe dislike of light (for instance in meningitis).

Phrenic Pertaining to the diaphragm.

Plasma cells Cells which form immunoglobulin.

Pleural effusion Effusion of fluid into the pleural cavity.

Pleurisy Inflammation of the pleural covering of the lungs.

Plexus In anatomical terms, a network of veins or nerves.

Pneumoconiosis A disease of the lungs caused by inhalation of certain dusts over long periods.

Pneumothorax Air within the pleural cavity.

Polyneuritis Involvement of many nerves by an inflammatory process.

Polyposis A condition in which a large number of polyps (mucosal outgrowths, usually with a stalk) cover the mucosa.

Postherpetic neuralgia A painful condition occurring after an attack of herpes zoster (shingles).

Proctoscope A tubular instrument for the examination of the anus and lower rectum.

Progestogen Substance possessing the activity of the corpus luteum hormone of the ovary.

Prophylaxis The prevention of disease.

Prostatism Symptoms of enlargement of the prostate gland.

Prosthesis An artificial part which may be used to replace one which has been removed — either externally (e.g. the breast or a limb, etc.) or internally (e.g. a heart valve or a hip joint, etc.).

Proteinuria The presence of protein in the urine.

Prothrombin Substance in the plasma formed in liver (by action of vitamin K) which is essential for blood clotting.

Protozoon An organism consisting of one cell.

Pruritus Itching.

Pulmonary embolism Pulmonary artery blockage by a clot carried from elsewhere in the blood until it lodges at this point.

Pulsus paradoxus Arterial pulse that is weaker during inspiration.

Pyaemia The presence of pus-producing bacteria in the blood leading to multiple abscesses.

Pyelitis Inflammation of the pelvis of the kidney.

Pyelogram Renal tract radiography (strictly — the renal pelvis).

Pyelography Radiographs of the renal tract.

Pyelonephritis Inflammation of the kidney.

Pylon The simplest temporary form of artificial limb.

Pyloric stenosis Narrowing of the pyloric opening between the stomach and the duodenum.

Pyloroplasty Surgical reshaping; in the case of the pylorus = enlarging of the opening. The suffix 'plasty' is derived from the Greek *plassein* = to mould. Hence it is used with a suitable prefix to indicate a refashioning (e.g. mammoplasty — of the breast; vesicoplasty — of the urinary bladder).

Pyrexia Fever.

Quadriplegia Paralysis of all four limbs.

Radicles The small vessels or tubes which unite to form a large one.

Radioactive scanning A technique in which a part of the body is systematically scanned by an apparatus sensitive to increased radio-activity. It thus locates the area of this increased activity.

Radioactivity Spontaneous disintegration of atoms accompanied by production of alpha, beta or gamma rays.

Radiosensitive Susceptibility to radiation.

Radiotherapy The treatment of disease by irradiation, for example, x-rays, gamma rays (usually malignant disease).

Referred pain Pain which, originating in an organ for which the brain has no body image, for example the heart or intestines, is referred to another part of the body for which there is a body image, and which shares the same nerve supply. The pain of a coronary thrombosis is thus felt in the left arm, of early appendicitis in the skin around the umbilicus, and of pharyngeal cancer in the ear.

Rejection The response on the part of a recipient to allograft tissue; the grafted tissue dies.

Relaxant Applied to drugs which paralyze voluntary muscles, and are commonly used during general anaesthesia (e.g. curare).

Resection Surgical removal of a part of the body or a tumour. ('Excision' is used with the same meaning.)

Respirator Machine for maintaining respiration by rhythmic inflation and deflation of the lungs.

Reticular formation Interlocking formations of nerve cells situated in the brainstem, belonging to the sensory system and intimately involved with the mechanism of maintenance of the state of consciousness.

Reticulosis Disease of the reticulo-endothelial system (that is, the lymph nodes, spleen and bone marrow). It is part of the body defence mechanism against infection.

Retinoblastoma A malignant tumour of the retina which occurs in infants and is congenital in origin.

Retrognathia Congenital recession of the jaws.

Rigor An extreme shivering fit.

Rodent ulcer Basal cell carcinoma which is locally invasive and does not metastasize.

Ryle's tube A narrow gauge rubber tube inserted into the stomach or duodenum for aspiration of contents or for artificial feeding.

Sagittal Vertical plane from the front to the back of the skull (or other part of the body).

Saline Salt solution. In the medical context unless otherwise stated, saline is a solution of 0.9 per cent sodium chloride.

Salpingitis Inflammation of the fallopian tube (salpinx).

Sarcoidosis A generalized disease affecting mainly skin, lymph nodes and lungs.

Scleroderma Disease characterized by thickening and fibrosis of the skin and subcutaneous tissues. It also involves the gastrointestinal tract, the lungs and the kidneys.

Seminoma A malignant tumour of the testis.

Sepsis A non-specific term for infection, usually local and with the production of pus.

Septa Thin partitions within or between anatomical structures.

Septicaemia Severe infection with large numbers of the causative bacteria multiplying and spreading in the bloodstream.

Sequestrum A piece of dead bone detached from healthy bone, as in the centre of an area of necrosis.

Shock Clinical state in which blood fails to perfuse the tissues.

Shunt Diversion of fluid, especially blood, through alternative pathway, for example in congenital heart disease, or when blood flows through parts of a lung which are not ventilated as in pneumonia.

Sigmoidoscopy Internal examination of rectum and sigmoid colon with a special illuminated tube.

Sinus A recess or track.

Sphincter The muscle whose function is to close a natural orifice.

Sphygmomanometer An instrument designed to measure the arterial blood pressure by inflating a cuff encircling the limb.

Spider naevi These are clusters of blood vessels in the skin radiating from a central red spot. They blanch on pressure and when the pressure is released can be seen to fill up again from the centre outwards.

Spina bifida A congenital failure of fusion of the lamina of the vertebra. Usually several vertebrae are affected. There may be nerve damage and thus serious interference with bladder function, locomotion, etc.

Spirometer An instrument used to measure such things as the volume of gas which a patient can breathe out after a deep breath in (i.e. the vital capacity).

Squamous cell carcinoma A carcinoma of scaly, or flattened, cells.

Stenosis Narrowing.

Steroids A class of chemical compounds including sex hormones, adrenal cortical hormones, cholesterol and cholic acid. They all have a nucleus of joined carbon rings.

Striae Lines on the abdomen due to stretching.

Stricture The narrowing of a natural passage.

Stridor A harsh vibrating sound produced in upper respiratory tract obstruction.

Sulphaemoglobinaemia The presence of sulphaemoglobin in the blood. Sulphaemoglobin is a greenish pigment formed by combination of sulphur with haemoglobin.

Suppuration An inflammatory condition with pus formation.

Surfactant Detergent-type fluid which lines alveoli of lungs and prevents them from sticking together if they become de-aerated.

Suture In surgery a stitch used to unite tissues during operation. In anatomy an immovable joint between two bones, especially in the skull.

Sympathetic nervous system A part of the nervous system (autonomic, or functionally independent) which regulates the activity of structures not under voluntary control, e.g. smooth muscle, etc.

Symphysis A relatively immobile joint consisting of cartilage between two bones.

Synergy Working together.

Syrinx A tube.

Systemic Refers to the circulation of blood around the body, as opposed to the lungs.

Systole The period during which the heart contracts.

Tachycardia Fast heart rate.

Talipes Club foot.

Telangiectasis Small collections of dilated capillary blood vessels in the skin.

Template A mould or cast.

Tenesmus Continual and painful feeling of wanting to open the bowel.

Tension pneumothorax Air under tension in the pleural space of the thoracic cavity.

Teratoma A type of tumour (may be benign or malignant) derived from more than one of the embryonic germinal layers.

Tetany Tonic contraction of muscles (usually associated with a deficiency of ionized calcium in the blood).

Thoracolaparotomy A surgical approach to the peritoneal cavity by a wound through the chest wall and diaphragm, with or without an extension of the wound through the abdominal wall.

Thoracotomy Operation by which the thoracic cavity is opened.

Thrill Vibration which can be felt by the hand.

Thrombocytopenia A deficit of platelets in the blood.

Thrombosis Clotting of blood in blood vessels during life.

Thrombus Blood clot.

Thymus An immunologically important gland situated in the upper anterior part of the thorax.

Thyroglossal cyst A cyst developing in the line of embryonic fusion between the thyroid gland and the base of the tongue.

Thyroid crisis Very acute thyrotoxicosis.

Thyroidectomy Excision of the thyroid gland.

Thyrotoxicosis A disease caused by excessive thyroid secretion in which there may be weight loss, extreme nervousness, sweating, tachycardia (q.v.), cardiac irregularities and heart failure.

Tomography The process of taking a radiograph of one plane of the body.

Toxoid A toxin deprived of its harmful properties but capable of producing immunity.

Tracheostomy Artificial opening made in the trachea.

Trisomy Three chromosomes in place of a pair giving one extra chromosome overall (that is, 47). By far the commonest is Trisomy 21 (Down's syndrome, mongolism).

Trocar An instrument which has a sharp point and is placed in the centre of a cannula to allow this to be introduced into a cavity.

Tulle gras A coarse-meshed gauze soaked with a soft paraffin preparation.

Tylosis palmarum A condition in which there is thickening of the superficial layer of the skin of the hands and feet.

Ultrasonic High-frequency sound waves (inaudible).

Uraemia Excessively high blood level of urea usually resulting from renal failure when other metabolic products are also retained in the body and cause a type of poisoning.

Urea A nitrogenous waste product normally eliminated by the kidney. Urea is produced mainly by metabolism of such substances as proteins.

Urethral caruncle A small fleshy excrescence at the female urethral meatus.

Vagotomy Division of the vagus nerves. The suffix 'otomy' is derived from the Greek *temnein* = to cut, hence it is used with the appropriate prefix to indicate surgical division (e.g. tenotomy — of a tendon; laparotomy — of the abdominal wall, etc.).

Varix (pl. varices) A pathologically dilated vein.

Vascular shutdown A state of vasoconstriction leading to diminished blood flow.

Vasoconstriction Diminution of the calibre of blood vessels associated with diminished flow of blood.

Vasodilatation An increase in calibre of blood vessels usually associated with an increase in flow of blood.

Venepuncture Puncture of a vein to extract blood or to inject a fluid.

Venography A radiograph of veins after injection of a radio-opaque dye.

Ventriculogram A radiograph of the cerebral ventricles. Contrast is obtained by filling them with air.

Vincent's angina An acute ulcerated and membranous infection of the tonsil.

Visceroptosis Falling or sagging of the abdominal viscera.

Viscid Semiliquid; having a glutinous consistency (viscous).

Volvulus Twisting of a part of the gut.

Xeroderma pigmentosum A condition characterized by reddening of the skin with blistering and pigmentation, on even very slight exposure to sunlight.

Index